The Science of Color

Second Edition

DEDICATED TO OUR MENTORS:

Mathew Alpern
Clarence H. Graham
Frances K. Graham
Anita E. Hendrickson
David H. Krantz
John Krauskopf
Alex E. Krill
R. Duncan Luce
Donald I. A. MacLeod
Davida Y. Teller
Brian A. Wandell
David R. Williams

The Science of Color

Second Edition

Edited by

Steven K. Shevell

Departments of Psychology and
Ophthalmology & Visual Science
University of Chicago

OSA®
Optical Society of America

ELSEVIER

Amsterdam • Boston • Heidelberg • London • New York •
Oxford • Paris • San Diego • San Francisco • Singapore •
Sydney • Tokyo

This book is printed on acid-free paper

First edition published 1953
Second edition 2003

Elsevier
The Boulevard, Langford Lane, Kidlington, Oxford OX5 1GB, UK
http://www.elsevier.com

ISBN 0–444–512–519

Library of Congress Catalog Number: 2003106330

A catalogue record for this book is available from the British Library

Cover illustration: The Farbenpyramide of J.H. Lambert (1772), from Chapter 1 in *The Origins of Modern Color Science* by J.D. Mollon. (Reproduced with permission of J.D. Mollon.)

Designed and typeset by J&L Composition, Filey, North Yorkshire
Printed and bound in Italy

03 04 05 06 07 PT 9 8 7 6 5 4 3 2 1

Contents

Preface

This second edition of *The Science of Color* focuses on the principles and observations that are foundations of modern color science. Written for a general scientific audience, the book broadly covers essential topics in the interdisciplinary field of color, drawing from physics, physiology and psychology. The jacket of the original edition of the book described it as 'the definitive book on color, for scientists, artists, manufacturers and students'. This edition also aims for a broad audience.

The legendary original edition was published by the Optical Society of America in 1953 and sold until 1999 after eight printings. It was written by a committee of 23, with contributions from the Who's Who of color including Evans, Judd, MacAdam, Newhall and Nickerson. This new edition was written by a smaller group of distinguished experts. Among the 11 authors are eight OSA fellows, five past or present chairs of the OSA Color Technical Group, the two most recent editors for color at the *Journal of the Optical Society of America A*, and four recipients of the OSA's prestigious Tillyer Medal. The authors also reviewed related chapters to strengthen sustantive content. While the field of color has spread too broadly since 1953 to say the new edition is 'the definitive book on color', the topics in each chapter are covered by recognized authorities.

The book begins by tracing scientific thinking about color since the seventeenth century. This historical perspective provides an introduction to the fundamental questions in color science, by following advances as well as misconceptions over more than 300 years. The highly readable chapter is an excellent introduction to basic concepts drawn upon later.

Every chapter begins with a short outline that summarizes the organization and breadth of its material. The outlines are valuable guides to chapter structure, and worth scanning even by readers who may not care to go through a chapter from start to finish. The outlines are also useful navigation tools for finding material at the reader's preferred level of technical depth.

A book of modest length must selectively pare its coverage. The focus here is on principles and facts with enduring value for understanding color. No attempt was made to cover color engineering, color management, colorant formulation or applications of color science. These are very important and rapidly advancing fields but outside the scope of this volume.

The authors are grateful to two experts who reviewed the complete text: Dr Mark Fairchild (Munsell Color Science Laboratory, Rochester Institute of Technology) and Dr William Swanson (SUNY College of Optometry). Their time and expertise contributed significantly to the quality of the chapters. Thanks are due also to Alan Tourtlotte, associate publisher at the OSA, for his determination and patience from conception to completion.

Many chapters were written with support from the National Eye Institute. The following grants are gratefully acknowledged: EY10016 (Brainard), EY 04440 (Lennie), EY 06678 (Packer), EY 00901 (Pokorny and Smith), EY 04802 (Shevell), EY 03164 (Wandell) and EY 04367 (Williams).

Steven K. Shevell
Chicago

Contributors

David H. Brainard
Department of Psychology
University of Pennsylvania
3815 Walnut Street
Philadelphia, PA 19104-6196
USA

Peter Lennie
Center for Neural Science
New York University
New York, NY 10003
USA

J.D. Mollon
Department of Experimental Psychology
University of Cambridge
Downing Street
Cambridge CB2 3EB
UK

Kurt Nassau
16 Guinea Hollow Road
Lebanon, NJ 08833
USA

Orin Packer
Department of Biological Structure
University of Washington
G514 Health Sciences Building, Box 357420
Seattle, WA 98195
USA

Joel Pokorny
Departments of Psychology and
Ophthalmology & Visual Science
University of Chicago
940 East Fifty-Seventh Street
Chicago, IL 60637
USA

Steven K. Shevell
Departments of Psychology and
Ophthalmology & Visual Science
University of Chicago
940 East Fifty-Seventh Street
Chicago, IL 60637
USA

Louis D. Silverstein
VCD Sciences, Inc.
9695 E. Yucca Street
Scottsdale, AZ 85260-6201
USA

Vivianne C. Smith
Departments of Psychology and
Ophthalmology & Visual Science
University of Chicago
940 East Fifty-Seventh Street
Chicago, IL 60637
USA

Brian A. Wandell
Department of Psychology
Stanford University
Stanford, CA 94305-2130
USA

David R. Williams
Center for Visual Science
University of Rochester
Rochester, NY 14627
USA

The Origins of Modern Color Science

J. D. Mollon

Department of Experimental Psychology
University of Cambridge, Downing Street, Cambridge
CB2 3EB, UK

Jove's wondrous bow, of three celestial dyes,
Placed as a sign to man amid the skies

Pope, *Iliad*, xi: 37

CHAPTER CONTENTS

The Science of Color
ISBN 0-444-512-519

Each newcomer to the mysteries of color science must pass through a series of conceptual insights. In this, he or she recapitulates the history of the subject. For the history of color science is as much the history of misconception and insight as it is of experimental refinement. The errors that have held back our field have most often been category errors, that is, errors with regard to the domain of knowledge within which a given observation is to be explained. For over a century, for example, the results of mixing colored lights were explained in terms of physics rather than in terms of the properties of human photoreceptors. Similarly, in our own time, we remain uncertain whether the phenomenological purity of certain hues should be explained in terms of hard-wired properties of our visual system or in terms of properties of the world in which we live.

1.1 NEWTON

Modern color science finds its birth in the seventeenth century. Before that time, it was commonly thought that white light represented light in its pure form and that colors were modifications of white light. It was already well known that colors could be produced by passing white light through triangular glass prisms, and indeed the long thin prisms sold at fairs had knobs on the end so that they could be suspended close to a source of light. In his first published account of his 'New Theory of Colors,' Isaac Newton describes how he bought a prism 'to try therewith the celebrated *Phaenomena* of *colours*' (Newton, 1671). In the seventeenth century, one of the great trade fairs of Europe was held annually on Stourbridge Common, near the head of navigation of the river Cam. The fair was only two kilometers from Trinity College, Cambridge, where Newton was a student and later, a Fellow. In his old age, Newton told John Conduitt that he had bought his first prism at Stourbridge Fair in 1665 and had to wait until the next fair to buy a second prism to prove his 'Hypothesis of colours'. Whatever the accuracy of this account and its dates – the fair in fact was cancelled in 1665 and 1666, owing to the plague (Hall, 1992) – the story emphasizes that Newton did not discover the prismatic spectrum: His contribution lies in his analytic use of further prisms.

Allowing sunlight to enter a small round hole in the window shutters of his darkened chamber, Newton placed a prism at the aperture and refracted the beam on to the opposite wall. A spectrum of vivid and lively colors was produced. He observed, however, that the colored spectrum was not circular as he expected from the received laws of refraction, but was oblong, with semi-circular ends.

Once equipped with a second prism, Newton was led to what he was to call his *Experimentum Crucis*. As before, he allowed sunlight to enter the chamber through a hole in the shutter and fall on a triangular prism. He took two boards, each pierced by a small hole. He placed one immediately behind the prism, so its aperture passed a narrow beam; and he placed the second about 4 meters beyond, in a position that allowed him to pass a selected portion of the spectrum through its aperture. Behind the second aperture, he placed a second prism, so that the beam was refracted a second time before it reached the wall (Figure 1.1). By rotating the first prism around its long axis, Newton was able to pass different portions of the spectrum through the second aperture. What he observed was that the part of the beam that was more refracted by the first prism was also more refracted by the second prism.

Moreover, a particular hue was associated with each degree of refrangibility: The least refrangible rays exhibited a red color and the most refrangible exhibited a deep violet color. Between these

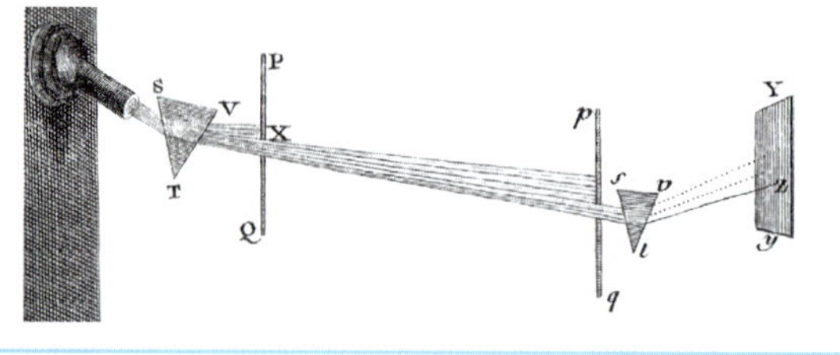

Figure 1.1 **An eighteenth-century representation of Newton's *Experimentum crucis*. As the left-hand prism is rotated around its long axis, the beam selected by the two diaphragms is constant in its angle of incidence at the second prism. Yet the beam is refracted to different degrees at the second prism according to the degree to which it is refracted at the first. (From Nollet's *Leçons de Physique Expérimentale*).**

two extremes, there was a continuous series of intermediate colors corresponding to rays of intermediate refrangibility. Once a ray of a particular refrangibility has been isolated in variants of the *Experimentum Crucis*, there was no experimental manipulation that would then change its refrangibility or its color: Newton tried refracting the ray with further prisms, reflecting it from various colored surfaces, and transmitting it through colored mediums, but such operations never changed its hue. Today we should call such a beam 'monochromatic': It contains only a narrow band of wavelengths – but that was not to be known until the nineteenth century.

Yet there was no individual ray, no single refrangibility, corresponding to white. White light is not homogeneous, Newton argued, but is a 'Heterogeneous mixture of differently refrangible Rays.' The prism does not modify sunlight to yield colors: Rather it separates out the rays of different refrangibility that are promiscuously intermingled in the white light of a source such as the sun. If the rays of the spectrum are subsequently recombined, then a white is again produced.

In ordinary discourse, we most often use the word 'color' to refer to the hues of natural surfaces. The color of a natural body, Newton argued, is merely its disposition to reflect lights of some refrangibilities more than others. Today we should speak of the 'spectral reflectance' of a surface – the proportion of the incident light that is reflected at each wavelength. As Newton observed, an object that normally appears red in broadband, white light will appear blue if it is illuminated by blue light, that is, by light from the more refrangible end of the spectrum.

The mixing of colors, however, presented Newton with problems that he never fully resolved. Even in his first published paper, he had to allow that a mixture of two rays of different refrangibility could match the color produced by homogeneous light, light of a single refrangibility. Thus a mixture of red and yellow make orange; orange and yellowish green make yellow; and mixtures of other pairs of spectral colors will similarly match an intermediate color, provided that the components of the pair are not too separated in the spectrum. 'For in such mixtures, the component colours appear not, but, by their mutual allaying each other, constitute a midling colour'(Newton, 1671). So colors that looked the same to the eye might be 'original and simple' or might be compound, and the only way to distinguish them was to resolve them with a prism. Needless to say, this complication was to give difficulties for his contemporaries and successors (Shapiro, 1980).

White presented an especial difficulty. In his first paper, Newton wrote of white: 'There is no one sort of Rays which alone can exhibit this. 'Tis ever compounded, and to its composition are requisite all the aforesaid primary colours' (Newton, 1671). The last part of this claim was quickly challenged by Christian Huygens, who suggested that two colors alone (yellow and blue) might be sufficient to yield white (Huygens, 1673). There do, in fact, exist pairs of monochromatic lights that can be mixed to match white (they are now called 'complementary wavelengths'), but their existence was not securely established until the nineteenth century (see section 1.7.1). Newton himself always denied that two colors were sufficient, but the exchange with Huygens obliged him to modify his position and to allow that white could be compounded from a small number of components.

In his *Opticks*, first published in 1704, Newton introduces a forerunner of many later 'chromaticity diagrams,' diagrams that show quantitatively the results of mixing specific colors (Chapters 3 and 7). On the circumference of a circle (Figure 1.2) he represents each of the seven principal colors of the spectrum. At the center of gravity of each, he draws a small circle proportional to 'the number of rays of that sort in the mixture under consideration.' Z is then the center of gravity of all the small circles and represents the color of the mixture. If two separate mixtures of lights have a common center of gravity, then the two mixtures will match. If, for example, all seven of the principal spectral colors are mixed in the proportions in which they are present in sunlight, then Z will fall in the center of the diagram, and the mixture will match a pure white. Colors that lie on the circumference are the most saturated ('intense and florid in the highest degree'). Colors that lie on a line connecting the center with a point on the circumference will all exhibit the same hue but will vary in saturation.

This brilliant invention is a product of Newton's mature years: It apparently has no

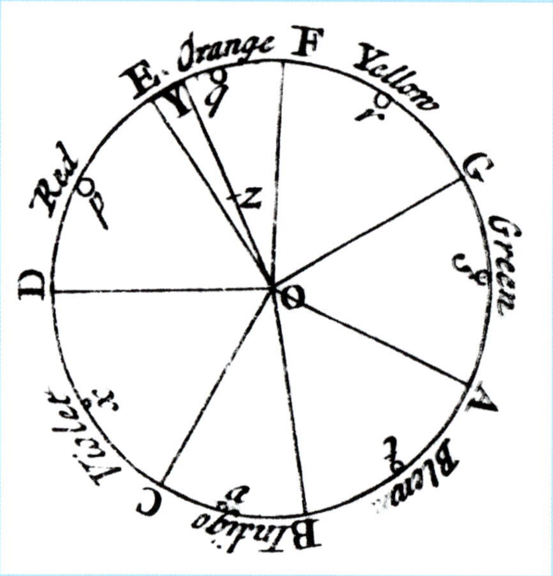

Figure 1.2 **Newton's color circle, introduced in his *Opticks* of 1704.**

antecedent in his published or unpublished writings (Shapiro, 1980). However, as a chromaticity diagram it is imperfect in several ways. First, Newton spaced his primary colors on the circumference according to a fanciful analogy with the musical scale, rather than according to any colorimetric measurements. Secondly, the two ends of the spectrum are apparently made to meet, and thus there is no way to represent the large gamut of distinguishable purples that are constructed by mixing violet and red light (although in the text, Newton does refer to such purple mixtures as lying near the line OD and indeed declares them 'more bright and more fiery' than the uncompounded violet). Thirdly, the circular form of Newton's diagram forbids a good match between, say, a spectral orange and a mixture of spectral red and spectral yellow – a match that normal observers can in fact make.

And in his text, Newton continues to deny one critical set of matches that his diagram does allow. The color circle implies that white could be matched by mixing colors that lie opposite one another on the circumference, but he writes:

> if only two of the primary Colours which in the circle are opposite to one another be mixed in an equal proportion, the point Z shall fall upon the centre O, and yet the Colour compounded of these two shall not be perfectly white, but some faint anonymous Colour. For I could never yet by mixing only two primary Colours produce a perfect white. Whether it may be compounded of a mixture of three taken at equal distances in the circumference, I do not know, but of four or five I do not much question but it may. But these are Curiosities of little or no moment to the understanding the Phaenomena of Nature. For in all whites produced by Nature, there uses to be a mixture of all sorts of Rays, and by consequence a composition of all Colours.
>
> (Newton, 1730)

In this unsatisfactory state, Newton left the problem of color mixing. To understand better his dilemma, and to understand the confusions of his successors, we must take a moment to consider the modern theory of color mixture. For the historian of science must enjoy a conceptual advantage over his subjects.

1.2 THE TRICHROMACY OF COLOR MIXTURE

The most fundamental property of human color vision is *trichromacy*. Given three different colored lights of variable intensities, it is possible to mix them so as to match any other test light of any color. Needless to say, this statement comes with some small print attached. First, the mixture and the test light should be in the same context: If the mixture were in a dark surround and the test had a light surround, it might be impossible to equate their appearances (see Chapter 4). Two further limitations are (a) it should not be possible to mix two of the three variable lights to match the third, and (b) the experimenter should be free to mix one of the three variable lights with the test light.

There are no additional limitations on the colors that are to be used as the variable lights, and they may be either monochromatic or themselves broadband mixtures of wavelengths. Nevertheless, the three variable lights are traditionally called 'primaries'; and much of the historical confusion in color science arose because a clear distinction was not made between the primaries used in color mixing experiments and the colors that are primary in our phenomenological experience. Thus, colors such as red and yellow are often called 'primary' because we recognize in them only one subjective quality, whereas most people would recognize in orange the qualities of both redness and yellowness.

The trichromacy of color mixture in fact arises because there are just three types of cone receptor cell in the normal retina. They are known as long-wave, middle-wave and short-wave cones, although each is broadly tuned and their sensitivities overlap in the spectrum (Chapter 3). Each type of cone signals only the total number of photons that it is absorbing per unit time – its rate of 'quantum catch.' So to achieve a match between two adjacent patches of light, the experimenter needs only to equate the triplets of quantum catches in the two adjacent areas of the observer's retina. This, in essence, is the trichromatic theory of color vision, and it should be distinguished from the fact of trichromacy. The latter was recognized, in a simplified form, during Newton's lifetime. But for more than a century before the three-receptor theory was introduced, trichromacy was taken to belong to a different domain of science. It was taken as a physical property of light rather than as a fact of physiology. This category error held back the understanding of physical optics more than has been recognized.

The basic notion of trichromacy emerged in the seventeenth century. Already in 1686, Waller published in the *Philosophical Transactions of the Royal Society* a small color atlas with three primary or simple colors. A rather clear statement is found at the beginning of the eighteenth century in the 1708 edition of an anonymous treatise on miniature painting (Figure 1.3):

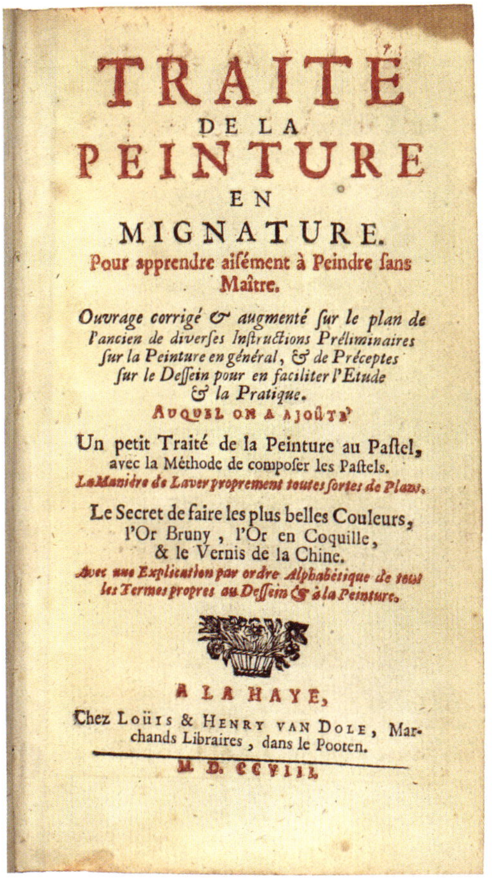

TRAITÉ
DE LA
PEINTURE
EN
MIGNATURE.
Pour apprendre aiſément à Peindre ſans Maître.
Ouvrage corrigé & augmenté ſur le plan de l'ancien de diverſes Inſtructions Préliminaires ſur la Peinture en général, & de Préceptes ſur le Deſſein pour en faciliter l'Etude & la Pratique.
AUQUEL ON A AJOÛTÉ
Un petit Traité de la Peinture au Paſtel, avec la Méthode de compoſer les Paſtels.
La Maniére de Laver proprement toutes ſortes de Plans.
Le Secret de faire les plus belles Couleurs, l'Or Bruny, l'Or en Coquille, & le Vernis de la Chine.
Avec une Explication par ordre Alphabétique de tous les Termes propres au Deſſein & à la Peinture.
A LA HAYE,
Chez LOÜIS & HENRY VAN DOLE, Marchands Libraires, dans le Pooten.
M. D. CCVIII.

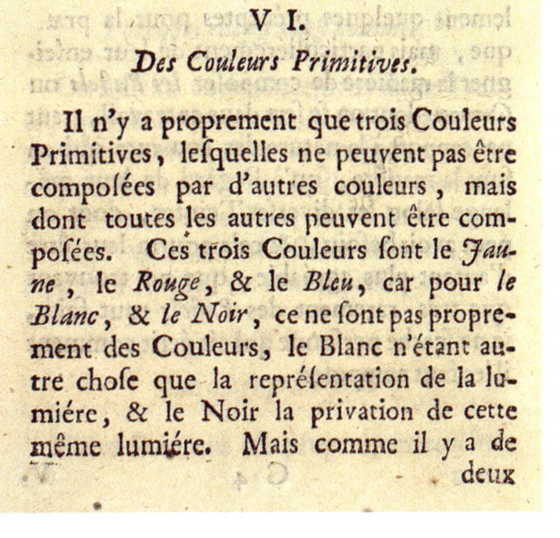

VI.
Des Couleurs Primitives.
Il n'y a proprement que trois Couleurs Primitives, leſquelles ne peuvent pas être compoſées par d'autres couleurs, mais dont toutes les autres peuvent être compoſées. Ces trois Couleurs ſont le *Jaune*, le *Rouge*, & le *Bleu*, car pour *le Blanc*, & *le Noir*, ce ne ſont pas proprement des Couleurs, le Blanc n'étant autre choſe que la repréſentation de la lumiére, & le Noir la privation de cette même lumiére. Mais comme il y a de deux

Figure 1.3 An early statement of trichromacy, from an anonymous treatise on miniature painting, published at The Hague in 1708.

> Strictly speaking there are only three primitive colors, that cannot themselves be constructed from other colors, but from which all others can be constructed. The three colors are yellow, red and blue, for white and black are not truly colors, white being nothing else but the representation of light, and black the absence of this same light.
>
> (Anonymous, 1708)

1.2.1 TRICHROMACY AND THE DEVELOPMENT OF THREE-COLOR REPRODUCTION

It is trichromacy – a property of ourselves – that makes possible relatively cheap color reproduction, by color printing, for example, and by color televisions and computer monitors (see Chapter 8). Three-color printing was developed nearly a century before the true nature of trichromacy was grasped. It was invented – and brought to a high level of perfection at its very birth – by Jacques Christophe Le Blon. This remarkable man was born in 1667 in Frankfurt am Main. It is interesting that Le Blon was working as a miniature painter in Amsterdam in 1708, when the anonymous edition of the *Traité de la Peinture en Mignature* was published at the Hague; and we know from unpublished correspondence, between the connoisseur Ten Kate and the painter van Limborch, that Le Blon was experimenting on color mixture during the years 1708–12 (Lilien, 1985).

In 1719, Le Blon was in London and he there secured a patent from George I to exploit his invention, which he called 'printing paintings.' Some account of his technique is given by Mortimer (1731) and Dossie (1758). To prepare each of his three printing plates, Le Blon used the technique of mezzotint engraving: a copper sheet was uniformly roughened with the finely serrated edge of a burring tool, and local regions were then polished, to varying degrees, in order to control the amount of ink that they were to hold. Much of Le Blon's development work went into securing three colored inks of suitable transparency; but his especial skill lay in his ability mentally to analyze into its components the color that was to be reproduced. Sometimes he used a fourth plate, carrying black ink. This manoeuvre, often adopted in modern color printing, allows the use of thinner layers of colored ink, so reducing costs and accelerating drying (Lilien, 1985).

In 1721, a company, The Picture Office, was formed in London to mass-produce color prints by Le Blon's method. Shares were issued at ten pounds and were soon selling at a premium of 150%, but Le Blon proved a poor manager and the enterprise failed. In 1725, however, he published a slender volume entitled *Coloritto*, in which he sets out the principle of trichromatic color mixing (Figure 1.4). It is interesting that he gives the same primaries in the same order (Yellow, Red, and Blue) as does the anonymous author of the 1708 text, and uses the same term for them, *Couleurs primitives*.

Notice that Le Blon distinguishes between the results of superposing lights and of mixing pigments. Today we should call the former 'additive color mixture' and the latter, 'subtractive color mixture.' Pigments typically absorb light predominantly at some wavelengths and reflect or transmit light at other wavelengths. Where Le Blon superposes two different colored inks, the light reaching the eye is dominated by those wavelengths that happen not to be absorbed by either of the inks. It was not until the nineteenth century that there was a widespread recognition that

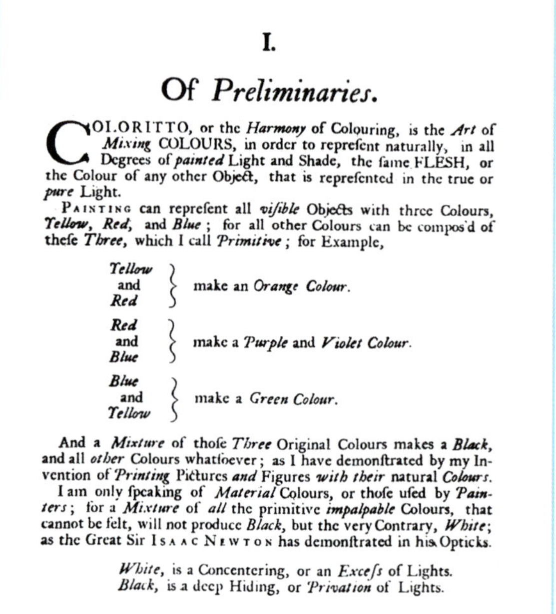

I.

Of *Preliminaries.*

COLORITTO, or the *Harmony* of Colouring, is the *Art* of *Mixing* COLOURS, in order to reprefent naturally, in all Degrees of *painted* Light and Shade, the fame FLESH, or the Colour of any other Object, that is reprefented in the true or *pure* Light.

PAINTING can reprefent all *vifible* Objects with three Colours, *Yellow*, *Red*, and *Blue*; for all other Colours can be compos'd of thefe *Three*, which I call *Primitive*; for Example,

Yellow and *Red* } make an *Orange Colour*.

Red and *Blue* } make a *Purple* and *Violet Colour*.

Blue and *Yellow* } make a *Green Colour*.

And a *Mixture* of thofe *Three* Original Colours makes a *Black*, and all *other* Colours whatfoever; as I have demonftrated by my Invention of *Printing* Pictures *and* Figures *with their* natural *Colours*.

I am only fpeaking of *Material* Colours, or thofe ufed by *Painters*; for a *Mixture* of *all* the primitive *impalpable* Colours, that cannot be felt, will not produce *Black*, but the very Contrary, *White*; as the Great Sir ISAAC NEWTON has demonftrated in his Opticks.

White, is a Concentering, or an *Excefs* of Lights.
Black, is a deep Hiding, or *Privation* of Lights.

Figure 1.4 **From J.C. Le Blon's *Coloritto* published in London in 1725.**

additive and subtractive mixture differ not only in the lightness or darkness of the product but also in the hue that may result (see section 1.7.1).

Le Blon himself explored a form of additive mixture. In his patent method of weaving tapestries, he juxtaposed threads of the primitive colors to achieve intermediate colors. An account is given by Cromwell Mortimer (1731):

> Thus Yellow and Red produce an Orange, Yellow and Blue a Green, Etc. which seems to be confirmed by placing two Pieces of Silk near together; viz. Yellow and Blue: When by intermixing of their reflected Rays, the Yellow will appear of a light Green, and the Blue of a dark Green; which deserves the farther Consideration of the Curious.

The phenomenon that Mortimer describes here is probably the same as the 'optical mixture' or 'assimilation' later exploited by Signac and the neo-impressionists (Rood, 1879; Mollon, 1992); and it still exercises the Curious (see Chapter 4). Some neural channels in our retina integrate over larger areas than do others, and this may be why, at a certain distance from a tapestry, we can see the spatial detail of individual threads while yet we pool the colors of adjacent threads. From Mortimer's account, it seems that Le Blon thought that the mixing was optical, and this will certainly be the case when the tapestry is viewed from a greater distance. However, a naturally-lit tapestry consisting of red, yellow, and blue threads can never simulate a white. For each of the threads necessarily absorbs some portion of the incident light, and in conventionally lit scenes we perceive as white only a surface that reflects almost all the visible radiation incident on it. In his weaving enterprise, Le Blon did not have the advantage of a white vehicle for his colors, such as he had when printing on paper. The best that he was able to achieve from adjacent red, yellow, and blue threads was a 'Light Cinnamon'. Similarly, since the three threads always reflect some light, it is impossible to simulate a true black within the tapestry. So Le Blon was obliged to use white and black threads in addition. And – Mortimer adds – 'tho' he found he was able to imitate any Picture with these five Colours, yet for Cheapness and Expedition, and to add a Brightness where it was required, he found it more convenient to make use of several intermediate Degrees of Colours.'

Sadly, Le Blon's weaving project did not prosper any better than the Picture Office. He was, however, still vigorous – at the age of 68 he fathered a daughter – and in 1737, Louis XV gave him an exclusive privilege to establish color printing in France. He died in 1741, but his printing technique was carried on by Jaques Gautier D'Agoty, who had briefly worked for him and who was later to claim falsely to be the inventor of the four-color method of printing, using three colors and black. Figure 1.5 – the first representation of the spectrum to be printed in color – was published by Gautier D'Agoty in 1752.

Le Blon himself did not acknowledge any contradiction between his practical trichromacy and Newtonian optics; but his successor, Gautier D'Agoty, was vehemently anti-Newtonian. He held that rays of light are not intrinsically colored or colorific. The antagonistic interactions of

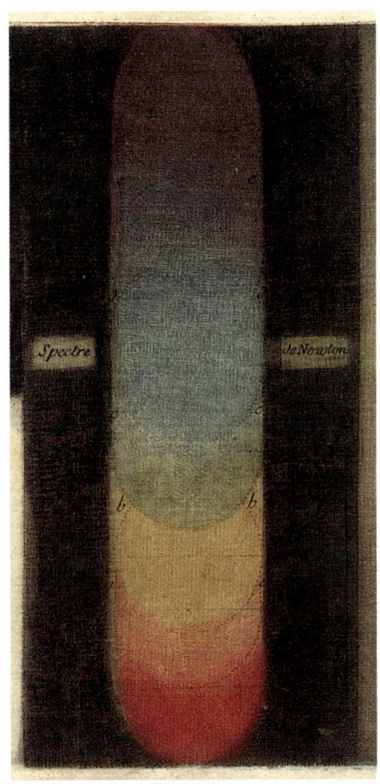

Figure 1.5 **The first representation of Newton's spectrum to be printed in color. From the *Observations sur l'Histoire Naturelle* of Gautier D'Agoty, 1752.**

light and dark (*'Les seules oppositions de l'ombre & de la lumiere, & leur transparence'*) produce three secondary colors, blue, yellow, and red, and from these, the remaining colors can be derived (Gautier D'Agoty, 1752).

1.2.2 TRICHROMACY IN OPPOSITION TO NEWTONIAN OPTICS

As the eighteenth century progressed, increasingly sophisticated statements of trichromacy were published, but their authors invariably found themselves in explicit or implicit opposition to the Newtonian account, in which there are seven primary colors or an infinity.

The anti-Newtonian Jesuit Louis Bertrand Castel (1688–1757) identified blue, yellow, and red as the three primitive colors from which all others could be derived. In his *Optique des Couleurs* of 1740, he gives systematic details of the intermediate colors produced by mixing the primaries. Father Castel was aware that phenomenologically there are more distinguishable hues between pure red and pure blue than between blue and yellow or between yellow and red – as is clear in the later Munsell system. By informal experiments he established a color circle of twelve equally spaced hues: Blue, celadon (sea-green), green, olive, yellow, fallow, nacarat (orange-red), red, crimson, purple, agate, purple-blue (Castel, 1740). These he mapped on to the musical scale, taking blue as the keynote, yellow as the third, and red as the fifth.

In his time, Castel was most celebrated for his scheme for a *clavecin oculaire* – the first color organ. For many years, the *clavecin oculaire* was a strictly theoretical entity, for Père Castel insisted that he was a *philosophe* and not an artisan. Nevertheless, there was much debate as to whether there could be a visual analogue of music. Tellemann wrote approvingly of the color organ, but Rousseau was critical, arguing that music is an intrinsically sequential art whereas colors should be stable to be enjoyed. Eventually, practical attempts seem to have been made to build a *clavecin oculaire* (Mason, 1958). A version exhibited in London in 1757 was reported to comprise a box with a typical harpsichord keyboard in front, and about 500 lamps behind a series of 50 colored glass shields, which faced back towards the player and viewer. The idea has often been revived in the history of color theory (Rimington, 1912).

One of the most distinguished trichromatists of the eighteenth century was Tobias Mayer, the Göttingen astronomer. He read his paper *'On the relationship of colors'* to the Göttingen scientific society in 1758, but only after his death was it published, by G.C. Lichtenberg (Forbes, 1971; Mayer, 1775; Lee, 2001). He argued that there are only three primary colors (*Haupfarben*), not the seven of the Newtonian spectrum. The *Haupfarben* can be seen in good isolation, if one looks through a prism at a rod held against the sky: On one side you will see a blue strip and on the other a yellow and a red strip, without any mixed colors such as green (Forbes, 1970). Here Mayer, like many other eighteenth-century commentators, neglects Newton's distinction between colors that look simple and colors that contain light of only one refrangibility. For an analysis of the 'boundary colors' observed by Mayer and later by Goethe, see Bouma (1947).

Mayer introduced a color triangle, with the familiar red, yellow, and blue primaries at its corners. Along the sides, between any two *Haupfarben*, were 11 intermediate colors, each being described quantitatively by the amounts of the two primaries needed to produce them. Mayer chose this number because he believed that it represented the maximum number of distinct hues that could be discerned between two primaries. By mixing all three primary colors, Mayer obtained a total of 91 colors, with gray in the middle. By adding black and white, he extended his color triangle to form a three-dimensional color solid, having the form of a double pyramid. White is at the upper apex and black at the lower.

A difficulty for Mayer was that he was offering both a chromaticity diagram and a 'color-order system.' The conceptual distinction between these two kinds of color space had not yet been made. A chromaticity diagram tells us only what lights or mixtures of lights will match each other. Equal distances in a chromaticity diagram do not necessarily correspond to equal perceptual distances. A color-order system, on the other hand, attempts to arrange colors so that they are uniformly spaced in phenomenological experience (see Chapters 3, 4 and 7).

One advance came quickly from J.H. Lambert, the astronomer and photometrist, who realized that the chosen primary colors might not be equal in their coloring powers (*la gravité spécifique des couleurs*) and would need to be given different weightings in the equations (Lambert, 1770). He produced his own color pyramid (Figure 1.6), realized in practice by mixing pigments with wax (Lambert,1772). The apex of the pyramid was white. The triangular base had red, yellow, and blue primaries at its apices, but black in the middle, for Lambert's system was a system of subtractive color mixture (section 1.7.1). He was explicit about this, suggesting that each of his primary pigments gained its color by absorbing light corresponding to the other two primaries. He made an analogy with colored glasses: If a red, a yellow, and a blue glass were placed in series, no light was transmitted.

Other eighteenth-century trichromatists were Marat (1780) and Wünsch (1792). Particularly anti-Newtonian was J.P. Marat, who, rejected by the *Académie des Sciences*, became a prominent figure in the French Revolution. He had the satisfaction of seeing several *académiciens* go to the guillotine, before he himself died at the hand of Charlotte Corday.

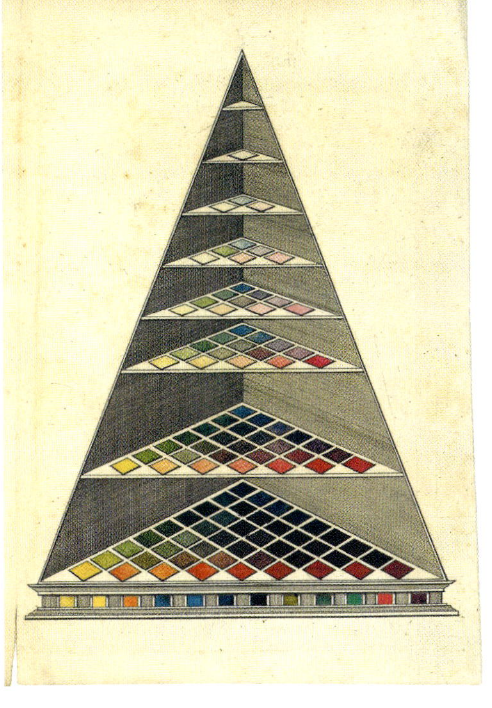

Figure 1.6 The *Farbenpyramide* of J.H. Lambert (1772). Reproduced with permission of J.D. Mollon.

1.2.3 THE MISSING CONCEPT OF A SENSORY TRANSDUCER

It has been said (Brindley, 1970) that trichromacy of color mixing is implicit in Newton's own color circle and center-of-gravity rule (see Figure 1.2). Yet this is not really so. If you choose as primaries any three points on the circumference, you can match only colors that fall within the inner triangle. To account for all colors, you must have imaginary primaries that lie outside the circle. And for Newton such imaginary primaries would have no meaning.

The reason is that Newton, and most of his eighteenth-century successors, lacked the concept of a tuned transducer, that is a receptor tuned to only part of the physical spectrum. It was generally supposed that the vibrations occasioned by a ray of light were directly communicated to the sensory nerves, and thence transmitted to the sensorium. Here are two characteristic passages from the *Queries* at the end of Newton's *Opticks*:

> *Qu* 12. Do not the Rays of Light in falling upon the bottom of the Eye excite Vibrations in the Tunica Retina? Which Vibrations, being propagated along the solid Fibres of the optick Nerves into the Brain, cause the Sense of seeing . . .
>
> *Qu.* 14. May not the harmony and discord of Colours arise from the proportions of the Vibrations propagated through the Fibres of the optick Nerves into the Brain, as the harmony and discord of Sounds arise from the proportions of the Vibrations of the Air? For some Colours, if they be view'd together are agreeable to one another, as those of Gold and Indigo, and others disagree . . .
>
> (Newton, 1730)

This was an almost universal eighteenth-century view: The vibrations occasioned by light were directly transmitted along the nerves. Since such vibrations could vary continuously in frequency, there was nothing in the visual system that could impose trichromacy. So the explanation of trichromacy was sought in the physics of the world.

Sometimes indeed, there was a recognition of the problem of impedance matching. Here is a rather telling passage from Gautier D'Agoty, written in commentary on his anatomical prints of the sense organs:

> The emitted and reflected ray is a fluid body, whose movement stimulates the nerves of the retina, and would end its action there, without causing us any sensation, if on the retina there were not nerves for receiving and communicating its movement and its various vibrations as far as our sense; but for this to happen, a nerve that receives the action of a ray composed of fluid matter (as is that of the fire that composes the ray) must also itself be permeated with the same matter, in order to receive the same modulation; for if the nerve were only like a rod, or like a cord, as some suppose, this luminous modulation would be reflected and could never accommodate itself to a compact and solid thread of matter . . .
>
> (Gautier D'Agoty, 1775)

An early hint of the existence of specific receptors can be found in a paper given to the St Petersburg Imperial Academy in July 1756 by Mikhail Vasil'evich Lomonosov. Both a poet and a scientist, Lomonosov established a factory that made mosaics and so he had practical experience of the preparation of colored glasses (Leicester, 1970). His paper concentrates on his physical theory of light. Space is permeated by an ether that consists of three kinds of spherical particle, of very different sizes. Picture to yourself, he suggests, a space packed with cannon balls. The interstices between the cannon balls can be packed with fusilier bullets, and the spaces between those with small shot. The first size of ether particle corresponds to salt and to red light; the second to mercury and to yellow light; and the third to sulfur and to blue light. Light of a given color consists in a gyratory motion of a given type of particle, the motion being communicated from one particle to another. In passing, Lomonosov suggests a physiological trichromacy to complement his physical trichromacy: the three kinds of particle are present in the 'black membrane at the bottom of the eye' and are set in motion by the corresponding rays (Lomonosov, 1757; Weale, 1957).

In the *Essai de Psychologie* of Charles Bonnet (1755) we find the idea of retinal resonators combined with a conventionally Newtonian account of light. Bonnet, however, supposed that for every degree of refrangibility there must be a resonator, just as – he suggested – the ear contains many different fibers that correspond to different tones. So each local region of the retina is innervated by fascicles, which consist of seven principal fibers (corresponding to Newton's principal colors); the latter fibers are in turn made up of bundles of fibrillae, each fibrilla being specific for an intermediate nuance of color. Bonnet was not troubled that this arrangement might be incompatible with our excellent spatial resolution in central vision.

In the last quarter of the eighteenth century, the elements of the modern trichromatic theory emerge. Indeed, all the critical concepts were present in the works of two colorful men, who lived within a kilometer of each other in the London of the 1780s. Each held a complementary part of the solution, but neither they nor their contemporaries ever quite put the parts together.

1.2.3.1 George Palmer

One of these two men was George Palmer. Gordon Walls (1956), in an engaging essay, described his fruitless search for the identity of this man. It was Walls' essay that first prompted my own interest in the history of color theory. In fact, Palmer was a prosperous glass-seller and, like Lomonosov, a specialist in stained glass (Mollon, 1985, 1993). He was born in London in 1740 and died there in 1795. His business was based in St Martin's Lane, but for a time in the 1780s he was also selling colored glass in Paris. His father, Thomas, had supplied stained glass for Horace Walpole's gothick villa at Strawberry Hill and enjoys a walk-on part in Walpole's letters (Cunningham, 1857).

George Palmer represents an intermediate stage in the understanding of trichromacy, for he was, like Lomonosov, both a physical and a physiological trichromatist. In a pamphlet published in 1777 and now extremely rare, he supposes that there are three physical kinds of light and three corresponding particles in the retina (Palmer, 1777b). In later references, he speaks of three kinds of 'molecule' or 'membrane'. The uniform motion of the three types of particle produces a sensation of white (Figure 1.7). His

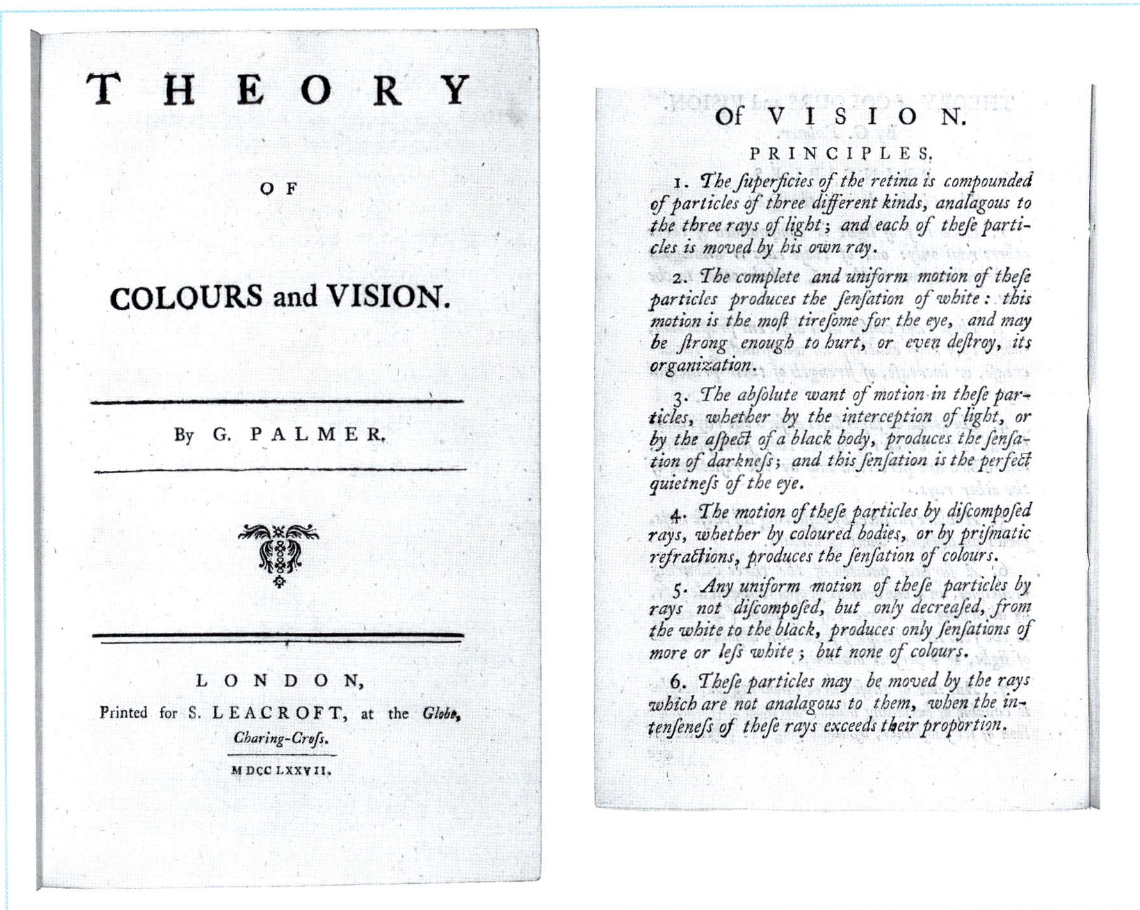

THEORY

OF

COLOURS and VISION.

By G. PALMER.

LONDON,

Printed for S. LEACROFT, at the *Globe*, *Charing-Croſs*.

MDCCLXXVII.

Of VISION.

PRINCIPLES.

1. *The ſuperficies of the retina is compounded of particles of three different kinds, analagous to the three rays of light; and each of theſe particles is moved by his own ray.*

2. *The complete and uniform motion of theſe particles produces the ſenſation of white: this motion is the moſt tireſome for the eye, and may be ſtrong enough to hurt, or even deſtroy, its organization.*

3. *The abſolute want of motion in theſe particles, whether by the interception of light, or by the aſpect of a black body, produces the ſenſation of darkneſs; and this ſenſation is the perfect quietneſs of the eye.*

4. *The motion of theſe particles by diſcompoſed rays, whether by coloured bodies, or by priſmatic refractions, produces the ſenſation of colours.*

5. *Any uniform motion of theſe particles by rays not diſcompoſed, but only decreaſed, from the white to the black, produces only ſenſations of more or leſs white; but none of colours.*

6. *Theſe particles may be moved by the rays which are not analagous to them, when the intenſeneſs of theſe rays exceeds their proportion.*

Figure 1.7 George Palmer's proposal that the retina contains three classes of receptor, in his *Theory of Colours and Vision* of 1777. Only four copies of this monograph are known to survive.

1777 essay attracted little support in Britain. The only review of this proto-trichromatic theory was one line in the *Monthly Review*: 'A *visionary* theory without *colour* of truth or probability.' In the French-speaking world, however, his ideas were better received: A translation of the pamphlet (Palmer, 1777a) attracted an extravagant review in the *Journal Encyclopédie*.

Once equipped with the idea of a specific receptor, Palmer ran with it. In 1781 in a German science magazine, his explanation of color blindness is discussed, although his name is there given mysteriously as 'Giros von Gentilly' while 'Palmer' is said to be a pseudonym (Voigt, 1781). He is reported to say that color blindness arises if one or two of the three kinds of molecules are inactive or are constitutively active (Mollon, 1997). In a later pamphlet published in Paris under his own name (Palmer, 1786), Palmer suggests that complementary color aftereffects arise when the three kinds of fiber are differentially adapted – an explanation that has been dominant ever since. To explain the 'flight of colors,' the sequence of hues seen in the afterimage of a bright white light, Palmer proposes that the different fibers have different time constants of recovery. And to explain the *Eigenlicht*, the faint light that we see in total darkness, he invokes residual activity in the fibers.

Another modern concept introduced by George Palmer is that of artificial daylight. In 1784, the Genevan physicist Ami Argand introduced his improved oil-burning lamp (Heyer, 1864; Schrøder, 1969). In its day, the Argand lamp revolutionized lighting. It is difficult for us today to appreciate how industry, commerce, entertainment, and domestic life were restricted by the illuminants available until the late eighteenth century. Argand increased the brilliance of the oil lamp by increasing the flow of air past the wick. He achieved this by two devices. First, he made the wick circular so that air could pass through its center, and second, he mounted above it a glass chimney. Unable, however, to secure suitable heat-resistant glass in France, he went to England in search of the flint glass that was an English specialty at the time. While he was gone, the lamp was pirated in Paris by an apothecary called Quinquet, who was so successful a publicist that his name became an eponym for the lamps. For a time, however, Quinquet had a partner, no other than George Palmer – and Palmer's contribution was clever: He substituted blue glass for Argand's clear glass, so turning the yellowish oil light into artificial daylight. Characteristically, this novel idea was set out in a pamphlet given away to customers (Palmer, 1785). The selling line was that artisans in trades concerned with color could buy the Quinquet–Palmer lamp, work long into the night, and so outdo their competitors. Palmer even proposed a pocket version that would allow physicians correctly to judge the color of blood or urine during the hours of darkness. The concept of artificial daylight appears again in a monograph by G. Parrot (1791).

George Palmer never took the final step of realizing that the physical variable is a continuous one. Living only streets away from him in 1780 was another tradesman, John Elliot, who postulated transducers sensitive to restricted regions of a continuous physical spectrum – but who never restricted the number of transducers to three (Mollon, 1987; in press).

1.2.3.2 John Elliot MD

Elliot was a man of a melancholic disposition, the opposite of the outgoing entrepreneur, George Palmer. It was said of him that he was of a sallow complexion and had the appearance of a foreigner, although he was born in Chard in Somerset in 1747. At the age of 14, he was bound apprentice to an apothecary in Spitalfields, London. At the expiry of his time, he became assistant in Chandler's practice in Cheapside and – if we are to believe the *Narrative of the Life and Death of John Elliot MD* (Anonymous, 1787) – it was during this period that he first established a romantic attachment to Miss Mary Boydell, whose many attractions included an Expectation – to be precise, an expectation of £30 000 on the death of her uncle, Alderman Boydell. Miss Boydell encouraged and then rejected the clever young apothecary. By 1780, Elliot was in business on his own, first in Carnaby Market and then, as he prospered, in Great Marlborough Street (Partington and McKie, 1941).

In his *Philosophical Observations on the Senses* (Elliot, 1780), he described simple experiments in which he mechanically stimulated his own eyes and ears, and was led to an anticipation of Johannes Mueller's 'Doctrine of Specific Nerve Energies' (Müller, 1840). Our sense organs, Elliot argued, must contain resonators – transducers – that are normally stimulated by their appropriate stimulus but can also be excited mechanically:

> there are in the retina different times of vibration liable to be excited, answerable to the time of vibration of different sorts of rays. That any one sort of rays, falling on the eye, excite those vibrations, and those only which are in unison with them . . . And that in a mixture of several sorts of rays, falling on the eye, each sort excites only its unison vibrations, whence the proper compound colour results from a mixture of the whole.
>
> (Elliot, 1780)

He develops his ideas in his *Elements of Natural Philosophy*, a work intended for medical students, which was first published in 1792 and then in a second edition in 1796. So modern is Elliot's account that it deserves quoting at length:

> The different colours, like notes of sound, may be considered as so many gradations of tone; for they are caused by vibrations of the rays of light beating on the eye, in like manner as sounds are caused by vibrations or pulses of the air beating on the ear. Red is produced by the slowest vibrations of the rays, and violet by the quickest . . .
>
> If the red-making rays fall on the eye, they excite the red-making vibrations in that part of the retina whereon they impinge, but do not excite the others because they are not in unison with them . . . From hence it may be understood that the rays of light do not cause colours in the eye any otherwise than by the mediations of the

> vibrations or colours liable to be excited in the retina; the colours are occasioned by the latter; the rays of light only serve to excite them into action. So likewise if blue- and yellow-making rays fall together on the same part of the retina, they excite the blue- and yellow-making vibrations respectively, but because they are so close together as not be distinguished apart, they are perceived as a mixed colour, or green; the same as would be caused by the rays in the midway between the blue- and yellow-making ones. And if all sorts of rays fall promiscuously on the eye, they excite all the different sorts of vibrations; and as they are not distinguishable separately, the mixed colour perceived is white; and so of other mixtures.
>
> We are therefore perhaps to consider each of these vibrations or colours in the retina, as connected with a fibril of the optic nerve. That the vibration being excited, the pulses thereof are communicated to the nervous fibril, and by that conveyed to the sensory, or mind, where it occasions, by its action, the respective colour to be perceived . . .
>
> (Elliot, 1786)

Elliot suggests that each of the several types of resonator is multiplied many times over, throughout the retina, the different types being completely intermingled. As we shall see later, his physiological insight was to lead him to the important physical insight that there might exist frequencies for which we have no resonators. Yet his life was to be brought to its unhappy end before he could make the final step of suggesting that there were only three classes of resonator in the retina.

The year 1787 found Elliot again obsessed with Miss Boydell and increasingly disturbed in his behavior. He bought two brace of pistols. He filled one pair with shot, and the other with blanks – or so the Defense claimed at the trial. On 9 July he came up behind Miss Boydell, who was arm in arm with her new companion, George Nichol. Elliot fired at Miss Boydell, but was seized by Nichol before he could shoot himself, as he apparently intended. By 16 July he was on trial at the Old Bailey. The prosecution insisted that the pistols had been loaded and that Miss Boydell had been saved only by her whalebone stays. The Jury found Elliot not guilty, but the Judge committed him to Newgate Gaol nevertheless, to be tried for assault (Hodgson, 1787). He died there on 22 July 1787.

1.2.3.3 Thomas Young

We have seen that all the conceptual elements of the trichromatic theory were available in the last quarter of the eighteenth century. However, the final synthesis was achieved only in 1801, by Thomas Young.

Young was born in Somerset in 1773, the eldest of ten children of a prosperous Quaker (Wood, 1954). His first scientific paper was on the mechanism of visual accommodation, a paper that secured his election to the Royal Society at the early age of 21. There is no evidence that Young himself ever performed systematic experiments on color mixing, but we do know that he was familiar with the evidence for trichromacy that had accumulated by the end of the eighteenth century. Intent on a medical career, he spent the academic year of 1795–96 at the scientifically most distinguished university in the realms of George III, the Georg-August University in Göttingen. We know from his own records that he there attended the physics lectures of G.C. Lichtenberg at 2 p.m. each day (Peacock, 1855); and from a transcript of these lectures got out by Gamauf (1811), we know that Young would have heard about the color-mixing experiments of Tobias Mayer, about the color triangle and the double pyramid formed from it, as well as about colored after-images and simultaneous color contrast.

After leaving Göttingen, Young spent a period at Emmanuel College, Cambridge, but by 1800 he was resident in London, having inherited the house and fortune of a wealthy uncle. In 1801, in a lecture to the Royal Society, he put forward the trichromatic theory of vision in a recognizable form. Adopting a wave theory of light, he grasped that the physical variable was wavelength and was continuous, whereas the trichromacy of color matching was imposed by the physiology of our visual system. The retina must contain just three types of sensor or resonator. Each resonator has its peak in a different part of the spectrum, but is broadly tuned, responding to a range of wavelengths.

> Now, as it is almost impossible to conceive each sensitive point of the retina to contain an infinite number of particles, each capable of vibrating in perfect unison with every possible undulation, it becomes necessary to suppose the number

> limited, for instance, to the three principal colours, red, yellow, and blue, of which the undulations are related in magnitude nearly as the numbers 8, 7, and 6; and that each of the particles is capable of being put in motion less or more forcibly, by undulations differing less or more from a perfect unison; for instance, the undulations of green light being nearly in the ratio of 6½, will affect equally the particles in unison with yellow and blue, and produce the same effect as a light composed of those two species: and each sensitive filament of the nerve may consist of three portions, one for each principal colour . . .
>
> (Young, 1802a)

Notice that in this first account Young does not refer explicitly to the trichromacy of color mixture; and he remains hesitant about the number of resonators. Later, in his article 'Chromatics' for *Encyclopaedia Britannica* (Young, 1817) he is firmer, now taking the three distinct 'sensations' to be red, green, and violet. The rays occupying intermediate places in the Newtonian spectrum excite mixed 'sensations,' so monochromatic yellow light excites both the red and green 'sensations' and monochromatic blue light excites the violet and the green 'sensations.' He is distinguishing here between the excitations of the nerves ('sensations of the fibres') and phenomenological experience: 'the mixed excitation producing in this case, as well as in that of mixed light, a simple idea only.' He realized – and it took others a long time to follow – that we cannot assume that the phenomenologically simplest hues (say, red, yellow, blue) necessarily correspond to the peak sensitivities of the receptors.

Thomas Young did not accurately know the spectral sensitivities of the three receptors, but he had overcome the category error that had held back color science since Newton. Clerk Maxwell was later to say, in a lecture to the Royal Institution: 'So far as I know, Thomas Young was the first who, starting from the well-known fact that there are three primary colours, sought for the answer to this fact, not in the nature of light, but in the constitution of man' (Maxwell, 1871).

1.3 INTERFERENCE COLORS

Yet Thomas Young's insight into sensory physiology was secondary to his contribution to color physics. Of his several legacies to modern science, none has been more significant than his generalized concept of interference. The colors of thin plates – the colors observed in soap bubbles and films of oil – had intrigued Hooke and Boyle and were measured systematically by Newton. But Newton, although he applied the concept of interference to explain the anomaly of tides in the Gulf of Tonking (Newton, 1688), and although he knew that the colors of thin films were periodic in character, did not make the leap that Thomas Young was to make a century later.

In order to quantify the conditions that gave rise to the colors of thin films, Newton pressed a convex lens of long focal length against a glass plate (Figure 1.8). Knowing the curvature of the convex surface, he could estimate accurately the thickness of the air film at a given distance from the point of contact. When white light was

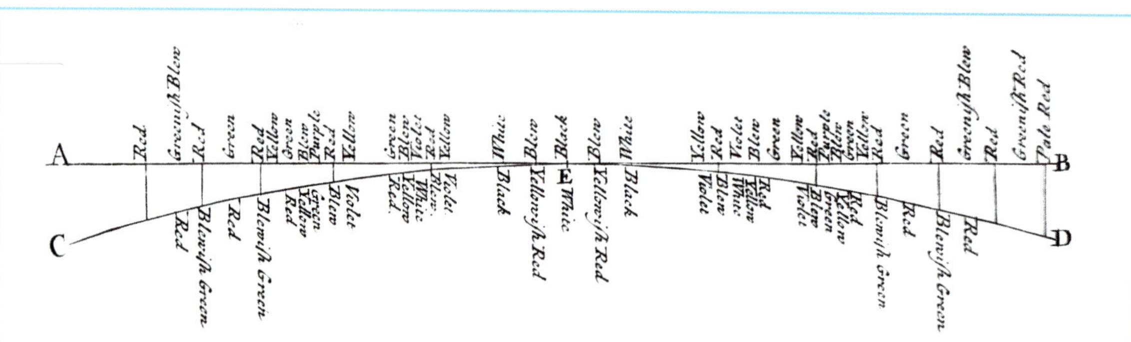

Figure 1.8 Newton's representation of the colors seen when a convex lens is pressed against a glass plate.

allowed to fall normally on the air film, Newton observed several series of concentric rings of color. If observations were made of light that had passed through both the lens and the plate, then colored rings were again seen, but these were complementary in hue to those seen by reflection from the plate. If light from only one part of the spectrum were used, then isolated bright bands were seen at certain distances from the central point. Newton supposed that each of the constituent colors of white light produced its own system of rings and that the colors seen with a white illuminant were due to the overlapping of the individual components. When using light of one color only, he could measure about 30 successive rings; and he found that in moving from one ring to the next, the corresponding thickness of the air film always increased by the same amount (Newton, 1730). Newton's own explanation was in terms of 'fits of easy reflection' and 'fits of easy transmission.' He supposed that a ray of light in a refracting medium alternates between two states ('fits'). In one state, the light is disposed to be reflected, in the other it is disposed to be transmitted. The rate of alternation between the two states varied with the color of the light (Shapiro, 1993).

Thomas Young was led to the concept of interference by his study of acoustics (Mollon, 2002). At Göttingen in 1796, to satisfy one of the requirements for his degree, he gave a lecture on the human voice (Peacock, 1855). Proceeding to Emmanuel College, Cambridge, he planned to prepare a paper on this subject, but 'found himself at a loss for a perfect conception of what sound was' and so set about collecting all the information he could, from books and from experiment (Young, 1804). A contemporary at Emmanuel wrote of him 'His rooms had all the appearance of belonging to an idle man . . . I once found him blowing smoke through long tubes.' He was soon to use the concept of interference to explain auditory beats – the waxing and waning of loudness that is heard as two tones of very similar pitch drift in and out of phase (Young, 1800).

Legend holds that Young was prompted to think about interference by observing the ripples generated by a pair of swans on the pond in Emmanuel College, and certainly he explicitly sets out such a lacustrine model in the pamphlet he wrote to defend his theory against the criticisms of Henry Brougham:

> Suppose a number of equal waves of water to move upon the surface of a stagnant lake, with a certain constant velocity, and to enter a narrow channel leading out of the lake. Suppose then another similar cause to have excited another equal series of waves, which arrive at the same channel at the same time, with the same velocity, and at the same time as the first. Neither series of waves will destroy the other, but their effects will be combined: if they enter the channel in such a manner that the elevations of one series coincide with those of the other, they must together produce a series of greater joint elevations; but if the elevations of one series are so situated as to correspond to the depressions of the other, they must exactly fill up those depressions, and the surface of the water must remain smooth; at least I can discover no alternative, either from theory or from experiment.
>
> (Young, 1804)

By his own account, it was only in May 1801 that Young realized that interference could explain the colors of thin plates. He supposed that light consisted of waves in an all-pervading ether. Different wavelengths corresponded to different hues, the shortest wavelengths appearing violet, the longest, red. In his initial model, however, the undulations were longitudinal – that is, along the line of the ray – rather than transverse, as Fresnel was later to show them to be.

In his Bakerian Lecture of November 1801, Young proposed that the colors of thin films depended on constructive and destructive interference between light reflected at the first surface and light reflected at the second: When the peak of one wave coincides with the trough of another, the two will cancel, but when the path length of the second ray is such that the peaks coincide for a given wavelength, then the hue corresponding to that wavelength will be seen (Young, 1802a). The first published account is in the *Syllabus* of his Royal Institution lectures:

> When two portions of the same light arrive at the eye by different routes, either exactly or very nearly in the same direction, the appearance or disappearance of various colours is determined by the greater or less difference in the lengths of the paths: the same colour recurring, when the intervals are multiples of a length, which, in the same

> medium, is constant, but in different mediums, varies directly as the sine of refraction.
>
> (Young, 1802b)

By applying his interference hypothesis to Newton's measurements of the colors of thin films, Young achieved the first accurate mapping of colors to the underlying physical variable. Figure 1.9 reproduces his table of the wavelengths that correspond to particular hues (Young, 1802a). Once converted from fractions of an inch to nanometers, the estimates closely resemble modern values. Particularly striking is the wavelength given for yellow, since it is in this region of the spectrum that hue changes most rapidly with wavelength. Young's value converts to 576 nm and this is within a nanometer of modern estimates of the wavelength that appears 'unique' yellow, the yellow that looks neither reddish nor greenish to an average eye in a neutral state of adaptation (Ayama *et al.*, 1987). His values for orange, green, and violet are very reasonable. The value for blue, 497 nm, is a longer wavelength than would be taken as the exemplar of blue today, but Newton's 'blew,' in a spectrum that had to accommodate indigo, may have been close to cyan, resembling the modern Russian *golyboi*. Indeed, we may have here an interesting explanation for Newton's statement that a mixture of spectral yellow and spectral blue makes green (Newton, 1671), a statement that has exercised historians of science (Shapiro, 1980).

It is in the same Bakerian lecture that Young made the first suggestion that interference also

Colours.	Length of an Undulation in parts of an Inch, in Air.	Number of Undulations in an Inch.	Number of Undulations in a Second.	Wavelength nm
Extreme -	.0000266	37640	458 millions of millions	
Red - -	.0000256	39180	477	650
Intermediate	.0000246	40720	495	
Orange - -	.0000240	41610	506	609
Intermediate	.0000235	42510	517	
Yellow -	.0000227	44000	535	576
Intermediate	.0000219	45600	555 (= 2^{48} nearly)	
Green - -	.0000211	47460	577	536
Intermediate	.0000203	49320	600	
Blue - -	.0000196	51110	622	497
Intermediate	.0000189	52910	644	
Indigo - -	.0000185	54070	658	469
Intermediate	.0000181	55240	672	
Violet - -	.0000174	57490	699	444
Extreme - -	.0000167	59750	727	

Figure 1.9 Thomas Young's table of the wavelengths corresponding to particular hues. Conversions to nanometers have been added to the right. (From his Bakerian Lecture published in 1802.)

accounts for the colors seen when light falls on striated surfaces (Young, 1802a). Young noted the systematic variation in hue as he rotated a pair of finely ruled lines at different angles to an incident beam, so anticipating the diffraction gratings that are today widely used in monochromators and spectroradiometers (Chapter 7).

As far as I am aware, the earlier literature holds no approximations to the Table of Figure 1.9. Thomas Young reached modern values in one leap. Yet it is important to realize that his accuracy is a tribute to the precision of Newton's measurements, made in the seventeenth century. Although Young's two-slit demonstration of optical interference (Young, 1807) has probably been even more influential in modern physics than Newton's prismatic experiments, it has to be said that Young was not by inclination an experimentalist. His first biographer, Hudson Gurney records:

> he was afterwards accustomed to say, that at no period of his life was he particularly fond of repeating experiments or even of very frequently attempting to originate new ones; considering that, however necessary to the advancement of science, they demanded a great sacrifice of time, and that when the fact was once established, that time was better employed in considering the purposes to which it might be applied, or the principles which it might tend to elucidate.
>
> (Gurney, 1831)

1.4 THE ULTRA-VIOLET, THE INFRA-RED, AND THE SPECTRAL SENSITIVITY OF THE EYE

Something else was clear to Thomas Young in 1801 and that was the continuity of visible and infra-red radiation. He writes: 'it seems highly likely that light differs from heat only in the frequency of its radiations' (Young, 1802a).

For most of the eighteenth century, there was little suspicion that radiation existed outside the visible spectrum. In part, we can attribute this innocence to the anthropocentric world-view that still prevailed: the Creator would not have filled space with radiation that Man could not perceive. A more specific explanation, however, is the absence – discussed above – of the physiological concept of a tuned transducer: If all frequencies are directly communicated to the nerves, then we should perceive all frequencies that exist.

Historians of science often attribute to James Hutton in 1794 the first suggestion of the existence of invisible rays beyond the red end of the spectrum. The first empirical demonstration was by William Herschel, the astronomer, the year before Thomas Young's Bakerian lecture (Herschel, 1800a). Figure 1.10 shows one of his experiments. He used a glass prism to form a solar spectrum on a graduated surface, and placed a thermometer with a blackened bulb at different positions within and beyond the spectrum, noting the rise of temperature. He placed further thermometers to one side of the spectrum to control for any change in ambient temperature (Herschel, 1800b). He systematically showed that the invisible rays are reflected, refracted and absorbed by different media, much as are the visible ones. Yet he concluded that the two kinds of ray are quite different in nature. He was misled by a category error.

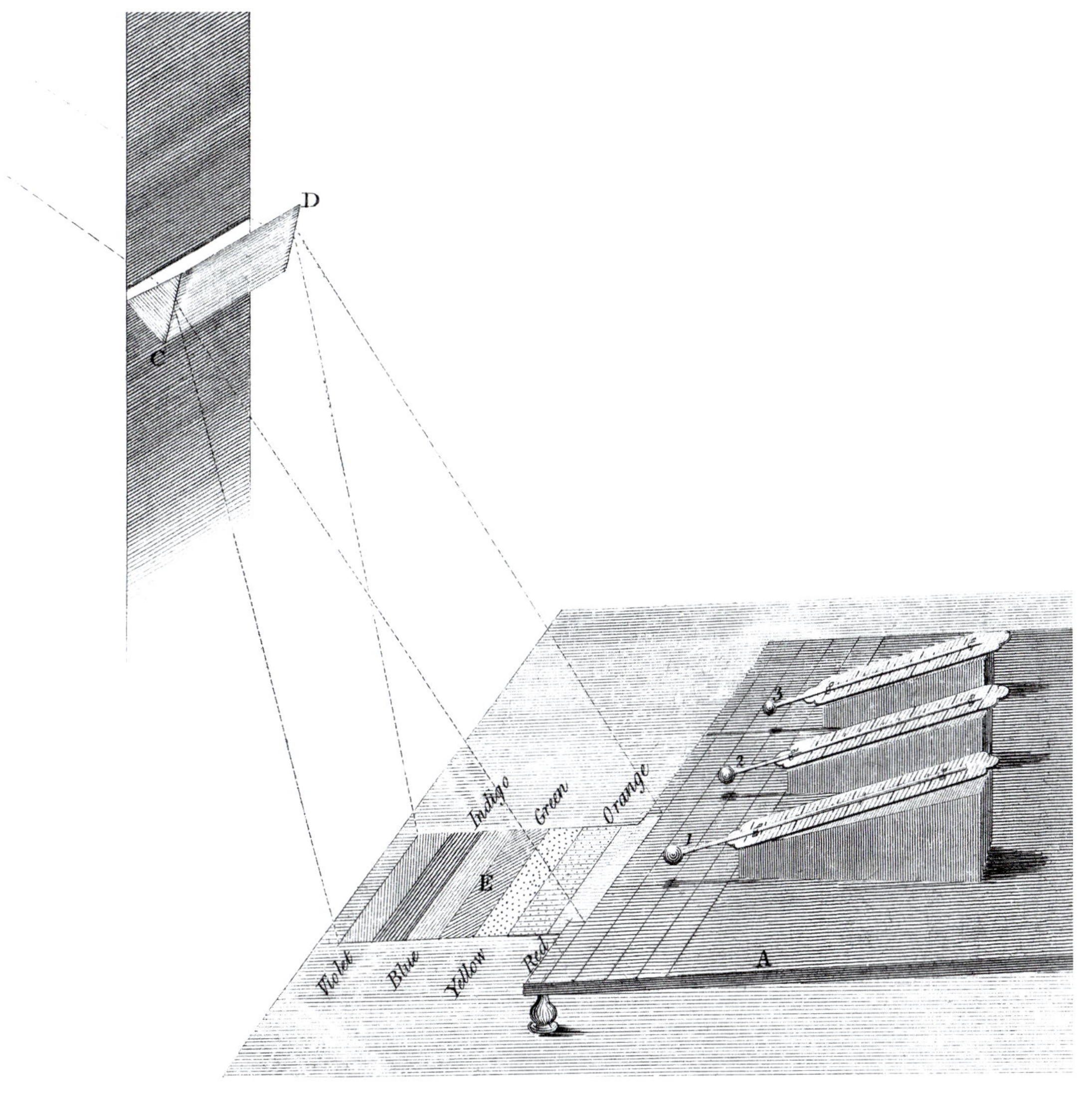

Figure 1.10 An experimental arrangement used by Herschel to investigate the infra-red. A rise in temperature is recorded by a thermometer placed beyond the visible spectrum.

Figure 1.11 shows Herschel's representation of the spectral efficiencies of the two types of ray. Certainly, he does deserve some credit for this plot. The very idea of a graph was still unusual in 1800; and this one may be the earliest ancestor of V_λ, the standard curve that represents the photopic sensitivity of the human eye (Chapter 3). The abscissa of Herschel's graph is refrangibility and will be dependent on the dispersive properties of the glass of the prism, as will the positions of the actual peaks. Notice that there is no ordinate for either of the two curves. For the thermal curve, it is the heating power as measured by the thermometer. To obtain the visual curve, Herschel scaled different colors by an acuity criterion, judging their ability to support the discrimination of spatial detail when light of different colors illuminated various objects under a microscope.

If he offered the second curve as a visual sensitivity curve, it would be rather impressive. But he doesn't. He offers it as a curve of the relative radiances of lights of different refrangibility, a spectral power distribution, and he offers a distinct curve for the calorific rays, which he supposes to be of a quite different quality. Operating with the wrong model of sensory transduction, Herschel is unable to grasp that the visible and invisible parts of the physical spectrum are continuous.

Yet the insight William Herschel lacked, had been provided in a work published 15 years earlier (Anonymous, 1786). The author of the latter work advances a vibratory theory of heat, and we can be sure of his identity, since it was printed with another essay that was rejected by the Royal Society. That careful body still retains the manuscripts that its referees rejected in the eighteenth century and hence we know that the author was John Elliot. And in a telling passage, Elliot writes:

> A writer on this subject has shewn (*Philosophical Observations on the Senses*, Etc) that colours may be excited in the eye, by irritating that organ, which do not at all depend on the rays of light . . . He therefore suggests that the rays of light excite colours in us only by the mediation of these internal colours. From whence it would follow, that if there are rays of light which have no

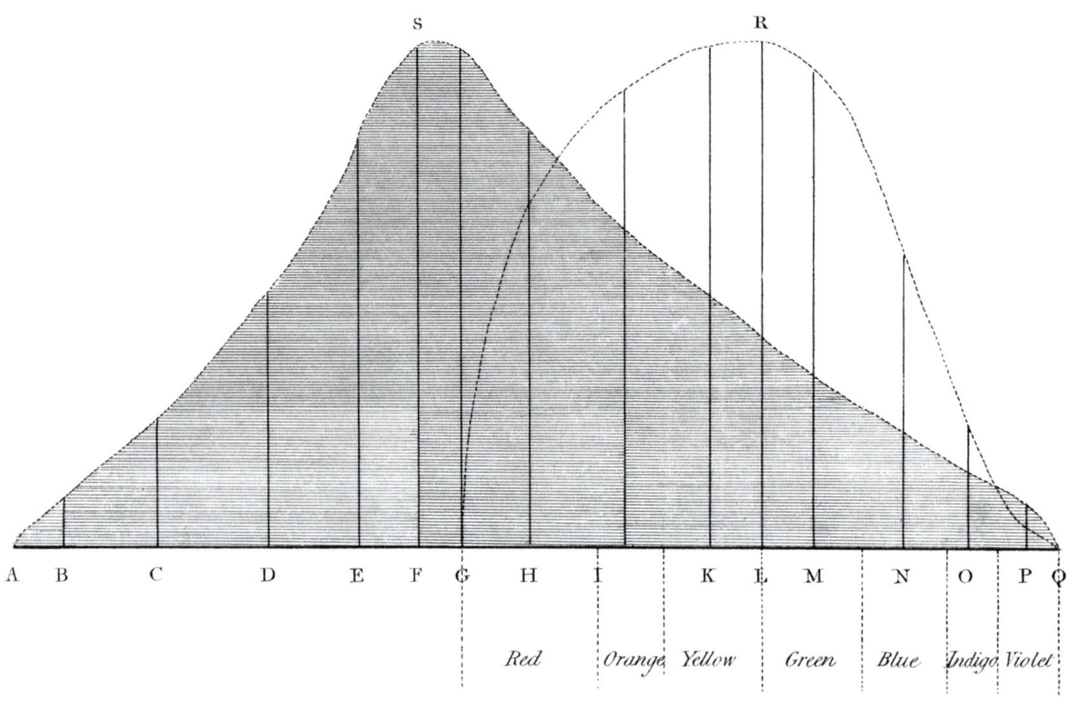

Figure 1.11 **Herschel's representation of the spectral efficiencies of what he supposed were two kinds of ray. *R* corresponds to visible radiation and *S* to the heat-making rays.**

answerable colours in the eye, those rays cannot be visible; that is, they cannot excite in us any sensation of colour.

Thus it was the concept of a tuned transducer that allowed Elliot to envisage the possibility of nonvisible radiation. There might be optical vibrations for which we have no answering resonators, as there may be acoustic vibrations that are too high or too low for us to hear. And down the side of one page, Elliot explicitly represents the visible spectrum extended in two directions, with only a limited space devoted to the seven Newtonian colors ROYGBIV (Figure 1.12). His diagram has had many successors.

Elliot also deserves credit as the father of spectroscopy, and he was the first to hint at the radiant spectrum of a black body and the concept of color temperature. He observed through a prism the spectrum of bodies as they were heated or allowed to cool. During cooling, for example, the peak of the band of radiation sinks downwards through from the blue to the red in the visible spectrum and out into the infra-red:

As the body in the third experiment cooled, it was pleasant to observe how, by degrees, the violet first, and then the indigo, blue, and the other inferior colours, vanished in succession, as if the spectrum were contracting itself towards its inferior part; and how the centre of the range seemed gradually to move from orange to red, and at length beneath it, as it sunk into the insensible part below R in the scheme, the superior part following it, till the whole range was out of sight, vanishing with red . . .

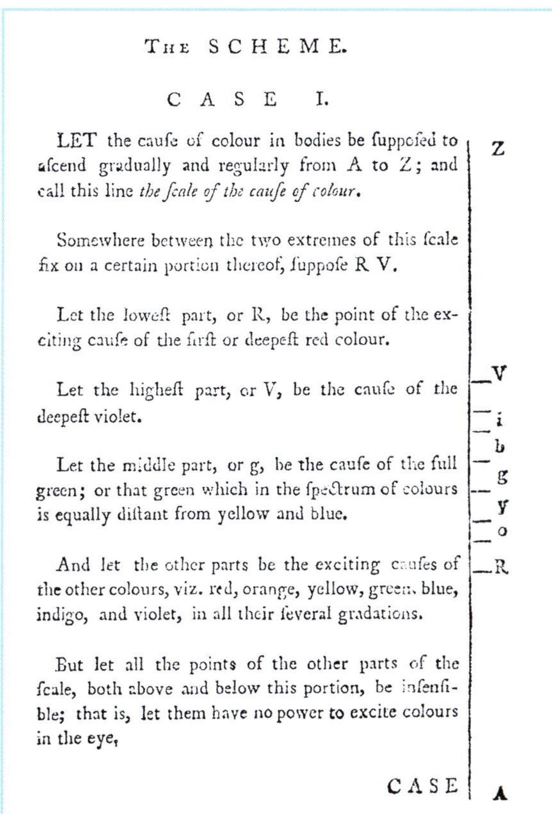
THE SCHEME.

CASE I.

LET the cauſe of colour in bodies be ſuppoſed to aſcend gradually and regularly from A to Z; and call this line *the ſcale of the cauſe of colour*.

Somewhere between the two extremes of this ſcale fix on a certain portion thereof, ſuppoſe R V.

Let the loweſt part, or R, be the point of the exciting cauſe of the firſt or deepeſt red colour.

Let the higheſt part, or V, be the cauſe of the deepeſt violet.

Let the middle part, or g, be the cauſe of the full green; or that green which in the ſpectrum of colours is equally diſtant from yellow and blue.

And let the other parts be the exciting cauſes of the other colours, viz. red, orange, yellow, green, blue, indigo, and violet, in all their ſeveral gradations.

But let all the points of the other parts of the ſcale, both above and below this portion, be inſenſible; that is, let them have no power to excite colours in the eye,

CASE

Figure 1.12 **The first representation of a spectrum that includes the ultra-violet and infra-red as well as the visible region. From John Elliot's *Experiments and observations on light and colours* of 1786. Elliot published the monograph anonymously.**

1.5 COLOR CONSTANCY, COLOR CONTRAST, AND COLOR HARMONY

When a given object is viewed in different illuminants, its apparent color changes much less than might be expected from the change in the spectral composition of the light that it reflects to our eye. The latter – the spectral flux reaching the eye – depends on both (a) the spectral composition of the illumination and (b) the object's spectral reflectance, its disposition to reflect some wavelengths more than others. It is the second of these that is of biological importance to us in recognizing the objects of our world; and the visual system appears able to discover, and compensate for, the color of the illumination in order to recover the surface property of the object. This relative stability of our color perception is called 'color constancy' (Chapter 4).

Color constancy cannot be accounted for by a simple model of three receptors and three corresponding nerves that each evoke particular sensations in the sensorium. Modern textbooks sometimes attribute such a model to Young, and so it is instructive to note that he was fully aware of color constancy. In his *Lectures* he writes:

when a room is illuminated either by the yellow light of a candle, or by the red light of a fire, a sheet of writing paper still appears to retain its whiteness; and if from the light of the candle we take away some of the abundant yellow light, and leave or substitute a portion actually white, the effect is

> nearly the same as if we took away the yellow light from white, and substituted the indigo which would be left: and we observe accordingly that in comparison with the light of a candle, the common daylight appears of a purplish hue.
>
> (Young, 1807)

In this compressed passage, Young not only describes color constancy, but also links it – as it has often been linked since – to the simultaneous contrast of color. An earlier passage from Young's *Syllabus* is equally telling:

> Other causes, probably connected with some general laws of sensation, produce the imaginary colours of shadows, which have been elegantly investigated and explained by Count Rumford. When a general colour prevails over the whole field of vision, excepting a part comparatively small, the apparent colour of that part is nearly the same as if the light falling on the whole field had been white, and the rays of the prevalent colour only had been intercepted at one particular part, the other rays being suffered to proceed.
>
> (Young, 1802b)

Young, however, was neither the first to observe color constancy nor the first to relate it to color contrast. The phenomenon itself was already described by the geometer Philippe De La Hire in 1694 in his monograph *Sur les diférens accidens de la Vuë*. We do not commonly realize, he says, that we see colors differently by daylight and by candlelight. For in a given illumination, we judge the array of colors as a whole (*l'on compare toutes les couleurs ensemble*). To appreciate the difference between objects illuminated by candlelight and those illuminated by daylight, what one must do is close the shutters of a room tightly during daylight hours and illuminate this room with candle light.

> . . . passing then into another place illuminated by sunlight, if one looks through the door of the room, the objects that are lit by candlelight will appear tinted reddish-yellow in comparison with those lit by the sun and seen concurrently. One cannot appreciate this when he is in the candle-lit chamber.
>
> (De La Hire, 1694/1730)

La Hire's monograph was published under the aegis of the Royal Academy of Sciences of Paris. A century later, the same Academy was to hear the most brilliant paper ever delivered on color constancy. The lecture was delivered in the spring of 1789, only weeks before the revolution began, and the author was another distinguished geometer, Gaspard Monge (Figure 1.13). It is a mark of the genius of this man that he held high office under administrations as diverse as the *ancien régime*, the *Comité de Salut Publique*, and the First Empire, owing no doubt to his skills as a military technologist.

To illustrate his lecture, Monge had hung a red cloth on the wall of a house opposite the west-facing windows of the meeting room of the Academy. He invited his fellow *académiciens* to view the red cloth through a red glass. The appearance of the cloth was counter-intuitive. Seen through a filter that transmitted predominantly red light, it might have been expected to continue to look a saturated red. But no, it looked pale, even whitish. The same was true when the assembled company inspected one of their fellows who happened that day to be wearing a red outfit. A yellow-tinted paper examined through a yellow glass looked absolutely white. Monge was aware that his illusion (we may call it the Paradox of Monge) was strongest when the scene was brightly lit and when there was an array of variously colored objects present in the scene, including objects that one knew to be naturally white. When all that was visible through the red glass was a red surface, the effect was abolished.

Monge related his illusion to a second phenomenon, that of colored shadows. In his day, colored shadows were already a familiar and antique phenomenon. They were briefly described, for example, in 1672 by Otto von

> Ainſi les jugemens que nous portons ſur les couleurs des objets ne paroiſſent pas dépendre uniquement de la nature abſolue des rayons de lumière qui en font la peinture ſur la rétine ; ils peuvent être modifiés par les circonſtances, & il eſt probable que nous ſommes déterminés plutôt par la relation de quelques-unes des affections des rayons de lumière, que par les affections elles-mêmes, conſidérées d'une manière abſolue.

Figure 1.13 **A critical passage from Gaspard Monge (1789), in which he insists on the relative nature of our color perception.**

Guericke of Magdeburg, the inventor of the vacuum pump. At the end of the eighteenth century, however, commentators were still uncertain as to whether they were perceptual phenomenon or had a physical basis. Von Guericke himself had supposed that they arose from the interaction of light and dark ('. . .*sicut gutta lactis & gutta atramenti ad invicem positae, in loco conjunctionis intermedio, coeruleum efficiunt colorem*'). Monge described how colored shadows can be seen in the morning of a fine day if one opens a window to allow diffuse skylight to enter a room and fall on a sheet of paper that is also illuminated by the light of a nearby candle. The shadow of a small object – where the paper is illuminated only by skylight – will look a rich blue. And yet if the candle is suddenly extinguished, the paper will look uniformly white, even though the region of the shadow has not physically changed. Very similar is an illusion communicated to Monge by Meusnier: If a room is illuminated by sunlight passing through a red curtain and if there is a small hole in the curtain that allows a beam of sunlight to fall on a sheet of white paper, then the patch of sunlight will not look white but rather will look 'a very beautiful green' (Monge, 1789).

To explain such illusions, and to explain the paradox of the red cloth, Monge suggested that our sensations of color do not depend simply on the physical light that reaches our eye from a given surface. Rather, we reinterpret this stimulus in terms of what we judge to be the illuminant falling on the scene: If we judge the illuminant to be reddish, then we shall perceive as greenish an object that physically delivers white light to the eye, since such an object is not delivering the excess of red light that a white surface ought to reflect in a reddish illuminant. Similarly, a red object in red illumination will look whitish to us because it delivers light of the same composition as the estimated illuminant.

In 1789, Thomas Young's Bakerian Lecture was more than a decade in the future, and Monge did not know what the physical variable was that distinguished the hues of the Newtonian spectrum, but he was clear that our perceptions of color in a complex scene do not depend *only* on that physical variable. In a passage that would be echoed two centuries later by Edwin Land, he wrote:

> So the judgements that we hold about the colors of objects seem not to depend uniquely on the absolute nature of the rays of light that paint the picture of the objects on the retina; our judgements can be changed by the surroundings, and it is probable that we are influenced more by the ratio of some of the properties of the light rays than by the properties themselves, considered in an absolute manner.

Monge is describing the process that today we should call 'color constancy,' the process that works largely unnoticed to allow us to judge the constant properties of surfaces in varying illuminants. Monge asked the question that has remained at the heart of studies of color constancy: How do we estimate the color of the illuminant in order to reinterpret the spectral stimulus reaching us from a given object? His answer reflects his primary interest in geometry. All surfaces reflect to our eye some light of the unmodified illuminant as well as light of the characteristic color of the object, the color that results from the object's absorption properties. At one extreme, a glossy object, like a stick of sealing wax, will exhibit highlights, regions of specular reflectance where the illuminant color predominates. Other regions of any object, whether glossy or not, will reflect varying proportions of illuminant and object colors, the proportions varying with the viewing angle and the indentations and protrusions of the surface. Here, Monge anticipates the theory of constancy advanced by Lee (1986): In a chromaticity diagram, the colors of each surface will lie along a line connecting the object color to the illuminant, and the illuminant chromaticity is defined by the intersection of such lines. Hurlbert (1998) has called this the 'chromaticity convergence' theory.

One of the first Americans to study color was Benjamin Thompson, Count Rumford. Writing to the Royal Society of London from Munich in April 1793, he described his experiments on colored shadows, experiments to which Thomas Young refers in the passage cited at the beginning of this section. He set up two matched Argand lamps (see section 1.2.3.1), 'well trimmed, and which were both made to burn with the greatest possible brilliancy.' The light they emitted was of the same color, for when they both illuminated a sheet of white paper and a small cylinder was interposed between the lamps and the paper, the two shadows of the cylinder were identical and colorless. Rumford mounted a blackened tube so that he could view in isolation the shadow cast by one of the two lamp beams. An assistant then introduced a yellow glass in front of this lamp. Observed through the tube, the shadow remained colorless, and indeed Count Rumford could not tell when the assistant passed the yellow glass in and out of the beam. Yet when he looked freely at the paper, the shadow was of a beautiful blue color, while the other was yellow. Here was uncontestable evidence that the cause of the colored shadows was not physical (Thompson, 1794). One other thing struck Rumford very forcibly in these experiments: Although the colors of the two shadows varied as the colors of the two illuminants were varied, there was always a perfect and very pleasing harmony between the colors of the paired shadows. Nowadays, we would note that the two colors are physical complementaries with respect to the light falling on the surrounding white paper: Each of the two shadows lacks part of the total illumination of the scene, and the missing part is present in the fellow shadow.

1.6 COLOR DEFICIENCY

1.6.1 INHERITED COLOR DEFICIENCY

We have seen that the normal human observer requires only three variables in a color-matching experiment (section 1.2). The common forms of inherited color deficiency are defined in terms of how they depart from standard color-matching behavior: 'Dichromats' can match all colors by mixing two primary lights, whereas 'anomalous trichromats' resemble normals in requiring three primaries in a color match but differ from the normal in the matches that they make. These inherited forms of color blindness are surprisingly frequent, affecting 8% of male Caucasian populations.

Yet the historical recognition of color deficiency came very late. This may reflect the imprecision of our common coinage of color words, and also the fact that the color blind seldom regret what they never have enjoyed, even reaching adulthood before an occupational test brings recognition. Robert Boyle, in his 'Uncommon Observations about Vitiated Sight' of 1688, described a 'Mathematician, Eminent for his skill in Opticks and therefore a very competent Relator of *Phaenomena*.' This subject made excellent use of his eyes in astronomical observations, but confused colors that appeared quite dissimilar to other men. Frustratingly Boyle does not tell us the particular colors that his subject confounded, but we may speculate on the identity of this mathematician and optician. Could we relate Boyle's brief description to Newton's remark that 'my own eyes are not very critical in distinguishing colours' (Newton, 1675/1757)?

Further cases of color deficiency were described with increasing detail in the English and French literature of the 1770s. Joseph Huddart (1777) gave an account of the shoemaker Harris, from a Quaker family of Maryport in Cumberland. Harris had good discrimination of form but poor color discrimination, a defect that he shared with his brother, a sea captain. Huddart writes of Harris:

> He observed also that, when young, other children could discern cherries on a tree by some pretended difference of colour, though he could only distinguish them from the leaves by their difference of size and shape. He observed also, that by means of this difference of colour they could see the cherries at a greater distance than he could, though he could see other objects at as great a distance as they; that is, where the sight was not assisted by the colour. Large objects he could see as well as other persons; and even the smaller ones if they were not enveloped in other things, as in the case of cherries among the leaves.

This is a telling passage, for it reveals the conditions under which we need color vision in the natural world. When a stationary target object is embedded in a background that varies randomly in form and lightness, it is visible only to an observer who can distinguish colors – that is, an observer who can discriminate surfaces by differences in their spectral reflectances (Mollon, 1989). As we shall see, the natural task of finding fruit in foliage was later to find its analogue in artificial tests for color deficiency (see section 1.7.4).

As the second half of the eighteenth century progressed, a wider public became aware that not everyone's perceptions of color were the same. In 1760 Oliver Goldsmith, who may himself have been color deficient, wrote of the inappropriateness of recommending the contemplation of paintings 'to one who had lost the power of distinguishing colors' (MacLennan, 1975). And by the 1780s color blindness was well enough known to be remarked on at the English court. Fanny Burney recounts in her journal an uncomfortable conversation with George III:

> He still, however, kept me in talk, and still upon music. 'To me,' said he, 'it appears quite as strange to meet with people who have no ear for music and cannot distinguish one air from another, as to meet with people who are dumb . . . There are people who have no eye for difference of colour. The Duke of Marlborough actually cannot tell scarlet from green!' He then told me an anecdote of his mistaking one of those colors for another, which was very laughable, but I do not remember it clearly enough to write it. How unfortunate for true virtuosi that such an eye should possess objects worthy of the most discerning – the treasures of Blenheim!'
>
> (Barrett, 1904)

So the existence of color deficiency was already well established when in 1794 the young John Dalton gave an account of his own dichromacy to the Manchester Literary and Philosophical Society. But Dalton's account was more analytic than anything that had gone before, and his later fame as a chemist meant that 'daltonism' became the term for color deficiency in many languages, including French, Spanish, and Russian. For him, the solar spectrum had two main divisions, which he called 'blue' and 'yellow.' 'My yellow,' he wrote, 'comprehends the red, orange, yellow and green of others' (Dalton, 1798). The red of sealing wax and the green of the outer face of a laurel leaf looked much the same to him, but scarlet and pink – which share a common quality for the normal observer – were quite different colors for Dalton, falling on opposite sides of neutral. In daylight the pink flowers of clover (*Trifolium pratense*) and of the red campion (*Lychnis dioica*) resembled the light blue of sky. What first prompted him to investigate his own vision was his observation that the flowers of the cranesbill, *Pelargonium zonale* (Figure 1.14), looked sky-blue by daylight but yellowish by candlelight (Lonsdale, 1874). Of his immediate acquaintances, only his own brother experienced this striking change. On further enquiry, however, he discovered that his defect of color perception was not so very rare: in one class of 25 pupils, he found two who agreed with him. He never, however, 'heard of one female subject to this peculiarity,' so giving the first indication that color deficiency is a sex-linked characteristic. We now know that it affects fewer than half of one percent of women.

John Dalton himself thought that his defect arose from a blue-colored medium within his eye. Since there was nothing odd to be seen by external observation of the anterior parts of his eye, he thought that it was likely be his vitreous humor that was blue, absorbing disproportionately the red and orange parts of the spectrum. To allow a test of this hypothesis, he directed that his eyes should be examined on his death.

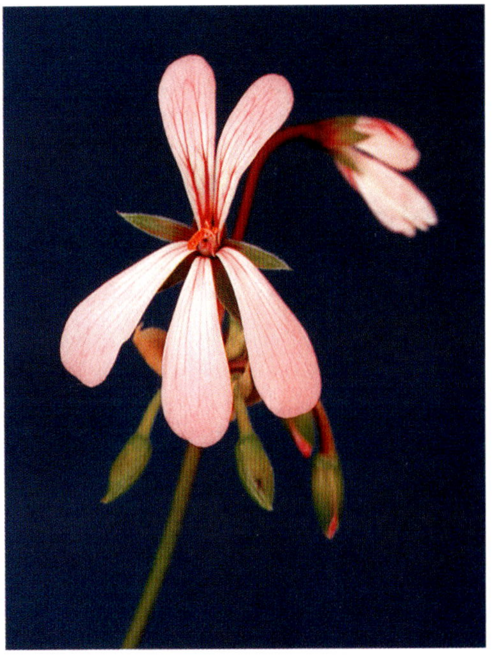

Figure 1.14 **The pink geranium or cranesbill, *Pelargonium zonale*. To John Dalton and his brother, the flower looked sky-blue by daylight but yellowish by candlelight. (Copyright: Department of Experimental Psychology, University of Cambridge, reproduced with permission.)**

He died aged 78 on 27 July 1844, and on the following day an autopsy was done by his medical attendant, Joseph Ransome. Ransome collected the humors of one eye into watch glasses and found them to be 'perfectly pellucid', the lens itself exhibiting the yellowness expected in someone of Dalton's age. He shrewdly left the second eye almost intact, slicing off the posterior pole and noting that scarlet and green objects were not distorted in color when seen through the eye (Wilson, 1845; Henry, 1854).

In fact, as we have seen (section 1.2.3.1), the correct explanation of most forms of inherited dichromacy had already been advanced by George Palmer (Voigt, 1781), when Dalton was only 15 years old. Palmer's suggestion was taken up in 1807 by Thomas Young. Listing Dalton's paper in the bibliography of his *Lectures on Natural Philosophy*, he remarks: 'He [Dalton] thinks it probable that the vitreous humour is of deep blue tinge: but this has never been observed by anatomists, and it is much more simple to suppose the absence or paralysis of those fibres of the retina, which are calculated to perceive red.'

Many distinguished commentators (e.g. Abney, 1913; Wright, 1967) have followed Young in assuming that it was the long-wavelength receptor that Dalton lacked. It is instructive to consider why this view was so persistent. First, in an often-cited phrase, Dalton described the red end of the solar spectrum as 'little more than a shade or defect of light.' Second, he saw no redness in pinks and crimsons, matching them to blues.

Let us take the two observations in turn. In the type of color blindness called 'protanopia,' where the long-wavelength cone is absent, a prominent sign is the foreshortening of the red end of the spectrum. In fact, the physicists Sir David Brewster and Sir John Herschel both questioned Dalton directly and both reported that he did not see the spectrum as foreshortened at long wavelengths (Brewster, 1842; Henry, 1854). In fact, even a deuteranope – someone lacking the middle-wave pigment – might speak of the long-wave end of the spectrum as dim, for the long-wave pigment in fact peaks in the yellow-green, and for a dichromat the long-wave end of the spectrum does not offer the *Farbenglut*, the extra brightness of saturated colors, that enhances the red end of the spectrum for the normal observer (Kohlrausch, 1923).

But what of the absence of redness in Dalton's experience of surfaces that the normal would call pink or scarlet? Does that mean he lacked long-wavelength cones? The trichromatic theory has historically often been combined with a primitive form of Mueller's Doctrine of Specific Nerve Energies: There are three receptors and three corresponding nerves, and centrally the nerves secrete red, yellow, and blue sensations or red, green, and blue sensations. It took a very long time for color science fully to free itself from this notion, and to this day generations of undergraduates are misled by lecturers and textbooks that speak of 'red,' 'green,' and 'blue' cones. Dalton helpfully specified several crimson and pink flowers that appeared blue to him. I have measured these flowers spectroradiometrically and have plotted their chromaticities in Figure 1.15. The two straight lines passing through the chromaticity of the daylight illuminant represent sets of chromaticities that match daylight for protanopes and deuteranopes respectively. Chromaticities that lie above the line will have the hue quality that the dichromat associates with long wavelengths, and chromaticities that lie below the line will have the quality that the dichromat associates with short wavelengths. For both types of dichromat the several pink and crimson flowers lie below the line and should have the same hue quality as blue sky. So Dalton's failure to see redness in these flowers is no basis for placing him in one category of dichromat or the other.

Shriveled fragments of Dalton's eye, preserved only in air, survive to this day in the possession of the Manchester Literary and Philosophical Society (Brockbank, 1944). In the 1990s the Society gave permission for small samples to be examined using the polymerase chain reaction, which allows the amplification of short stretches of DNA defined by primer sequences specific to particular genes. This exercise in molecular biography yielded only copies of the gene that encodes the long-wave photopigment of the retina and never the gene that encodes the middle-wave photopigment (Hunt *et al.*, 1995; Mollon *et al.*, 1997). So Dalton appears to have been a deuteranope, and not the protanope lacking 'red' cones, as so often supposed.

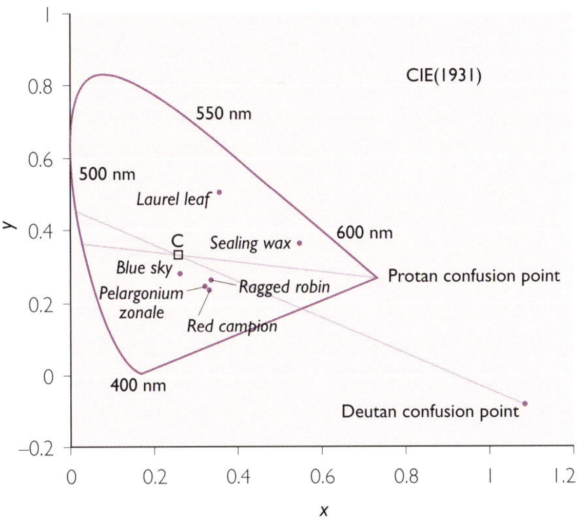

Figure 1.15 The CIE (1931) chromaticity diagram (see section 1.7.1 and Chapter 3). Plotted in the diagram are several flowers that looked blue to Dalton: the cranesbill (*Pelargonium zonale*), red campion (*Lychnis dioica*) and ragged robin (*Lychnis floscuculi*). Also plotted are sealing wax and the upper side of a laurel leaf, which Dalton judged to be very similar in color. The open square in the center of the diagram represents Illuminant C, a standard approximation to daylight. Passing through this point are two lines, one (a 'protan confusion line') representing the set of chromaticities that would be confused with white by a dichromat who lacks the long-wave cones, and the other (a 'deutan confusion line') representing the set of chromaticities that would be confused with white by a dichromat who lacks the middle-wave cones. For both kinds of dichromat, the pink flowers lie on the blue side of the neutral line, whereas sealing wax will have the opposite quality. Dalton (1798) himself wrote '*Red* and *scarlet* form a genus with me totally different from pink'.

1.6.2 ACQUIRED DEFICIENCIES OF COLOR PERCEPTION

Color discrimination can deteriorate during a person's lifetime, owing to ocular diseases (such as glaucoma), or to systemic conditions that affect the eye and optic pathways (such as diabetes and multiple sclerosis), or to strokes, cerebral inflammations, and head injuries. What one loses, one notices and regrets. So it might be expected that acquired deficiencies would have been recorded historically before the inherited deficiencies.

Certainly, a self-report of altered color vision occurs as early as 1671 in the *Traité de Physique* of Jacques Rohault (Figure 1.16). Since it leads him to suspect the existence of congenital color anomalies, the passage is worth translating in full:

> Yet I would venture to insist that just as it often happens that the same food tastes quite different to two different people, similarly it can be that two men have very different sensations when looking at the same object in the same way; and I am the more convinced of this because I have an experience of it that is wholly personal to me: For it happening once that my right eye was weakened and injured, by looking for more than twelve hours through a telescope at the contest of two armies, which was going on a league away; I now find my vision so affected that when I look at yellow objects with my right eye, they do not appear to me as they used to do, nor as they now appear when I observe them with the left. And what is remarkable is that I do not notice the same variation in all colors but only in some, as for example in green, which appears to come close to blue when I observe it with the right eye. This experience of mine makes me believe that there are perhaps some men who are born with, and retain all their life, the disposition that I currently have in one of my eyes, and that there perhaps are others who have the disposition that I enjoy in the other: However, it is impossible for them or anyone else to be aware of this, because each is accustomed to call the sensation that a certain object produces in him by the name that is already in use; but which, being common to everyone's different sensations, is nonetheless ambiguous.

Rohault's textbook was widely circulated in several editions, and so it may not be coincidence that the following decade brought a flurry of case reports – of varying sophistication. Stephan Blankaart, in a Dutch collection of medical reports, briefly described a woman who, after suffering a miscarriage, 'saw objects as black' but later recovered (Blankaart, 1680). In 1684 'the great and experienced Oculist' Dawbenry Turbervile wrote from Salisbury to the Royal Society: 'A Maid, two or three and twenty years old, came to me from *Banbury*, who could see very well, but no colour beside *Black* and *White*' (Turbervile, 1684). But Turbervile then spoils his already slight report by adopting an emissive theory of vision: 'She had such Scintillations by night (with the appearances of Bulls, Bears Etc.) as terrified her

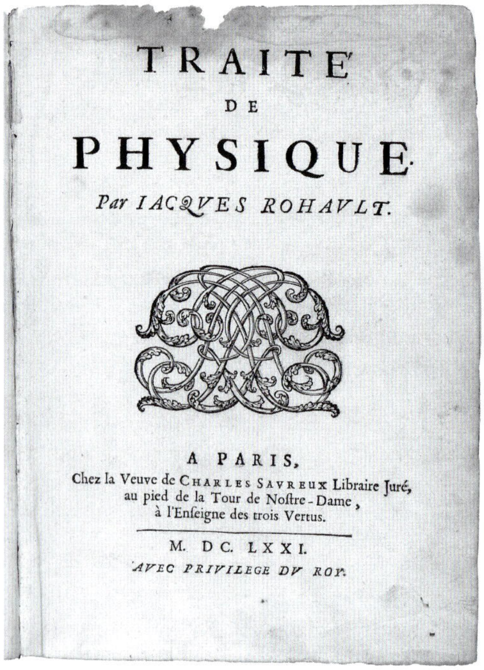

Figure 1.16 **The treatise of physics of Jacques Rohault (1671), in which he describes an acquired disturbance of his own color vision.**

very much; she could see to read sometimes in the great darkness for almost a quarter of an hour.' He is implying that the 'Scintillations' – the subjective sensations of light that now would be called 'phosphenes' – corresponded to actual light. This misinterpretation of phosphenes lingered until the nineteenth century and was one of the factors that prompted the young Johannes Mueller to develop his 'Doctrine of Specific Nerve Energies.'

Whatever we make of Turbervile's Maid from Banbury, we can only admire Robert Boyle's account of a suspiciously similar case, published in his *Vitiated Sight* of 1688. The subject was a gentlewoman 'about 18 or twenty years old' when Boyle had examined her. After an unidentified illness treated with blisters, she had lost her sight entirely. Slowly light sensation and then form vision returned, but color perception remained impaired. Like the Maid from Banbury 'she is not unfrequently troubled with flashes of Lightning, that seem to issue out like Flames about the External Angle of her Eye, which often make her start, and put her into Frights and Melancholy Thoughts' (Boyle, 1688). With materials that came to hand, Boyle established that she could read and had good acuity, but was unable to identify reds, greens or blues. He adds – in a passage both poetic and insightful – 'when she had a mind to gather Violets, tho' she kneel'd in that Place where they grew, she was not able to distinguish them by the Colour from the neighbouring Grass, but only by the Shape, or by feeling them.' Banbury is but 25 km from Boyle's home in Oxford; and Boyle, always troubled by poor eyesight, himself consulted Turbervile. Almost certainly, Boyle and Tubervile describe the same case, but Boyle's is much the better account.

1.7 THE GOLDEN AGE (1850–1931)

Our survey has shown that many of the concepts of modern color science were in place by the middle of the nineteenth century. The following decades saw a golden era, when colorimetry emerged as a quantitative science and when color perception held a more prominent place in scientific discussion and in public debate than it has held before or since.

1.7.1 COLOR MIXTURE

When Hermann Helmholtz published his first papers on color in 1852, he was already celebrated for his essay on the conservation of force, his measurements of the speed of neural conduction, and his invention of the ophthalmoscope. Born in Potsdam in 1821, he had become professor at Königsberg in 1849. One of his first contributions to color science was to clarify the distinction between the subtractive mixture of pigments and the additive mixture of colored lights (Helmholtz, 1852). He conceived of a pigment as a series of semi-transparent layers of particles acting as filters to light that is reflected from the underlying layers. Consider a mixture of yellow and blue pigments. A bright yellow pigment will reflect red, yellow, and green light, whereas a blue pigment will reflect green, blue, and violet. Some light, Helmholtz suggested, will be reflected by particles at the surface, and this component will include a large range of wavelengths and will be close to white in its composition. Light that is reflected from deeper layers, however, will be subject to absorption by both blue and yellow particles; and so the light that is returned to the eye will be dominated by wavelengths that are not absorbed by either component – in this case, wavelengths from the green region of the spectrum.

Helmholtz offered a striking illustration of the difference between additive and subtractive mixture. He painted the center of a disk with a mixture of yellow and blue pigment, but in the outer part of the disk he painted separate sectors with the same individual component pigments. When the disk was spun, the center looked dark green, as painterly tradition required, but the circumference looked lighter and grayish. In the former case, the perceived color depends on residual rays that are reflected after the physical mixture of pigments. In the latter case, the two broadband components are effectively combined at the retina, owing to the temporal integration of successive stimuli within the visual system.

It is reassuring, however, and instructive, to see a genius err. And so we can note that Helmholtz's 1852 paper contains an empirical error and a conceptual error. He reports his results for the additive mixture of spectral, narrow-band, colors. He formed two prismatic spectra that overlay each other at 90°, so that all combinations of monochromatic lights were present in the array; and he then viewed small regions of the array in isolation. His empirical error was to conclude that there was only one pair of spectral colors, yellow and indigo-blue, that were complementaries in that they would mix additively to form a pure white; from other combinations, the best that he could achieve was a pale flesh color or a pale green – a report that recalls Newton's phrase 'some faint anonymous Colour.' The failure of Helmholtz to identify more than one pair of complementaries may merely reflect difficulty in isolating the appropriate small regions of the array. But his conceptual error in the 1852 paper is instructive. By mixing red and a mid-green, he was unable to match a monochromatic yellow in saturation. This result is correct and the reason for it is that a mid-green light stimulates all three cones, whereas a monochromatic yellow stimulates only the long- and middle-wave cones. Helmholtz was led, however, explicitly to reject what he understood to be Young's trichromatic theory. If yellow is the color seen when red and green sensations are concurrently excited, he argued, then exactly the same color should be produced by the simultaneous action of red and green rays. Because green is a phenomenologically simple hue, he does not entertain the possibility that monochromatic green light excites more than one class of fiber.

The failure of Helmholtz to find more than one pair of complementaries drew a response from the mathematician Hermann Grassmann. Grassmann (1853) began with the assumption that color experience is three-dimensional, being fully described by the attributes of hue, brightness, and saturation. These three attributes of sensation correspond, he suggested, to the three physical variables of wavelength (or frequency), intensity (or amount of light), and purity (the ratio of white to monochromatic white in a mixture). By assuming from the start that vision was three-dimensional and by adding the assumption that phenomenological experience never changed discontinuously as one of the physical variables was changed, Grassmann was able to show that each point on the color circle ought to have a complementary. Helmholtz now adopted a better method of mixing spectral lights and found that the range of wavelengths between red and greenish-yellow had complementaries in the range between greenish-blue and violet (Helmholtz, 1855; Figure 1.17). A range of greens, however, do not have complementaries that lie within the spectrum: Their complementaries are purples, i.e. mixtures of lights drawn from the red and violet ends of the spectrum. Moreover, complementary lights of equal brightness do not necessarily mix to yield white: The ratio needed in the mixture may be very unequal. For example, in the mixture of yellow-green and violet that matches white, the violet component will be of much lower brightness than the yellow-green component. If the center-of-gravity principle for mixing is to be preserved and if the weightings of the component lights are to be in terms of subjective luminosity, then a chromaticity diagram like that of Figure 1.18 is required. The range of purples is represented by a straight line connecting the two ends of the locus of spectral colors.

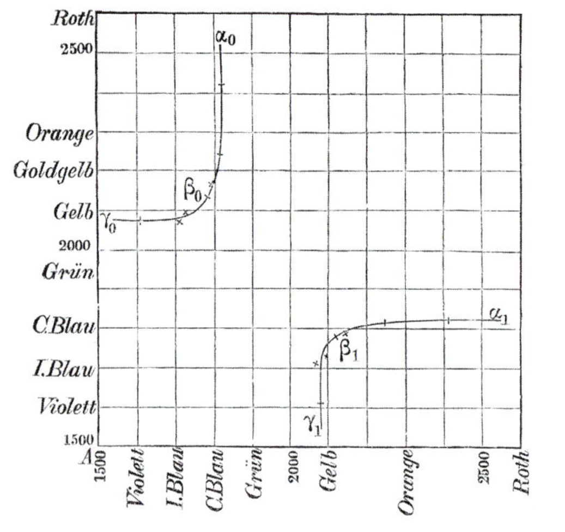

Figure 1.17 **Helmholtz's graph of the wavelengths that are complementaries, i.e., the wavelengths that will form white when mixed in a suitable ratio.**

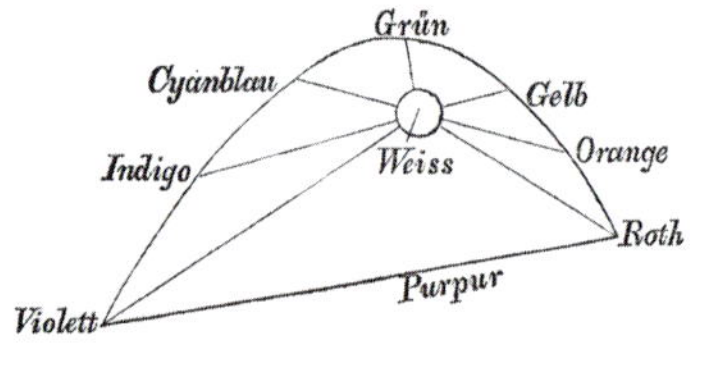

Figure 1.18 **The first chromaticity diagram to have a modern form, prepared by Helmholtz on the basis of his measurements of complementaries.**

In the same year, 1855, the 24-year-old James Clerk Maxwell took Young's theory several steps further (Maxwell, 1855a, 1855b). He made his experiments on additive mixture by means of a spinning top that carried superposed disks (Figure 1.19). The disks, cut from colored papers, were slit along a radius, so that Clerk Maxwell could expose a chosen amount of a given color by slipping one disk over another. He used two sets of disks, one set of twice the diameter of the other. The inner disks were typically formed by white and black and, when spun, they exhibited a gray corresponding to how much of each paper was exposed. In the outer ring, he typically used sectors of three different colors. Clerk Maxwell experimentally adjusted the proportions of the three colors of the outer ring until, being spun, they gave a gray that was equivalent to the gray

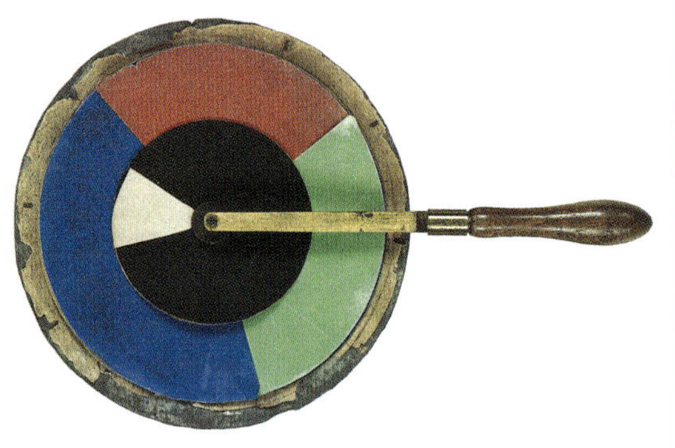

Figure 1.19 **The color-mixing top of James Clerk Maxwell. The instrument survived in the collection of the Cavendish Laboratory, Cambridge. This photograph was taken in 1982. (Copyright: Department of Experimental Psychology, Cambridge University, reproduced with permission.)**

seen in the inner area. Once the match was achieved, Clerk Maxwell used the perimeter scale to read off the space occupied by each paper in hundredths of a full circle. Suppose the outer colors were vermilion (V), ultramarine (U), and emerald green (EG), and the center papers snow white (SW) and black (Bk). Then he would write an equation of the following form:

$$.37\ V + .27\ U + .36\ EG = .28\ SW + .72\ Bk$$

Suppose that we take the three outer colors as our standard colors. By replacing one of the outer colors by some test color, Clerk Maxwell could obtain a series of equations that contained two of the standard colors and the test color. Then, by bringing the test color to the left-hand side of the equation, and bringing the three standard colors to the right, he could represent the test color as the center of gravity of three masses, whose weights are taken as the number of degrees of each of the standard colors.

By 1860 Clerk Maxwell had constructed a device that allowed him to match daylight with mixtures of three monochromatic lights (Maxwell, 1860). This allowed him to express the spectrum in terms of three primaries and to plot against wavelength the amounts of the three primaries required to match any given wavelength (Figure 1.20). The latter curves are the forerunners of later 'color matching

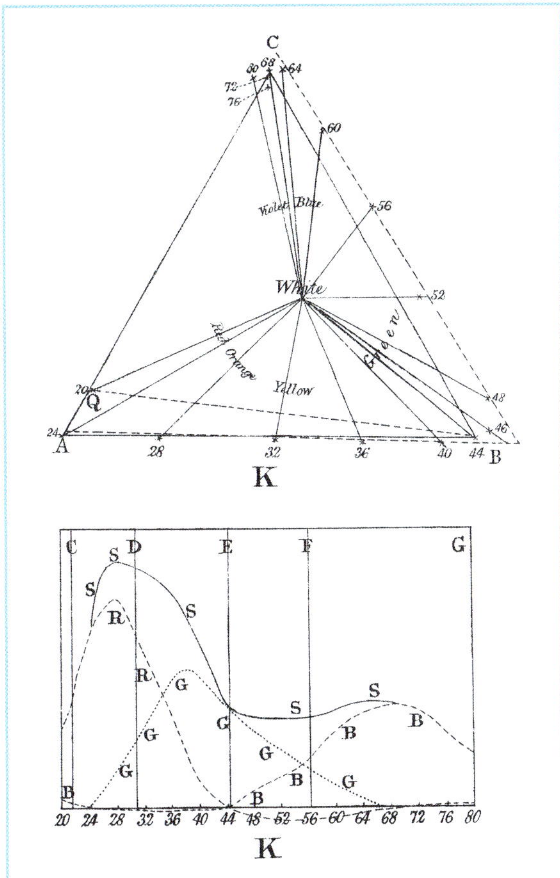

Figure 1.20 **The first empirical color-matching functions. The data shown are for Clerk Maxwell's wife, Katherine. The lower plot represents the proportions of the red, green and blue primaries needed to match a given wavelength. The spectrum runs from red on the left to violet on the right. The upper plot is a chromaticity diagram based on the same color-matching data. The locus of the spectral colors is expressed in terms of the proportions of the three primaries used in the experiment.**

functions.' In the same paper, Clerk Maxwell noted that the matches he made with central vision did not hold when he observed them indirectly. This discrepancy, and also the discrepancy between his central matches and those of his wife, he attributed to the yellow spot of the central retina, which selectively absorbs light in the wavelength range 430–90 nm.

Fresh determinations of the color matching functions were made in the 1920s by Guild, using a filter instrument, and by Wright, using monochromatic stimuli. When the two sets of results were expressed in terms of a common set of primaries, they were found to agree extremely well, and they were taken as the basis for a standard chromaticity diagram adopted by the Commission Internationale d'Éclairage (CIE) in 1931. This CIE system has remained the principal means of specifying colors for trade and commerce (Chapter 3). W.D. Wright has left us a personal account of its origins, in an Appendix to Kaiser and Boynton (1996).

1.7.2 THE SPECTRAL SENSITIVITIES OF THE RECEPTORS

We have seen that a chromaticity diagram allows any light to be specified in terms of three arbitrary primary lights: All that we need to know is the relative amount of each primary that is required to match the test light. It is then straightforward to re-express the chromaticity of the test light in terms of a new set of primary lights, since we know how much of each of the old primaries is required to match each of the new primaries. But somewhere in the diagram there should be a set of three points that have a special status: These would be the lights – if they existed – that stimulated only one individual class of Young's receptors. Clerk Maxwell in 1855 was firm in saying that such lights do not exist in the real world. He draws a version of Newton's color circle within a larger triangle and writes:

> Though the homogeneous rays of the prismatic spectrum are absolutely pure in themselves, yet they do not give rise to the 'pure sensations' of which we are speaking. Every ray of the spectrum gives rise to all three sensations, though in different proportions; hence the position of the colours of the spectrum is not at the boundary of the triangle, but in some curve CRYGBV considerably within the triangle . . . All natural colours must be within this curve, and all ordinary pigments do in fact lie very much within it.
>
> (Maxwell, 1855b)

Clerk Maxwell himself proposed how it might be possible experimentally to establish the positions of the individual receptors in a chromaticity diagram – and thus to express each wavelength of the spectrum in terms of the relative excitation it produces in the three receptors. It is necessary to assume that the color blind retain two of the normal receptors and lack a third. In 1855 Clerk

Maxwell was aware of only one class of color blind subjects, those he thought to lack the long-wave receptor. Using his technique of spinning disks, he showed that these dichromatic subjects needed only four colors (including black) in their equations (Maxwell, 1855a). With the red, green, and blue standard colors of Figure 1.21, for example, a dichromat generated the equation

$$.19G + .05B + .76\ Bk = 1.00\ R,$$

that is, a full red was equivalent to a dark blue-green mixture. Along the line Redβ (see Figure 1.21), the subject can match all chromaticities merely by varying the amount of black in the mixture: In other words, provided we equate the different chromaticities in lightness, he cannot discriminate among them. Such a line would today be called a 'dichromatic confusion line.' To distinguish chromaticities on this line, the normal must be using the receptor that the dichromat lacks. All that varies along the line is the degree of excitation of the receptor that is missing in the color blind. If we establish a second confusion line (e.g. $\gamma\delta$ in the diagram), then the point D, where Redβ and $\gamma\delta$ intersect, gives the position in the chromaticity diagram of the missing receptor. Physical lights can then be re-expressed in terms of the relative excitations of the three receptors.

This approach, which Clerk Maxwell proposed in 1855, has remained a prominent psychophysical method for estimating the spectral sensitivities of the retinal receptors. Arthur König (Figure 1.22), a colleague of Helmholtz, obtained color-matching functions for normals, protanopes and deuteranopes, and derived the sensitivities shown in Figure 1.23 (König and Dieterici, 1892). Notice that the peak of König's long-wave receptor lies in the yellow region of the spectrum. Twentieth-century color-matching functions allowed fresh estimates of the receptor sensitivities (e.g. Nuberg and Yustova, 1955; Wyszecki and Stiles, 1967). An important advance came from precise measurements of the confusion lines of tritanopes, those rare dichromats who lack the short-wave receptor (Wright, 1952). However, even amongst those who favored a trichromatic theory, receptor sensitivities derived by Clerk Maxwell's method did not secure universal acceptance until late in the twentieth century. Convergent evidence came from the work of W.S. Stiles, who measured thresholds for monochromatic increments on monochromatic fields. By varying systematically either the wavelength of the test flash or that of the adapting field, he was able to show that the sensitivity of an individual cone channel is primarily determined by

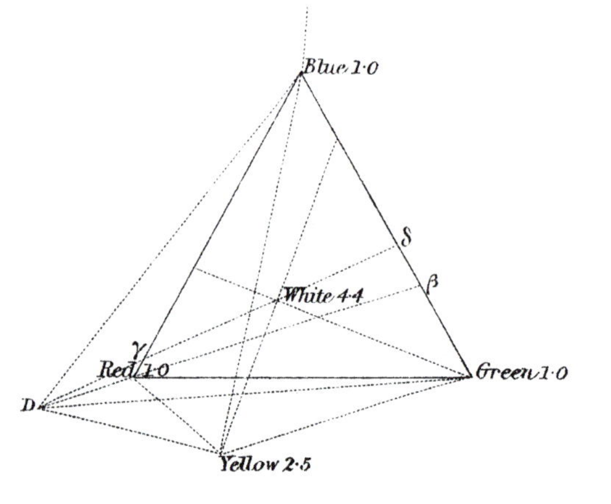

Figure 1.21 **Clerk Maxwell's diagram showing how the position in the chromaticity diagram of one of the retinal receptors can be estimated from the confusions made by a dichromat.**

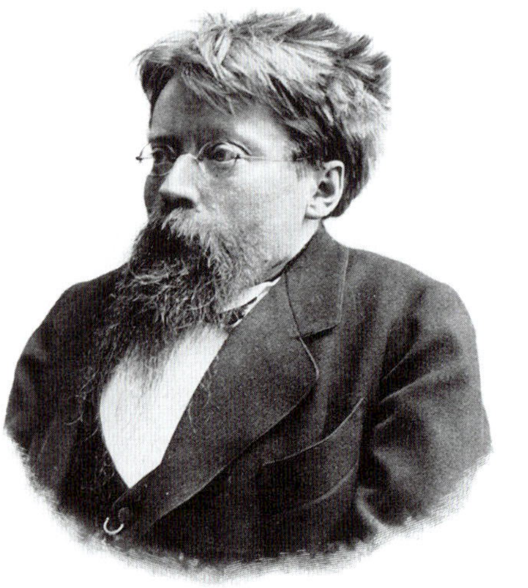

Figure 1.22 **Arthur König (1856–1901), a protégé of Helmholtz. König suffered from a progressive and painful deformity of the spine.**

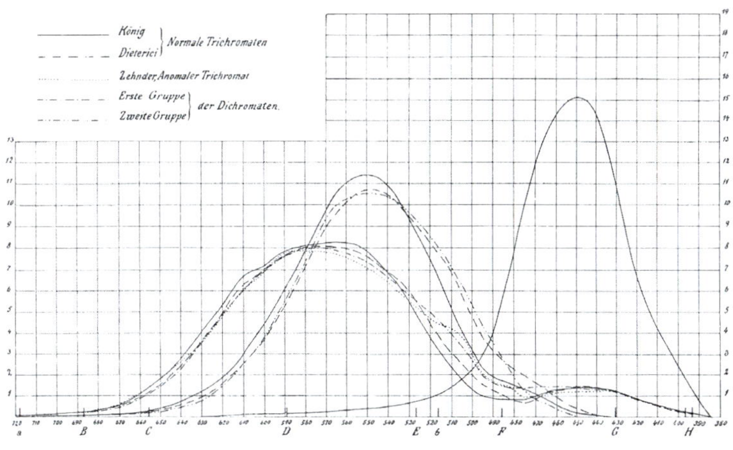

Figure 1.23 The first realistic estimates of the sensitivities of the retinal receptors. The spectrum is plotted with long wavelengths to the left. The solid and dashed curves show the estimates of the receptors of normal observers. (From König and Dieterici, 1892.)

the photons absorbed by that channel alone; and thus he was able to estimate the spectral sensitivities of the cones, estimates that resembled those obtained by Clerk Maxwell's method (Stiles, 1939). Objective measurements of the cone pigments were later obtained by the method of reflection densitometry (Rushton, 1965) and by direct microspectrophotometric and electrophysiological measurements of single cones.

1.7.3 ANOMALOUS TRICHROMACY

Clerk Maxwell died of cancer in 1879, when still only forty-eight. His successor in the Cavendish chair of physics at Cambridge was Baron Rayleigh, who took the post only because the agricultural depression had temporarily spoiled his plans of maintaining a large private laboratory on his family estate at Terling Place (Strutt, 1924). In 1881, Lord Rayleigh described how he had discovered that three of his wife's brothers – including Arthur Balfour, later British Prime Minister and author of the 'Balfour Declaration' – differed from him in matching monochromatic yellow light with a mixture of red and green. The mixture set by Rayleigh himself looked 'almost as red as red sealing wax' to his brothers-in-law, who set a match with only half as much red in it. A fourth brother was normal, as were the three sisters. Others in Rayleigh's circle, including J.J. Thompson (his successor as Cavendish Professor), similarly required a much smaller ratio of red to green in the match than did the normal observer, while two further observers required *more* red in the match, in the ratio 2.6 to 1 relative to the normal. Yet several of these deviant observers had fine discrimination in the red–green range and could not be conventionally described as color blind (Rayleigh, 1881).

The class of observers identified by Rayleigh were soon being called 'anomalous trichromats' (König and Dieterici, 1886). Rayleigh himself suggested that they were very common, and we now know that they constitute some 6% of the male population. However, the distinguished Dutch ophthalmologist Donders showed that the anomalous observers with good discrimination (such as the Balfour brothers) were relatively uncommon, and that an anomalous match was more often associated with reduced discrimination of color (Donders, 1884). He also obtained 'Rayleigh equations' for a population of over 50 normal observers and noted the large variation in their individual matches.

Donders standardized the wavelengths used for the Rayleigh equation: The red and green components of the mixture were provided by the lithium line at 670 nm and the thallium line at 535 nm, and this mixture was to be matched to the orange light of the sodium line at 589 nm. Remarkably, Donders' red and orange wavelengths have been retained to this day as standards for the Rayleigh equation (e.g. German standard DIN 6160). The green component was later moved to the mercury line at 546 nm, since this gives a mixture that is closer to the orange in saturation.

1.7.4 TESTS FOR COLOR DEFICIENCY

There is never any end to the invention of new color tests, but nearly all the main principles emerged in the period 1870–1930. The introduction of tests for mass screening was prompted by the use of color signaling on the rapidly expanding railroads (Wilson, 1855; Jennings, 1896). At Lagerlunda in Sweden, in the early hours of 15 November 1875, nine people died when two express trains collided on a single-line track (Nettleship, 1913). The engineer of the late-running northbound express apparently did not recognize a red light waved by the stationmaster at Bankeberg station, for he slowed and then restarted forwards without the stationmaster's order. A lineman ran with a red lamp after the train, but a carriage oiler, in the front van, is said to have called out to the engineer that he saw the 'line-clear' signal. Two or three minutes later, as it steamed up the incline to the bridge over the Lagerlund river, the train met the southbound express (Figure 1.24). The engineer and the oiler of the northbound train were among the dead, but Professor F. Holmgren of Upsala raised the possibility that one or other had been color blind. He campaigned for the screening of all railway employees. The superintendent of the Upsala–Gefle line provided Holmgren with a private rail car and he proceeded down the line, halting at each station and gatekeeper's house to test every employee. Some 4.8% of the personnel, including a stationmaster and an engineer, were found to be color-deficient (Holmgren, 1877).

Holmgren sought a test that did not require the naming of colors, since the daltonian's use of color terms will often disguise an inability to discriminate. Instead, Holmgren required the sorting of colored wools: 'it is necessary to leave to the activity of the hands the task of revealing the nature of sensation.' The examiner places on the table a sample skein, green for the first test and purple for the second. Nearby, is a jumbled pile of skeins of varying color and lightness. The subject is asked to pick from the pile the skeins that have the same hue. Daltonians quickly reveal themselves by picking from the pile not only the skeins that a normal would pick, but also 'confusion colors' characteristic of this form of deficiency.

Concurrently, in Germany, Stilling introduced the first 'pseudoisochromatic plates,' which pres-

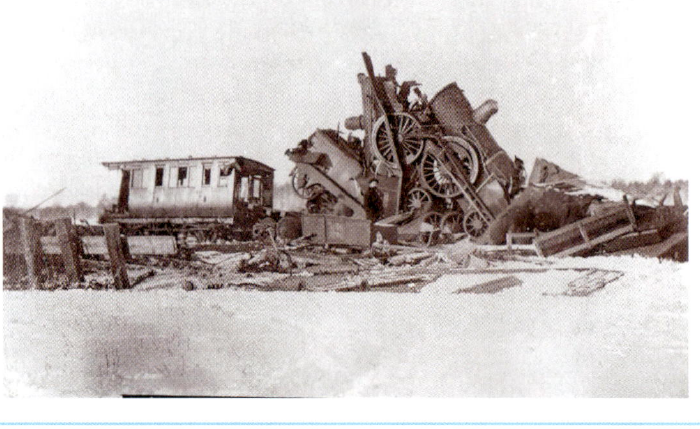

Figure 1.24 **The fatal consequence of color blindness? The scene after the Lagerlunda collision of November 1875. (Reproduced by permission of Sveriges Järnvägsmuseum.)**

ent a target digit or letter of one color embedded in a background of another color. Initially, an attempt was made to print solid figures of one chromaticity on an equally light background of a second chromaticity, the chromaticities being ones confused by the color blind. It was quickly found, however, that it was impossible to print figure and ground in such a way as to eliminate all edge artifacts. Moreover, a figure and ground that were equally light for one daltonian were not necessarily so for another. Stilling solved these problems by two ingenious manoeuvres (Stilling, 1877). First, he broke the target and the field into many small patches, each with its own contour; and secondly, instead of attempting to equate the lightness of target and field, he varied the lightness of the individual patches (Figure 1.25). So neither edge artifacts nor luminance differences could be used as cues to discriminate the target from the background. The target can be detected only by color discrimination, and the task resembles the natural task that challenges the color blind, that of finding fruit amongst dappled foliage.

Stilling's pseudoisochromatic plates are all of the 'disappearing' type, so called because the target becomes invisible for a particular type of color-deficient observer. A clever later variant was the 'transformation plate', where the normal and the color-deficient give alternative readings. This is achieved by linking the elements of the array by one neural signal for the normal and by a different one for the daltonian: For example, on an orange background, the normal might link bluish-green elements with yellow-green elements, whereas, for the daltonian, the more salient linkage might be between the bluish-green elements and plum-colored ones, or between elements of similar lightness. Early examples of transformation plates dating from 1916 are seen in the test of Podestà, who was *Marine-Generaloberarzt* of the Germany Navy. This test has passed into the graveyard that accommodates many forgotten color tests, but it is the most baroque set of plates ever produced, and it is particularly clever because some of the alternative readings are also antonyms (Figure 1.26). The following year, the Japanese ophthalmologist Ishihara published the first edition of a set of plates that included disappearing and transformation plates, as well as plates in which the daltonian sees a digit that is masked for the normal by random color variation (Ishihara, 1917). Despite many rivals, the pseudoisochromatic plates of Ishihara became – and remain today – the dominant instrument for routine screening of color vision. They readily detect dichromats and all but a tiny minority of anomalous trichromats. In part, this sensitivity is achieved not by testing color discrimination but by pitting one perceptual organization against a second.

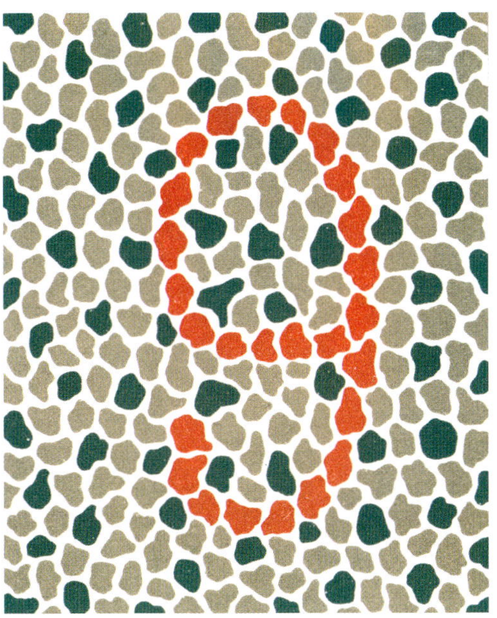

Figure 1.25 **An example of a pseudoisochromatic test for color deficiency. (From Stilling, 1877.)**

Whereas the Ishihara plates are used for screening, the *classification* of color deficiency depends on another instrument introduced early in the twentieth century: the anomaloscope of Nagel (1907). This optical device is essentially a reverse spectroscope: Lights from three slits pass through a prism, and an ocular lens focuses them on the subject's pupil. In the standard model, the slits isolate the wavelengths chosen by Donders for the Rayleigh equation (see section 1.7.3). The subject sees a field subtending 2 degrees: One half-field is illuminated by orange light and the second by the red-green mixture. One control varies the ratio of red to green light in the mixture, and a second adjusts the luminance of the orange light. Dichromats

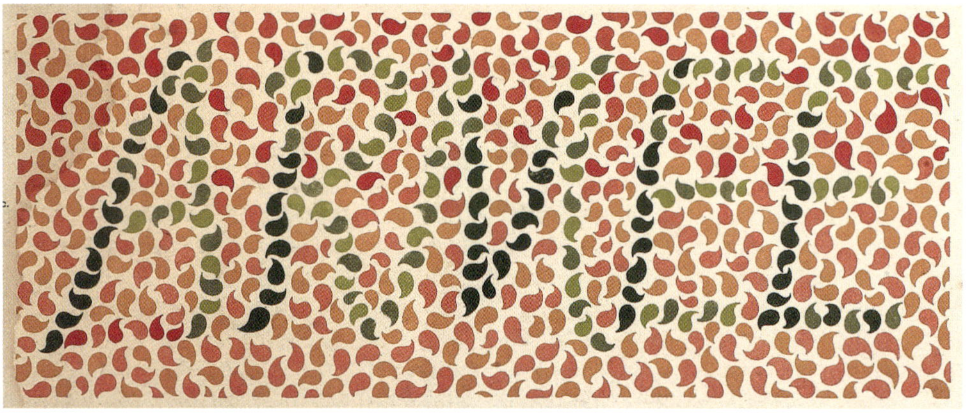

Figure 1.26 **A transformation plate from the test of Podestà (1916). The normal reads 'Armee' but the dichromat reads the antonym, 'Zivil'.**

reveal themselves by matching the orange field with any mixture of red and green, and protanopes and deuteranopes can be distinguished by the amounts of orange lights they require to match different red-green mixtures. Anomalous trichromats are classified by their Rayleigh equations as 'protanomalous' (requiring excess red) or 'deuteranomalous' (requiring excess green). Their power of discrimination (and that of those with normal equations) can be gauged by the *range* of matches that they accept.

An insight into the early days of color testing can be had by reading the entertaining history of Mr Trattles, a British seaman who was denied his First Mate's certificate after earlier passing the Holmgren test (Boltz, 1952). His case was discussed in both Houses of Parliament, and Winston Churchill, then President of the Board of Trade, defended Holmgren's test (Hansard, 1909). On the basis of spectral luminosity measurements at Imperial College, the physicist William Abney declared Trattles a protanope. Trattles finally secured his certificate after he had been taken down the Thames one winter's night on a steamer and had successfully identified navigation lights in the presence of witnesses. He was probably protanomalous, but there is no record that he was ever tested with Nagel's new invention. The Trattles case well illustrates the intense public interest in color perception in the period before the First World War.

1.7.5 COLOR AND EVOLUTION

The Origin of Species was published in 1859, and in the following decades, Darwinism spread to all branches of biology. The father of visual ecology is undoubtedly a Canadian, Grant Allen, later infamous for his feminist novel *The Woman Who Did*. In 1879 he argued systematically that color perception in animals had co-evolved with color signals in plants. His own summary cannot be bettered:

> Insects produce flowers. Flowers produce the colour-sense in insects. The colour-sense produces a taste for colour. The taste for colour produces butterflies and brilliant beetles. Birds and mammals produce fruits. Fruits produce a taste for colour in birds and mammals. The taste for colour produces the external hues of humming-birds, parrots, and monkeys. Man's frugivorous ancestry produces in him a similar taste; and that taste produces the various final results of the chromatic arts.
>
> (Allen, 1879)

Donders (1883) explicitly suggested that human trichromacy evolved from an earlier dichromatic state and had appeared first in females. The basis of the evolution was the successive differentiation of a visual molecule. The American psychologist Christine Ladd-Franklin (Figure 1.27) made evolution central to her own theory of color perception. She proposed:

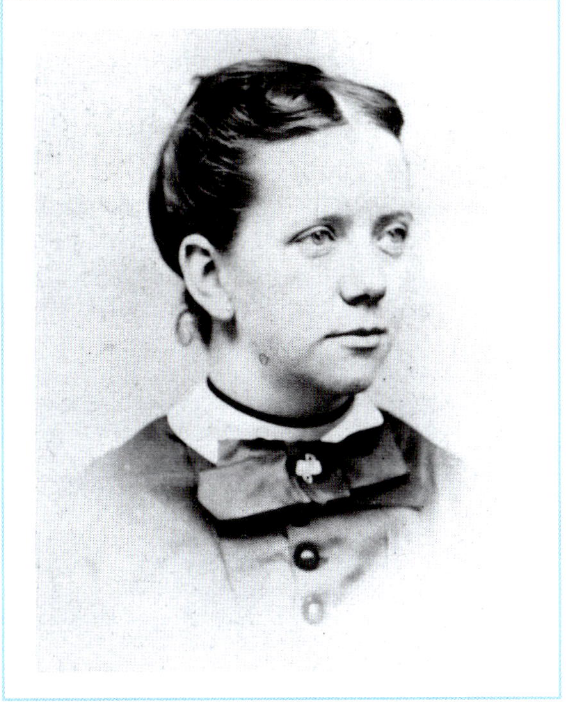

Figure 1.27 **Christine Ladd-Franklin (1847–1930). A graduate of Vassar, Ladd-Franklin studied vision in Göttingen and Berlin, and developed an evolutionary account of color perception (Copyright © Special Collections, Vassar College Library, reproduced with permission).**

> that the substance which in its primitive condition excites the sensation of grey becomes in the first place differentiated into two substances, the exciters of yellow and blue respectively, and that at a later stage of development the exciter of the sensation of yellow becomes again separated into two substances which produce respectively the sensations of red and green.
>
> (Ladd-Franklin, 1892)

Mrs Ladd-Franklin's chemistry is of its time, and she assumes too close a link between her receptor molecules and sensations. But her *sequence* anticipates the modern view of the evolution of primate photopigments: Molecular genetics suggest that the long- and middle-wave pigments became differentiated relatively recently in primate evolution, whereas the common ancestor of these molecules diverged from the short-wave pigment at a much earlier, pre-mammalian stage (Nathans *et al.*, 1986).

1.8 NERVES AND SENSATIONS

The work of Helmholtz, Clerk Maxwell and König did not secure universal acceptance of a three-receptor theory. A prominent opponent was the physiologist Ewald Hering, who took his start from color sensations. There are four hues in our experience – red, green, yellow, and blue – that look phenomenologically simple, whereas other hues, such as orange or purple, look to us mixed in quality. We can see the redness and the blueness in a purple, whereas we cannot mentally dissect a pure red or a pure blue. Moreover, the simple hues are organized into two antagonistic pairs (*Gegenfarben*): red and green, and yellow and blue. The qualities of a given pair are ones that do not normally occur together. Hering proposed that each pair of *Gegenfarben* was associated with the dissimilation or assimilation of a specific visual substance in the eye or visual system (Hering, 1878).

For much of its history, the trichromatic theory had the disadvantage of being tied to a simple Müllerian doctrine in which there were three types of visual nerve corresponding to the three receptors. Granted, as early as 1869 J.J. Chisholm, a physician from Charleston, South Carolina, suggested that 'there are special nerve fibres, for the recognition of special colours, independent of those used in the clear definition of objects'(Chisholm, 1869). And the same suspicion was expressed by Thomas Laycock (1869), who wrote: 'the optic nerve may subserve to at least three differentiations – namely, form, colour, and as a nerve of touch simply'. Only in the twentieth century, however, did the idea emerge that some nerve fibers might be excited by one type of photoreceptor and inhibited by others (Adams, 1923). A nerve that signaled the ratio of quantum catches in different classes of cone would be directly signaling chromaticity, rather than signaling the absolute level of quantum catch in one class of photoreceptors. The cones themselves are color blind (section 1.2), responding with a signal of the same sign to a broad spectral band; but a nerve that responds to the ratio of cone excitations does represent chromaticity as such.

In the 1960s, by micro-electrode recording from the lateral geniculate nucleus (LGN) of the primate visual system, neurons were revealed that did draw inputs of opposite sign from different classes of cone (De Valois *et al.*, 1967). Such cells gave an excitatory response to one part of the spectrum and an inhibitory response to another part. Moreover, the cells appeared to fall into four classes, on the basis of (a) whether their excitatory response was at short wavelengths or at long and (b) where in the spectrum the excitatory response crossed over to inhibition. Many commentators were ready to identify these spectrally antagonistic cells with the yellow–blue and red–green opponent processes of Hering. Brindley (1970) was one of very few skeptics. In textbooks it became a commonplace to say that that theory of Helmholtz held at the level of receptors while the theory of Hering applied at a post-receptoral level. In fact, there turned out to be little correspondence between: (a) the directions in color space that uniquely stimulate individual types of chromatically antagonistic cells in the primate LGN, and (b) the red–green and blue–yellow axes of phenomenological color space (Derrington *et al.*, 1984).

In surveying the history of color science, we have seen that confusion arose when information from one domain was used to constrain models in a different domain. The properties of our subjective color space still remain to taunt us today. We do not know the status that should be given to the phenomenological observations of Hering and we do not know how to incorporate them into a complete account of color science.

FURTHER READING

The following works are recommended:

Crone, R.A. (1999) *A History of Color*. Dordrecht: Kluwer Academic.
Gage, J. A. (1993) *Colour and Culture*. London: Thames and Hudson.
MacAdam, D. (1970) *Sources of Color Science*. Cambridge, MA: MIT Press.
Turner, R.S. (1994) *In the Eye's Mind: Vision and the Helmholtz–Hering Controversy*. Princeton, NJ: Princeton University Press.

The following analytic bibliographies are valuable:

Bell, J. (1926) *Colour-blindness. Eugenics Laboratory Memoirs, XXIII*. Cambridge: Cambridge University Press.
Helmholtz, H. von (1896) *Handbuch der Physiologischen Optik*, 2nd edn. Hamburg: Voss.
Plateau, J. (1877) Bibliographie analytique des principaux phénomènes subjectifs de la vision. *Mémoires de l'Académie royale des sciences, des lettres et des beaux-arts de Belgique*, volume 42.
Sutcliffe, J.H. (1932) *British Optical Association Library and Museum Catalogue*. London: BOA.

A chronological bibliography of color is maintained by the Grupo Argentino del Color at the web site: http://www.fadu.uba.ar/sicyt/color/bib.htm

REFERENCES

Abney, W. (1913) *Researches in Colour Vision and the Trichromatic Theory*. London: Longmans, Green Co.
Adams, E.Q. (1923) A theory of color vision. *Psychological Review*, 30, 56–76.
Allen, G. (1879) *The Colour-Sense: Its Origin and Development*. London: Trübner & Co.
Anonymous (1708) *Traité de la peinture en mignature*. La Haye (The Hague): van Dole.
Anonymous (1786) *Experiments and observations on light and colours: to which is prefixed the analogy between heat and motion*. London: J. Johnson.
Anonymous (1787) *A Narrative of the Life and Death of John Elliot M.D. containing an account of the rise, progress, and catastrophe of his unhappy passion for Miss Mary Boydell; a review of his writings. Together with an Apology, written by himself*. London: Ridgway.
Ayama, M., Nakatsue, T., and Kaiser, P.K. (1987) Constant hue loci of unique and binary balanced hues at 10, 100, and 100 Td. *Journal of the Optical Society of America A*, 4, 1136–44.
Barrett, C. (ed.) (1904) *Diary and Letters of Madame D'Arblay*. London: Macmillan.
Blankaart, S. (1680) *Collectanea Medico-Physica oft Hollands Jaar-Register Der Genes- en Natuur-kundige Aanmerkingen van gantsch Europa*. Amsterdam: Johan ten Hoorn.
Boltz, C.L. (1952) *A Statue to Mr. Trattles*. London: Butterworths.
Bonnet, C. (1755) *Essai de psychologie; ou considérations sur les opérations de l'âme, sur l'habitude et sur l'education*. London.
Bouma, P.J. (1947) *Physical Aspects of Colour*. Eindhoven: Philips.
Boyle, R. (1688) *Some Uncommon Observations about Vitiated Sight*. London: J. Taylor.
Brewster, D. (1842) *Letters on Natural Magic, addressed to Sir Walter Scott, Bart*. London: J. Murray.
Brindley, G. S. (1970) *Physiology of the Retina and Visual Pathway*. London: Arnold.
Brockbank, E.M. (1944) *John Dalton*. Manchester: Manchester University Press.
Castel, L. (1740) *L'Optique des couleurs*. Paris: Briasson.
Chisholm, J.J. (1869) Colour blindness, an effect of neuritis. *Ophthalmic Hospital Reports*, pp. 214–15.
Cunningham, P. (ed.) (1857) *The Letters of Horace Walpole, Earl of Orford*. London: Richard Bentley.

Dalton, J. (1798) Extraordinary facts relating to the vision of colours. *Memoirs of the Literary and Philosophical Society of Manchester*, 5, 28–43.

De La Hire, P. (1694) Dissertation sur les différens accidens de la vuë. *Mémoires de l'Académie Royale des Sciences*, 9, 530–634.

De Valois, R.L., Abramov, I., and Jacobs, G.H. (1967) Analysis of response patterns of LGN cells. *Journal of the Optical Society of America*, 56, 966–77.

Derrington, A.M., Krauskopf, J., and Lennie, P. (1984) Chromatic mechanisms in lateral geniculate nucleus of macaque. *Journal of Physiology (London)*, 357, 241–65.

Donders, F.C. (1883) *Nog eens: de kleurstelsels, naar aanleiding van Hering's kritiek*. Utrecht: G. Metzelaar.

Donders, F.C. (1884) Equations de couleurs spectrales simples et de leurs mélanges binaires, dans les systèmes normal (polychromatique) et anormaux (dichromatiques). *Archives Néerlandaises des sciences exactes et naturelles*, 19, 303–46.

Dossie, R. (1758) *The Handmaid to the Arts*. London: J. Nourse.

Elliot, J. (1780) *Philosophical Observations on the Senses of Vision and Hearing*. London: J. Murray.

Elliot, J. (1786) *Elements of the Branches of Natural Philosophy Connected with Medicine*. London: J. Johnson.

Forbes, E.G. (1970) Tobias Mayer's theory of colour-mixing and its application to artistic reproductions. *Annals of Science*, 26, 95–114.

Forbes, E.G. (1971) *Tobias Mayer's Opera Inedita*. London: Macmillan.

Gamauf, G. (1811) *Lichtenberg über Luft und Licht nach seinen Vorlesungen herausgegeben. Erinnerungen aus Lichtenbergs Vorlesungen über Erxlebens Anfangsgründe der Naturlehre*. Vienna and Trieste: Geistinger.

Gautier D'Agoty, J.F. (1752) *Observations sur l'Histoire Naturelle, sur la Physique et sur la Peinture, avec des Planches imprimées en couleur*. Paris: Delaguette.

Gautier D'Agoty, J.F. (1775) *Exposition anatomique des organes des sens, jointe a la névrologie entiere du corps humain et conjecture sur l'électricité animale*. Paris: Demonville.

Grassmann, H.G. (1853) Zur Theorie der Farbenmischung. *Annalen der Physik*, 89, 69–84.

Guericke, O. v. (1672) *Experimenta Nova (ut vocantur) Madeburgica de Vacuo Spatio*. Amstelodami: Janssonium.

Gurney, H. (1831) *Memoir of the Life of Thomas Young, M.D., F.R.S.* London: John and Arthur Arch.

Guyot, G.-G. (1769) *Nouvelles récréations physiques et mathématiques*. Paris: Gueffier.

Hall, A.R. (1992) *Isaac Newton*. Oxford: Blackwell.

Hansard (1909) *The Parliamentary Debates of the United Kingdom*. London: HMSO.

Helmholtz, H. (1852) Über die Theorie der zusammengesetzten Farben. *Annalen der Physik*, 87, 45–66.

Helmholtz, H. (1855) Über die Zusammensetzung von Spectralfarben. *Annalen der Physik*, 94, 1–28.

Henry, W.C. (1854) *Memoirs of the life and scientific researches of John Dalton*. London: Cavendish Society.

Hering, E. (1878) *Zur Lehre vom Lichtsinne. Sechs Mittheilungen an die Kaiserliche Akademie der Wissenschaften in Wien*. Vienna: Carl Gerold's Sohn.

Herschel, W. (1800a) Investigation of the Powers of the prismatic Colours to heat and illuminate Objects; with remarks that prove the different Refrangibility of radiant Heat. To which is added, an Inquiry into the Method of viewing the Sun advantageously with Telescopes of large Apertures and high magnifying Powers. *Philosophical Transactions of the Royal Society*, 90, 255–83.

Herschel, W. (1800b) Experiments on the Refrangibility of the Invisible Rays of the Sun. *Philosophical Transactions of the Royal Society*, 90, 284–92.

Heyer, T. (1864) *Ami Argand*. Geneva: Gruaz.

Hodgson, E. (1787) *The Trial of Doctor John Elliot, for Feloniously Shooting at Miss Mary Boydell*. London: Hodgson.

Holmgren, F. (1877) *Color-blindness in its Relation to Accidents by Rail and Sea*. Washington: Smithsonian Institute.

Huddart, J. (1777) An account of Persons who could not distinguish Colours. *Philosophical Transactions of the Royal Society*, 67, 260–5.

Hunt, D.M., Dulai, K.S., Bowmaker, J.K., and Mollon, J.D. (1995) The chemistry of John Dalton's color blindness. *Science*, 267, 984–8.

Hurlbert, A.C. (1998) Computational models of colour constancy. In V. Walsh and J. Kulikowski (eds), *Perceptual Constancy: Why Things Look as They Do*. Cambridge: Cambridge University Press.

Hutton, J. (1794) *A Dissertation upon the Philosophy of Light, Heat and Fire*. Edinburgh.

Huygens, C. (1673) An Extract of a Letter Lately Written by an Ingenious Person from Paris, Containing Some Considerations upon Mr. Newtons Doctrine of Colors, as Also upon the Effects of the Different Refractions of the Rays in Telescopical Glasses. *Philosophical Transactions of the Royal Society*, 8, 6086–7.

Ishihara, S. (1917) *Series of Plates Designed as Tests for Colour-blindness*. Tokyo.

Jennings, J.E. (1896) *Color-Vision and Color-Blindness. A Practical Manual for Railroad Surgeons*. Philadelphia: F.A. Davis.

Kaiser, P.K. and Boynton, R.M. (1996) *Human Color Vision*. Washington, DC: Optical Society of America.

Kohlrausch, A. (1923) Theoretisches und Praktisches zur heterochromen Photometrie. *Pflügers Arch. Gesamte Physiol. Menschen Tiere*, 200, 216–19.

König, A. and Dieterici, C. (1886) Die Grundempfindungen und ihre Intensitätsvertheilung im Spectrum. *Sitzungsberichte Preuss. Akad. Wissenschaften, Berlin*, pp. 805–29.

König, A. and Dieterici, C. (1892) Die Grundempfindungen in normalen und anomalen Farbensystemen und ihre Intensitätsverteilung im Spektrum. *Zeitschrift für Psychologie*, 4, 241–347.

Ladd-Franklin, C. (1892) A new theory of light sensation. *International Congress of Psychology, 2nd Congress*. London, Kraus Reprint, 1974.

Lambert, J.H. (1770) Mémoire sur la Partie Photométrique de l'Art du Peintre. *Histoire de L'Académie Royale des Sciences et Belles-Lettres. Année MDCCLXVIII*, 24, 80–108.

Lambert, J.H. (1772) *Beschreibung einer mit dem Calauschen Waschse ausgemalten Farbenpyramide, wo die Mischung jeder Farbe aus Weiss und drey Grundfarben angeordnet, dargelegt und derselben Berechnung und vielfacher Gebrauch angewiesen wird durch J. H. Lambert.* Berlin: Hande and Spener.

Laycock, T. (1869) *Mind and Brain*. New York: Appleton.

Lee, B.B. (2001) Colour science in Göttingen in the 18th Century. *Color Research and Application*, 26, S25–S31.

Lee, H.-C. (1986) Method for computing the scene-illuminant chromaticity from specular highlights. *Journal of Optical Society of America, A3*, 1694–9.

Leicester, H.M. (1970) *Mikhail Vasil'evich Lomonosov on the Corpuscular Theory*. Cambridge, MA: Harvard University Press.

Lilien, O.M. (1985) *Jacob Christoph Le Blon*. Stuttgart: Anton Hiersemann.

Lomonosov, M.V. (1757) *Oratio de origine lucis*. Petropoli: Typis Academiae Scientiarum.

Lonsdale, H. (1874) *The Worthies of Cumberland. Volume 5. John Dalton*. London: Routledge.

MacLennan, M. (1975) *The Secret of Oliver Goldsmith*. New York: Vantage Press.

Marat, J.P. (1780) *Découvertes de M. Marat sur la Lumière; Constatées par une suite d'Expériences nouvelles*. Paris: Jombert.

Mason, W. (1958) Father Castel and his color clavecin. *Journal of Aesthetics and Art Criticism*, 17, 103–16.

Maxwell, J.C. (1855a) Experiments on Colour, as perceived by the Eye, with remarks on Colour-blindness. *Transactions of the Royal Society of Edinburgh*, 21, 275–98.

Maxwell, J.C. (1855b) On the theory of colours in relation to colour-blindness. *Researches on colour-blindness*. G. Wilson, pp. 153–9.

Maxwell, J.C. (1860) On the theory of the compound colours and the relations of the colours in the spectrum. *Philosophical Transactions of the Royal Society*, 150, 57–84.

Maxwell, J.C. (1871) On colour vision. *Proceedings of the Royal Institution of London*, pp. 260–71.

Mayer, T. (1775) *Opera Inedita*. Göttingen: J.C. Dieterich.

Mollon, J. D. (1985) L'Auteur énigmatique de la théorie trichromatique. *Actes du 5eme Congrès*. Paris, Association Internationale de la Couleur.

Mollon, J.D. (1987) John Elliot MD (1747–87). *Nature*, 329, 19–20.

Mollon, J.D. (1989) 'Tho' she kneel'd in that Place where they grew ...'. *Journal of Experimental Biology*, 146, 21–38.

Mollon, J.D. (1992) Signac's secret. *Nature*, 358, 379–80.

Mollon, J.D. (1993) George Palmer. *The Dictionary of National Biography* (ed. C. S. Nicholls). Oxford: Oxford University Press, pp. 509–10.

Mollon, J.D. (1997) '..aus dreyerley Arten von Membranen oder Molekülen': George Palmer's legacy. *Colour Vision Deficiencies XIII* (ed. C.R. Cavonius). Dordrecht: Kluwer.

Mollon, J.D. (2002) The origins of the concept of interference. *Philosophical Transactions of the Royal Society A*, 360, 1–13.

Mollon, J.D. (in press) John Elliot (1747–87). *New Dictionary of National Biography* (ed. H.C.G. Matthew). Oxford: Oxford University Press.

Mollon, J.D., Dulai, K.S., and Hunt, D.M. (1997) Dalton's colour blindness: an essay in molecular biography. *John Dalton's Colour Vision Legacy* (eds C. Dickinson, I. Murray and D. Carden). London: Taylor and Francis, pp. 15–33.

Monge, G. (1789) Mémoire sur quelques phénomènes de la vision. *Annales de Chimie*, 3, 131–47.

Mortimer, C. (1731) An Account of Mr. James-Christopher Le Blon's Principles of Printing, in Imitation of Painting and of Weaving Tapestry, in the same manner as Brocades. *Philosophical Transactions of the Royal Society*, 37, 101–7.

Müller, J. (1840) *Handbuch der Physiologie des Menschen*. Coblenz: H. Ischer.

Nagel, W.A. (1907) Zwei Apparate für die Augenärzliche Funktionsprüfung. Adaptometer und kleines Spektralphotometer (Anomaloskop). *Zeitschrift für Augenheilkunde*, 17, 201–22.

Nathans, J., Thomas, D., and Hogness, D.S. (1986) Molecular genetics of human color vision: The genes encoding blue, green, and red pigments. *Science*, 232, 193–202.

Nettleship, E. (1913) *On Cases of Accident to Shipping and on Railways due to Defects of Sight*. London: Adlard and Son.

Newton, I. (1671) A Letter of Mr. Isaac Newton, Professor of the Mathematicks in the University of Cambridge; Containing His New Theory about Light and Colors: Sent by the Author to the Publisher from Cambridge, Febr. 6. 1671/72; In Order to be Communicated to the R. Society. *Philosophical Transactions of the Royal Society*, 6, 3075–87.

Newton, I. (1675/1757) Newton's second paper on color and light, read at the Royal Society in 1675/6. *History of the Royal Society of London*. T. Birch. London, Millar, vol. 3, pp. 247–305.

Newton, I. (1688) *Philosophiae Naturalis Principia Mathematica*. London: Joseph Streater.

Newton, I. (1730) *Opticks, or a Treatise of the Reflections, Refractions, Inflections & Colours of Light*. London: Wm. Innys.

Nuberg, N.D. and Yustova, E.N. (1955) Issledovanie cvetovogo zrenija dikhromatov. *Trudy Gosudarstvennogo Opticheskogo Instituta*, 24, 33–93.

Palmer, G. (1777a) *Théorie des couleurs et de la Vision*. Paris: Prault.

Palmer, G. (1777b) *Theory of colours and vision*. London: S. Leacroft.

Palmer, G. (1785) *Lettre sur les moyens de produire, la nuit, une lumière pareille à celle du jour*. Paris: 'Chez l'Auteur, rue Meslé, No. 18'.

Palmer, G. (1786) *Théorie de la Lumière, applicable aux arts, et principalement à la peinture*. Paris: Hardouin et Gattey.

Parrot, G.F. (1791) *Traité contenant la manière de changer notre lumière artificielle de toute espèce en une lumière semblable à celle du jour.* Strasbourg: J.G. Treuttel.

Partington, J.R. and McKie, D. (1941) Sir John Eliot, Bart. (1736–86), and John Elliot (1747–87). *Annals of Science*, 6, 262–7.

Peacock, G. (1855) *Life of Thomas Young MD, FRS*. London: John Murray.

Podestà, H. (1916) *Wandtafeln zur Prüfung des Farbensinnes und Erkennung der Farbensinnstörungen*. Hamburg: Friederischsen.

Rayleigh, L. (1881) Experiments on colour. *Nature*, 25, 64–6.

Rimington, A.W. (1912) *Colour-music. The Art of Mobile Colour*. London: Hutchinson.

Rood, O.N. (1879) *Modern Chromatics with Applications to Art and Industry*. London: Kegan Paul.

Rushton, W.A.H. (1965) Chemical basis of colour vision and colour blindness. *Nature*, 206, 1087–91.

Schrøder, M. (1969) *The Argand Burner*. Odense: Odense University Press.

Shapiro, A.E. (1980) The evolving structure of Newton's theory of white light and color. *Isis*, 71, 211–35.

Shapiro, A.E. (1993) *Fits, Passions and Paroxysms*. Cambridge: CUP.

Stiles, W.S. (1939) The directional sensitivity of the retina and the spectral sensitivities of the rods and cones. *Proceedings of the Royal Society B 127*, pp. 64–105.

Stilling, J. (1877) *Die Prüfung des Farbensinnes beim Eisenbahn- und Marine-personal*. Cassel: Theodor Fischer.

Strutt, R.J. (1924) *John William Strutt: Third Baron Rayleigh*. London: Edward Arnold.

Thompson, B. (1794) An Account of some Experiments upon coloured Shadows. By Lieutenant-General Sir Benjamin Thomson, Count of Rumford, F.R.S. In a Letter to Sir Joseph Banks, Bart. P.R.S. *Philosophical Transactions of the Royal Society*, 84, 107–18.

Turbervile, D. (1684) Two Letters from the great, and experienced Oculist, Dr. Turbervile of Salisbury, to Mr. William Musgrave S.P.S. of Oxon, containing several remarkable cases in Physick, relating chiefly to the Eyes. *Philosophical Transactions of the Royal Society*, 14, 736–7.

Voigt, J.H. (1781) Des herrn Giros von Gentilly Muthmassungen über die Gesichtsfehler bey Untersuchung der Farben. *Magazin für das Neueste aus der Physik und Naturgeschichte (Gotha)*, 1, 57–61.

Walls, G.L. (1956) The G. Palmer Story. *Journal of the History of Medicine*, 11, 66–96.

Weale, R.A. (1957) Trichromatic ideas in the seventeenth and eighteenth centuries. *Nature*, 179, 648–51.

Wilson, G. (1845) The life and discoveries of Dalton. *British Quarterly Review*, 1, 157–98.

Wilson, G. (1855) *Researches on colour-blindness, with a supplement on the danger attending the present system of railway and marine coloured signals.* Edinburgh: Sutherland & Knox.

Wood, A. (1954) *Thomas Young, Natural Philosopher 1773–1829*. Cambridge: Cambridge University Press.

Wright, W.D. (1952) The characteristics of tritanopia. *Journal of the Optical Society of America*, 42, 509–21.

Wright, W.D. (1967) *The Rays are not Coloured*. London: Hilger.

Wünsch, C. E. (1792) *Versuch und Beobachtungen über die Farben des Lichts*. Leipzig: Breitkopf.

Wyszecki, G. and Stiles, W.S. (1967) *Color Science*. New York: Wiley.

Young, T. (1800) Outlines of experiments and inquiries respecting sound and light. *Philosophical Transactions of the Royal Society*, 90, 106–50.

Young, T. (1802a) The Bakerian Lecture. On the Theory of Light and Colours. *Philosophical Transactions of the Royal Society of London*, 92, 12–48.

Young, T. (1802b) *A syllabus of a course of lectures on natural and experimental philosophy*. London: Royal Institution.

Young, T. (1804) *Reply to the animadversions of the Edinburgh reviewers on some papers published in the Philosophical Transactions*. London: Longman & Co.

Young, T. (1807) *A course of lectures on natural philosophy and the mechanical arts*. London: J. Johnson.

Young, T. (1817) Chromatics. *Supplement to the Encyclopaedia Britannica*, 3, 141–63.

2 Light, the Retinal Image, and Photoreceptors

Orin Packer[1] and David R. Williams[2]

[1] Department of Biological Structure
G514 Health Sciences Building, Box 357420, University of Washington, Seattle WA 98195, USA

[2] Center for Visual Science
University of Rochester, Rochester, NY 14627, USA

CHAPTER CONTENTS

The Science of Color
ISBN 0–444–512–519

2.1 INTRODUCTION

This chapter discusses the sequence of events, beginning with the stimulus, that ultimately leads to the generation of signals in photoreceptors. We will first describe the physical attributes of the light emanating from the object that are important for human vision. Next, we will examine the transmittance of light through the optics of the eye and the formation of the retinal image. Finally, we will discuss the sampling of the light distribution in the retinal image by the mosaic of photoreceptors.

2.2 THE LIGHT STIMULUS

All quantitative analyses of human visual performance, whether in the domain of color vision or otherwise, require meaningful ways to describe the light stimulus. The number of descriptions from which to choose is large, sometimes bewilderingly so. The appropriate description to use in a given situation depends on such factors as the spatial, temporal, and spectral properties of the stimulus. It also depends on whether you want to provide a purely physical description of the stimulus or take into account known properties of human vision to estimate the visual effect of the stimulus. Here we provide a brief conceptual discussion of the specification of light stimuli. More complete descriptions can be found in Appendix A and in Wyszecki and Stiles (1982).

Light stimuli can be described with any of four classes of measurement: actinometry, radiometry, photometry, and colorimetry. Actinometry and radiometry characterize light in physical terms that are independent of the properties of the human visual system. Actinometry measures light in units of photons. Radiometry measures light in energy units. Photometry and colorimetry quantify light stimuli in terms of the effect they have on vision. Colorimetry reduces the many-valued spectrum of a light stimulus, usually defined in radiometric terms, to three numbers that describe its effect on the short (S), middle (M), and long (L) wavelength sensitive cone photoreceptors. Photometry reduces the many-valued spectrum of a light stimulus to a single number that estimates its visual effectiveness. Both colorimetry and photometry are based on a standard observer whose response to light of different wavelengths is representative of the normal population of observers. Here we confine our discussion to the standard observer's response to luminance since colorimetry is discussed in a later chapter.

For many applications in visual science, such as specifying the light level of a CRT display in a psychophysical experiment, photometric measurements alone are adequate. In color science, radiometry or actinometry are used when it is important to preserve spectral information, as in the case of characterizing light absorption by the ocular media or photopigment, or when the spectral response of an observer is expected to differ from that of the photometric standard observer. Most light-measuring devices display measurements in radiometric rather than actinometric units. Actinometry is often used in the context of light absorption by the retina since the minimum amount of light required to isomerize a photopigment molecule is a single photon.

2.2.1 RADIOMETRY

In addition to choosing whether to use actinometry, radiometry, or photometry, you must decide how best to describe light in space and time. For example, as illustrated in Table 2.1, if you use radiometry, you must also decide among energy, power, intensity, exitance, irradiance, or radiance, each of which is appropriate in a different situation. Radiant energy, expressed in joules (J) is simply the total energy emitted by a stimulus. This specification is used relatively infrequently because it provides no information about how that energy is distributed in space or time. Radiant power or flux, specified in joules s^{-1} or watts, specifies how the energy is distributed in time. Figure 2.1 shows that radiant intensity, specified in watts steradian^{-1}, specifies the direction and the angular density with which power is emitted from a source. It is often used to describe point sources. Irradiance, specified in watts m^{-2}, specifies how much power falls on each location of a surface. It is often used to describe the spatial density of power falling on a surface when direction and angular density does not need to be taken into account. Exitance is identical to irradiance except that it refers to power being emitted from rather than falling on a surface. Lastly, radiance, specified in watts per steradian per meter squared, combines the properties of both radiant intensity and irradiance to specify the direction and angular density of the power falling on each point of a surface.

Each of these radiometric terms has a parallel term in actinometry and photometry. The equivalent terms for each class of measurement correspond to rows of Table 2.1. The actinometric and photometric equivalent values can be converted from radiometric units using rules described in Appendix A below. Lastly, since most lights are broadband, it will often be necessary to describe their wavelength composition. This can be done by adding the word spectral and the subscript λ to any of the actinometric or radiometric units, such as spectral photon flux irradiance, $E_{p\lambda}$.

Table 2.1 Descriptions of light stimuli in three systems of measurement, actinometry, radiometry, and photometry. The name of the measurement, its units and the symbol by which it will be referred to in this paper are listed in each cell

	Actinometry	Radiometry	Photometry
Amount of light	Photon dose photons $\mathbf{Q_p}$	Radiant energy joules (J) $\mathbf{Q_e}$	Luminous energy lumens·s $\mathbf{Q_v}$
Amount per unit time	Photon flux photons·s^{-1} $\mathbf{P_p}$	Radiant power or flux J·s^{-1} = watts (W) $\mathbf{P_e}$	Luminous power or flux lumens (lm) $\mathbf{P_v}$
Amount per unit time per unit solid angle	Photon flux intensity photons·s^{-1}·sr^{-1} $\mathbf{I_p}$	Radiant intensity W·sr^{-1} $\mathbf{I_e}$	Luminous intensity lm·sr^{-1} = candelas (cd) $\mathbf{I_v}$
Amount per unit time per unit area	Photon flux irradiance photons·s^{-1}·m^{-2} $\mathbf{E_p}$	Irradiance W·m^{-2} $\mathbf{E_e}$	Illuminance lm·m^{-2} = lux (lx) $\mathbf{E_v}$
Amount per unit time per unit solid angle per unit area	Photon flux radiance photons·s^{-1}·sr^{-1}·m^{-2} $\mathbf{L_p}$	Radiance W·sr^{-1}·m^{-2} $\mathbf{L_e}$	Luminance lm·sr^{-1}·m^{-2} = cd·m^{-2} $\mathbf{L_v}$

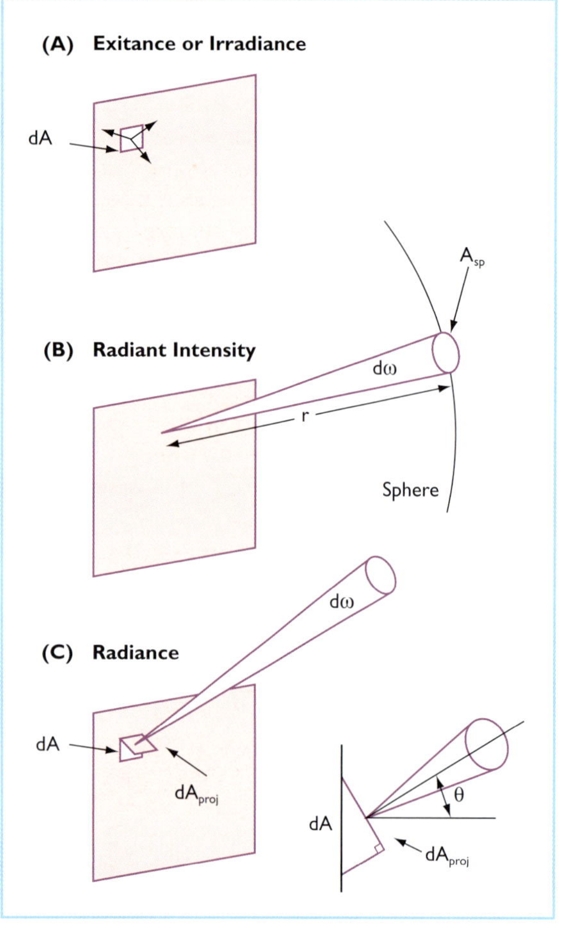

Figure 2.1 The geometry of the basic radiometric quantities: (A) exitance and irradiance; (B) radiant intensity; (C) radiance; *dA* is a patch of surface of infinitesimal size. dA_{proj} is the patch of surface visible from the direction of observation. dω is a solid angle of infinitesimal size. *r* is the radius of a sphere. A_{sp} is the area of the sphere cut off by the solid angle dω. θ is the angle between a surface normal and the direction in which the radiance measurement is made.

2.2.2 PHOTOMETRY

Radiometry and actinometry provide useful physical descriptions of light stimuli that are completely independent of the properties of the human visual system. However, when specifying stimuli seen by the eye, we often need to describe how visually effective a stimulus is. The radiance of a light stimulus is often a poor predictor of its brightness. Photometry was developed to provide quantitative descriptions of light stimuli that are visually meaningful.

The photometric system is based on the standard observer, an imaginary individual whose visual system has an agreed upon and precisely defined spectral sensitivity, chosen to mimic the spectral sensitivity of the average human visual system. Specific individuals measured under specific conditions may have significantly different spectral sensitivities than the standard observer. Moreover, the perception of brightness by human observers is affected by other factors, such as saturation, which means that the photometric system should not be construed as providing a highly accurate measure of the subjective sensation of brightness in an individual. Though these differences have been the basis for more than one career in visual science, the photometric system is an approximate method to predict how bright a wide variety of stimuli are to individual human observers.

At high light levels where cones normally operate, the standard observer's spectral sensitivity is given by the photopic luminous efficiency function, $V(\lambda)$ and was derived from psychophysical measurements of heterochromatic photometry (Wyszecki and Stiles, 1982). At low light levels where rods normally operate, the standard observer takes on a different spectral sensitivity, the scotopic luminous efficiency function, $V'(\lambda)$ that was derived from brightness matches of stimuli viewed in rod vision and measurements of threshold under dark-adapted conditions as a function of wavelength. Several variants of these functions are useful for color scientists and they are explained in Appendix A. All of these luminous efficiency functions are plotted here in Figure 2.2, and tabulated in Table 2.3 which is found in Appendix A.

The photometric system also takes into account another property of the eye, pupil size. When luminance (measured in candelas m^{-2}) is multiplied by the area of the pupil in mm^2, the product is the troland value. The troland is widely used in color science because it reflects, better than luminance alone, the visual effectiveness of a stimulus seen through a pupil of a particular size.

2.2.3 ACTINOMETRY OF THE RETINAL IMAGE

The previous sections have described methods for defining the stimulus external to the eye.

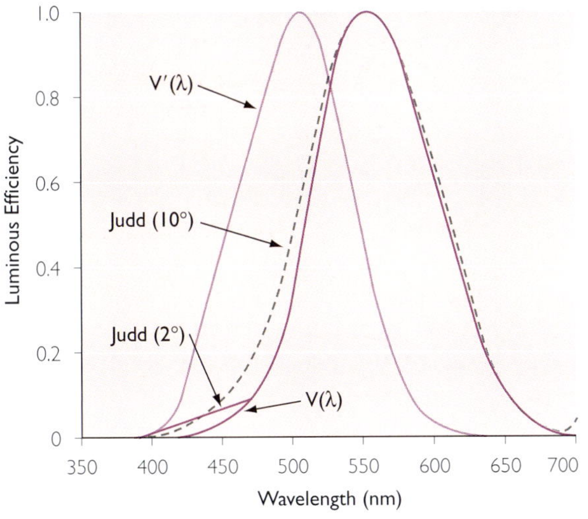

Figure 2.2 The commonly used luminous efficiency functions of vision defined by the Commission Internationale de L'Eclairage (CIE).

Some of these, such as retinal illuminance, incorporate some of the properties of the eye such as its overall spectral sensitivity and pupil size. We next show how one can quantify the light in the image formed on the retina.

Photometry provides an estimate of the visual effectiveness of stimuli by assuming that the eye at a given light level has a single spectral sensitivity, that of a standard observer. Of course, normal human color vision is governed by activity in three separate classes of cone photoreceptor, each with its own spectral sensitivity. Photometry is therefore of no use for quantifying the effect of visual stimuli on individual cone classes. Colorimetry, on the other hand, says a lot about what happens at the three cone types and is discussed in another chapter. One might also choose to use radiometry for this purpose, but the absorption of light by photopigment involves discrete events in which single photons isomerize single molecules of pigment. For this reason, actinometry is the most natural system to use. To apply actinometry to the retinal image, we must first have a model that allows us to predict the dimensions of the retinal image. When this is done it becomes possible to compute the retinal photon flux irradiance and from that, the photon flux arriving at any area of the retina. The reader who wishes to follow the logic of these calculations will find them in Appendix A.

2.2.4 EXAMPLES OF RETINAL PHOTON FLUX

In Table 2.2, we have applied calculations based on the previous concepts to examples of visual

Table 2.2 Common light levels expressed in different measurement systems

	Actinometric		Radiometric	Photometric (photopic, 6mm pupil)	
	Absorbed photon flux P_p (photons·s^{-1})		Radiance L_e (W·sr^{-1}·m^{-2})	Luminance Lv (cd·m^{-2})	Trolands
Source[1]	M cone	Rod			
Sun (from sea level)	2.38E+12	1.92E+12	1.30E+07	3.16E+09	8.93E+10
Projector filament	2.38E+10	1.92E+10	1.30E+05	3.16E+07	8.93E+08
Tungsten filament	1.51E+09	1.22E+09	8.21E+03	2.00E+06	5.65E+07
White paper in sunlight	3.00E+07	2.42E+07	1.64E+02	3.98E+04	1.13E+06
Blue sky	1.89E+06	1.53E+06	1.03E+01	2.51E+03	7.10E+04
Rod saturation	2.38E+05	1.92E+05	1.30E+00	3.16E+02	8.93E+03
Typical office desktop	9.50E+04	7.66E+04	5.18E−01	1.26E+02	3.56E+03
Reading	2.38E+04	1.92E+04	1.30E−01	3.16E+01	8.93E+02
Feeble interior lighting	2.38E+03	1.92E+03	1.30E−02	3.16E+00	8.93E+01
Lower end of mesopic	7.54E+01	6.08E+01	4.11E−04	1.00E−01	2.83E+00
Absolute threshold[2]		3.5E−01	4.35E−06	1.33E−03	3.73E−02
Absolute threshold[2]		2.00E−04	2.47E−09	7.5E−07	2.12E−05

[1] Makous (1998).
[2] See text for an explanation of the two absolute thresholds.

stimuli and important light levels that span the intensity range of human vision. Each light level is expressed in terms of radiance, luminance, troland value, and absorbed photon flux. Since most interesting stimuli are broadband, we calculated spectral photon flux irradiance, $E_{p\lambda}$, and spectral photon flux, $P_{p\lambda}$, by applying the calculations to each wavelength in the stimulus and summing the results. We made the assumption that the stimuli have equal energy at all wavelengths and that the diameter of the pupil of the eye is 6 mm. Lastly, we took into account the efficiency with which the retina actually uses photons by correcting for the Stiles–Crawford effect ($\rho = 0.05$), absorption of photons by the optical media (Table I(2.4.6) from Wyszecki and Stiles, 1982), absorption of photons in the photopigment (Baylor *et al.*, 1987) and the efficiency with which absorbed photons actually isomerize photopigment (0.67; Dartnall, 1968). We will come back to these topics in more detail later. For the moment the important point is that the actinometric numbers represent the number of photons that actually isomerize photopigment molecules, not just those that are incident on the cornea.

The absolute thresholds at the bottom of the table require some additional explanation. The first absolute threshold was calculated for the case of a small (22' diameter), short (10 ms), monochromatic (507 nm) stimulus imaged at the eccentricity of maximum rod density (Hallett, 1987). It would deliver about 100 quanta to the cornea and ten or fifteen of those would actually be absorbed by the 1600 rods illuminated by the stimulus. The vast majority of rods will not absorb any photons at all during the short stimulus presentation. We calculated what stimulus luminance would deliver 10 absorbed quanta to this field in 10 ms as well as the absorbed photon flux for each rod. This particular example represents the stimulus conditions that require the fewest photon absorptions to reach threshold. The second absolute threshold is for a large, long stimulus that exceeded both the spatial summation area and the temporal integration time of the visual system. In this case, luminance threshold is as low as 7.5×10^{-7} candelas/m^2 (Pirenne, 1962). However, the number of absorbed photons required to reach threshold would be much higher than for the small, short stimulus.

2.3 SOURCES OF LIGHT LOSS IN THE EYE

Light is lost to reflection and absorption as it passes through the optics of the eye to the retina. These losses need to be accounted for when the spectral properties of the light reaching the photopigment are important, such as for designing stimuli for psychophysical experiments. For most purposes, light losses due to reflection from the surfaces of the ocular media are minimal. However, the media preferentially absorb a substantial proportion of the short wavelength light. This gives the lens, for example, a distinctly yellow appearance.

2.3.1 LIGHT LOSS DUE TO REFLECTION

Light losses due to reflection from the surfaces of the optical media are small and largely wavelength-independent. The largest reflectance for normally incident illumination occurs at the front surface of the cornea, where about 3 percent of the light is reflected. This reflection is large because of the substantial difference in the refractive indices of air and cornea. Reflections from other optical surfaces total less than 0.3 percent of the incident light (Boettner and Wolter, 1962). Although small, the specular reflections or Purkinje images from the front and back surfaces of the cornea and lens can be used to noninvasively track the direction of gaze (Cornsweet and Crane, 1973) and to measure the spectral transmittance of the ocular media in situ (van Norren and Vos, 1974).

2.3.2 LIGHT LOSS DUE TO ABSORPTION

The ocular media (Figure 2.3), comprised of the cornea, aqueous humor, lens, vitreous humor, retinal vasculature, and macular pigment, are a cascaded series of color filters. Their transmission spectra have been measured both in excised tissue and in situ. The data presented in Figure 2.4(A) are based on measurements of freshly enucleated eyes.

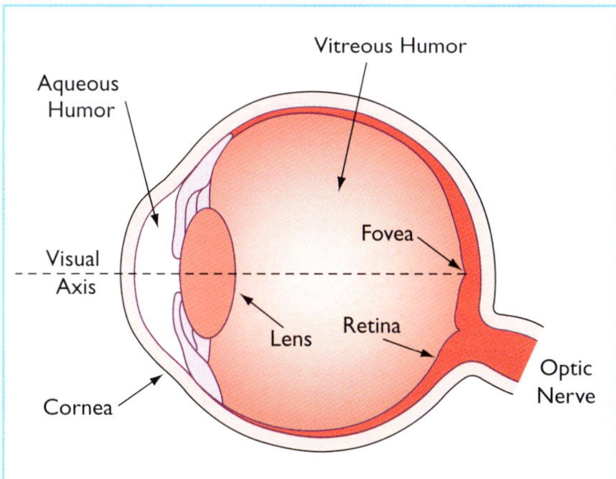

Figure 2.3 A schematic drawing of a cross-section through the human eye showing the parts that are important to our discussion. (After Ruddock, 1972.)

2.3.2.1 The cornea

Across the visible spectrum, the cornea is nearly transparent (Figure 2.4A), absorbing less than 10% of the incident light at 800 nm and less than 20% of the incident light at 400 nm. However, in the ultra-violet at wavelengths less than 300 nm, corneal absorption increases to more than 99%. This absorption has little impact on vision, because the lens and macular pigment absorb short wavelengths even more efficiently, but it may serve to protect the lens from excessive short-wavelength exposure.

2.3.2.2 The aqueous and vitreous humors

The aqueous and vitreous humors absorb less than 10% of the incident illumination at all wavelengths between 400 and 800 nm (Figure 2.4A) and are the most transparent of the optical media.

2.3.2.3 The lens

The pigments of the lens absorb short wavelengths very strongly (Figure 2.4A). In fact, lens absorption is so dominant that it is often substituted for the total absorption of the ocular media at visible wavelengths. In the young adult, lens absorption is very high at wavelengths less than 390 nm, but is < 10% between 450 and 900 nm. Absorption has been measured in excised lenses, by comparing the spectral sensitivities of eyes with and without lenses, and by taking the ratio of the intensities of the Purkinje images originating from the front and back surfaces of the lens (van Norren and Vos, 1974).

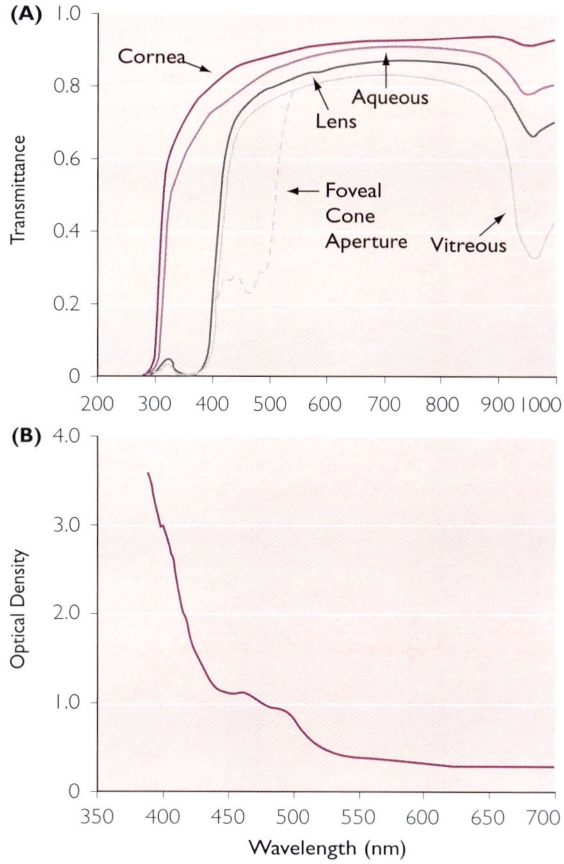

Figure 2.4 The transmittance and optical density of the ocular media. (A) The proportion of photons transmitted as a function of wavelength. The data are replotted from Boettner and Wolter (1962) based on measurements of freshly enucleated eyes. Each curve is the transmittance at the rear surface of the labeled structure, therefore showing the cumulative effects of all the layers up to that point. The amount of light scattered in the preparation that is collected by the detector can alter estimates of transmittance. These data were collected through the axial part of the pupil over a 170° acceptance angle, which minimizes light lost to scattering and produces a relatively high estimate of transmittance. (B) The optical density of the optics of the human eye as a function of wavelength. This curve is the sum of the density of the anterior optics except the lens from Boettner and Wolter (1962), the density of the lens from van Norren and Vos (1974) and the density of the macular pigment from Wyszecki and Stiles (1982).

Unlike other ocular filters, lens transmission changes as a function of age. At birth, the human lens contains a short wavelength absorbing pigment that decreases in concentration during the first 5 years or so of early childhood (Cooper and Robson, 1969). After age 30, there is an increase in the amount of light scattered within the lens which reduces transmission at all wavelengths. In addition, there is an increase in the density of pigments that absorb strongly at short wavelengths as well as an increase in lens thickness.

Although there is considerable individual variability, Figure 2.5 shows the average spectral lens density for a young (20 years) and an old (80 years) observer. The effects of age are greatest at short wavelengths. Between ages 20 and 60, lens density for 400 nm light increases 0.12 log units per decade on average. After age 60, the density increase accelerates to 0.4 log units per decade on average.

2.3.2.4 The retinal vasculature

The retinal vasculature is a meshwork of capillaries within the retina. Optically it lies between the cornea and the photoreceptors and filters the light reaching the retina. Figure 2.6 (Snodderly *et al.*, 1992) shows the vasculature of a macaque monkey including a central avascular zone with a diameter of about 600 μm. The human avascular zone is smaller, ranging from 120 to 600 μm (Bird and Weale, 1974), although some people may have very fine capillaries even at the center of fixation.

With increasing eccentricity from the edge of the avascular zone, capillary coverage increases to about 40% (Figure 2.7, left scale). From capillary coverage and volume, we calculated (Figure 2.7, right scale) that light incident on the photoreceptors is filtered by a vasculature that, if it were uniform, would be equivalent to a layer of blood about 2 μm in thickness at eccentricities exceeding 1 mm.

Figure 2.8 shows that, like the lens and macular pigment, the vasculature filters most strongly at short wavelengths. The spectral properties of blood are dominated by hemoglobin which absorbs most strongly between 400 and 450 nm. The shape of the absorption band between 520 and 590 nm depends on the degree of oxygenation of the hemoglobin (van Kampen and Zijlstra, 1983).

Using the Beer–Lambert law, the transmittance of the vascular filter can be calculated from the hemoglobin spectrum, the effective concentration of hemoglobin in blood (~10 mm/liter, van Norren and Tiemeijer, 1986), and the

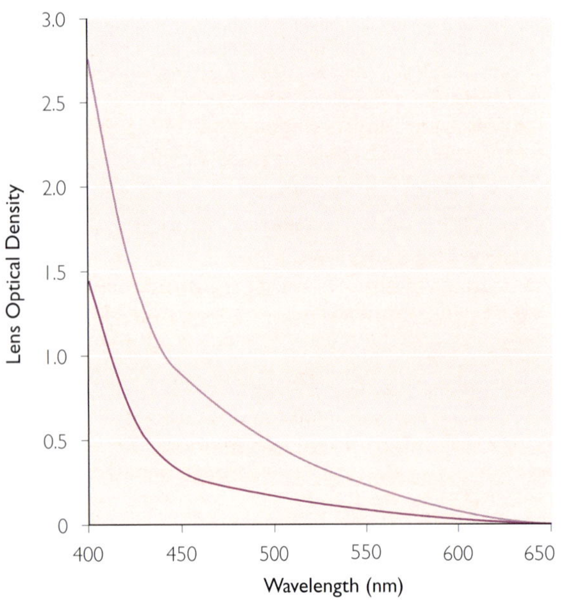

Figure 2.5 **The optical density of the lens of the human eye as a function of age. The upper curve represents the lens density of an average 80-year-old. The lower curve represents the lens density of an average 20-year-old. (Calculated from Table 1 of Pokorny *et al.*, 1987.)**

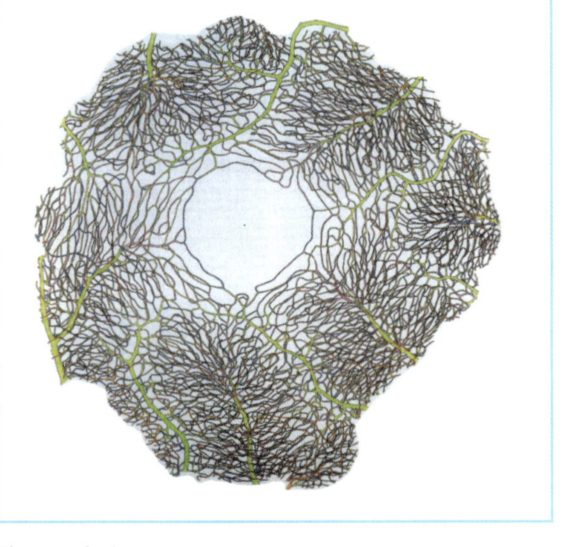

Figure 2.6 **An image of the capillary network of the macaque monkey retina. (From Snodderly *et al.*, 1992. Copyright © 1992 by the Society for Neuroscience.)**

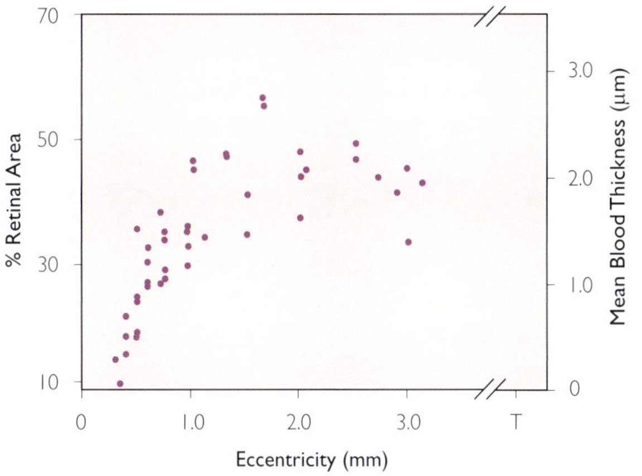

Figure 2.7 The distribution of retinal capillaries. The left axis shows the percentage of retinal area covered by capillaries as a function of eccentricity in millimeters. The right axis shows the thickness of the blood layer that would result if the capillary volume at each eccentricity were reformed into a single layer. *T* represents the far temporal periphery. (Retinal coverage and capillary volume are from Snodderly *et al.*, 1992. Copyright © 1992 by the Society for Neuroscience.)

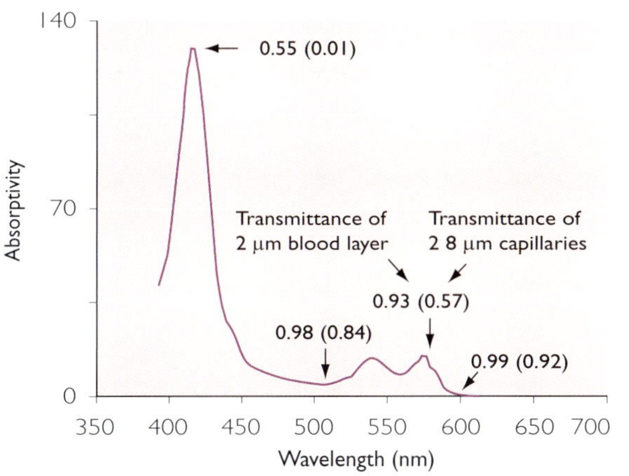

Figure 2.8 The absorption spectrum of oxyhemoglobin, the primary absorbing element of the blood. The curve is replotted from van Kampen and Zijlstra (1983). For our purposes the absorptivity scale is arbitrary. The numbers not enclosed in parentheses represent the transmittance of a 2 μm thick layer of blood. The numbers in parentheses represent the transmittance of two overlapping 8 μm capillaries.

thickness of the blood layer. In Figure 2.8, the transmittances of a 2 μm thick blood layer at several key wavelengths are shown on the oxyhemoglobin spectrum. Transmittance would be significantly reduced only at wavelengths between 400 and 450 nm.

Of course, the retinal vasculature is not a single layer of uniform thickness. The capillaries lie between the pupil and the photoreceptors and cast shadows whose widths are larger than the capillaries themselves. If the distance of the capillary from the photoreceptor is 50 μm and the pupil diameter is 6 mm, the shadow would be 2 or 3 times the width of the capillary. This is roughly equivalent to multiplying capillary coverage by two or three. At eccentricities greater than 1 mm, this would imply complete retinal coverage, while at eccentricities less than 1 mm, some photoreceptors would be shaded while others would not. To take an extreme example, a photoreceptor directly under two overlapping 8 μm capillaries would receive only 57% of the 555 nm light (Figure 2.8, transmittances in parentheses) received by a neighbor lying under a gap between capillaries. At short wavelengths this difference would be larger. The invisibility of the vasculature in normal viewing presumably is due to local retinal gain changes, cortical adaptation, and the failure to represent retinal regions beneath the denser vessels (Adams and Horton, 2002).

2.3.2.5 The macular pigment

The final filter, the macular pigment, is also integral to the retina, absorbing most strongly from 400 to 550 nm with a peak near 458 nm (Figure 2.9A). Macular pigment is a combination of the isomeric carotenoids zeaxanthin and lutein (Bone *et al.*, 1985) which are closely related to the xanthophyll pigments found in leaves. These pigments are obtained from the diet and transported to the retina.

Macular pigment concentration falls with increasing eccentricity from a peak at the center of the fovea, to an asymptotic level at 3° (~1 mm) of eccentricity (Figure 2.9B). Although not visually important, a measurable concentration of pigment can be found even in far peripheral retina. Macular pigment concentration also shows a high degree of individual variability. Although a spectral absorbance function with a peak density of 0.5 log units is plotted in Figure 2.9(A), individual peak densities range from 0 in some albinos (Abadi and Cox, 1992) to over 1.2 log units.

Macular pigment density also varies from layer to layer within the retina. The highest concentrations are found in the fibers of Henle (photoreceptor axons) (Snodderly *et al.*, 1984a),

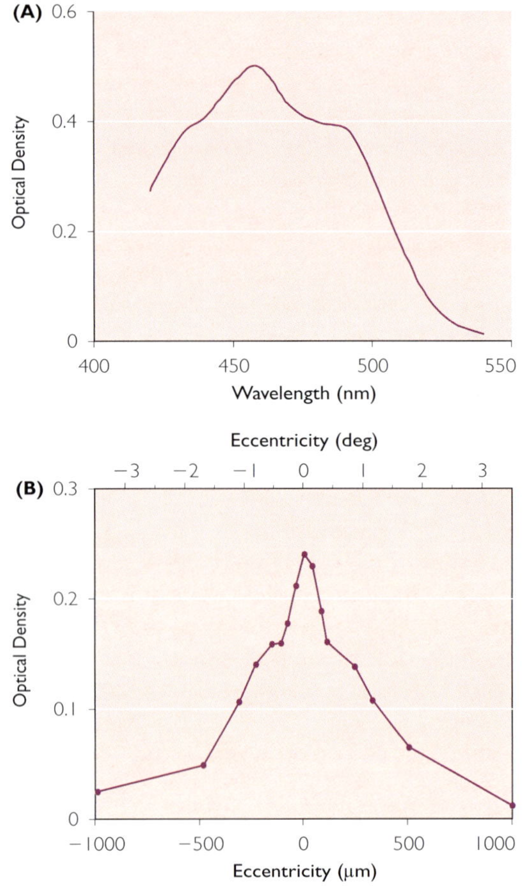

Figure 2.9 The optical properties of the macular pigment. (A) Macular pigment absorbance peaks at a wavelength of 458 nm. Absolute density varies considerably from individual to individual. Replotted from Bone *et al.* (1992) (B). The amount of macular pigment is highest at the center of the fovea and falls with increasing eccentricity. (Replotted from Snodderly *et al.*, 1984b.)

with smaller concentrations occurring in the inner plexiform layer. Macular pigment can be detected prenatally and increases in concentration during early life, but remains unchanged after 9 years of age (Werner *et al.*, 1987).

2.3.2.6 Total filtering by prereceptoral factors

For many purposes, such as for calibrating the spectral properties of light reaching the photoreceptors, the ocular media are most conveniently thought of as a single color filter (Figure 2.4B). The ocular filter is nearly opaque in the ultraviolet at wavelengths below 400 nm. Across the range of visible wavelengths, optical density decreases with increasing wavelength. In the infrared, absorption remains low out to about 900 nm.

It is important to realize that Figure 2.4(B) represents the average optical density of many eyes. As we have already seen, both lens and macular pigment density vary substantially from person to person. Most of the variability in lens density occurs at wavelengths below 450 nm (for a review see van Norren and Vos, 1974), while most of the variability in macular pigment density occurs between 400 and 525 nm. When a highly accurate estimate of ocular media density is required, especially at short wavelengths, each subject should be measured. A good method for estimating ocular transmittance is to compare measured scotopic spectral sensitivity to the absorption spectrum of rhodopsin (Weale, 1954; Pulos, 1989).

2.3.3 EFFECTS OF PRERECEPTORAL FILTERING ON COLOR MATCHING

Prereceptoral filtering does have a measurable effect on color matching. Because most of us have three classes of cone photoreceptors in our retinas, each with a different spectral sensitivity, we can, subject to certain restrictions, match an arbitrary light by mixing the proper amounts of three primary lights that are widely separated in color space. The relative amounts of the primaries required defines a color match. Because color matches depend on the relative numbers of photons absorbed by the three classes of cones, individual differences in macular pigment and lens density should be reflected in these color matching functions. Indeed, color matches to a standard white stimulus are spread out in color space along a line that connects the white point with the spectrum locus between 570 and 580 nm (Stiles and Burch, 1958). Varying the density of the lens and macular pigment shifted predicted color matches in a similar way (Wyszecki and Stiles, 1982). In one particularly striking example, the differences between two sets of color matches made in a single observer 21 years apart were consistent with yellowing of the lens. Factor analysis also identifies lens and macular pigment density differences as major sources of variability in the 10° and 2° color-matching data of Stiles and Birch (Webster and MacLeod,

1988). Estimates of the standard deviations of the differences were consistent with the variability of direct measurements of lens and macular pigment density. It is possible to normalize color-matching data so that observers with identical underlying photopigment sensitivities, but different ocular filters, have the same matches when monochromatic stimuli are used (Wright, 1928–29).

2.3.4 EFFECTS OF PRERECEPTORAL FILTERING ON COLOR APPEARANCE

Since spectral filtering by the optic media changes the relative numbers of photons absorbed by the three classes of cones, we might expect the ocular media to alter color appearance in the same way that short-wavelength blocking sunglasses do. However, neural mechanisms may well recalibrate color vision (Pokorny and Smith, 1977; Mollon, 1982; MacLeod, 1985; Neitz *et al.*, 2002) when confronted with changes in ocular filtering over time or retinal location. By a number of measures, color appearance is reasonably stable with increasing age despite the yellowing of the ocular media. For example, although they report that stimuli appear less chromatic, older observers assign the same hue names to stimuli as do younger observers (Schefrin and Werner, 1990).

The signals from the three classes of cones are almost immediately reorganized into opponent color channels. In the 'red–green' channel, signals from the L cones oppose signals from the M cones and in the 'blue–yellow' channel, signals from the combined L and M cones oppose signals from the S cones. One way of assessing color appearance is to measure the wavelengths at which the signals from the opposing cone types balance. The balance of the red–green chromatic channel, as measured by the wavelengths that correspond to unique blue and unique yellow, remains constant with age (Werner and Schefrin, 1993). The location of the white point is also quite constant. On the other hand, the wavelength of unique green, a measure of the balance point of the blue–yellow channel, shifts towards shorter wavelengths (Schefrin and Werner, 1990). This is in the direction expected by yellowing of the optical media but the size of the shift is sometimes smaller than would be expected from the media changes.

If color appearance is to remain constant with age, there must be compensation for this yellowing as well as for any changes in the sensitivities of the cone mechanisms or their postreceptoral pathways (Werner and Steele, 1988). Sensitivity measured by brightness matching increases with age for short and middle wavelengths. This suggests that neural gain can increase to overcome decreases in the amount of light reaching the retina. Perfect compensation for optical yellowing would require higher gain increases at shorter wavelengths. The most recent evidence (Kraft and Werner, 1999) suggests that this does in fact occur to some extent, although in those subjects with the highest lens densities compensation is not complete.

Neural mechanisms might also recalibrate color vision to maintain a constant color appearance from place to place on the retina. For example, macular pigment density is much higher in central than peripheral retina. Peripheral retina is more sensitive to short wavelengths than the fovea when measured with flicker photometry (Weale, 1953; Abramov and Gordon, 1977) and this increased sensitivity may be due to reduced filtering by macular pigment.

2.3.5 PROTECTIVE EFFECTS OF PRERECEPTORAL FILTERING

It has long been thought that short wavelength light may induce the formation of cataracts in the lens. The role that natural light exposure plays remains a contentious issue. It is clear, however, that artificially high levels of ultra-violet radiation cause cataracts in laboratory animals (Dolin, 1994). The high corneal density at wavelengths below 300 nm probably protects the lens.

Short wavelength light is also capable of causing photooxidative damage to the retinal pigment epithelium (Ham *et al.*, 1982), and possibly the S and M cones (Sperling *et al.*, 1980; Sykes *et al.*, 1981; Haegerstrom-Portnoy, 1988; Werner *et al.*, 1989). Strong filtering by the lens between 300 and 400 nm and by the macular pigment below 500 nm likely protects the retina against the photochemical effects implicated in retinal diseases such as age-related macular degeneration (Snodderly, 1995). The carotenoid pigments of the retina are also thought to chemically block photooxidative reactions that are damaging to the retina (Burton and Ingold, 1984).

2.4 SOURCES OF BLUR IN THE RETINAL IMAGE

In addition to reducing the intensity of the light reaching the retina, the optics of the eye blur the retinal image. The quality of this image depends on diffraction at the pupil, aberrations in the cornea and lens, light scatter in the optical media, and the optical properties of the retina itself. We first describe the effects of diffraction and aberrations in the eye, ignoring for the moment the effects of light scatter and optical properties of the retina. Diffraction and aberrations are well-characterized with Fourier optics. For an excellent treatment of Fourier optics in imaging systems, see Goodman (1996).

2.4.1 THE GENERALIZED PUPIL FUNCTION AND IMAGE FORMATION

When an observer fixates a star, a bundle of parallel light rays impinge on the eye, as shown in Figure 2.10. Each ray takes a different path through the optics and where it eventually intersects the retina depends on the eye's optical quality. If the observer's eye were free of aberrations, all the rays, no matter where they entered the pupil, would converge to a compact point at the center of the fovea, as shown in Figure 2.10(A). The cornea and lens of such an eye would require just the right optical surfaces and refractive indices to bend each ray so they all converge to a single point. Real eyes always have some aberrations so that at least some of the incident parallel rays fail to converge perfectly, resulting in a blurred image of the star. The retinal image of a single point of light, such as a distant star, corresponds to the impulse response or point spread function (PSF) of the eye's optics, shown in Figure 2.10(B) for a perfect eye. The point spread function provides a complete description of image quality at that retinal location for a given wavelength of light. Indeed, if the point spread function is known at a retinal location, one can calculate the retinal image for any object imaged in monochromatic light at that location.

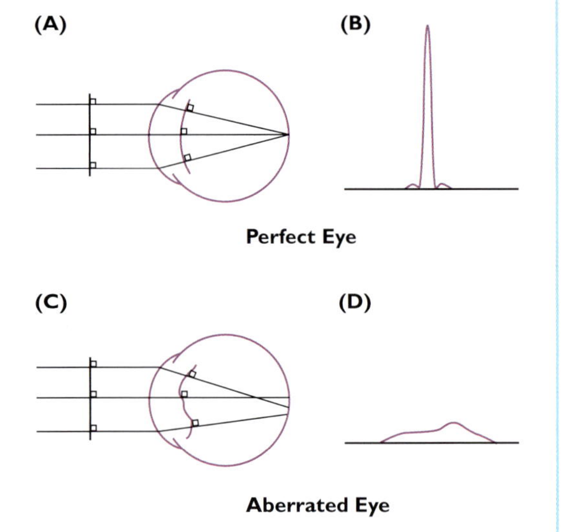

Figure 2.10 **(A) Parallel rays from a point source converge to a single point on the retina of an ideal eye. Expressed in terms of wave optics, a planar wave front is transformed to a spherical wave front by the eye's optics and then collapses to a point. (B) The light distribution of the retinal image of a point source, which is blurred only by diffraction at the pupil. (C) The path of rays in an aberrated eye. The wave front inside the eye is distorted from the ideal spherical shape. The difference between the aberrated and the ideal wave front is the wave aberration. (D) The blurred light distribution of the retinal image caused by the presence of aberrations in the eye.**

The following wave optics interpretation of image formation complements the ray description. In Figure 2.10(A), each of the parallel light rays arriving from the star can be thought of as indicating the direction in which the wave front is travelling. If, starting at some position on the optical axis, we connected the nearest points on each wave that had the same phase, the resulting surface, called a wave front, would be a plane. The optics of a perfect eye transform this planar wave front from the star into a spherical wave front. The spherical wave front, in turn, collapses upon itself to form a crisp point of light on the retina. To form the spherical wave front, the perfect eye delays light travelling through the center of the pupil relative to that travelling through the edge so that each takes exactly the same time to reach the retinal location where the image is formed. In the aberrated eye shown in Figure 2.10(C), the wave front is not delayed by the proper amounts as it passes through the optics and the actual wave front inside the eye departs from the ideal spherical wave front. Because it is misshapen, it fails to collapse to a crisp point at the retina as shown in Figure 2.10(D). The errors in the delays could arise from several sources, such as a misshapen cornea or lens. For our purposes, it is sufficient to sum all the errors experienced by a photon passing through the cornea and lens and assign the sum to the point in the entrance pupil of the eye through which the photon passed. The errors could be expressed in units of time, but it is more convenient to express them in a unit of distance, such as micrometers, indicating how far the distorted wave front departs at each point in the entrance pupil from the ideal wave front. A map of the eye's entrance pupil that plots the error at each entry point is called the eye's wave aberration. The wave aberration includes all the eye's aberrations at a particular wavelength of light that ultimately influence image quality at a particular location on the retina.

The eye's optics not only influence the time it takes photons to reach the retina from different directions, they also influence the number of photons arriving at the retina from different directions. For example, the iris absorbs practically all the light that strikes it, precluding any light from arriving from directions outside the pupil. The generalized pupil function is an extension of the wave aberration that captures both the delay properties of the eye's optics and their transmittance. The power of the generalized pupil function is that, if it is known, it is possible to calculate the point spread function, which as we said before is a complete description of image quality. This allows us to determine directly the impact of the wave aberration and pupil diameter on retinal image quality. A quantitative description of the generalized pupil function can be found in Appendix B.

2.4.2 DIFFRACTION

We can illustrate the power of the generalized pupil function by first considering the case of an aberration-free eye which blurs the retinal image only because of diffraction by the pupil. We already saw in Figure 2.10(B) that even in an eye with perfect optics, the light from the star is not imaged as a single point. Rather the image is a bright central point surrounded by dimmer rings. This occurs because light spreads or diffracts whenever it passes through a circular aperture such as the pupil. Thus, diffraction is the ultimate limit on image quality in any optical system. The degree of spreading is greater for smaller pupils and shorter wavelengths of light.

Figure 2.11(A) shows the wave aberration for an aberration-free eye. Figure 2.11(E) again shows that the image of an infinitely small point of light (PSF) has the form of a central point surrounded by rings. This is called an Airy disk and can be described quantitatively by

$$I(r) = [2J_1(\pi r) / \pi r]^2$$

where $I(r)$ is normalized intensity as a function of distance r from the peak and J_1 is a Bessel function of the first kind. The radius of the PSF, r_o, expressed in radians and measured from the peak to the first point at which the intensity is zero, is given by

$$r_o = 1.22\lambda/a$$

where λ is the wavelength of light and a is the diameter of the circular pupil. Because the width of the diffraction-limited PSF is proportional to wavelength and inversely proportional to pupil diameter, the retinal image quality of this ideal eye is optimum at large pupil sizes and short wavelengths. Converting radians to degrees, we find that for a 3 mm pupil, the radius of the PSF is 0.62' of arc at 440 nm and 0.98' of arc at 700 nm. At 555 nm, the radius is 1.2' of arc for a 2 mm pupil and 0.29 for an 8 mm pupil. The width of this function is sometimes characterized by the full width at half height, which happens to have almost the same value as the radius.

2.4.3 MONOCHROMATIC ABERRATIONS

In any real eye, optical performance is worse than predicted by diffraction because of imperfections in the optics. Figure 2.11(B), (C), and (D) are wave aberrations for three typical human eyes. The wave aberration is different for each eye. The corresponding PSFs (Figure 2.11F,

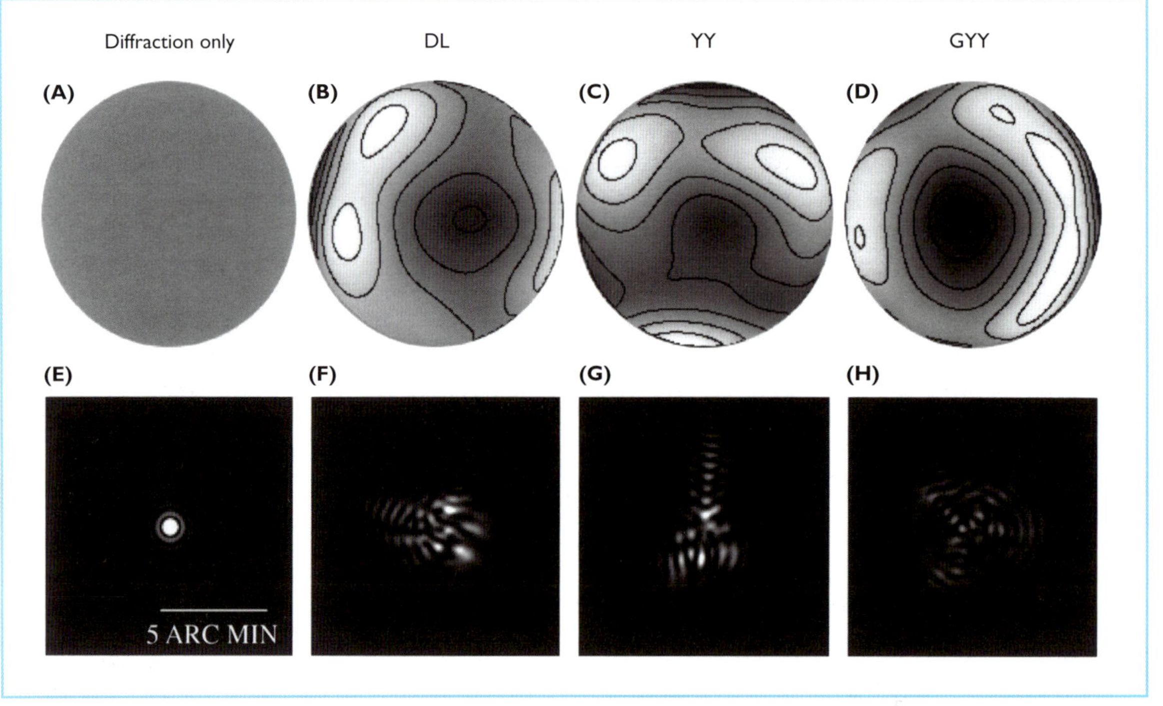

Figure 2.11 **(A) The wave aberration of a perfect eye. (B–D) The wave aberrations of three normal human eyes. Pupil size was 6 mm, defocus and astigmatism have been removed. (E) The PSF of a perfect eye in which image quality is limited only by the diffraction of light. (F–H) The PSFs corresponding to the wave aberrations of the three human eyes shown in B–D.**

G, and H) are considerably broader than the aberration-free PSF for the same 6 mm pupil size. Aberrations obscure the Airy disc pattern due to diffraction and produce a larger and more complex light distribution.

Figure 2.12 illustrates how the PSF changes with pupil diameter for a typical human eye. In the normal eye, the greater spatial detail transmitted by the large pupil is offset by the losses caused by aberrations. Aberrations generally affect the light rays that enter the edge of the pupil more strongly than they affect rays entering the center of the pupil. At small pupil sizes, aberrations are insignificant and diffraction dominates. The PSF takes on the characteristic shape of the Airy pattern, with a wide core and little light in the skirt around it. In bright light, the pupil size is typically about 3 mm or less in diameter, in which case the full width at half height of the PSF is approximately 0.8 minutes of arc, corresponding to about twice the width of a cone at the foveal center. At larger pupil sizes aberrations dominate. The PSF then has a small core but reveals an irregular skirt that corresponds to light distributed over a relatively large retinal area.

The wave aberration can be described as the sum of a number of component aberrations such as defocus, astigmatism, coma, spherical aberration, as well as other aberrations that do not have common names. The wave aberration can be decomposed into these constituent aberrations in much the same way that Fourier analysis can decompose an image into spatial frequency components. It is convenient to use Zernike polynomials as the basis functions instead of sines and cosines, because Zernike polynomials have the same shape as the eye's pupil. Figure 2.13 shows the Zernike modes that are most commonly found in human eyes. In general, the largest aberrations correspond to slow variations in error across the pupil. The largest monochromatic aberration of the eye is typically defocus followed by astigmatism. These are the only aberrations that spectacles correct. However, normal eyes have many

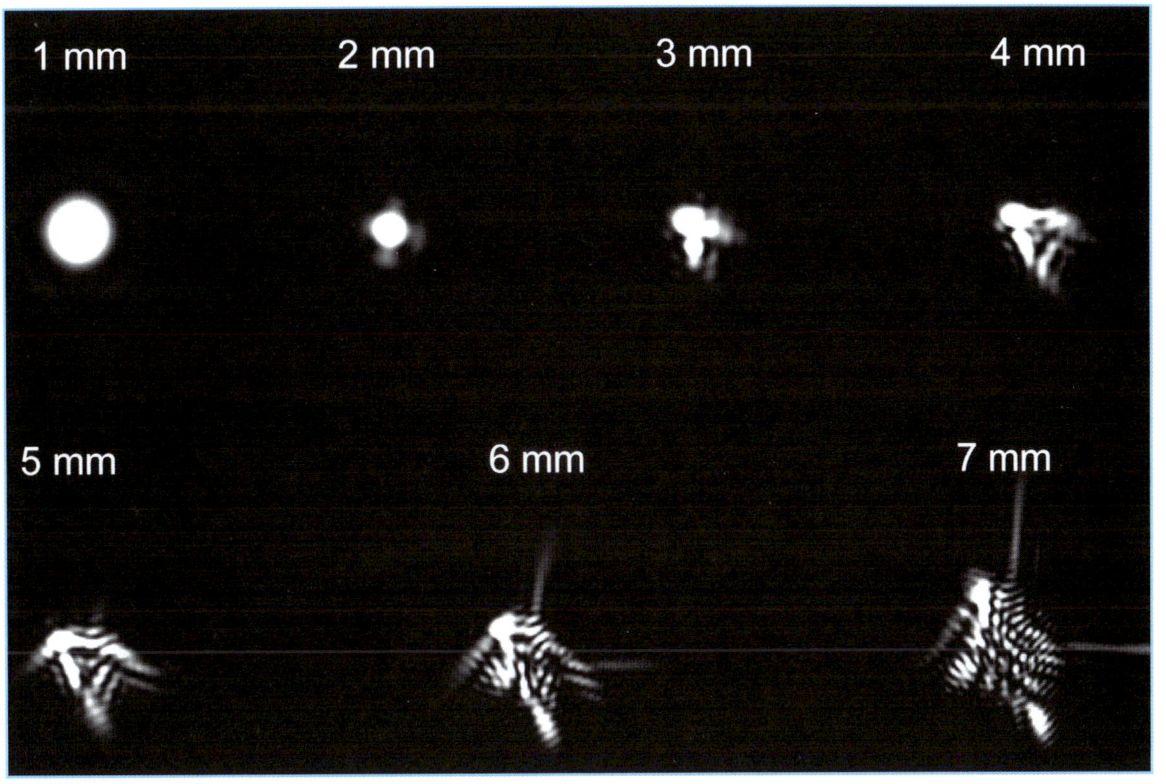

Figure 2.12 **The dependence of the PSF on pupil diameter for a typical human eye. At small pupil sizes, diffraction dominates. For large pupils aberrations are the primary cause of retinal image blur. (Courtesy of Austin Roorda.)**

monochromatic aberrations besides defocus and astigmatism. Generally speaking, aberrations that correspond to more rapidly varying errors across the pupil have smaller amplitudes and make a smaller contribution to the total wave aberration.

Defocus is often expressed in diopters, which correspond to the reciprocal of the focal length in meters of the lens necessary to restore good focus.

2.4.3.1 Computing retinal image quality

Figure 2.14 shows that a retinal image can be calculated for some arbitrary object either in the spatial domain by convolving the light distribution of the object with the point spread function of the eye, or in the spatial frequency domain by multiplying the object spectrum by the optical transfer function. In practice, this calculation is usually more efficient in the frequency domain. The optical transfer function required for this calculation can itself be calculated from either the point spread function or the generalized pupil function. A more quantitative description of these calculations is found in Appendix B.

When these calculations are applied to an eye with perfect diffraction-limited optics and a 3 mm pupil illuminated with 632.8 nm light, the incoherent optical cutoff is 82.7 cycles/degree. The solid curves in Figure 2.15 show modulation transfer functions (MTFs) for a diffraction-limited eye with pupil diameters ranging from 2 through 7 mm calculated for a wavelength of 555 nm.

Figure 2.15 also shows the mean monochromatic MTFs (long dashed lines) computed from the wave aberration measurements for 14 eyes made with a Hartmann-Shack wavefront sensor (Liang and Williams, 1997). With increasing pupil diameter, the difference between the diffraction-limited and real MTFs grows, due to the decrease in the contribution of diffraction to retinal blur and the increase in the role of aberrations.

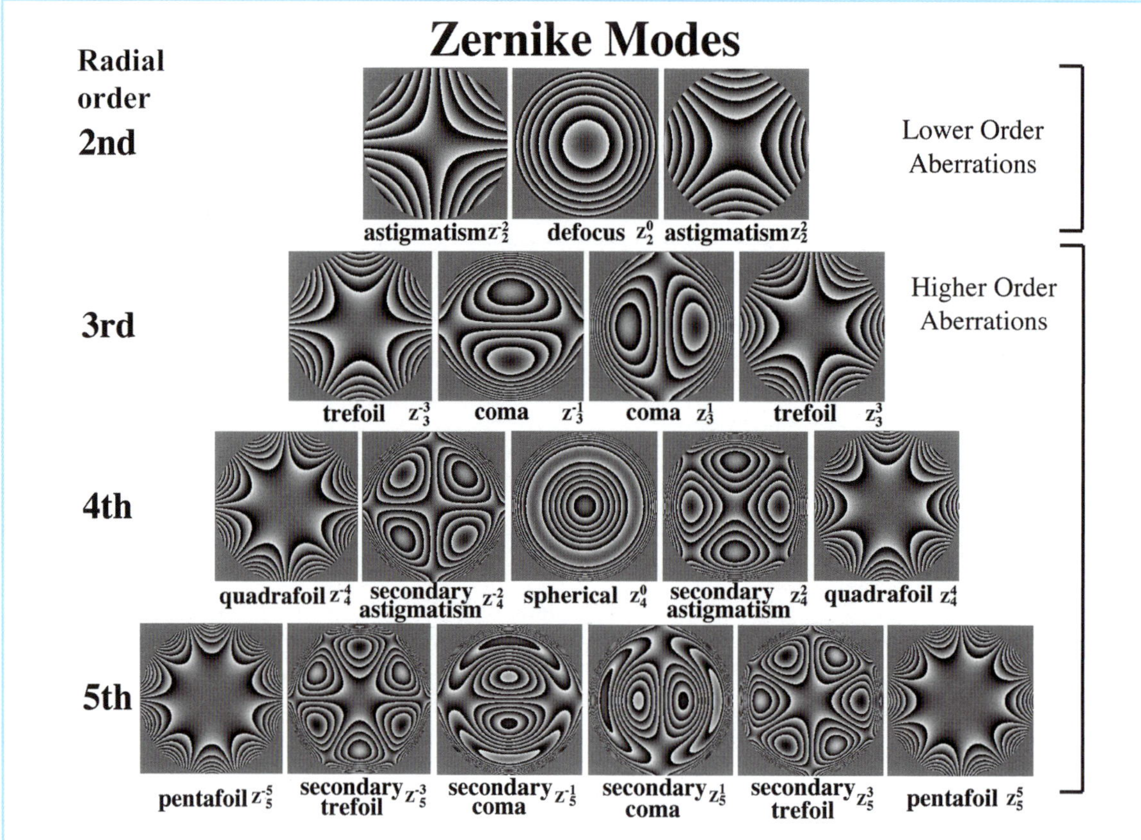

Figure 2.13 The pyramid showing each of the Zernike modes in radial orders 2 through 5, along with their names and their designation (OSA Standard). Tip, tilt, and piston, which would normally cap the pyramid, have been excluded because they do not influence image quality. (Courtesy Jason Porter.)

For small pupil sizes, the MTF is high at low spatial frequencies owing to the absence of light in the skirt of the PSF. For large pupil sizes, however, the MTF is reduced at low spatial frequencies due to the large skirt in the PSF that aberrations produce. However, at high frequencies, the MTF is higher than that for small pupils due to the narrower core of the PSF. The implication of this is that, although a 2–3 mm pupil is commonly said to represent the best tradeoff between diffraction and aberrations, there is no single optimum pupil size. The optimum size depends on the task. Smaller pupils minimize optical aberrations for visual tasks involving low spatial frequencies. Larger pupils transmit high spatial frequencies for tasks that involve fine spatial detail even though they suffer more aberrations. If the goal is to resolve very fine features in images of the retina, then larger pupils transfer more contrast.

Retinal image quality is often represented by the MTF alone in spite of the fact that a complete description also requires the phase transfer function (PTF). The PTF has received less attention than the MTF simply because early methods of measuring the optical quality of the eye, such as laser interferometry and the double pass technique, lose phase information (Artal *et al.*, 1995). However, image quality in the human eye depends on the phase transfer function when the pupil is large. Furthermore, accurate phase information is important for the perception of complex scenes (Piotrowski and Campbell, 1982).

2.4.4 CHROMATIC ABERRATIONS

The largest aberrations in human eyes are defocus and astigmatism, followed by the aggregate effect of all the remaining, higher order mono-

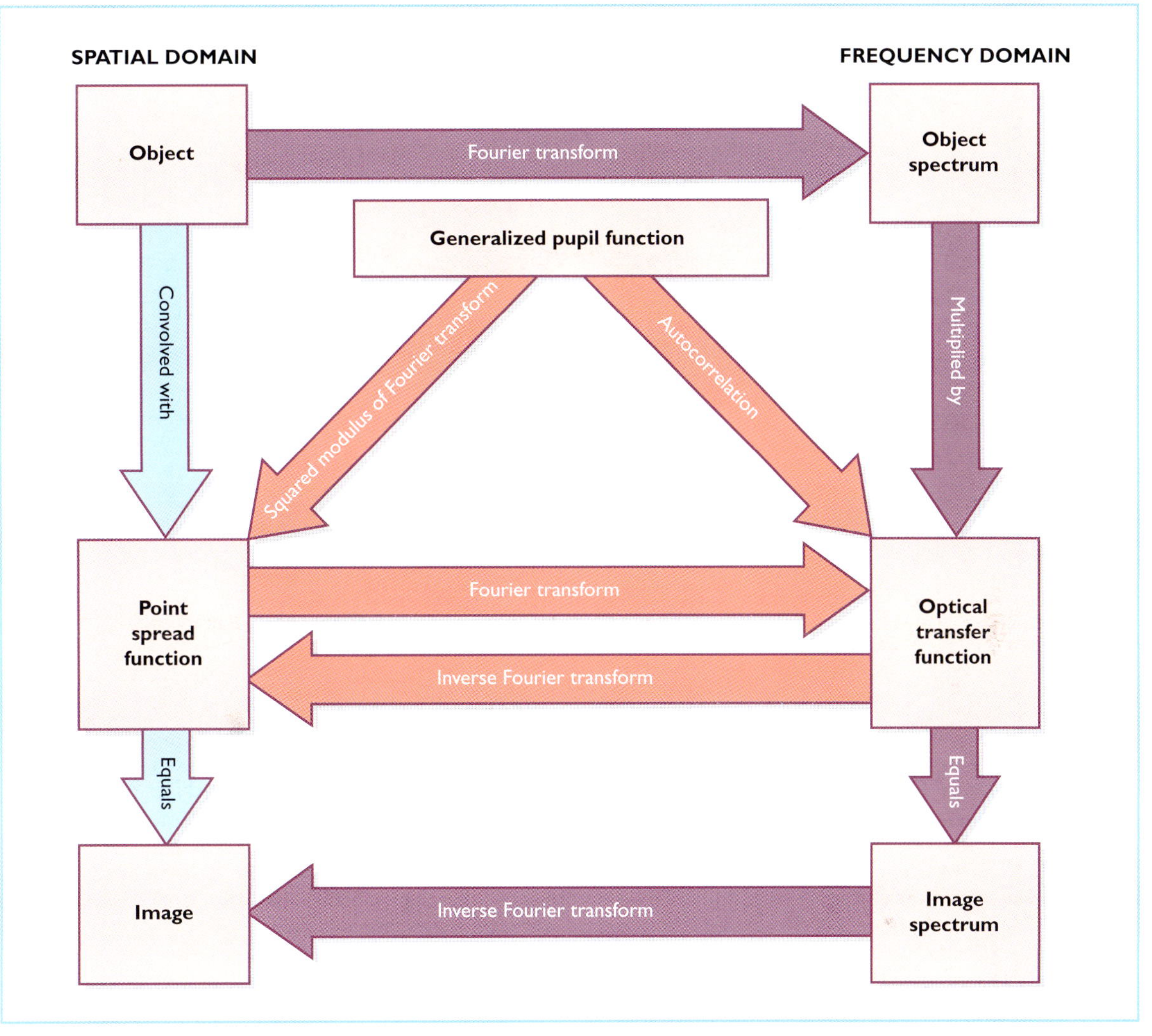

Figure 2.14 **A roadmap for Fourier optics illustrating two paths for computing the retinal image of an object when the point spread function of the eye (PSF), or equivalently, the optical transfer function (OTF), is known. The computation indicated with blue arrows is carried out entirely in the spatial domain. The convolution of the light distribution of the object with the PSF gives the retinal image directly. The more efficient computation in the spatial frequency domain is illustrated with purple arrows. In that case, the product of the object spectrum and the optical transfer function is the image spectrum, from which the image itself can be obtained by inverse Fourier transformation. The roadmap also indicates how the PSF and the OTF can be obtained from the generalized pupil function.**

chromatic aberrations. Chromatic aberration is not as large as the combined effect of the higher order aberrations and its influence on vision is less pronounced. Chromatic aberration arises because the refractive index of the ocular media, like all common optical media, increases with decreasing wavelength. Consequently, any light rays incident on the cornea except those perpendicular to its surface will, upon passing into the eye, be bent more if the wavelength is short than if it is long. This chromatic dispersion causes both the plane of best focus and the retinal location of the image of a monochromatic point source to depend on wavelength. The same simplified model of the eye that was used to describe retinal image size (see Figure 2.43 in Appendix A) can also serve as the basis for the analysis of chromatic aberration (Thibos, 1987).

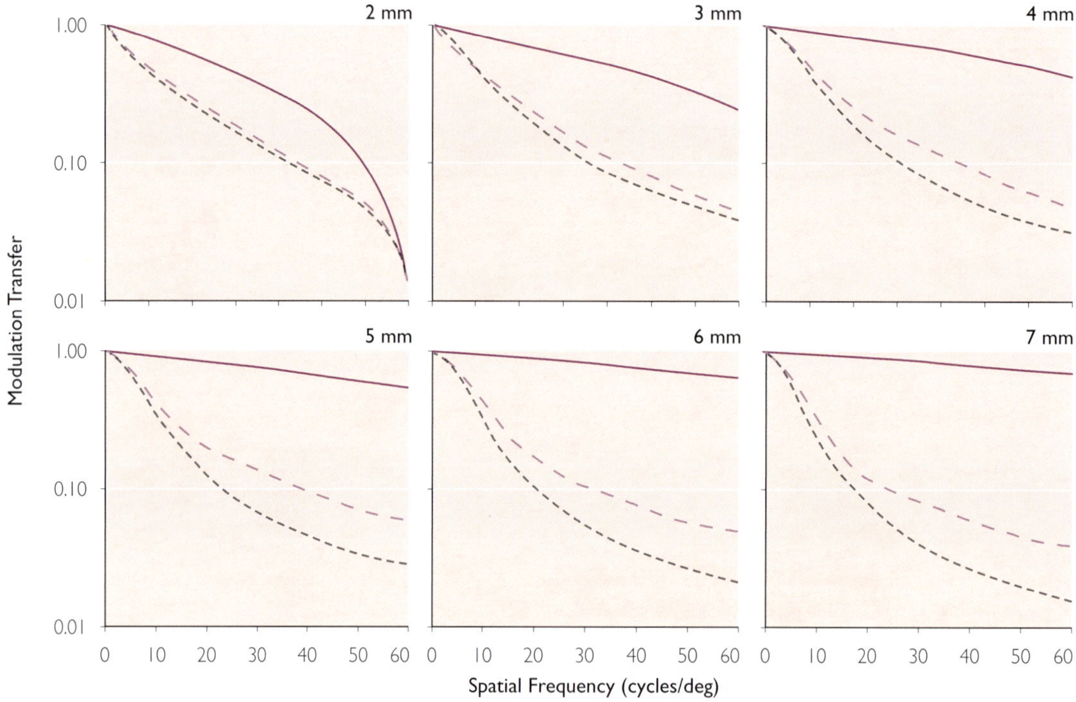

Figure 2.15 **Modulation transfer functions calculated for eyes with pupils ranging from 2 through 7 mm. In each panel, the solid line shows the MTF for an eye whose optics suffer only from diffraction, λ = 555 nm. The long dashed lines show the mean monochromatic MTFs of 14 normal human eyes. MTFs were computed from wave aberration measurements obtained with a Hartmann–Shack wavefront sensor and a 7.3 mm pupil (Liang and Williams, 1997). The short dashed lines show the MTFs expected in white light taking into account the axial but not the transverse chromatic aberration of the eye. The eye was assumed to be accommodated to 555 nm and its spectral sensitivity was assumed to correspond to the photopic luminosity function.**

The MTFs were calculated without defocus and astigmatism by setting the appropriate Zernike terms in the wave aberration to zero. This is not quite the same as finding the values of defocus and astigmatism that optimize image quality as one does in a conventional clinical refraction. Had such an optimization been performed, the white light and monochromatic MTFs would have been more similar. (Courtesy Geun-Young Yoon.)

2.4.4.1 Axial chromatic aberration

Figure 2.16 shows how a point source lying on the optic axis of the eye is imaged on the retina. If the point source consists of two wavelengths, the short wavelength light is brought to a focus nearer to the lens than the long wavelength light. When the point source is effectively at infinity and the eye is in focus for long wavelengths, the short wavelength light will be broadly distributed in a blur circle. If the point is moved nearer the eye such that the short wavelength light is well focused, then the long wavelength light will be blurred. This wavelength-dependent displacement in the axial position of best focus is called axial or longitudinal chromatic aberration.

Figure 2.17 shows the chromatic difference of focus of the eye, which has been measured extensively. There is almost no variation from observer to observer because all eyes are made of essentially the same materials with the same chromatic dispersion. From 400 to 700 nm the total chromatic difference of focus is ~2.25 diopters.

Axial chromatic aberration causes the wave aberration of the eye to depend on the wavelength of light. To a first approximation, the only Zernike polynomial that depends strongly on wavelength is the defocus term, with all the other aberrations retaining similar amplitudes when expressed in micrometers.

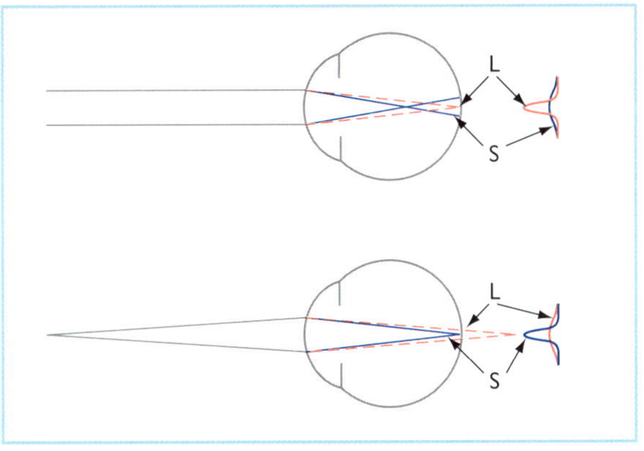

Figure 2.16 The geometrical optics of axial chromatic aberration. At the top, an eye focused on a point source at infinity brings long wavelength light (L, red lines) to a sharp focus on the retina producing a peaked light distribution. Short wavelength light (S, blue lines) is brought to a focus in front of the retina producing a large blur circle on the retina. At the bottom, the eye is focused on a point source close to the eye. The short wavelength light is brought to a sharp focus, but long wavelengths focus behind the retina.

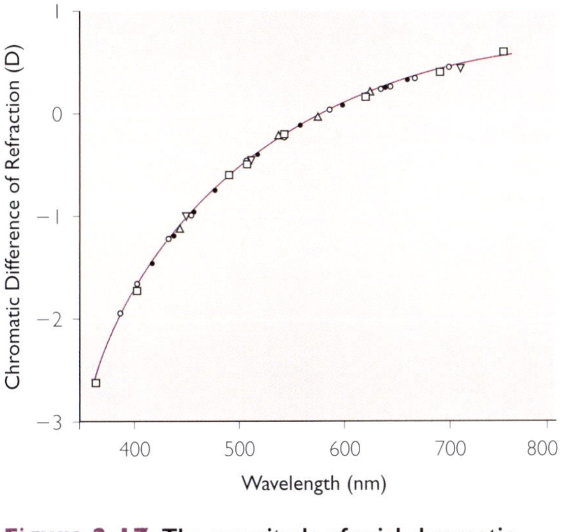

Figure 2.17 The magnitude of axial chromatic aberration in diopters as a function of wavelength averaged over several studies (replotted from Charman, 1995). Different symbols represent data from different studies.

2.4.4.2 What wavelength does the eye focus on?

Because of axial chromatic aberration, only a single wavelength of a broadband stimulus can be in best focus at any given time. It is common to assume that the eye focuses somewhere in the middle of the spectrum, in the vicinity of 555 nm where the eye is most sensitive at photopic light levels. For broadband stimuli, this would minimize the loss in retinal image contrast seen by the L and M cones that mediate detailed pattern vision. However, the wavelength that is in focus also depends on the distance of the object being viewed. The eye has an accommodative lag, which means that the actual distance that is in optimal focus lies between the object distance and the resting point of accommodation. The resting point varies from eye to eye but on average lies at a distance of about 1 m (Charman, 1995). For objects that are nearer than the resting point, the wavelength in best focus shifts toward the short-wavelength end of the spectrum. For objects that are further than the resting point, the wavelength in best focus shifts toward the long-wavelength end of the spectrum.

2.4.4.3 Why isn't axial chromatic aberration very deleterious?

Since the total range of chromatic aberration across the visible spectrum corresponds to a little over 2 diopters of defocus, the blur it produces ought to have important effects on spatial vision. However, Campbell and Gubisch (1967) found that contrast sensitivity for monochromatic yellow light was only slightly greater than contrast sensitivity for white light. Visual performance on spatial tasks usually depends very little on the S cones, the cone class that would generally experience the greatest retinal image blur due to axial chromatic aberration. Moreover, the proximity of the L and M absorption spectra means that the deleterious effects of axial chromatic aberration will be similar for both cone types. The reduced spectral sensitivity of the eye at short and long wavelengths also reduces the deleterious effects of chromatic aberration. In fact, the 2 diopters of defocus produced by chromatic aberration will have an effect on image quality similar to 0.15 diopters of monochromatic defocus, an amount that is generally not detectable (Bradley *et al.*, 1991). Figure 2.15 compares the MTFs in monochromatic (long dashed curves) and broadband (short dashed curves) light.

It has been suggested (Walls, 1963; Nussbaum *et al.*, 1981) that the short wavelength absorbing pigments of the ocular media play an important role in limiting blur from chromatic aberration. Reading and Weale (1974) modeled chromatic aberration in the eye and found that the optimum filter for reducing the deleterious effects of chromatic aberration on spatial vision in daylight would have spectral characteristics very similar to those of the macular pigment. However, the effect of spectral filtering in the ocular media on the modulation transfer function is relatively small. A less widely recognized reason that chromatic aberration is not more deleterious is that it is overwhelmed by the numerous monochromatic aberrations. These aberrations, most of which spectacles fail to correct, dilute the impact of axial chromatic aberration (Marcos *et al.*, 1999; Yoon and Williams, 2002).

2.4.4.4 Transverse chromatic aberration

The axial chromatic aberration illustrated in Figure 2.16 shows only the restricted case of a point lying on the optic axis of the eye. In general, the point source will lie off the optic axis. For example, if the fovea is displaced from the optic axis, as it is in many eyes, then chromatic dispersion causes a lateral displacement of the retinal image as well as an axial displacement (Figure 2.18). The image of a point lies closer to the optic axis in short wavelength light than it does in long wavelength light. This lateral displacement is called transverse or lateral chromatic aberration. Transverse chromatic aberration can manifest itself either as a lateral displacement of a single point in a scene, as illustrated in Figure 2.18, or as a magnification difference of an extended object. The amount of transverse chromatic aberration at the fovea depends strongly on the position of the pupil of the eye relative to the nodal point. If the pupil lay at the nodal point, there would be no transverse chromatic aberration. Usually, the natural pupil is well aligned with respect to the achromatic axis (Rynders *et al.*, 1995), so that transverse chromatic aberration does not typically reduce image quality in the fovea. However, a lateral shift of the pupil of only one millimeter would be expected to smear the spectrum from 400 to 700 nm across 8 minutes of arc (Thibos *et al.*, 1990). This corresponds to a 180 degree phase reversal of a 3.75 cycles/degree grating. Thus, when small artificial pupils are used during psychophysical experiments involving chromatic gratings, alignment must be very good indeed.

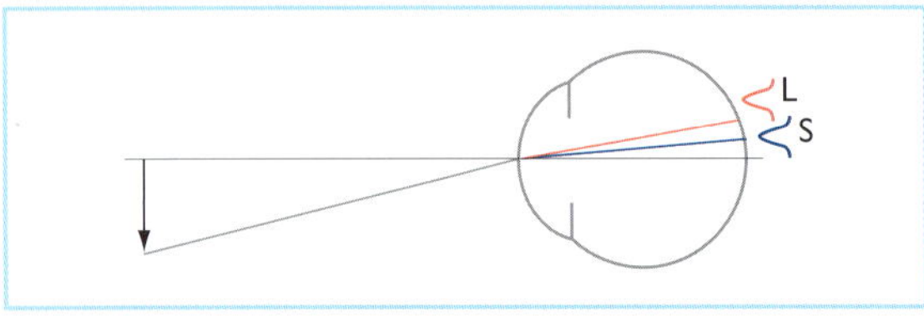

Figure 2.18 **The geometrical optics of transverse chromatic aberration. An arrow which subtends a substantial angular extent is being imaged on the retina. The position of the image of the tip of the arrow depends on wavelength, being closer to the optical axis for short wavelength light (S, blue lines) than for long wavelength light (L, red lines). Thus, the image of a white object will tend to be smeared.**

The existence of transverse chromatic aberration causes a stereoscopic phenomenon called chromostereopsis in which objects at the same distance from the observer, but of different spectral radiance, appear to lie in different depth planes. By displacing retinal images with different spectral radiance, transverse chromatic aberration erroneously creates binocular disparity in the left and right eye images, which is interpreted by the brain as a difference in depth (Einthoven, 1885).

2.4.4.5 Techniques to avoid chromatic aberration

In color vision experiments, particularly those in which isoluminant stimuli are produced, it is often very important to eliminate luminance artifacts in the stimulus caused by chromatic aberration. For example, an isoluminant grating can be produced by adding together gratings of short- and middle-wavelength light. If the amplitudes of the two gratings are adjusted to have equal luminance, the combined stimulus will look like interleaved red and green stripes. However, when viewed at a very high spatial frequency near the resolution limit, the colors of the grating disappear and one sees only an achromatic grating. While the inability to resolve the colored stripes is consistent with a lower bandwidth for chromatic mechanisms (Sekiguchi *et al.*, 1993b), the residual achromatic grating is probably a result of chromatic aberration in the eye. Axial chromatic aberration ensures that at least one grating will be out of focus and will therefore have reduced contrast, which can result in a luminance modulation as spatial frequency is increased. At the same time, transverse chromatic aberration can shift one grating relative to the other on the retina, which also creates a luminance modulation in the retinal image.

There are several ways to avoid or reduce chromatic aberration. If stimuli are produced in multiple channels of a Maxwellian view system, axial chromatic aberration can be corrected by adjusting the optical distances so that stimuli of different wavelengths are in focus simultaneously. Another approach is to use an achromatizing lens specifically designed to correct axial chromatic aberration of the eye (Bradley *et al.*, 1991). Small pupils can also be used to increase the depth of focus of the eye, reducing axial chromatic aberration. It is worth noting though that unless the achromatizing lens or small pupil is perfectly aligned it may make matters worse.

The use of interference fringes is an extreme example of using a small pupil to increase the depth of focus (Sekiguchi *et al.*, 1993a). Interference fringes are high contrast sinusoidal gratings formed on the retina by shining two laser beams through the pupil of the eye and allowing them to interfere with each other. Since all the light enters the eye through two tiny separated pupils, depth of focus is very high. The use of stimuli confined to low spatial frequencies minimizes the visual consequences of transverse chromatic aberration. At moderate spatial frequencies, the magnification and phase of the short- and long-wavelength gratings can be independently adjusted to compensate for transverse chromatic aberration, although this becomes progressively more difficult with increasing spatial frequency (Sekiguchi *et al.*, 1993a).

2.4.5 SCATTER

In addition to losses due to diffraction and optical aberrations, retinal image contrast is reduced by light scatter in the anterior optics and retina (Vos, 1963). The sources of scattered light in the eye that contribute to the contrast reduction of the retinal image are (1) forward scatter from the cornea, (2) forward scatter from the lens, (3) forward scatter from the retina, and (4) back scatter from the fundus. Roughly a quarter of the scatter comes from the cornea, another quarter from the retina, and the remaining half from the lens. Since most of the forward scattering is by relatively large particles, the scattered light in the eye does not show a strong wavelength dependence (Wooten and Geri, 1987).

Scatter reduces contrast principally by adding a veiling illumination to the retinal image that reduces the ratio of the intensities of the lightest and darkest regions. In the normal eye at high light levels, scatter is not a major source of image blur. It becomes important primarily in situations where the observer is detecting a relatively dim object in the presence of a glare source. A good example from daily life is the driver who fails to detect a pedestrian in the roadway as a result of glare from oncoming headlights. Scattering tends to increase with age and can sometimes make it difficult for older people to drive at night even though by many measures, such as acuity, their vision remains quite good (Westheimer and Liang, 1995). Performance on certain psychophysical experiments can also be measurably degraded by scatter, although the amount is quite dependent on stimulus conditions. For example, the detection threshold of a small spot of light is noticeably raised by surrounding it with a bright annulus. The amount of scatter can be estimated by measuring the illuminance of a superimposed background required to degrade detection of the small spot to the same level caused by the annulus. Under similar conditions, the scattered illuminance ranges from 1 to 28% of the illuminance of the retinal image (Shevell and Burroughs, 1988). The smaller values are for conditions in which the annulus is farther away from the spot being detected and thus scatters less light over it. In general, it is important to consider whether scatter is likely to be a problem for some particular experiment. For a given stimulus configuration, the amount of scattering can often be measured.

2.5 PHOTORECEPTOR OPTICS

Once light passes through the anterior optics of the eye and forms a retinal image, photoreceptors transduce it into a neural signal. The morphology of photoreceptors gives them properties similar to fiber optic waveguides. Figures 2.19(A) and (C) are vertical sections through the human retina (Curcio *et al.*, 1990) that reveal the morphology of foveal and peripheral photoreceptors. The normally transparent layers have been stained to make the structure visible. In the living eye, light would have passed through these sections of retina from the bottom to the top. After passing through the cell layers of the inner retina, light is funneled through the photoreceptor inner segments, the large tapered profiles in the middle of each image, and into the photopigment filled outer segments, the thread-like profiles at the top of each image. In the fovea (Figure 2.19A), all of the photoreceptors are cones, while in peripheral retina (Figure 2.19C), narrow cylindrical rods fill in around the large tapered cones. We will now examine the individual photoreceptor as an optical element in order to see how its aperture affects sensitivity and spatial resolution, how self-screening within the photopigment-filled outer segment affects spectral sensitivity, and how the morphological properties of individual photoreceptors confer directional sensitivity.

2.5.1 THE PHOTORECEPTOR APERTURE

Light first interacts with rods and cones at the photoreceptor apertures, which are shown face on (Figures 2.19B and D) with the aid of a Nomarski microscope. The aperture is located at the level of the inner segments where the indices of refraction inside and outside of the photoreceptors diverge enough that the rods and cones begin to capture light (arrows in Figures 2.19A and C). Evidence for this comes from observations of the retina using Nomarski optics which show that the photoreceptors first become distinct from their matrix at this level. Additionally, the psychophysically measured aperture covaries with inner segment diameter and not outer segment diameter as a function of retinal eccentricity (Chen *et al.*, 1993). The size of the

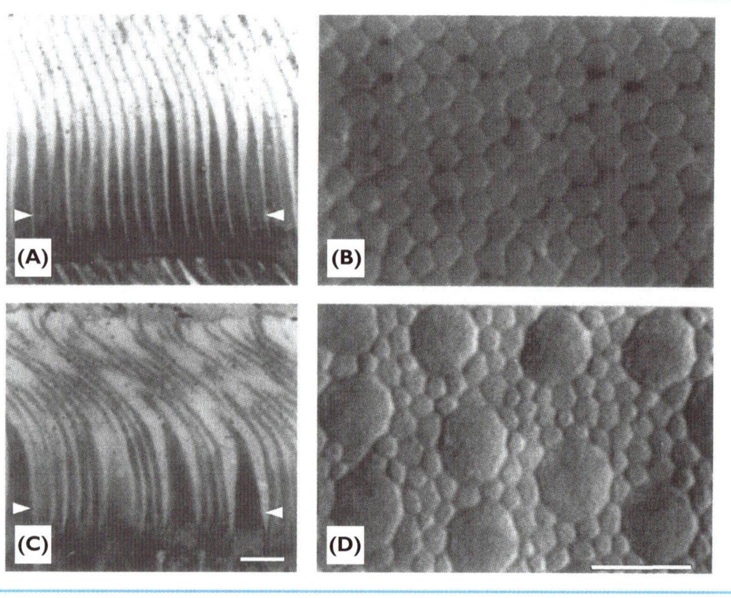

Figure 2.19 **The human retina viewed in histological vertical sections and face on using a Nomarski microscope (from Curcio et *al.*, 1990). (A) Vertical section through the fovea. The large funnel-shaped profiles are cone inner segments. The thin fibers at the top are the pigment-filled outer segments. The shearing in the outer segments is a tissue-processing artifact. In the intact retina, light would pass through from bottom to top. (B) Nomarski image of the foveal center. All of the profiles are cone inner segments. (C) Vertical section of mid-peripheral retina. Filling in between the cones are the thinner more cylindrical rods. (D) Nomarski image of mid-peripheral retina. The large profiles are cones and the smaller profiles are rods. The scale bars are 10 μm. The white arrows indicate the level at which the inner segments become optically distinct. (Copyright © 1990 *Journal of Comparative Neurology*. Reprinted by permission of Wiley-Liss, Inc., a subsidiary of John Wiley & Sons, Inc.)**

photoreceptor aperture is important because cones need to reliably detect small differences in retinal image contrast while at the same time preserving important spatial detail. These attributes are not easy to accommodate in a single detector. Spatial resolution is lower for a large aperture because the aperture pools all of the photons that fall on it, and in the process, averages away spatial detail. Sensitivity, on the other hand, is higher for a large aperture that can collect more photons. We will now examine this tradeoff between high spatial resolution and high sensitivity.

2.5.1.1 Anatomical and psychophysical measurements

Figure 2.20 shows that in the macaque monkey, cone inner segments are about 2.5 μm in diameter at the center of the fovea, about 8 μm at 20° of eccentricity, and over 11 μm at the edge of temporal retina. Rod inner segments (not shown) also increase in diameter from about 1.5 μm at their eccentricity of first appearance just outside the foveola to over 4 μm near the temporal edge of the retina.

The size of the foveal cone aperture has also been estimated psychophysically. MacLeod *et al.* (1992) formed interference fringes on the retina and estimated foveal cone aperture size from the demodulation of a distortion product as a function of spatial frequency. Measured in this way, the cone aperture was about half the anatomical diameter. This measurement probably represents a lower bound on the true size of the cone aperture. This difference between the anatomical and functional measurements suggests that the anatomical is larger than the functional aperture.

2.5.1.2 Spatial filtering

For the purposes of evaluating spatial filtering and photon capture, the photoreceptor is often modeled as a circular aperture. The diffraction limit of the largest aperture estimate, the 2.5 μm anatomical aperture, of a foveal cone is ~150 cycles/degree at midspectral wavelengths. Thus, the cone aperture is capable of preserving much finer detail than exists in the retinal image because the optics of the eye filter out spatial frequencies above about 60 cycles/degree. Therefore, under normal viewing conditions, the spatial resolution of the eye is not limited by filtering at the cone aperture (Williams, 1985).

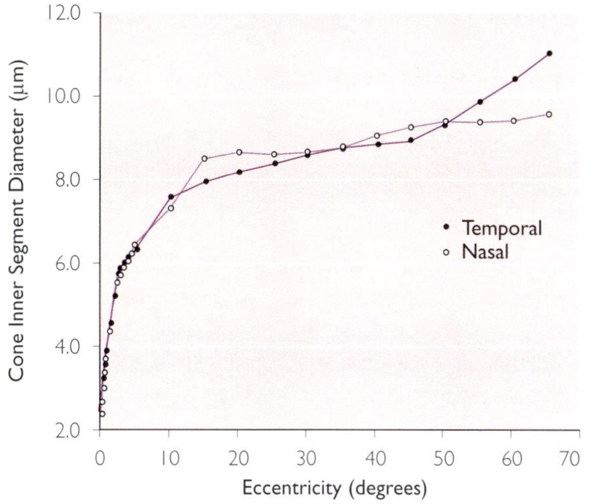

Figure 2.20 **Inner segment diameter of macaque monkey cones as a function of retinal eccentricity in degrees along the horizontal meridian. ● represent nasal retina. ○ represent temporal retina. Inner segment diameter in macaque and human does not differ substantially. (After Packer *et al.*, 1989. Copyright © 1989 *Journal of Comparative Neurology*. Reprinted by permission of Wiley-Liss, Inc., a subsidiary of John Wiley & Sons, Inc.)**

Peripheral cone apertures are larger and thus filter high spatial frequencies more strongly. Even so, aperture filtering does not match optical filtering until cone inner segment diameter reaches 6 μm, which occurs in macaque retina at an eccentricity of about 4°. Even at the edge of the retina, spatial frequencies up to 20 cycles/degree would be preserved. However, the aperture does reduce the contrast of spatial frequencies that alias (see below) (Miller and Bernard, 1983) and the close match between the spatial frequencies that alias and filtering by the aperture suggests that detection and resolution of gratings in peripheral retina is limited by aperture filtering (Thibos *et al.*, 1987).

2.5.1.3 Contrast detection

The ability to detect contrast is a fundamental property of the visual system and depends on the strength of the visual signal relative to any noise that contaminates it. The main source of noise in the visual optics is due to the quantum nature of light. The result of this quantum nature is that the number of photons that isomerize the photopigment molecules in a photoreceptor outer segment will vary from interval to interval. This variability makes it difficult to distinguish between two stimuli of only slightly different light output. The probability that a particular number of photons will isomerize photopigment molecules during a given interval is described by a Poisson distribution,

$$p(n) = a^n/e^x n!$$

where p is the probability of counting exactly n photoisomerizations given that, over many repetitions of the measurement, an average of x photoisomerizations occur. The standard deviation of the distribution of photoisomerizations about x is the square root of x. For example, to reliably detect an intensity difference between two lights 84% of the time, there should be a separation of 1 standard deviation in the mean number of photoisomerizations produced. Using this criterion, the smallest contrast that can be reliably distinguished, c, will be

$$c = \sqrt{x}/x$$

In the case of a single foveal cone, a 100 troland stimulus produces approximately 1100 photoisomerizations/s (Makous, 1997). Assuming only photon noise, a 50 ms stimulus (approximately equal to the temporal integration time), would produce ~55 photoisomerizations, which is sufficient to detect contrasts of ~14%. Thus, individual foveal cones are not highly reliable contrast detectors at low photopic luminances. The visual system is capable of detecting 0.5% contrast or less under ideal circumstances, and that requires at least 40 000 photoisomerizations. This could be accomplished by increasing retinal light levels to 8×10^5 trolands during that 50 ms interval or by combining the signals of multiple photoreceptors. The visual system relies on spatial pooling of signals from many photoreceptors to achieve high contrast sensitivity at low spatial frequencies.

In summary, individual foveal cones support excellent spatial resolution but are good detectors of contrast only at higher light levels. Although the cone aperture is much smaller than required for good spatial resolution, we will see later that cone sampling also benefits from small, tightly packed cone apertures. Thus the resolution-sensitivity tradeoff has been resolved in favor of high spatial resolution. At lower light levels, where spatial resolution is limited by photon scarcity anyway, signals from many photoreceptors need to be combined to improve sensitivity.

2.5.2 AXIAL PHOTOPIGMENT DENSITY

Good visual sensitivity requires that the photons captured by the cone apertures isomerize as much photopigment as possible. Efficient photon usage is promoted by the ability of photoreceptors to funnel light through long photopigment filled outer segments. This ability is a result of waveguide properties. Figure 2.21 is a transmission image of peripheral macaque retina. The retina was illuminated from the normal direction and the photoreceptors funneled the light through the inner and outer segments. Each bright spot is an image of the outer segment tip of a photoreceptor. The image on the left is focused on the tips of the cones, while the image on the right is focused on the tips of the rods. The intensity of the light emerging from the rod outer segment tips averages 1.7 times the intensity of the light incident on the rod aperture. This is direct evidence that even the rods, which are less funnel shaped than the cones, have the ability to trap and even concentrate light within their outer segments.

Once the light is confined, long outer segments give a photon a better chance of interacting with a pigment molecule. Outer segment length varies as a function of retinal location (Polyak, 1957; Hendrickson and Yuodelis, 1984), being longest (45 μm) at the center of the fovea and shortest in the far periphery. The simplest geometrical calculation predicts that outer segment axial density is the product of outer segment length and the specific density of photopigment (0.16/μm, Baylor *et al.*, 1984). In the fovea, measurements made with retinal densitometers, which collect light that has passed through the photopigment twice, are never this high (0.72), seldom exceed 0.4 and are commonly as low as 0.05. This is probably because retinal densitometry doesn't take into account stray light such as reflection from the membrane surfaces of the outer segments disks (van de Kraats *et al.*, 1996) or from the junctions between the inner and outer segments. In peripheral

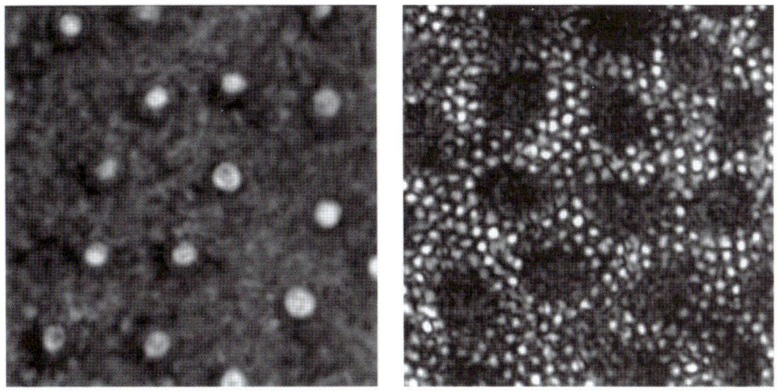

Figure 2.21 **Transmittance image of an excised patch of macaque monkey retina. The retina is being illuminated from the normal direction and viewed under a light microscope that is focused in the plane of the outer segment tips. The image on the left is focused on the cones. The image on the right is focused on the rods. (From Packer *et al.*, 1996. Copyright © 1996 by the Society for Neuroscience)**

retina, on the other hand, photopigment transmittance imaging (Packer *et al.*, 1996) has measured axial photopigment densities that are consistent with the simple calculation.

2.5.3 SELF-SCREENING AND COLOR MATCHING

In addition to improving the efficiency with which the retina absorbs photons, high axial photopigment density also broadens the spectral absorptance of photopigment. This, in turn, broadens the underlying spectral sensitivities of the photoreceptors and slightly changes our color vision as assessed by such measurements as color matching.

The dependence of the photopigment spectrum on optical density is known as self-screening. Self-screening results because the fraction of light absorbed depends on wavelength and because absorption can never exceed 100% of the illuminating light. Assume, for example, that a column of pigment is illuminated axially by a broadband light and that the column of pigment absorbs all of the light at 560 nm but only a small fraction at 450 nm and 650 nm. If more pigment is added, the column still absorbs 100% of the light at 560 nm. However, it absorbs a larger proportion of the light at long and short wavelengths causing the absorption curve to flatten. The spectrum of the photopigment contained in an outer segment of a particular length can be calculated from the Beer–Lambert law, where

$$t(\lambda) = 10^{-dce(\lambda)}$$

and t is the proportion of incident light transmitted (transmittance) as a function of wavelength (λ), d is the path length through the pigment, c is pigment concentration and e is the absorptivity of the pigment as a function of wavelength.

This equation shows that the changes in spectral sensitivity due to self-screening can be due either to changes in the length of the path that light takes through the pigment or to changes in the concentration of the pigment. Outer segment length remains constant at any particular retinal location, but light level can substantially affect the concentration of unbleached pigment molecules. Figure 2.22 shows that the spectral absorptance function of an L cone (spectra from Baylor *et al.*, 1987) narrows when its optical density changes from 0.4 log units following dark adaptation to 0.01 log units following exposure to a very high light level. This change in the shape of the absorptance spectrum is reflected in the color matching functions which are not the same for a moderate light level like 1000 trolands as they are for a very high light level like 100 000 trolands (Wyszecki and Stiles, 1980).

Conversely, photopigment density and absorption spectra have been estimated from color

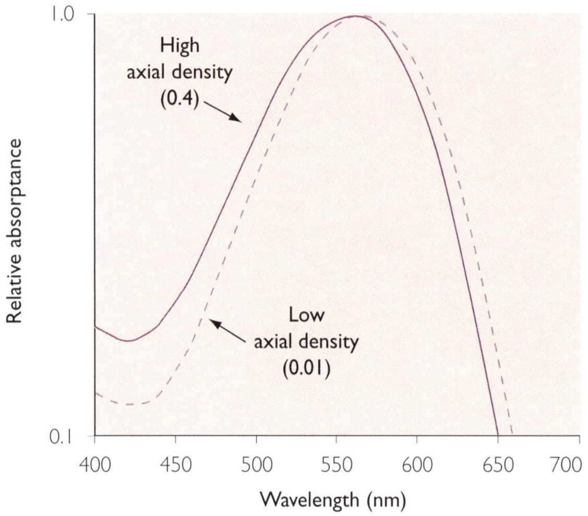

Figure 2.22 The relative absorption spectra of L cone photopigment at high and low concentrations. The broader curve represents axial densities that might be typical of fully dark adapted conditions. The narrower curve represents axial densities that might be typical of fully light adapted conditions. (L cone spectra are from Baylor *et al.*, 1988.)

matches made before and after bleaching by calculating the density and spectra that are most consistent with the changes in the matches (Burns and Elsner, 1985; MacLeod and Webster, 1988).

2.5.4 DIRECTIONAL SENSITIVITY

Another property conferred on vision by the optical properties of individual photoreceptors is directional sensitivity. Figure 2.23 shows that a beam of light illuminating a photocell produces the same meter reading regardless of whether the beam travels through the center of a lens and hits the detector straight on or enters the edge of a lens and hits the same location at an angle. This detector is not directionally sensitive.

However, light reaching a given point on the retina through the center of the pupil is more visually effective than the same light reaching the same point through the edge of the pupil. Thus, the retina is directionally sensitive.

2.5.4.1 The Stiles–Crawford effect of the first kind

Retinal directional sensitivity was first measured psychophysically by Stiles and Crawford (1933) and is called the Stiles–Crawford effect of the first kind (SCI).

Figure 2.24 shows SCI data collected from a group of subjects foveally viewing a 670 nm 0.6° test field at a retinal illuminance of 40 td (Applegate and Lakshminarayanan, 1993). The log-relative sensitivity of three points in the pupil can be determined by following the dashed lines between pupil and graph. The peak of the SCI is located 0.2 mm superior and 0.5 mm nasal

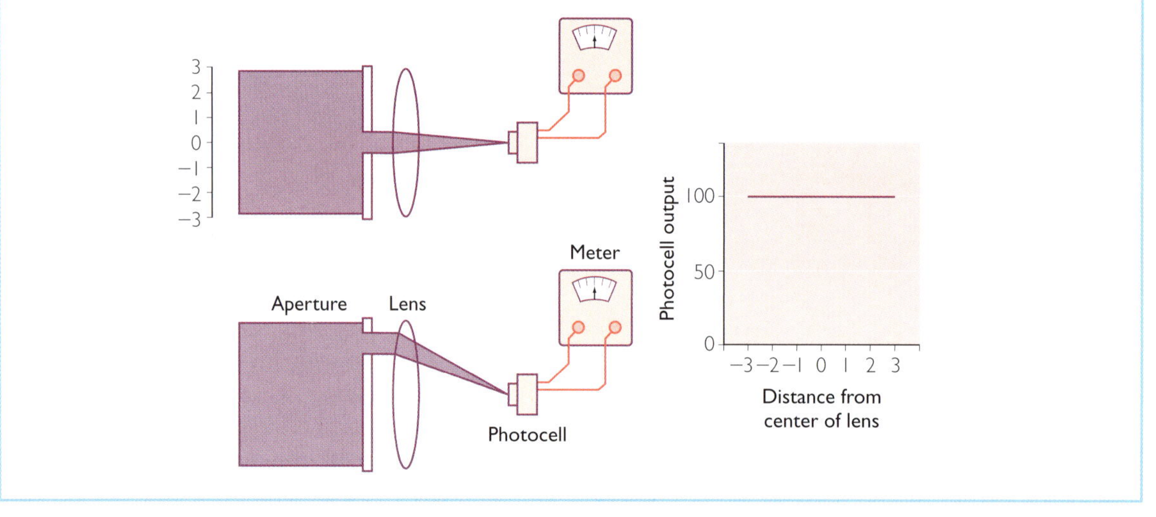

Figure 2.23 Schematic illustrating the lack of directional sensitivity of a simple silicon light detector. (From Rodieck, 1973.)

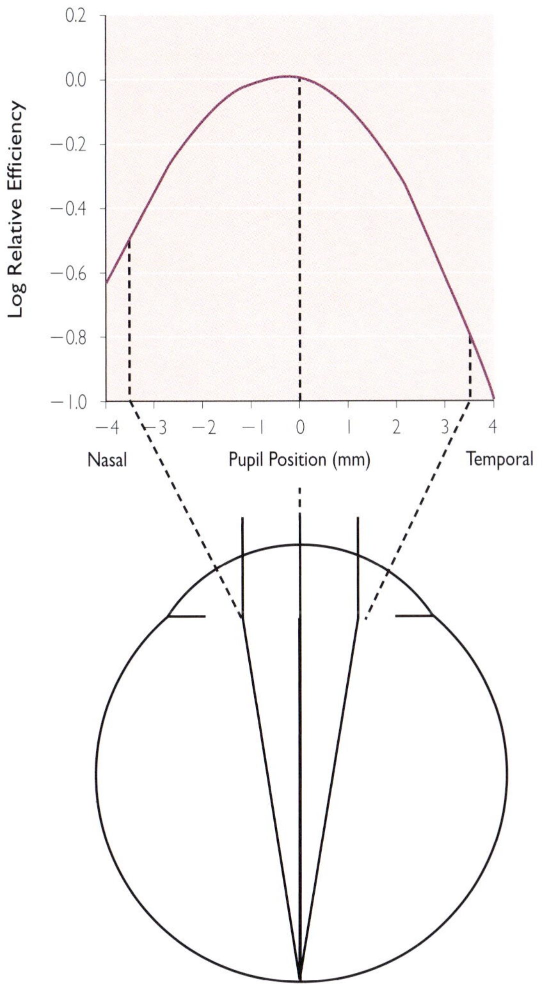

Figure 2.24 **Schematic diagram of the Stiles–Crawford effect of the first kind. The upper graph shows the log relative efficiency with which light is used as a function of the location in the pupil at which it enters the eye. Three points on the function are represented by rays entering the pupil of the eye. (The parameters of the Stiles–Crawford function are from Applegate and Lakshminarayanan, 1993.)**

to the center of the pupil. In order to quantify the degree of directional sensitivity, the data were fit with a parabola of the form

$$\log \eta = \log \eta_{max} - \rho(x - x_{max})^2$$

where η is the sensitivity at x mm from the center of the pupil, and rho (ρ) describes the width of the parabola. Larger values of ρ correspond to greater directional sensitivity (narrower parabolas). The average ρ value of these data was 0.05. A parabolic fit to the data is reasonably accurate for pupils smaller than 6 mm in diameter. Although most studies of the SCI have modeled their data using the parabola shown above, directional sensitivity is more accurately described in terms of a Gaussian (Safir *et al.*, 1970). For those who prefer the Gaussian model, the parabolic ρ value can be expressed in terms of the half-width at half-height of a Gaussian using the following equation.

$$\mathrm{HWHH} = (0.3/\rho)^{0.5}$$

The directional sensitivity measured by the SCI depends on a number of parameters (for an excellent review see Enoch and Lakshminarayanan, 1991). When the stimulus is detected by cones, the directional sensitivity remains relatively constant as a function of luminance. However, when luminance is low and rods are detecting the stimulus, directional sensitivity is much less pronounced. Directional sensitivity also depends on wavelength (Stiles, 1939), being greatest at the ends of the spectrum and least between 500 and 600 nm. Directional sensitivity also depends on retinal location, being lowest for a small stimulus imaged at the center of the fovea, highest in the perifovea and lower again in the far periphery. Broader directional sensitivity at the center of the fovea (Burns *et al.*, 1997) likely reflects the long, thin, slightly tapered morphology of the centralmost cones. This is consistent with the fact that rods, which have similar morphology, exhibit little directional sensitivity.

2.5.4.2 Fundus reflectometry

In addition to psychophysics, which measures the directional sensitivity of absorbed photons, it is also possible to measure the directional properties of light reflected from the retina. Although most incident light is absorbed in either the retina or the pigment epithelium, one out of every 10^3 or 10^4 incident photons is reflected from the retina and back out of the pupil (Rushton, 1965). Some of these reflected photons fall between photoreceptors and are reflected back from the extracellular space between photoreceptors, while others are incident on photoreceptor apertures and are reflected back down the axis of the photoreceptor. Those reflected photons that missed the photoreceptors have little directional character and uniformly fill the pupil, while those photons reflected back down the axes of the photoreceptors leave the eye near the center of the pupil (van Blockland and van Norren, 1986). Each photoreceptor thus acts like a tiny flashlight, emitting light in a cone whose width depends on its optical properties (Snyder, 1969). Furthermore, all of the flashlights are pointed towards the center of the pupil (Laties and Enoch, 1971; Roorda and Williams, 2002). Thus, the directional sensitivity of the retina can be estimated by measuring the width of the intensity profile of the light leaving the eye through the center of the pupil.

Directional sensitivity measurements made with fundus reflectometry have foveal ρ values that are on average about twice those measured psychophysically. The Stiles–Crawford effect is a psychophysical measurement of the directionality of photons incident on the photoreceptors and absorbed by photopigment, while fundus reflectometry measures the directionality of photons reflected from the retina. Two factors explain a large fraction of the differences in directional sensitivity measured with the two techniques (He *et al.*, 1999). First, part of the light captured by cone inner segments leaks out of the outer segments and is not waveguided back out of the photoreceptor that captured it. This reflected light has less power contained in higher order modes (see next section) and as a result is emitted in a narrower cone. Second, individual cones are so small that the light reflected back from them is coherent. Slight differences in cone length introduce phase differences in the light from neighboring cones. The resulting interference narrows the angular extent of the light in the pupil. Thus although both the behavioral and optical methods of measuring the directional sensitivity of the retina tap into the waveguide behavior of photoreceptors, the property responsible for retinal directional sensitivity, they do so in slightly different ways.

2.5.4.3 The photoreceptor as an optical waveguide

The SCI is known to be retinal in origin and mediated by the waveguide properties of photoreceptors (Enoch and Lakshminarayanan, 1991). An optical waveguide has a core of high refractive index surrounded by a cladding of lower refractive index. In a photoreceptor, the cytoplasm of the inner and outer segments serves as the high index core and the cell membrane and surrounding fluid serve as the cladding. Because photoreceptors have diameters near the wavelength of light, their optical behavior is better explained using wave optics rather than geometrical optics (Toraldo di Francia, 1949).

Light waves incident on a photoreceptor aperture propagate along the length of the inner and outer segments. These waves constructively and destructively reflect from the cell membrane, setting up stationary energy patterns or modes in and around the photoreceptor. These modes are analogous to the standing waves set up in a vibrating string. The parameter

$$V = \pi d/\lambda \, (n_1^2 - n_2^2)^{0.5}$$

indicates which modes can be supported by a cylindrical waveguide, where d is diameter, λ is wavelength, and n_1 and n_2 are the indices of refraction of the core and cladding respectively. When V is large, several modes may exist simultaneously. Images of modal patterns observed in vertebrate photoreceptors can be found in Enoch and Lakshminarayanan (1991). The energy of a mode exists both inside and outside of the photoreceptor, but only the energy within the photoreceptor interacts with photopigment. As V increases, the proportion of energy within the photoreceptor increases relative to that outside.

Each mode is associated with a particular pattern of directional sensitivity. As the angle of incidence of the illuminating light increases, less energy is coupled into a mode. If the photoreceptor supports multiple modes, increasing the angle of incidence causes the higher order modes to be more efficiently stimulated. For any given V, the higher order modes also have a smaller percentage of their energy within the photopigment. Therefore, since the directional sensitivity of the photoreceptor is the sum of the sensitivities of the individual modes, increasing the angle of incidence reduces the amount of light that can interact with the photopigment.

Models which incorporate these features and

which can be used to predict the directional sensitivity of photoreceptors include those of Snyder and Pask (1973a,b), Wijngaard (1974), and Starr (1977). However, a definitive model of the waveguide properties of rods and cones has yet to be formulated.

2.5.4.4 What purpose does directional sensitivity serve?

A potentially important purpose for directional selectivity is to improve the optical quality of the eye. The directional sensitivity of photoreceptors combined with their orientation towards the center of the pupil would limit light collection to those photons that enter the eye near the optical axis, eliminating the more highly aberrated peripheral rays. However, calculations suggest that directional sensitivity produces only modest improvements in retinal image contrast (Atchison *et al.*, 1998) for eyes that are in good focus. Although the Stiles–Crawford effect is retinal in origin, its effect on image quality at any single point on the retina is due to the reduction in the pupil size produced by the reduced effectiveness of the light entering the edges of the pupil. Also, the softening of the aperture margin caused by the Stiles–Crawford effect tends to enhance modulation transfer at low spatial frequencies. The effect of the SCI on image quality can be calculated by appropriately modifying the amplitude term of the generalized pupil function (see section 2.4.1). Figure 2.25 shows that the effect of the SCI on retinal image quality is minor for small pupils when retinal images are in good focus. In addition, the cones of the central-most retina, which ought to gain the largest advantage from improved optical quality, are not very directionally sensitive. On the other hand, when the retinal image is not in good focus due to accommodative lag, or other aberrations, the benefits of the SCI on retinal image quality is larger (Mino and Okano, 1971; Legge *et al.*, 1987; Zhang *et al.*, 1999). Additionally, this analysis neglects the deleterious effects of light that passes through and is scattered by the sclera as well as light that is scattered by the fundus. These sources of stray light cast a uniform veil across the retina, reducing retinal image contrast, and the Stiles–Crawford effect probably plays a useful role in preventing this light from being absorbed by photoreceptors. An alternative explanation for direction selectivity is that it is a consequence of advantages that accrue by confining photopigment to small diameter outer segments. Smaller outer segments might have reduced metabolic costs to build and maintain. It is possible that the waveguide properties allow equivalent quantum catch rates in smaller, less costly outer segments, and that the antennae properties of cones observed in the pupil simply follow passively from advantages of funneling.

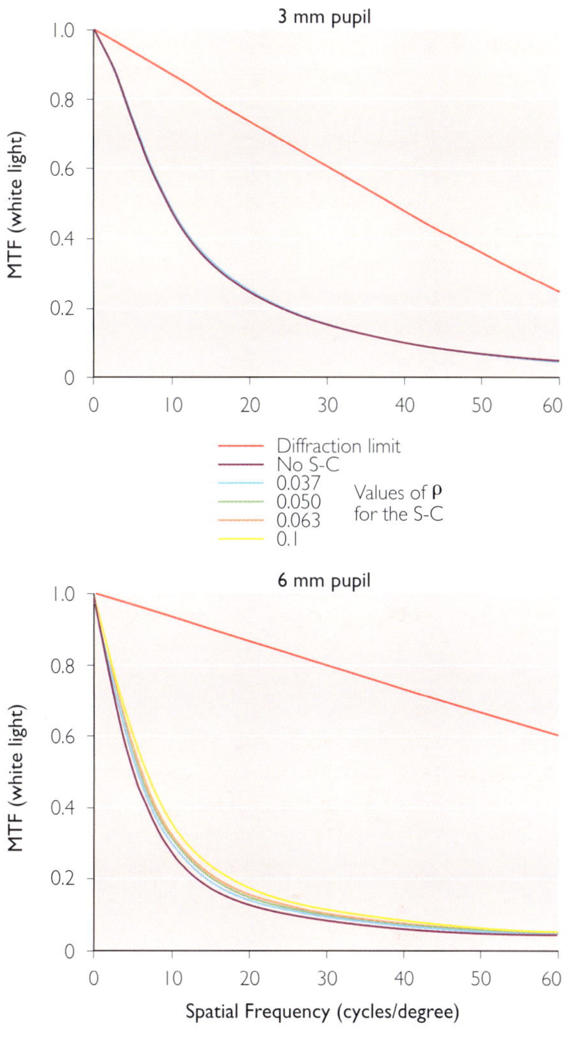

Figure 2.25 **The effect of the Stiles–Crawford effect on image quality. Modulation transfer is plotted as a function of spatial frequency for 3 and 6 mm pupils. MTFs were calculated for ρ values ranging from 0 to 0.1. A ρ of 0 represents no SCI. A ρ of 0.05 is a typical value, while a ρ of 0.1 represents a very pronounced SCI.**

Directional sensitivity tailors the effective pupils for rod and cone vision to their different functions. Rods need to collect photons from the entire pupil in order to maximize sensitivity, a task that would be hindered by a smaller effective pupil. Cones, on the other hand, presumably operate better with a smaller effective pupil that can reject the most oblique photons that result from retinal scattering. This allows them to operate with a higher spatial resolution and a better signal to noise ratio. Thus, differences in directional sensitivity allow the rods and cones operating together under mesopic conditions to have different effective pupil sizes that are better matched to the different roles they play.

2.5.4.5 The Stiles–Crawford effect of the second kind

In addition to changes in the efficiency with which photons are captured as a function of angle of incidence, there is also a shift in the hue and saturation of monochromatic lights (Stiles, 1937; Hansen, 1946). This is called the Stiles–Crawford effect of the second kind (SCII). This hue shift is of the order of a few nanometers with the direction depending on wavelength, as shown in Figure 2.26 (Enoch and Stiles, 1961). At both short and long wavelengths, the hue of the oblique beam shifts towards the hue of longer wavelengths, while at mid-wavelengths, the hue of the oblique beam shifts towards the hue of shorter wavelengths. In addition, wavelengths longer than about 515 nm appear slightly desaturated when they arrive at the retina obliquely, while wavelengths between 515 and 480 nm appear supersaturated. The size of the shift and the wavelengths at which it reverses direction vary substantially from observer to observer.

According to the laws of color matching (Grassman, 1853; Krantz, 1975), the hue of a stimulus depends on the relative numbers of

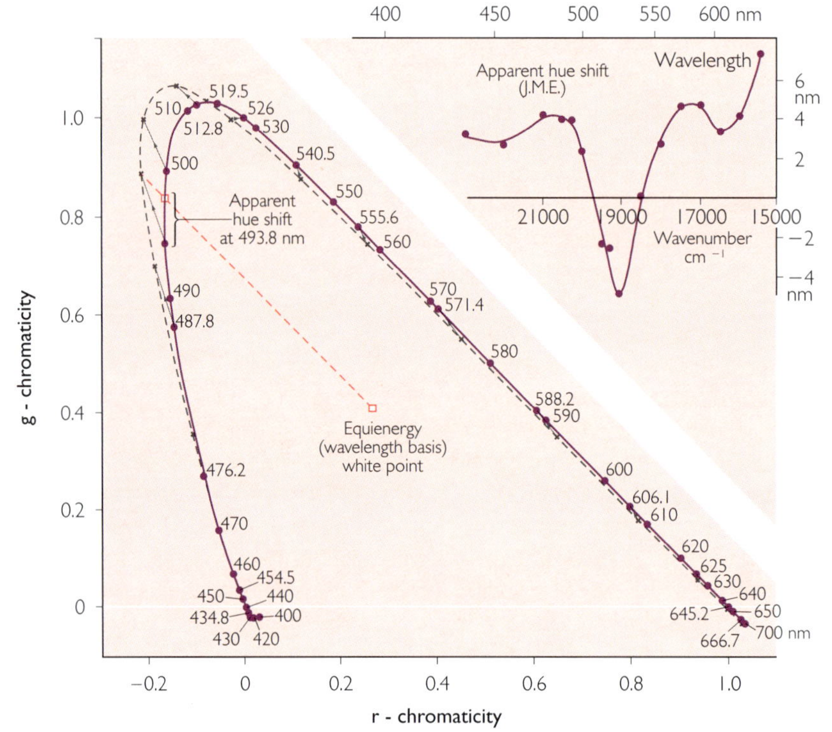

Figure 2.26 **The Stiles–Crawford effect of the second kind (SCII). The top right graph shows the hue shift in nanometers as a function of wavelength. The chromaticity diagram shows the shift in saturation. The chromaticity of lights entering the center of the pupil is shown as a solid line. The chromaticity of lights entering the edge of the pupil and making a 10° angle of incidence with the retina is shown by the dotted line. (From Enoch and Stiles, 1961.)**

photopigment absorptions in the three classes of cones. Therefore, an explanation of the SCII would seem to require a change in the relative numbers of absorptions as a function of angle of incidence. The explanation must be based on factors no more central than photopigment absorption itself. There are two ways of changing the relative numbers of absorptions as a function of the angle of incidence. The first is by changing the spectral sensitivities of the photopigments. The second is by changing the relative amounts of light reaching the photopigment of the different cone types. The mechanisms invoked to implement these possibilities are self-screening and photoreceptor directional sensitivity.

Self-screening is a way to change the spectral sensitivities of existing photopigments. At the moderate light levels of most SC experiments, the concentration of photopigment remains reasonably constant. Therefore, pigment density changes must be due to changes in the effective path length of light passing through the photopigment. Waveguide theory predicts that increasing the angle of incidence of the illumination shortens the average pathlength through the photopigment, since an increasing fraction of photons will leak out of the outer segment before they travel its entire length. Thus, at oblique incidence, an average photon will encounter fewer photopigment molecules and self-screening will cause the spectral sensitivity function to be narrower than at normal incidence.

If the directional sensitivities of the cone types differ, due to small but systematic differences in refractive index or morphology, then the relative numbers of photons captured and funneled into photopigment might change as a function of angle of incidence, altering the relative numbers of photon absorptions in the three cone types.

In an effort to understand the SCII, self-screening and waveguide effects have been invoked separately and in combination (for a review see Alpern, 1986). There has even been one attempt to explain the SCII effect on the basis of prereceptoral factors alone (Weale, 1981). To a first approximation, self-screening can explain most of the hue shift, although Alpern suggests that the breakdown in color matches between normally incident primaries and obliquely incident test fields when intensity is scaled may require additional explanation.

2.6 PHOTORECEPTOR TOPOGRAPHY AND SAMPLING

In the previous section, we discussed the optical and morphological characteristics that shape the information processing capacity of individual photoreceptors. However, photoreceptors do not work in isolation. Rather, they are organized into mosaics that tile the retina and convert the continuous distribution of light in the retinal image into a set of discrete samples. We will now expand our discussion to include a description of the topographic organization of these photoreceptor mosaics and consider how mosaic topography affects the quality of the sampled representation of the retinal image. We will begin by describing the topographic features and visual implications of the photoreceptor mosaic as a whole. The division of the cone mosaic into interleaved short (S), middle (M), and long (L) wavelength sensitive cone submosaics and the implications of this for color vision will follow.

2.6.1 PHOTORECEPTOR TOPOGRAPHY OF THE MOSAIC AS A WHOLE

2.6.1.1 Cone topography

Color and spatial vision at high light levels is subserved by 4–5 million cones (Osterberg, 1935; Curcio *et al.*, 1990) that are distributed unevenly across the retina. Perhaps the most striking feature of photoreceptor topography is the radial symmetry with which both rods and cones are distributed around the fovea. Superimposed on the basic radial pattern, however, are asymmetries. The first is a 'cone streak' (Figure 2.27A) reminiscent of the visual streak found in the retinas of some lower vertebrates. This streak extends along the horizontal meridian from midtemporal retina to the nasal periphery and includes the fovea which is specialized for high spatial acuity. Cone density peaks at an

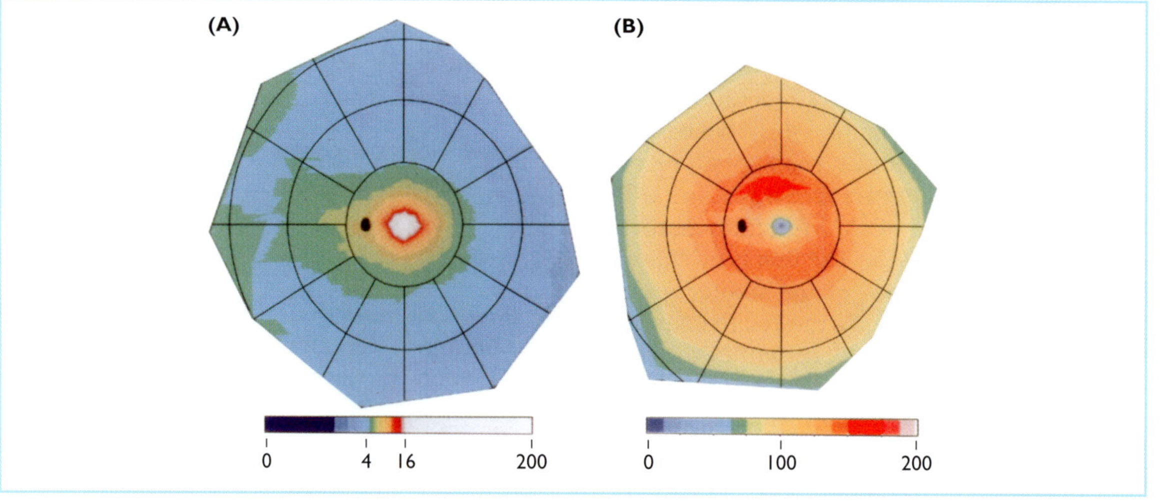

Figure 2.27 **Color topographic maps of cone (A) and rod (B) numerical density. The density scale, shown under each map, is photoreceptors/mm² × 1000. Blue represents low densities and red represents high densities. In A, areas in white exceed 16 000 photoreceptors/mm². The rings are spaced at intervals of about 20°. The fovea is at the center of the inner ring. Nasal and temporal retina are to the left and right of the fovea respectively. (From Curcio *et al.*, 1990. Copyright © 1990 *Journal of Comparative Neurology*. Reprinted by permission of Wiley-Liss, Inc., a subsidiary of John Wiley & Sons, Inc.)**

average of 200 000 cones/mm² at the center of the fovea, then falls sharply to one half maximum at <0.2° of eccentricity, to one-tenth maximum at 1° of eccentricity and to 5000 cones/mm² or less near the edge of the retina (Figure 2.28). Cone distribution is also nasotemporally asymmetric. Overall, there are about 25% more cones in nasal than temporal retina. This asymmetry is not apparent near the fovea, but becomes more pronounced with increasing eccentricity.

Foveal cones are set in a lattice which has an approximately triangular packing arrangement (see Figure 2.19B). The mean center to center spacing of the central-most cones has been measured anatomically at 2.24 μm (27' of arc) and interferometrically (see below) in the living human eye at 2.7 μm (32' of arc) (Williams, 1988). The 60° symmetry of the triangular lattice was apparent in both types of measurements. Triangular packing allows the foveal cones to maximize the proportion of retinal surface covered with photoreceptor apertures while retaining their round shape. Even so, in the macaque monkey, anatomical measurements indicate that ~15% of the retinal surface is space between cone inner segments (Packer *et al.*, 1989). In fact, the resulting 15% loss of photons between cones is probably a lower limit since the cone aperture measured psychophysically is smaller yet, predicting larger spaces between cones. Further evidence that photons do, in fact, fall between cones comes from images of the cone mosaic made after neutralizing the optical aberrations of the eye (see below, Figure 2.36). In the original images, cones are bright spots separated by dark regions. Even in the presence of residual optical blurring that redistributes photons from the bright spots into the dark areas, photons still disappear into the spaces between cones. Not all of the photons that fall between photoreceptors are lost to vision, however, since some pass through the walls of neighboring outer segments into photopigment or pass through the walls of neighboring inner segments at an angle shallow enough to be recaptured (Chen and Makous, 1989).

2.6.1.2 Rod topography

Interspersed around the cones of the human retina are about 90 million rods (Osterberg, 1935; Curcio *et al.*, 1990) which subserve vision at low light levels (see Figure 2.19D). The region of highest rod density is in a 'rod ring' around the fovea at an eccentricity of about 12° (3.6 mm) (Figure 2.27B). In the average eye, the peak rod density of 180 000 rods/mm² occurs on the rod ring in superior retina just to the nasal side of the fovea. Rods are absent at the center of the human fovea and sparse at the center of the monkey fovea (Packer *et al.*, 1989). The absence of foveal rods can be demonstrated by noting that a dim spot of light in a dark room is more easily detected a few degrees away from the center of fixation where rod density is high. In the human retina, the diameter of the rod-free zone, defined to be the region with fewer than 1000 rods/mm^2 averages 1.25° (0.375 mm). At the edge of the retina, rod density declines to 40–60 thousand rods/mm^2. Rod density along the horizontal meridians as a function of eccentricity is plotted in Figure 2.28(C).

Because the rod sampling rate is so high, especially in peripheral vision, and their signals are immediately pooled, the discrete nature of the rod mosaic is not very important for spatial vision. However, the rod system operates at low light levels where every photon counts. Therefore, the tight packing of the rods minimizes the intervening spaces into which photons could be lost. We have estimated the proportion of photons lost by measuring the proportion of light absorbed in a patch of rod-dominated peripheral monkey retina similar to that shown in Figure 2.21. The proportion of light absorbed across the whole patch was calculated by taking the ratio of the light transmitted before and after bleaching the photopigment and averaging across all of the pixels in the image. The axial absorptance of individual rods was estimated by averaging only the pixels corresponding to rod outer segment tips. The ratio of the proportion of incident photons absorbed by a patch of retina and the axial absorptance of the individual rods in that patch suggests that at least 30% of the photons incident on peripheral retina are lost between the rods.

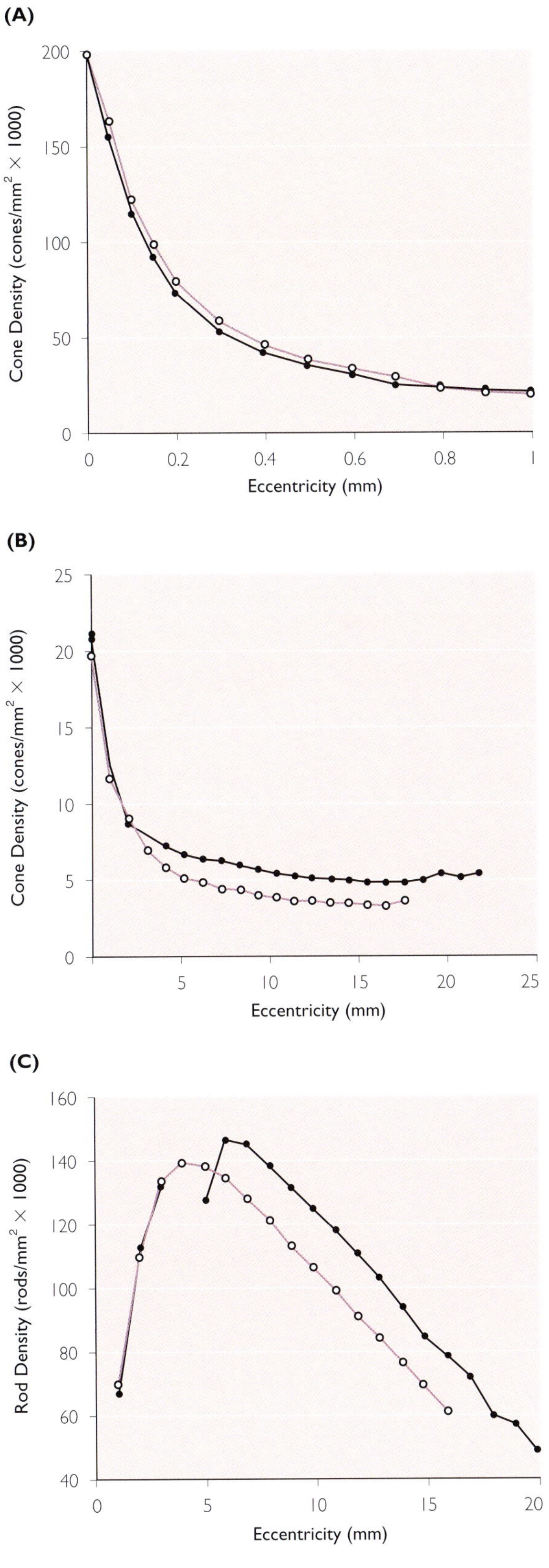

Figure 2.28 **Photoreceptor density along the horizontal meridian of the human retina. Filled symbols are nasal retina. Open symbols are temporal retina. (A) Cone density (cones × 1000/mm^2) from the foveal center to 1 mm of eccentricity. (B) Cone density (cones × 1000/mm^2) from 1 to 22 mm of eccentricity. (C) Rod density (rods × 1000/mm^2). In central retina, the conversion factor 0.29 mm/degree will convert retinal eccentricity in millimeters to retinal eccentricity in visual degrees. (From Curcio et al., 1990. Copyright © 1990 *Journal of Comparative Neurology*. Reprinted by permission of Wiley-Liss, Inc., a subsidiary of John Wiley & Sons, Inc.)**

2.6.2 PHOTOMETRIC QUANTUM EFFICIENCY

Ideally, all of the photons incident on the cornea would be transduced into visual signals. In fact, however, only a small proportion of the incident photons are visually effective. There are several sources of photon loss in the ocular media. Some photons are absorbed by pigments in the anterior optics of the eye, others fall uselessly between the photoreceptors, and yet others pass through the photopigment without isomerizing a pigment molecule. In order to estimate the combined effects of all the sources of light loss, it is possible to calculate the proportion of quanta incident on the cornea that actually isomerizes a photopigment molecule and is transduced into a neural signal. This proportion represents the optical efficiency of the visual system and is called photometric quantum efficiency (Pelli, 1990).

Photometric quantum efficiency has traditionally been estimated from the product of (1) the fraction of photons incident on the cornea that are transmitted by the ocular media, (2) the fraction of photons arriving at the retina that are captured by photoreceptors, (3) the fraction of captured photons that are absorbed by photopigment, and (4) the fraction of absorbed photons that isomerize photopigment molecules (0.67; Dartnall, 1968). Estimates of photometric quantum efficiency at absolute threshold based on the product of the above factors range between 11% and 48% in rod-dominated peripheral retina (Sharpe, 1990). We made a more direct measurement of the proportion of incident light actually absorbed by the retina in an attempt to eliminate some of the uncertainties inherent in estimating the optical properties of individual photoreceptors. Photometric quantum efficiency was ~12%, near the lower end of the range of the earlier estimates. Thus, the combined losses in the anterior optics and photoreceptor mosaic are no less than 50% and probably closer to 90%.

If photometric quantum efficiency at absolute threshold were the same as the overall quantum efficiency of vision at absolute threshold, then all of the information loss in the visual system could be attributed to the anterior optics and the photoreceptor mosaic. However, all measurements of the overall quantum efficiency of vision at absolute threshold are less than 10% (Barlow, 1977; Hallett, 1987; Pelli, 1990). Therefore, photometric quantum efficiency is higher than the overall quantum efficiency of vision which shows that neural processing further degrades the visual signal over and above the losses incurred in the anterior optics and the retina. Assuming an overall quantum efficiency of 10% at absolute threshold and a photometric quantum efficiency of 12%, the efficiency with which the neural visual system can process the visual information and detect the stimulus can be as high as 80%. In other words, the physical limit to performance is dominated by the quantal nature of light. However, if the stimulus is made larger or of longer duration or presented on a background, overall quantum efficiency may drop by several orders of magnitude while photometric quantum efficiency remains about the same, implying that neural efficiency must also drop by several orders of magnitude. In short, under most conditions, the physical limit to performance is dominated not by the quantum nature of light but by inefficiency in neural processing.

2.6.3 SAMPLING THEORY

The fidelity with which the nervous system can represent the retinal image depends critically on the sampling characteristics of the photoreceptor mosaic. According to the sampling theorem (Shannon, 1949), to reconstruct a one-dimensional signal from a set of samples, the sampling rate must be equal to or greater than twice the highest frequency in the signal. Applying this theorem to the cone mosaic, with a given spacing between receptors, the highest spatial frequency that is adequately sampled, known as the Nyquist limit, is half the sampling frequency of the mosaic. Of course the cone mosaic is a two-dimensional sampling array, for which there is a corresponding two-dimensional sampling theorem (Pettersen and Middleton, 1962). In fact, it is not straightforward to extrapolate from the one-dimensional case illustrated here to the two-dimensional sampling performed by the cone mosaic because of the many ways in which the spatial frequency response plane can be tiled by frequency domains. Nevertheless, in the interests of brevity, we will adopt the basic intuitions derived from the one-dimensional case.

Figure 2.29 shows that when a row of cones samples a sine wave, there is no way to tell whether the samples are from a low frequency being sampled by an adequate number of photoreceptors or from a higher frequency that is being undersampled. When a retinal image is undersampled by the photoreceptor mosaic, those spatial frequencies above the Nyquist limit are misinterpreted by the visual system as low frequencies called aliases. These aliases are impossible to distinguish from naturally occurring low spatial frequencies and therefore distort the sampled representation of the retinal image.

The product of the spatial frequency spectrum of a visual scene and the modulation transfer function of the eye's optics determine the spatial frequency spectrum of the retinal image. The spatial frequency spectra of natural visual scenes vary but generally have amplitudes that decline as the inverse of spatial frequency (Field, 1987). This fact by itself helps the visual system avoid aliasing. Figure 2.30 shows the relationship between the eye's modulation transfer function for various pupil sizes and the foveal cone Nyquist limit. It is only where the modulation transfer function exceeds the Nyquist limit that aliasing could arise. The figure shows that, under normal viewing conditions, human foveal vision is quite well protected from the effects of aliasing because the optics of the eye filter out those spatial frequencies above ~60 cycles/degree that exceed the Nyquist limit of the foveal cone mosaic. This relationship between optics and mosaic is often described as one in which they are matched, first articulated by Helmholtz (1896). While this is approximately true for the fovea, we will see later that the optics are substantially superior to the grain of the peripheral mosaic and especially that of subsequent neural sampling arrays en route to the brain. Indeed, even in foveal vision, experiments in which adaptive optics (see below) are used to improve the optics of the normal eye (Liang *et al.*, 1997; Yoon and Williams, 2002) indicate that vision can be improved somewhat by improving the optics, without incurring obvious negative consequences of aliasing.

An especially effective way to investigate aliasing is with the use of laser interferometry, which bypasses the blurring effects of the eye's optics (Williams, 1985). Under these conditions, aliasing can be exploited to study the topography of the photoreceptor mosaic in the living human eye (Williams, 1988). When two beams from a single laser overlap, they interfere with each other, producing an interference fringe with a sinusoidal luminance profile whose spatial frequency depends on beam separation. By shining the two beams through the pupil of the eye, a

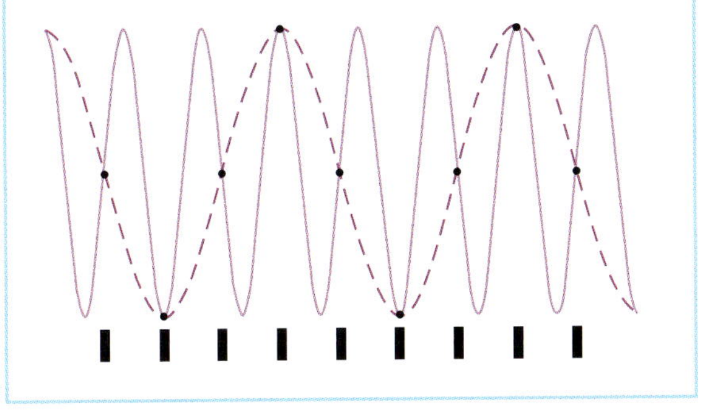

Figure 2.29 **Aliasing when a sine wave is sampled by a one-dimensional array of photoreceptors (black cylinders at the bottom). It is impossible to tell whether the photoreceptor responses are the result of sampling each cycle of a low frequency (dashed curve) with two photoreceptors per cycle or the result of sampling a high frequency (solid curve) with a fewer number of samples per cycle.**

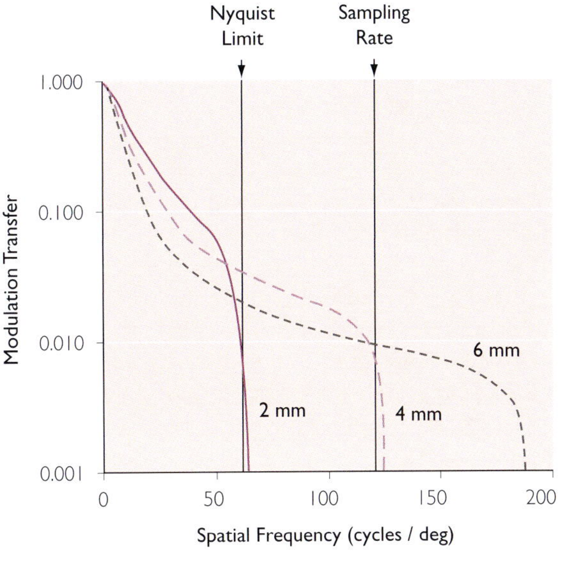

Figure 2.30 **The relationship between the eye's modulation transfer in white light and foveal cone sampling. Modulation transfer as a function of spatial frequency in cycles/degree is shown for 2, 4, and 6 mm pupils. Only where the MTF exceeds the foveal cone Nyquist limit will aliasing occur.**

sinusoidal grating is formed on the retina. Because the beams are largely unaffected by the optics, the spatial frequency of the high contrast interference fringe is limited only by the size of the pupil. In the case of an 8 mm pupil, the cutoff exceeds 200 cycles/degree. Under these conditions, many observers report seeing a low frequency moiré pattern not present in the original image (Byram, 1944, Campbell and Green, 1965; Williams, 1985). These studies support earlier observations by Bergmann (1858), who reported seeing aliasing-like effects when viewing gratings normally, without the benefit of interferometry.

A highly regular array of sampling elements produces aliases that are also highly regular, while aliasing by a disordered array takes the form of noise. In the case of the foveal cones, the packing geometry is regular enough to produce moiré patterns that look like zebra stripes. In some observers, the zebra stripes are clear enough to be sketched (Figure 2.31). The spacing of the photoreceptors can then be measured by noting the spatial frequency at which the zebra stripes have the coarsest appearance. This occurs when fringe spacing is matched to the spacing of the rows of the cone mosaic. In the human fovea, the spatial frequency at which the zebra stripes appear coarsest corresponds to twice the cone Nyquist frequency or about 120 cycles/degree. In a few observers, the foveal cone mosaic has enough regularity to exhibit the rotational symmetry inherent in a triangular lattice. In these observers, zebra stripe coarseness varies as a function of the orientation of the interference fringe relative to the cone mosaic, being greatest every 60° when the bars of the fringe align with the rows of photoreceptors.

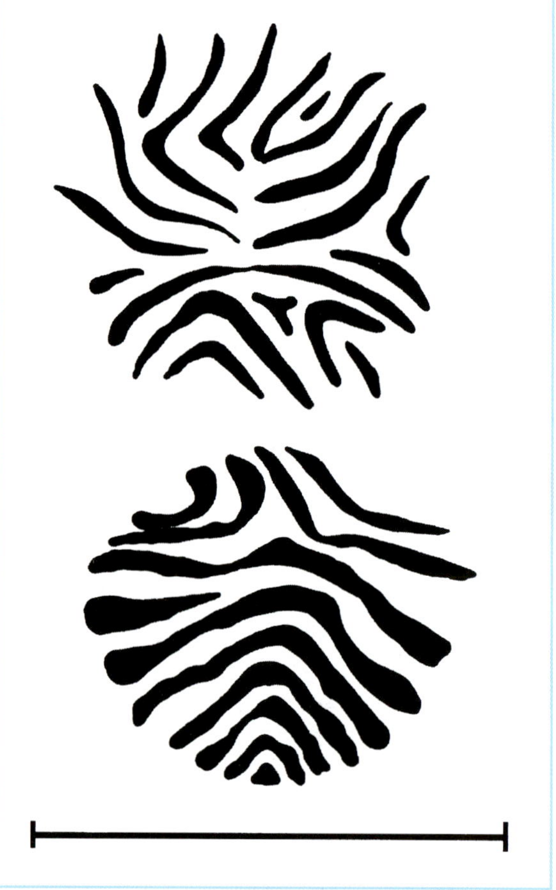

Figure 2.31 **A sketch of the moiré patterns seen by two observers while viewing a high contrast 120 cycles/degree interference fringe. The scale bar represents 1 degree of visual angle. (From Williams, 1985.)**

2.6.4 OFF-AXIS IMAGE QUALITY AND RETINAL SAMPLING

Under normal viewing conditions, foveal vision is protected from aliasing by optical filtering. However, Figure 2.32 shows that the same is not true for peripheral vision because optical bandwidth declines only slowly with increasing eccentricity (Jennings and Charman, 1981; Navarro *et al.*, 1993; Williams *et al.*, 1996) while the center to center spacing of the cones increases rapidly. At just a few degrees of retinal eccentricity, the Nyquist limit of the cone mosaic (dashed line) drops below the optical cutoff (filled symbols). We have used as an estimate of the optical cutoff, the spatial frequency at which the modulation transfer function drops to 0.10, using the data of Williams *et al.* (1996) for a 3 mm pupil. Energy at spatial frequencies above the Nyquist limit but below the optical cutoff can then produce detectable aliasing under normal viewing conditions (Smith and Cass, 1987; Thibos *et al.*, 1987; Anderson and Hess, 1990; Galvin and Williams, 1992; Artal *et al.*, 1995; Thibos *et al.*, 1996).

The parvocellular ganglion cell mosaic, which subserves our detailed spatial vision, also samples

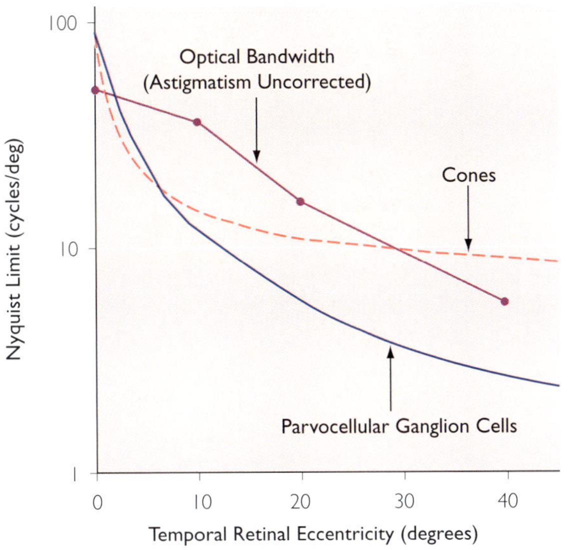

Figure 2.32 The Nyquist limit of the cone and parvocellular ganglion cell mosaics (Curcio *et al.*, 1990; Curcio and Allen, 1990) as a function of retinal eccentricity in degrees. Also plotted is the optical bandwidth as a function of eccentricity from Williams *et al.* (1996: Fig. 6a). The optical bandwidth is taken as the spatial frequency at which modulation transfer has dropped to 0.10. Pupil size was 3 mm and the modulation transfer function was obtained when the eye was focused at the circle of least confusion, without correction for astigmatism. The sampling density of the mosaics falls off much more quickly than the bandwidth of the optics, setting up the possibility of aliasing at eccentricities exceeding a few degrees.

the retinal image by collecting signals from the cones that make up its receptive fields. The sampling characteristics of the parvocellular ganglion cell mosaic can be estimated from ganglion cell density (Curcio and Allen, 1990) which declines much more rapidly with retinal eccentricity than that of the cone mosaic. This makes the peripheral retina even more susceptible to ganglion cell aliasing than to cone aliasing. Figure 2.32 shows that the Nyquist limit of the parvocellular ganglion cell mosaic (solid line) crosses the optical cutoff at about 2° of eccentricity. At eccentricities exceeding 5°, there is energy in the retinal image at spatial frequencies above the Nyquist limits of both the cone and parvocellular ganglion cell mosaics (Williams *et al.*, 1996).

In spite of these sampling mismatches, peripheral aliasing is not a particularly troubling phenomenon. There are several possible reasons for this. First, although peripheral aliasing can be detected in the laboratory, its salience depends quite strongly on the optical quality of the eye.

Aberrations of the peripheral optics such as oblique astigmatism do reduce the power of those spatial frequencies that would otherwise alias. Additionally, disorder in the cone and ganglion cell sampling arrays (Yellott, 1982, 1983), lateral chromatic aberration (Thibos, 1987), defocus caused by accommodative lag, and the relative lack of high spatial frequencies in natural scenes (Field, 1987; Galvin and Williams, 1992) all combine to minimize the effects of peripheral aliasing on visual experience. In fact, Snyder *et al.* (1986) argue convincingly that evolution should drive the cutoff of the eye's optics to frequencies higher than the Nyquist limit. This is because the resulting improvement in image contrast at spatial frequencies below the Nyquist limit more than offsets the deleterious effects of any aliasing of spatial frequencies above the Nyquist limit. Along similar lines, it is at least theoretically possible that functional coupling through the gap junctions known to interconnect cones could be used by the visual system to improve sensitivity to lower spatial frequencies without significantly reducing visual resolution or increasing the deleterious effects of aliasing (Hsu *et al.*, 2000).

2.6.5 S CONE TOPOGRAPHY

Up to this point, we have evaluated the sampling characteristics of the cone mosaic as a whole. This is reasonable when considering the effects of cone sampling on luminance tasks since the spectral sensitivities of the L and M cones, which together subserve luminance vision and comprise more than 90% of all retinal cones, overlap extensively. As far as detailed form vision is concerned, to a first approximation, the L and M cone submosaics operate as a single dense mosaic. Of course this isn't strictly true. For one thing, there are gaps in the L/M cone mosaic caused by S cones. Moreover, the difference in the L and M cone spectra makes the mosaic susceptible to chromatic aliasing. Chromatic aliasing can occur in the retina because only a single type of photoreceptor samples the retinal image at any given location (see Figure 2.19 above). This means that at a local spatial scale, the retina is color blind. This is unlike color film which samples each location in the image with three emulsions, each of which is sensitive to a different part of the visible spectrum. The L, M, and S cones submosaics are interleaved with each other so that the sampling density of each submosaic is necessarily lower than the sampling density of the mosaic as a whole. Chromatic aliasing, therefore, can arise at lower spatial frequencies than the Nyquist limit for the mosaic as a whole.

The sampling characteristics of the S cone submosaic provide a useful way to introduce the problem of chromatic aliasing because S cones sample the retinal image so sparsely. S cones have morphological, histological and immunocytochemical differences that allow them to be distinguished from L and M cones and labeled in situ (deMonasterio *et al.*, 1981, 1985; Ahnelt *et al.*, 1987; Wikler and Rakic, 1990; Curcio *et al.*, 1991). Figure 2.33(A) shows a patch of macaque monkey retina stained with a Procion dye that selectively labels S cones. The S cone distribution has also been studied psychophysically in the living human eye (Williams *et al.*, 1981; Williams and Collier, 1983).

S cones are absent at the center of the fovea at eccentricities less than 50 μm (10' of arc), reach a peak numerical density of about 2000 cones/mm^2 at an eccentricity of 100–300 μm (20–60') and then gradually decline in density with increasing eccentricity (Figure 2.33B). At the eccentricity of peak S cone density, center to center spacing averages about 22 μm (4'), increasing in the periphery to 40 μm (8') or more. Measured anatomically (Curcio *et al.*, 1991), the S cones account for about 7% of all cones and are sparsely distributed in peripheral retina. Individual S cones tend to be more evenly spaced across the retina than would be expected from a random distribution in the macaque monkey, though they are packed in a less orderly fashion in human retina (Bumsted *et al.*, 1996; Roorda and Williams, 1999). There also is apparently a species difference in the S cone distribution at the foveal center, with the human usually showing a region on the order of 20' of arc in diameter that is devoid of S cones. This S cone-free area is not so apparent in the monkey.

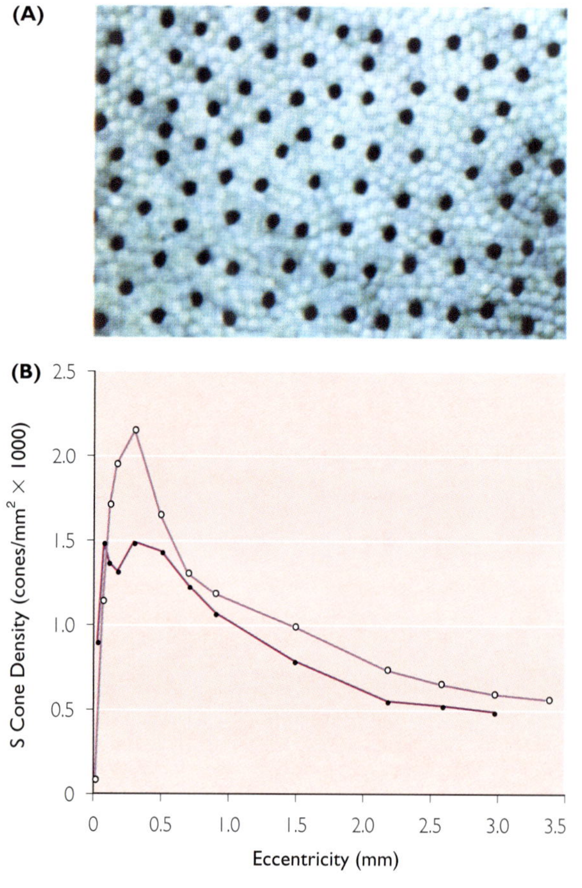

Figure 2.33 The S cone mosaic of the macaque monkey retina. (A) The S cones (dark profiles) have been stained with a Procion dye (from deMonasterio *et al.*, 1981). (B) The S cone numerical density profile as a function of eccentricity along the horizontal meridian. Filled symbols are nasal retina. Open symbols are temporal retina. In central retina, the conversion factor 0.29 mm/degree will convert retinal eccentricity in millimeters to retinal eccentricity in visual degrees. (From Curcio *et al.*, 1991. Copyright © 1991 *Journal of Comparative Neurology*. Reprinted by permission of Wiley-Liss, Inc., a subsidiary of John Wiley & Sons, Inc.).

2.6.6 IMPLICATIONS OF S CONE SAMPLING

Because the sampling density of the S cone submosaic is lower than the density of the mosaic as a whole, spatial resolution under conditions in which it operates independently must be lower than the spatial resolution of the composite mosaic. It is possible to create such isolating conditions by superimposing a violet grating on a bright, long wavelength background that suppresses the sensitivity of the L and M cones to the grating. Under these conditions, most psychophysical data suggest that S cone acuity is 10–15 cycles/degree, somewhat higher than the 7 cycles/degree predicted by anatomical measurements (Stromeyer *et al.*, 1978). Thus, the S cones are sparse enough that their resolution is ¼ to ⅙ that of the luminance mechanism fed by L and M cones.

In situations where the S cone mechanism detects contrast independently, its submosaic ought to produce an alias at spatial frequencies lower than those required to produce aliasing for the mosaic as a whole. The S cone submosaic has a Nyquist limit much lower than the optical cutoff of 60 cycles/degree. Therefore, under S cone isolating conditions, there is a substantial band of spatial frequencies that would be undersampled and subject to aliasing. Williams and Collier (1983) demonstrated that a violet grating on a yellow adapting background looks like a grating up to a spatial frequency of 10–15 cycles/degree. However, at spatial frequencies beyond the resolution limit and up to 20 to 35 cycles/degree, the grating can still be distinguished from a uniform background. In this frequency range, the grating looks like two-dimensional spatial noise, consistent with aliasing by an irregular S cone submosaic. Brewster's colors (see below) are another manifestation of S cone aliasing (Williams *et al.*, 1991). However, the mismatch between the S cone sampling rate and the highest spatial frequencies in the retinal image is reduced by chromatic aberration. Chromatic aberration is especially effective at blurring the short wavelengths to which the S cones are most sensitive. Figure 2.34 shows the effect of chromatic aberration on the modulation transfer for each of the three cone types. Contrast loss is much larger for the S cones. For a 3 mm pupil, modulation transfer is reduced to 10% at the Nyquist frequency of the S cone submosaic which is represented by the vertical line at a spatial frequency of 10 cycles/degree. This effect gets larger as pupil size increases and the larger off-axis aberrations come into play. For a 6 mm pupil, modulation transfer is reduced to only ~5% at the Nyquist frequency of the S cone submosaic. While our calculations suggest that chromatic

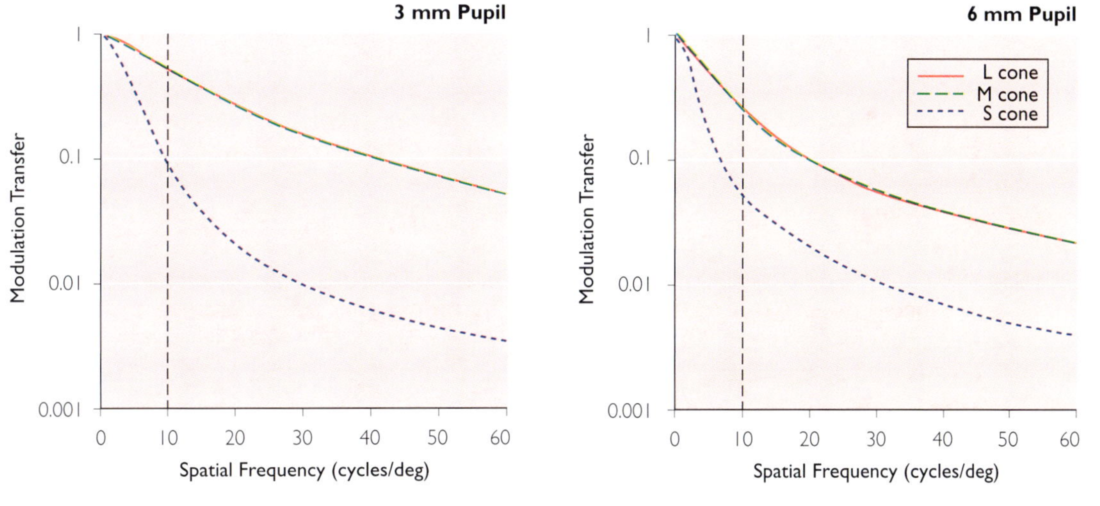

Figure 2.34 The calculated modulation transfer function for a white light stimulus at pupil sizes of 3 and 6 mm based on the wave aberrations of 14 normal eyes. The MTFs were calculated for each of the three cone classes using the full amount of astigmatism and adjusting focus for each subject to optimize M and L cone MTFs at 16 cycles/deg in white light, assuming this is approximately what an accommodating subject would do. This value of defocus was then used to compute the S cone MTF. Axial but not transverse chromatic aberration was included in the calculation. To bring the S cone MTF into register with the L and M cone MTFs requires a rescaling of spatial frequency by a factor of about 3 for a 6 mm pupil and a factor of 4 for a 3 mm pupil. The vertical line at 10 cycles/deg is taken to be the approximate Nyquist limit of the S cone mosaic, which is about 6 times lower than the Nyquist limit for the M/L cone mosaic. Thus the optics of the eye, once chromatic aberration is included, protect the S cone mosaic from aliasing, though not quite as effectively as they do the M and L cones. (Courtesy Geun-Young Yoon.)

aberration protects the S cone mosaic from aliasing, the issue is not without controversy (McLellan *et al.*, 2002).

Chromatic aberration and the properties of natural scenes are apparently sufficient to prevent S cone submosaic aliasing from intruding in our daily visual experience. It is especially striking that the absence of S cones from the central 20' of arc of the fovea in most humans is not subjectively obvious to us since it renders us tritanopic within the most acute portion of our visual field (Williams *et al.*, 1981). The brain must be equipped with sophisticated interpolation circuitry capable of hiding this gaping chromatic blind spot from us (Brainard and Williams, 1993).

2.6.7 L AND M CONE TOPOGRAPHY

For the photoreceptor mosaic as a whole, rods and cones are easily localized and can be distinguished on the basis of their morphology. In the case of the S cone submosaic, there are sufficient histological and immunocytochemical differences to allow differential staining. However, there are no known morphological differences between the L and M cones on which to base a discrimination. It is only recently that their topography has been revealed.

Several methods have provided information about the relative numbers of L and M cones in the mosaic, including microspectrophotometry (MSP), photopigment transmittance imaging, suction electrode recording, genetic analysis, and psychophysics (see Packer *et al.*, 1996 for important references). Analysis of the mRNA content of the retina has been quite useful in determining the relative numbers of L and M cones in patches of retina as well as classifying individual cones (Hagstrom *et al.*, 2000). The cones contain the L and M photopigment genes on their X chromosomes. When photopigment is manufactured by the cone, messenger RNA (mRNA) carries the instructions from the genes in the nucleus to the site where the photopigment is assembled. Each cone expresses only a single type of photopigment. In addition, each cone apparently makes about the same amount of mRNA. Therefore, a measurement of the relative amounts of L and M mRNA gives an estimate of the relative numbers of L and M cones. Very sensitive techniques have been developed for measuring the type of mRNA produced in a single cone or the relative amounts of mRNA produced in a patch of retina. Results using this technique show that there are differences in the L/M ratio as a function of retinal location. L cones are more numerous near the edge of the retina than they are near the fovea in humans (Hagstrom *et al.*, 1997). There is also a tendency for higher ratios in temporal retina in the macaque monkey (Deeb *et al.*, 2000).

Even without identifying individual cone types in the mosaic, it is obvious that the L and M cone submosaics cannot be crystalline in their packing geometry. Figures 2.19(B) and (D) show that the composite lattice is not perfectly regular. Therefore, the L and M submosaics must exhibit at least as much spatial disorder as the composite lattice. This disorder is especially large outside the fovea where rods and S cones begin to intrude. In addition to disorder in the physical positions of the cones, the interleaving of the L and M submosaics is far from regular. Mollon and Bowmaker (1992) used axial MSP to distinguish the L and M cones in several small patches of monkey fovea and found that the L and M cone assignment could not be distinguished from that of a random distribution. Packer *et al.* (1996) examined the L and M cone topography of larger patches of peripheral monkey retina using photopigment transmittance imaging, a technique that can classify the L and M cones on the basis of the photopigment they contain. Figure 2.35 is a composite image that shows a patch of peripheral retina. Color has been assigned to the image based on measurements of the photopigment transmittance in the patch. The color was assigned to indicate the appearance of the retina were it possible to view it under the microscope without bleaching all of the photopigment in the process. Viewed under these conditions, the L, M, and S cones have bluish, purplish, and yellowish hues respectively, while rods are reddish. Examples of L cones, M cones, and rods are indicated with arrows. It is obvious even from this small image that the L and M cones are not assigned in a highly ordered way. Analysis of a larger patch of peripheral retina showed a tendency for like-type cones to clump though the sample size was small.

Recently, noninvasive measurements of the positions of L and M cones in the central retina

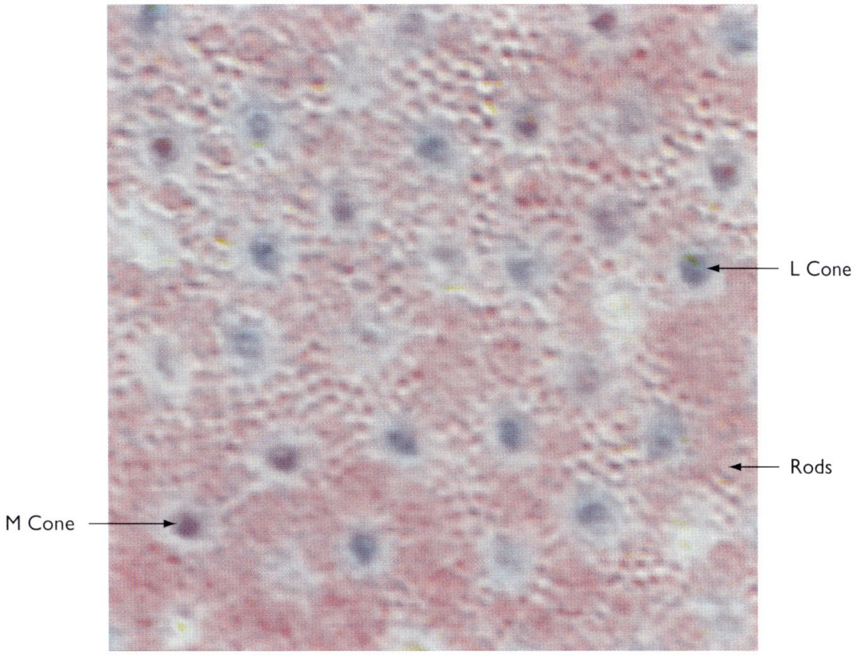

Figure 2.35 A color composite image of a patch of retina rendered to reveal its true colors. The larger sparse cells are cones and the small reddish profiles filling in around them are the rods. Purple colored cells are M cones. Blue colored cells are L cones. Yellowish colored cells are likely to be S cones. This image was created in our laboratory from photopigment transmittance images of a patch of peripheral macaque retina.

of the living human eye have been made by using adaptive optics to neutralize the aberrations of the ocular media (Roorda and Williams, 1999). This allows individual foveal cones to be resolved and, with retinal densitometry, classified on the basis of their photopigment type. Figure 2.36 shows images of the foveal cone mosaic of two human eyes and one macaque eye in which identified cones have been overlaid with a colored dot that represents its photopigment type. The relative number of L and M cones differs greatly between the two eyes. In two patches of retina, one from the nasal and one from the temporal fovea, subject JW had a mean ratio of L to M cones of 3.79 whereas AN had a ratio of 1.15. Subject JW was not selected for this experiment based on any prior knowledge of his color vision. However, AN was selected because previous measurements of his spectral electroretinogram (ERG), a technique for measuring the electrical activity of the retina using external electrodes, had suggested that he was unusually middle-wavelength sensitive, which was confirmed by our imaging observations (Brainard *et al.*, 2000). Though the selection of subjects was not random, the large individual difference between the two is consistent with the variability found using psychophysical methods (Rushton and Baker, 1964; Vimal *et al.*, 1989), spectral ERG (Jacobs and Neitz, 1993; Jacobs and Deegan, 1997; Carrol *et al.*, 2002), microspectrophotometry (Bowmaker and Dartnall, 1980; Dartnall *et al.* 1983), and mRNA analysis (Hagstrom *et al.*, 1997; Yamaguchi *et al.*, 1997).

In short, we now have complete descriptions of the L and M cone topography for a small number of locations in the retinas of a small number of individuals. We do not yet know the extent of individual variability or the extent to which topography may depend on retinal location. The available data suggest that the L to M ratio is quite variable from individual to individual. L and M cones are arranged in a highly disordered manner which is either perfectly random or very close to it. There is no evidence that the L and M submosaics are interleaved in a way that would distribute each cone type evenly across the retina in a regular pattern.

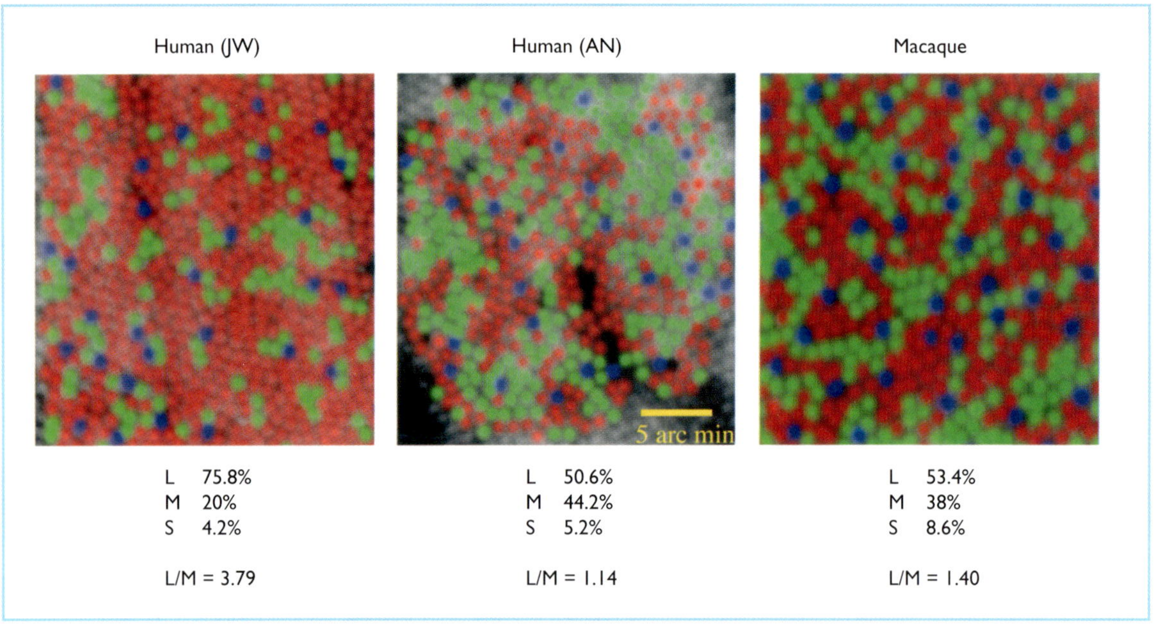

Figure 2.36 Images of living photoreceptor mosaic from two humans and one monkey taken through the optics of the eye. Adaptive optics neutralized the aberrations that would ordinarily prevent the resolution of individual photoreceptors. The red dots overlie the L cones, green dots overlie the M cones and blue dots indicate S cones. Numbers below each image represent the relative percentages of the L, M and S cones as well as the L/M ratio. (Reprinted by permission from *Nature* (Roorda and Williams, 1999). © Copyright 1999, Macmillan Publishers Ltd.)

2.6.8 IMPLICATIONS OF L AND M CONE SAMPLING

2.6.8.1 Photopic luminosity and color appearance

The large individual differences in L to M cone ratio show that evolution has not driven all eyes toward some optimum proportion of M and L cones. It is striking how little difference the ratio of L to M makes for color vision, except when the ratio becomes very extreme. Rushton and Baker (1964) provided evidence that variations in the relative amounts of M and L pigments assessed with retinal densitometry were correlated with variations in the shape of the photopic luminosity function measured with flicker photometry. It seems likely that an individual's photopic luminosity function directly reflects L and M cone numerosity. Deeb *et al.* (2000) showed that the weights of cone inputs to H1 cells and parasol ganglion cells in monkey retina depend on the ratio of cone numerosity in the mosaic, assessed with mRNA analysis. Brainard *et al.* (2000) showed that the eye's spectral sensitivity assessed with a flicker ERG method also reflected cone numerosity as measured with the adaptive optics imaging method of Roorda and Williams (1999). All the same, it is worth keeping in mind that these effects are small. Due to the similarity of the M and L cone spectra, the photopic luminosity function changes relatively little with large changes in L to M cone ratio (cf. Jacobs and Deegan, 1997).

Color appearance, at least for low spatial frequencies where aliasing is not an issue, seems to depend rather little if at all on the L to M ratio (Jordan and Mollon, 1993; Miyahara *et al.*, 1998; Neitz *et al.*, 2002). Brainard *et al.* (2000) showed that the wavelength of unique yellow, measured in the same two individuals imaged by Roorda and Williams, differed by less than 2 nm, despite the 3.3-fold difference in L to M cone ratio. The wavelength of unique yellow varies much too little in the population to be consistent with the variation in L and M cone ratio. This suggests that the zero crossing of the red–green opponent mechanism is set by some other factor than cone numerosity. Perhaps, as Pokorny and Smith (1977) proposed, setting the zero point to correspond to the ambient chromaticity of natural scenes would be a more efficient choice for the visual system, since it would minimize the metabolic cost of transmitting variations in redness and greenness.

Neitz *et al.* (2002) have provided compelling evidence for the plasticity of color vision, showing that experience can modify the boundary between red and green.

2.6.8.2 L and M cone resolution

Because the sampling densities of the L and M cone submosaics are lower than the density of the mosaic as a whole, one might expect to find both a reduction in the acuity of the separate L and M cone submosaics as well as evidence for chromatic aliasing, just as we did for the S cone submosaic. However, there is apparently no substantial reduction in acuity observed in studies in which chromatic adaptation was used to isolate either the L or M cone submosaic. There is no measurable difference in contrast sensitivity or acuity when the L and M cones are isolated compared to conditions in which they operate together (cf. Brindley, 1953; Williams, 1991). This is true even when using laser interference fringes to exclude blurring by the optics of the eye. To be sure, resolution will decline when the density of cones in the submosaic becomes sparse enough. The S cone submosaic is a case in point. Nonetheless, relatively large density losses have no obvious effects on grating acuity (Geller *et al.*, 1992). This is almost certainly due to the disordered arrangement of L and M cones which creates small clumps of like-type cones whose spacing is much less than the average spacing of that submosaic. These clumps may be sufficiently large and common to subserve better than expected acuity, especially with extended stimuli such as large patches of grating. Only when one cone class is greatly underrepresented, as in some heterozygous carriers for congenital x-linked protanopia, is resolution clearly affected in cone isolating conditions (Miyahara *et al.*, 1998). Presumably, visual stimuli that are more localized, such as vernier targets, would be better suited to reveal a deficit due to the coarser grain of the separate L and M cone submosaics.

Just as resolution is not much affected when the L and M cone mosaics are isolated, neither are the foveal aliasing effects seen at very high frequencies with interference fringes. Subjects report that the zebra stripe patterns look essentially the same under all conditions of chromatic adaptation, except for changes in apparent contrast. Also, the spatial frequency at which the foveal moiré pattern is coarsest shows little or no change even under the most extreme conditions of chromatic adaptation that can be arranged while still keeping the percept suprathreshold (Williams *et al.*, 1991). In fact, simulations show that the invariant appearance of zebra stripes is actually what you would expect, even if chromatic adaptation is successful at completely desensitizing one submosaic and sparing the other.

Consider a regular lattice, and the same lattice with two thirds of the receptors randomly deleted (Figure 2.37). The complete mosaic corresponds to the condition where the L and M cones both see equal contrasts and can work together. The mosaic with random deletions is meant to simulate the situation when the fringe contrast exceeds threshold for the M cone mosaic alone. When these two lattices sample a grating stimulus whose bars have a spacing near that of the rows of receptors, the moiré patterns are quite similar. Therefore, the similarity of foveal zebra stripe patterns under conditions of extreme chromatic adaptation is consistent with the sampling properties of the separate submosaics.

2.6.8.3 Chromatic aliasing

Nonetheless, the existence of independent L and M submosaics does predict another form of aliasing, similar to that described for the S cone mosaic. Submosaic or chromatic aliasing is a common artifact in imaging systems. The brightly colored moiré patterns that result when a color CCD camera images the fine grooves machined in the gears of Figure 2.38 are a good example. Because the three classes of light sensors in the camera are arranged in regular array the moiré pattern is vividly chromatic.

The visual system, on the other hand, is remarkably resistant to the effects of chromatic aliasing. In those cases in which it can be detected at all, it is subtle and fleeting. One of the earliest reports of chromatic percepts related to the topographic organization of the cone mosaic comes from Holmgren (1884), who noticed that the hue

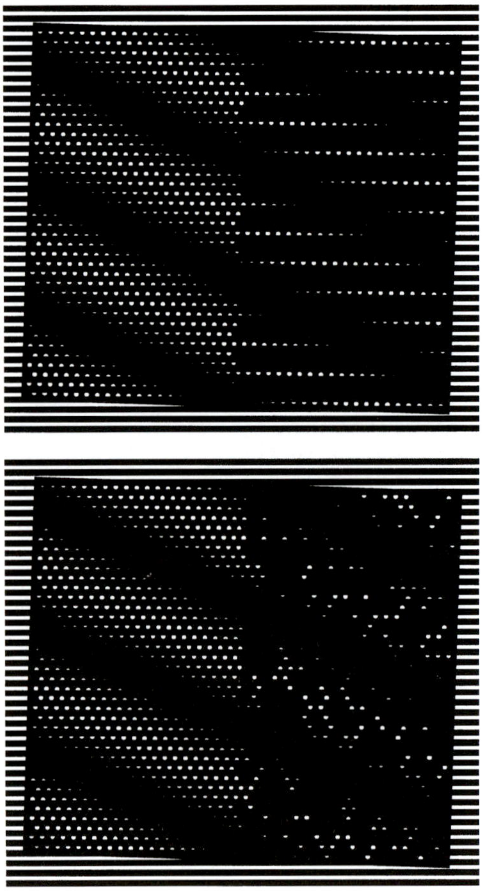

Figure 2.37 **A simulation showing the invariant appearance of zebra stripes in the face of random and regular receptor loss. On the left side of each panel a regular lattice is undersampling a horizontal grating. Because of sampling regularity, the alias is a striped pattern. On the right side of each panel, two thirds of the sampling elements have been deleted. In the top panel the deletions were done in a regular pattern. In the bottom panel, the deletions were random. The aliases look similar in all cases. (After Williams, 1991.)**

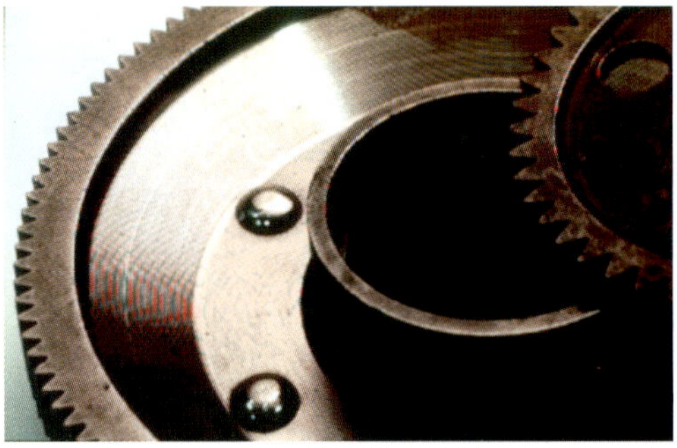

Figure 2.38 **Chromatic aliasing produced by a color camera imaging fine spatial detail in the machined gears that is above the Nyquist limit of its three sensor arrays. Because the sensors in each array are highly ordered, the alias takes the form of a highly chromatic moiré pattern. (From Williams *et al.*, 1993.)**

of stars varied from instant to instant, a fact he attributed to selective excitation of different cone classes as the point of light moved across the mosaic. Psychophysicists have since exploited this observation by using small spots (cf. Krauskopf, 1978; Cicerone and Nerger, 1989; Vimal *et al.*, 1989) to map the organization of the L and M cone submosaics. However, this color percept is never very salient because the optics of the eye blur the point of light across several cones. It has recently become possible to use adaptive optics (Liang, Williams and Miller, 1997) to reduce the diameter of the spots of light to less than the diameter of an individual cone. Under these conditions, the chromatic percept is greatly strengthened.

Many observers report seeing a splotchy pattern of desaturated colors while viewing high contrast patterns such as black and white lines with spatial frequencies between 10 and 40 cycles/degree (Brewster, 1832; Skinner, 1932; Luckiesh and Moss, 1933; Erb and Dallenbach, 1939). Williams *et al.* (1991) have named this effect, Brewster's colors, after the first to have described them.

When subjects are asked to match Brewster's colors with a computer screen displaying a pattern of spatially similar chromatic splotches (Williams *et al.*, 1991), they choose a direction in color space along which only L and M cones are modulated when the eye is in good focus (Figure 2.39A, right). When the eye is defocused by −1 to −1.5 diopters, observers choose a direction along which only the S cones are modulated (Figure 2.39A, left). Apparently, at best subjective focus, short wavelengths are strongly blurred by the optics (Figure 2.39B). Therefore, the L and M cones are strongly modulated while the S cones see a nearly uniform field. When the eye is defocused by −1 to −1.5 diopters, the opposite is true. Therefore, the hue of the Brewster's colors is consistent with the cone types being modulated.

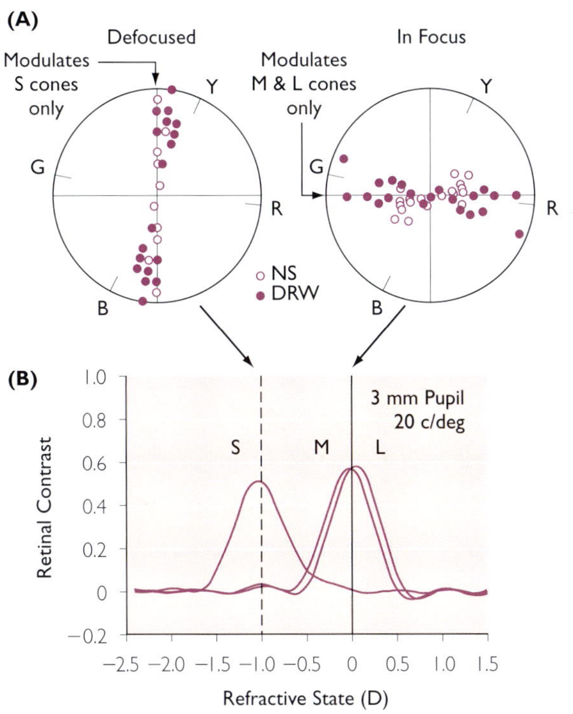

Figure 2.39 An explanation of Brewster's colors. (A) The circles represent the isoluminant color plane of color space. A stimulus whose chromaticity varies along the yellow–blue (YB) axis modulates S cones only while a stimulus that varies along the red–green (RG) axis modulates only L and M cones. The data points represent the matches made by two observers (NS and DRW) to chromatic noise images that were designed to mimic the perception of Brewster's colors. When the eye was in focus, Brewster's colors appeared to be red and green and observer's matches fell along the RG axis. When the eye was defocused by −1, −1.25, or −1.5 diopters, the Brewster's colors appeared yellow and blue and matches fell along the YB axis. (B) A plot of retinal contrast as a function of refractive state. When the eye is defocused by −1 diopters, the grating that elicits Brewster's colors stimulates only the S cones as indicated by the dashed vertical line. When the eye is in good focus at 0 diopters, the grating stimulates only the L and M cones as indicated by the solid vertical line. This analysis ignores the influence of monochromatic aberrations in the eye, which will reduce the large differences in contrast predicted in B. (From Williams *et al.*, 1991, with permission.)

Furthermore, a simulation of trichromatic sampling using the spatial coordinates of cones from a real photoreceptor mosaic followed by bilinear interpolation predicts the splotchy chromatic appearance reported by observers. For a 20 cycle/degree achromatic grating defocused by −1 diopters, the model predicts violet and greenish-yellow splotches consistent with modulation of S cones only (Figure 2.40, left). When the eye is brought to best focus, the model predicts red and green splotches consistent with the modulation of L and M cones only (Figure 2.40, right). At low spatial frequencies, the model predicts that a grating will be seen with little or no chromatic artifacts. Thus, Brewster's colors are submosaic aliases whose hues depend on which cone types are undersampling the high contrast target.

The spatial grain of the M and L cone submosaics is well hidden in normal viewing, and models like that illustrated above tend to produce more aliasing than is usually observed in normal viewing. Neither grating acuity nor the aliasing effects produced by high contrast interference fringes on cone isolating backgrounds reveals it. The invisibility of the separate M and L submosaics under these extreme conditions makes it unlikely that the grain of the submosaics degrades spatial vision under ordinary viewing conditions. The subtle and fleeting Brewster's colors that are observed when viewing high contrast black and white patterns are the only known visible manifestation. The visual system has apparently evolved the capacity for red–green color discrimination without any substantial cost for spatial vision under natural viewing conditions. A number of factors conspire to make the L to M ratio relatively unimportant. The statistics of natural scenes make high contrast, high spatial frequency signals rare events, optical blurring in the eye reduces the potential for aliasing, and clever postreceptoral processing based on prior information about natural visual scenes may also tend to hide the apparently haphazard organization of the trichromatic mosaic.

2.7 SUMMARY

In this chapter, we have discussed the sequence of events that ultimately leads to the generation of signals in photoreceptors. Many of these events can be summarized in the form of an ideal observer (Geisler, 1989). This ideal observer calculates the best possible contrast sensitivity at each stage of visual processing given the information present in a stimulus such

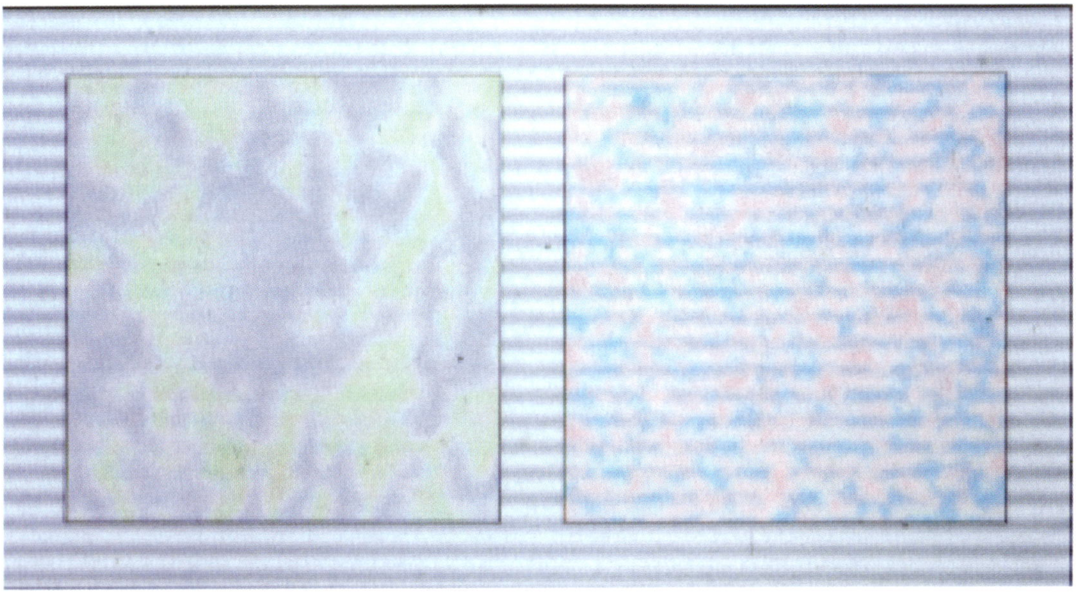

Figure 2.40 **A simulation of Brewster's colors. A high contrast black and white grating of 20 cycles/deg is sampled by a mosaic whose cone positions are taken from an image of a real photoreceptor mosaic. Bilinear interpolation was used as a simple method to reconstruct an image from the cone signals. The L to M cone ratio was set to 2 and 10% of the cones were randomly assigned to be S cones. (Left) Result of sampling with −1 diopter of defocus and a random assignment of L and M cones. (Right) Result with the eye at best focus. (From Williams *et al.*, 1991, with permission.)**

as a sinusoidal grating. Although contrast sensitivity does not account for all of the factors that we have talked about, such as the perceived patterns of aliases, it summarizes many of the important steps. Figure 2.41 shows that the first factor that limits the performance of the ideal observer is the quantum nature of light. The field size required to present a fixed number of cycles of a visual stimulus decreases linearly with increasing spatial frequency. Stimulus area as well as the number of stimulus photons thus decreases as the square root of spatial frequency. Since the variance of photon noise equals the mean number of photons, the resulting decrease in the signal to noise ratio also follows a square root relationship which gives the contrast sensitivity function a slope of −1. A second major factor that limits visual performance is light loss, whose signature is a simple downward shift in the contrast sensitivity function. Light loss occurs in the optical media, between photoreceptors, as a result of the finite axial density of the photopigment, and as a result of photoisomerization inefficiency following absorption. A third major factor that limits visual performance is spatial frequency-dependent filtering, whose signature is a change in the shape of the contrast sensitivity function. Filtering occurs in the optics, at the pupil, and at the cone aperture. In this schematic, we have assumed that the optics of the eye were bypassed by the use of interference fringes. As a result, optical filtering is not explicitly shown although it would have a similar but greater effect than cone blurring. Even after taking all of the optical factors into account, however, there remains a substantial gap between the best possible performance of the ideal observer and the actual performance of a human subject. These additional losses must be attributed to neural processing.

We can get some clues as to where these losses occur by representing the response of the visual system at each stage of visual processing by a point spread function (Sekiguchi *et al.*, 1993b). Wider point spread functions indicate more information loss. Due to optical blurring, the

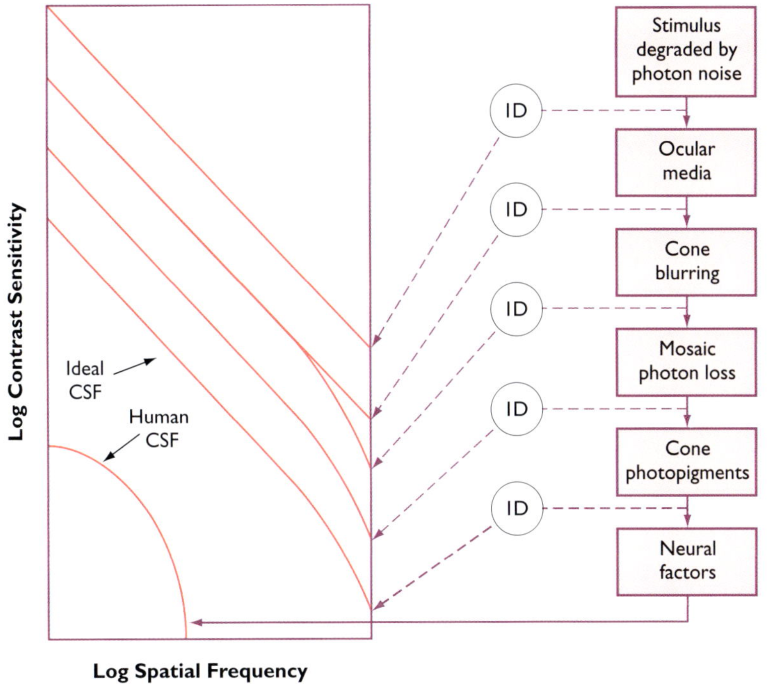

Figure 2.41 **Contrast sensitivity of an ideal observer at each stage of visual processing beginning with the quantum nature of light and ending with the cone mosaic. The ideal observer's contrast sensitivity is always higher than the actual contrast sensitivity of a human observer. (From Williams *et al.*, 1993.)**

smallest possible retinal point spread function under normal viewing conditions has a full width at half height of about 0.8' of arc (Figure 2.42). The cone apertures have very narrow point spread functions that cause little additional blurring. The idea of the point spread function can be extended to neural processing by expressing psychophysical measurements in terms of a neural point spread function. In the case of isochromatic stimuli, the point spread function has a width similar to that of the optical point spread function. The neural machinery needed to detect luminance differences is very efficient and introduces only a little additional blurring. On the other hand, the width of the point spread function associated with the detection of isoluminant gratings is nearly twice that of the optical point spread, suggesting additional information losses in those neural mechanisms that process chromatic information over and above the optical factors that we have considered here.

2.8 APPENDIX A: QUANTIFYING THE LIGHT STIMULUS

2.8.1 RADIOMETRY

2.8.1.1 Radiant energy

The most fundamental radiometric quantity is radiant energy, Q_e, expressed in joules (J). The subscript e indicates a radiometric quantity. Radiant energy is simply a measure of the total amount of light. The equivalent quantity in actinometry is the number of photons in the stimulus. In visual science, radiant energy is not a commonly used quantity because it does not tell us how concentrated the light is in space or time. It is sometimes used to describe very small and brief stimuli. This is because the visual effect of a stimulus that is smaller than the eye's spatial summation area and shorter than the eye's integration

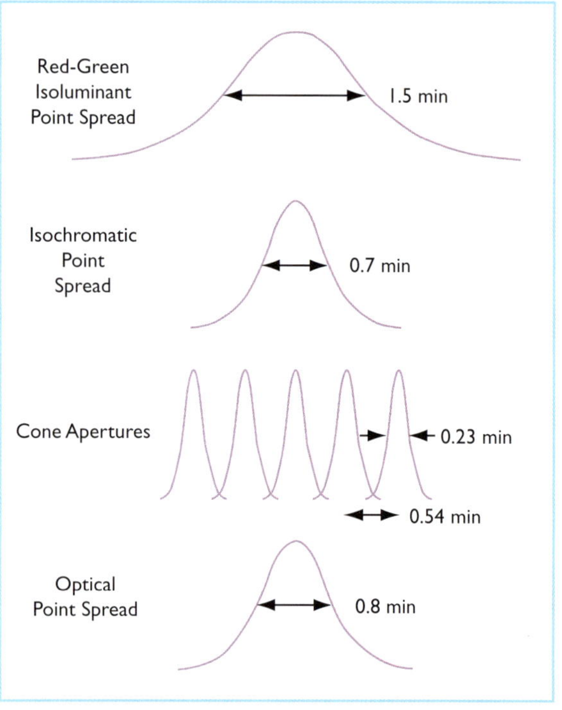

Figure 2.42 A comparison of the widths of optical point spread functions representing blurring by the optics and the cone apertures with neural point spread functions representing the effects of neural blurring on psychophysical isoluminant and isochromatic discriminations. (From Williams *et al.*, 1993.)

time does not depend on how the light is distributed in space and time. A famous example comes from the classic experiment of Hecht, Shlaer, and Pirenne (1942), who estimated that only about 10 photons must be absorbed in the visual pigment for an observer to reliably detect a small, brief flash under optimal conditions.

2.8.1.2 Radiant power

Radiant power, P_e, which is sometimes called radiant flux, is a measure of the concentration of energy in time and is given by

$$P_e = dQ_e/dt$$

where dQ_e is the energy during an infinitesimally small period of time, dt. Radiant power is expressed in watts, where one watt is equal to 1 joule s^{-1}. The actinometric equivalent is photon flux, expressed in photons s^{-1}.

The use of derivatives in the expression above allows us to define the radiant power at any instant in time, so that we can chart how the radiant power changes over time. For a time-varying signal, in the limit dQ_e/dt approaches a constant value for smaller and smaller values of dt.

2.8.1.3 Exitance and irradiance

Though the definition of radiant power allows it to be specified at any point in time, it does not allow the radiant power to be specified at any point in space. Consider a surface, such as that illustrated in Figure 2.1A that emits light some of which ultimately enters the pupil of the eye. The surface might emit light either because it is scattering or reflecting light that falls on it, or it might be self-luminous such as a CRT screen. In either case, the radiant power emitted will generally vary from point to point. The exitance, E_e, of the surface is a measure of the radiant power emitted from a given location on the surface, allowing us to describe surfaces that are not uniform. The exitance is given by

$$E_e = d^2Q_e/dtdA = dP_e/dA$$

where dA is an infinitesimally small area of the surface. Note that the definition of exitance resembles that for radiant power except for the addition of dA in the denominator. The units for exitance are joules s^{-1} m^{-2} which is equal to watts m^{-2}.

Irradiance, which has exactly the same units as exitance, refers to the radiant power falling on, or irradiating, a point on a surface rather than exiting from it. The photometric equivalent of irradiance is illuminance. In visual science, irradiance is much more commonly used than exitance. We more often want to specify how much light is falling on a photosensitive surface such as the retina, a silicon photodetector, or a photographic emulsion. We will return to the irradiance of the retinal image later. Irradiance is the quantity to use if you want to describe the spatial density of the radiant power falling on a surface but you do not need to specify the distribution of directions the light is coming from.

2.8.1.4 Radiant intensity

The radiant power emitted by a surface can depend on the direction the light propagates away from the surface. For example, if the surface were a mirror illuminated by a laser, the radiant power emitted from the mirror would depend strongly on direction. Virtually all the photons would stream off in a single direction and the eye would see nothing unless the pupil were positioned to intercept the reflected beam. The radiant intensity, I_e, is the radiant power emitted in a particular direction into the infinitesimally small solid angle, $d\omega$, and is given by

$$I_e = d^2Q_e/dtd\omega = dP_e/d\omega$$

Radiant intensity is expressed in units of watts per steradian. Note that the definition of radiant intensity resembles that for radiant power with the addition of $d\omega$ in the denominator.

Figure 2.1(B) shows the geometry underlying the concept of solid angle. The solid angle, ω, expressed in steradians, sr, is the three-dimensional analog of angles defined in two dimensions and expressed in radians. Imagine a point on a surface that is radiating light into a hemisphere with radius, r. A cone with its vertex at the point on the surface intersects the hemisphere, defining an area, A_{sp}. Solid angle is given by the expression

$$\omega = A_{sp}/r^2$$

Very often in light measurement, we need to calculate the solid angle subtended by planar objects. If r is greater than 1.75 times the radius of the object, the area of the planar object can be substituted for the area of the surface of a sphere with an error of less than 10%. In describing the solid angle of visual stimuli, we usually express visual angle in degrees. To convert from deg^{-2} to steradians, it is useful to know that one square degree equals 3.05×10^{-4} steradians.

In the expression for radiant intensity above, $d\omega$ is an infinitesimally small solid angle around a specific direction in which radiant power propagates. Just as irradiance allows you to describe the spatial density of radiant power, radiant intensity allows you to describe the angular density of radiant power. Radiant intensity, or its photometric equivalent, luminous intensity, is usually used to describe small stimuli such as point sources though it is defined for extended sources as well.

2.8.1.5 Radiance

Exitance and irradiance both incorporate location but not direction; radiant intensity incorporates direction but not location. Radiance is a particularly useful quantity that allows us to describe the radiant power in a particular location and propagating in a particular direction. Radiance, L_e, is given by

$$\begin{aligned} L_e &= d^3Q_e/dtd\omega dA\cos\theta \\ &= d^2P_e/d\omega dA\cos\theta \\ &= dI_e/dA\cos\theta \end{aligned}$$

where d^2P_e is the radiant power emitted into solid angle $d\omega$ by an infinitesimal area on the surface dA. The units of radiance are watts per steradian per meter squared. The equivalent photometric quantity is luminance, which will be defined later.

The $\cos\theta$ in the denominator, when multiplied by dA, defines the area of the surface visible from the direction of observation rather than the actual area of the surface, as shown in Figure 2.1(C). θ is the angle formed between the surface normal and the direction in which the radiance measurement is made. To understand the significance of this, consider a good diffuse reflector such as a white piece of paper. If we measure the radiant intensity of the paper in units of watts sr^{-1} as a function of θ, it will decline as a cosine function of increasing angle simply because the projected area of the paper declines in this way. This is known as Lambert's law and diffusers that obey this law, which are common in nature, are said to be Lambertian. However, the radiance of the paper will remain unchanged because the projected area appears in the denominator of the definition of radiance. The radiant intensity, which is in the numerator, declines in exactly the same way as the projected area with increasing angle, leaving radiance constant. Other properties of radiance that make it a particularly valuable quantity will be discussed later.

2.8.1.6 Spectral radiance

Most visual stimuli in color science have radiant power distributed across a broad range of wavelengths. The definition of radiance, or any other radiometric quantity for that matter, can be modified slightly so that we can express the radiance in a very narrow range of wavelengths. The spectral radiance is the radiance within a narrow range of wavelengths $d\lambda$ and usually has units of watts per nanometer per meter squared per steradian. Spectral radiance, $L_{e\lambda}$, is given by:

$$L_{e\lambda} = d^4Q_{e\lambda}/dtd\omega dA_{proj}d\lambda$$

2.8.1.7 Wavelength, frequency, and wavenumber

In color science, light is most commonly described in terms of its wavelength. The wavelength of light, λ, in meters, is given by,

$$\lambda = c/\nu$$

where c is the speed of light in a vacuum, 3.0×10^8 m s^{-1}, and ν is the frequency of light in cycles/second (Hz). Wavenumber, which is the reciprocal of wavelength and is usually expressed in cm^{-1}, is sometimes used. Frequency is less frequently used, though there is reason to prefer it over either wavelength or wave number. The velocity of light in a medium is the velocity in a vacuum divided by the refractive index of the medium, so that light slows down when traveling through matter. Likewise, both wavelength and wavenumber depend on refractive index, whereas the frequency does not. When we state the wavelength of a visual stimulus, we are usually referring to the wavelength the light would have had were it propagating in a vacuum. In fact, when the light enters the eye its wavelength is only about ¾ the wavelength it would have had in a vacuum. A second reason to favor frequency is that the shape of photopigment absorption spectra with different peak frequencies is roughly constant on a frequency axis, but not a wavelength axis. Despite these advantages, for the convenience of all of us who were trained to think in terms of wavelength instead of frequency, we will use wavelength here.

2.8.2 PHOTOMETRY

When specifying stimuli seen by the eye, we often want to use a description that conveys how visually effective a stimulus is since the radiance of a light stimulus is often a poor predictor of its brightness. Photometry was developed to address these issues. At the heart of the photometric system, whose standards are maintained by the Commission Internationale de l'Eclairage (CIE), is the standard observer, an imaginary individual whose visual system has an agreed upon and precisely defined spectral sensitivity, chosen to mimic the spectral sensitivity of the average human visual system.

The standard observer's photopic spectral sensitivity is given by the luminous efficiency function, $V(\lambda)$. This function, which has a maximum of 1 at 555 nm, was derived from several sets of psychophysical measurements based on heterochromatic photometry (see Wyszecki and Stiles, 1982 for details). At low light levels where rods normally operate, the standard observer takes on a different spectral sensitivity, the scotopic luminous efficiency function, $V'(\lambda)$. The $V'(\lambda)$ function, which has the maximum value of 1 at 507 nm, was derived from brightness matches of stimuli viewed in rod vision and measurements of threshold under dark-adapted conditions as a function of wavelength.

The scotopic and photopic luminous efficiency functions are normalized to one at their maxima. In 1924, the CIE adopted a standard photopic luminous efficiency function, while in 1951, they adopted a standard scotopic efficiency function. These remain the standard functions in use today. However, there are several variants of these functions that are useful for color scientists. Judd (1951) proposed a revision of the photopic luminous efficiency function that is more sensitive at short wavelengths and a more accurate description of actual human visual performance. This revision now has official recognition as a supplement to the CIE 1924 function. Both the CIE 1924 function and Judd's supplement are valid for field sizes less than about 4 degrees. The CIE has adopted another photopic luminous efficiency function for larger, 10 degree fields. All these luminous efficiency functions are shown in Figure 2.2, and tabulated in Table 2.3.

2.8.2.1 Converting radiometric units to photometric units

Any radiometric measure can be converted to the corresponding photometric measure by computing the effect of the stimulus defined in

Table 2.3 The CIE luminous efficiency functions of vision

Wavelength	$V\lambda$	$V'\lambda$	Judd 2°	Judd 10°
380	3.9e−05	0.000589	0.0004	1.40e−05
390	0.00012	0.00221	0.0015	0.000283
400	0.000396	0.00929	0.0045	0.002
410	0.00121	0.0348	0.0093	0.0088
420	0.004	0.0966	0.0175	0.0214
430	0.0116	0.1998	0.0273	0.0387
440	0.023	0.328	0.0379	0.0621
450	0.038	0.455	0.0468	0.0895
460	0.06	0.567	0.06	0.1282
470	0.091	0.676	0.091	0.1852
480	0.129	0.793	0.129	0.2536
490	0.208	0.904	0.208	0.3391
500	0.323	0.982	0.323	0.4608
510	0.503	0.997	0.503	0.6067
520	0.71	0.935	0.71	0.7618
530	0.862	0.811	0.862	0.8752
540	0.954	0.65	0.954	0.962
550	0.995	0.481	0.995	0.9918
560	0.995	0.329	0.995	0.9973
570	0.952	0.208	0.952	0.9556
580	0.87	0.121	0.87	0.8689
590	0.757	0.0655	0.757	0.7774
600	0.631	0.0332	0.631	0.6583
610	0.503	0.0159	0.503	0.528
620	0.381	0.00737	0.381	0.3981
630	0.265	0.00334	0.265	0.2835
640	0.175	0.0015	0.175	0.1798
650	0.107	0.000677	0.107	0.1076
660	0.061	0.000313	0.061	0.0603
670	0.032	0.000148	0.032	0.0318
680	0.017	7.15e−05	0.017	0.0159
690	0.00821	3.53e−05	0.00821	0.0077
700	0.0041	1.78e−05	0.0041	0.0372

radiometric terms on the CIE standard observer. Luminous power or flux is the photometric quantity that corresponds to radiant power. The fundamental unit of luminous power is the lumen (lm), which corresponds to the watt in radiometry. There are two kinds of lumens, photopic and scotopic. At photopic light levels,

$$P_v = K_m \int P_{e\lambda}(\lambda)V(\lambda)\, d\lambda$$

where P_v is the photopic luminous power in lumens (lm), K_m is a constant equal to 683 lm W^{-1}, $P_{e\lambda}$ is the spectral radiant power, and $V(\lambda)$ is the photopic luminous efficiency function. At scotopic light levels,

$$P'_v = K'_m \int P_{e\lambda}(\lambda)V'(\lambda)\, d\lambda$$

where P'_v is the photopic luminous power in lumens (lm) and K'_m is equal to 1700 lm W^{-1}.

Multiplying the luminous efficiency function by the spectral radiant power weights the spectral radiant power depending on the visual effectiveness of each wavelength. Integrating the product produces a single number that estimates the combined effect on vision of the radiant power at all wavelengths. If the light source is monochromatic, the integral can be omitted and one can convert in either direction between photometric and radiometric quantities. However, for broadband lights, it is not possible to recover a spectral radiometric distribution if only the corresponding photometric quantity is known. While the equations above are written to convert radiant power to luminous power, one could convert any radiometric quantity, such as radiance to its photometric equivalent, which is luminance, simply by substituting the appropriate quantity for $P_{e\lambda}$ in the equations above.

2.8.2.2 The troland

The goal of the photometric system is to take into account a property of the eye, namely its spectral sensitivity, when quantifying stimuli seen by the visual system. In that same spirit, the troland was invented to take into account the effect of the eye's pupil. For a stimulus of fixed luminance, the illuminance of the retinal image, expressed in lumens per square meter of retina, will increase in proportion to the area of the pupil. If you have measured the luminance of a visual stimulus and you know the area of the observer's pupil while viewing the stimulus, the photopic troland value, T, expressed in trolands, is given by

$$T = L_v\, p$$

where L_v is the luminance in cd m^{-2} and p is the area of the pupil in mm^2. Scotopic trolands are similarly computed but using luminance values based on the scotopic luminous efficiency function.

The above definition of the troland is convenient when you use a light meter that reads the luminance of a surface such as a CRT screen. Some light meters are not equipped with lenses. These also can also be used to calculate troland values. In that case, the photodetector surface is placed in the plane where the observer's pupil would normally lie. In Maxwellian view systems, where this technique is frequently used, the photodetector surface is placed conjugate to the artificial pupil so that all the light that would ordinarily pass into the eye is collected by the detector. The illuminance measurement provided by the detector can be converted to luminous power simply by multiplying by the area of the detector, being careful to express the area in the same units as those incorporated in the readout units. (In many devices, the size of the photodetector is exactly 1 cm^2 and the readout units are expressed in luminous power cm^{-2} so that the displayed number gives the luminous power directly.) Then, the troland value, T, is given by

$$T = P_v\, \omega^{-1}\, 10^6$$

where P_v is the luminous power in lumens and ω is the solid angle subtended by the stimulus at the eye's nodal point (which will be defined below). If the light is monochromatic, and you made your measurement of the light entering the pupil in irradiance units instead of illuminance units, then the troland value, T, is given by

$$T = 683\, P_e\, V_\lambda\, \omega^{-1}\, 10^6$$

where P_e is radiant power in watts.

The troland value is often referred to as retinal illuminance, but this usage is technically incorrect. As we will see later, the actual retinal illuminance depends not just on the luminance of the stimulus and the area of the pupil as the definition of troland value suggests, but also on the focal length of the eye and the transmittance of the ocular media.

Neither the troland value nor the actual retinal illuminance take into account the directional sensitivity of the retina, or the Stiles–Crawford effect. This effect, described in section 2.5.4, means that the visual effectiveness of a stimulus depends on the distribution of luminous power in the pupil and not simply on the total amount. Nonetheless, the troland value is a useful quantity and is widely used in color science today.

2.8.2.3 More obscure photometric units

There are a large number of terms for describing light that can be found in the literature and are not discussed here. These include luxons, nits, footcandles, apostilbs, blondels, and talbots. Should you encounter these terms and need to convert them into the quantities that are commonly accepted by vision scientists, their definitions can be found in Wyszecki and Stiles (1982). They are not repeated here in the hope that this might help to discourage their use.

2.8.2.4 Light meters

Commercial devices for measuring light have a bewildering number of names, and these names are often used without a great deal of consistency. For our purposes, there are basically four types of instruments: radiometers, spectroradiometers, photometers, and colorimeters. The capabilities of these four instruments are often combined into a single device.

Radiometers measure light in terms of radiometric units. An example of a simple radiometer is a silicon photodiode with a filter in front of it to make the overall energy-based sensitivity of the device flat across the visible spectrum. The device spatially integrates all the light falling on the photosensitive surface of the photodiode. Such devices essentially measure the irradiance of the light falling on them with typical units of microwatts cm^{-2}. More sophisticated versions of these devices can integrate irradiance over a user-specified time interval, so that radiant energy in a flash of light can be measured. Photometers measure light in photometric units. The simple photodiode discussed above can be converted from a radiometer to a photometer by replacing the filter in front of it with a specific yellow–green appearing filter that gives the detector a spectral sensitivity similar to the photopic luminous efficiency function. Such a device measures illuminance, usually in lux (lx), which is the photometric equivalent of irradiance. One lux is equivalent to one lumen m^{-2}.

Both radiometers and photometers of this kind can be used to measure other quantities besides irradiance and illuminance. For example, suppose you want to measure the luminous intensity of a light source such as an LED with the photometer. If the light falls uniformly across the photodetector, you could multiply the measured illuminance by the area of the detector to compute the total luminous power it is receiving. The luminous intensity is then the luminous power divided by the solid angle subtended by the detector at the source. (This is equivalent to dividing the measured illuminance of the source by the square of the distance of the photodetector from the source.) The units of luminous intensity are candelas (cd) where one candela is equal to one lumen sr^{-1}. Alternatively, you can compute the luminance of a source such as a CRT from the measured illuminance. You would place a mask over all areas of the CRT except a small uniform patch whose luminance you would like to measure. The luminance of the patch can be calculated by dividing the luminous intensity, calculated as described above, by the projected area of the patch in square meters. The units of luminance are candelas m^{-2}.

Some radiometers and photometers are equipped with a lens and a viewfinder. The region of the scene in the viewfinder over which the light measurement is made is indicated, usually by a black dot. These devices make radiance/luminance measurements as simple as pressing a button because they image the object onto the photodetector. Ignoring transmission losses in the lens, the radiance (and luminance) of the image of a surface within the solid angle subtended by the lens, is the same as that of the surface itself (see Boyd, 1983 for a proof). This means that such devices can read out radiance (and luminance in the photometric versions) directly without the user having to measure any distances or projected areas.

Whereas the devices described above integrate light at different wavelengths, arriving at single number, spectroradiometers measure radiant power at multiple wavelengths. This is usually accomplished by using a diffraction grating to spread the light from the region of interest into a spectrum that is sampled by a one-dimensional array of detectors. The spectral radiance distribution can be computed from the distribution of radiant power across the detectors. These devices are quite useful in color science because they provide the basic data from which all radiance and luminance computations can be performed. In addition, these devices, when equipped with the appropriate software, can behave as colorimeters, calculating the chromaticity coordinates of surfaces.

2.8.3 ACTINOMETRY

2.8.3.1 Converting radiometric units to actinometric units

Any radiometric quantity, such as radiant power, irradiance, or spectral radiance, can be converted to the corresponding actinometric quantity by applying Planck's Law, which states that the energy in a single photon, Q, is

$$Q = h\nu$$

where ν is the frequency of the light and h is Planck's constant, 6.6262×10^{-34} J s. The number of photons, Q_p, is given by

$$Q_p = 5.0341 \times 10^{15} \lambda Q_e$$

where Q_e is radiant energy expressed in joules and λ is the wavelength of light measured in nanometers. The subscript p stands for photon and indicates an actinometric quantity. This equation would hold not only for radiant energy and photons but also for any corresponding pair of radiometric and actinometric quantities, such as radiance and photon flux radiance.

In color science, spectral sensitivity curves from psychophysical experiments are sometimes plotted using an energy basis on the ordinate and at other times using a quantum basis. The shapes of the curves depend on which basis is used, with the quantum basis version always higher at the short wavelength end of the spectrum. If you want to convert a quantum-based spectral sensitivity curve expressed in photons s^{-1} deg^{-2} to an energy-based curve expressed in watts deg^{-2}, divide by $5.0341 \times 10^{15} \lambda$, if you want to convert from an energy to a quantum basis, multiply by $5.0341 \times 10^{15} \lambda$.

2.8.4 ACTINOMETRY OF THE RETINAL IMAGE

2.8.4.1 The reduced eye

To apply actinometry to the retinal image, we must first have a model of the eye that allows us to predict with reasonable accuracy the dimensions of the retinal image. Figure 2.3 shows a cross-section through the human eye, indicating the most important features for our purposes. The passage of rays through this structure is complex, in part because of the gradient index properties of the human lens, which have not been completely characterized. Numerous schematic eyes have been designed to capture the imaging properties of real eyes (see Wyszecki and Stiles, 1982 for details). We will use a simplified model of the eye, called the reduced eye (Elmsley, 1952), which does an adequate job of predicting the dimensions of the retinal image despite its inaccuracies in some other respects.

The reduced eye, shown in Figure 2.43, consists of a single convex surface which does the refracting work of the cornea and lens in the real eye. This is not quite as gross a violation of reality as it might first appear. In the real eye, the first surface of the cornea accounts for about 80% of the refracting power of the total eye, with the lens mainly responsible for focusing the eye on objects at different distances. This spherical surface has a radius of curvature, PN, of 5.56 mm. The reduced eye has a pupil, which is located, for simplicity in a plane containing the principal point, P.

In the real eye, the retinal image is formed in a medium with a higher refractive index than that outside the eye. Correspondingly, the reduced eye has a refractive index, n', inside of ⁴⁄₃ and a refractive index, n, outside of 1. This influences the posterior focal length of the eye which influences the size, and therefore, the actinometry of the retinal image. The distance between the refractive surface at P and the retina at R is the posterior focal length of the eye, f', which has a value of 22.22 mm.

Suppose the reduced eye is viewing an object that is very distant from the eye. We can locate the position of the retinal image of a point on the object by considering two rays from the object point. Since the object is very far away these rays will be effectively parallel as they impinge on the eye, as shown in Figure 2.43. Consider first the ray that intersects the optic axis at P, where it makes an angle θ with respect to the optic axis outside the eye. The law of refraction, also known as Snell's Law, states that the angle the ray makes inside the eye, θ', will be given by

$$\sin\theta' = (n/n') \sin\theta$$

For small values of θ and substituting the refractive indices assumed for the reduced eye, this can be rewritten

$$\theta' = \theta/n' = 0.75\theta$$

Again for small angles, the size of the retinal image, S_r, is given by

$$\tan \theta' = \tan (0.75\theta) = S_r/f'$$

Substituting the reduced eye value for f' solving for S_r, we have, approximately

$$S_r = 0.291\theta$$

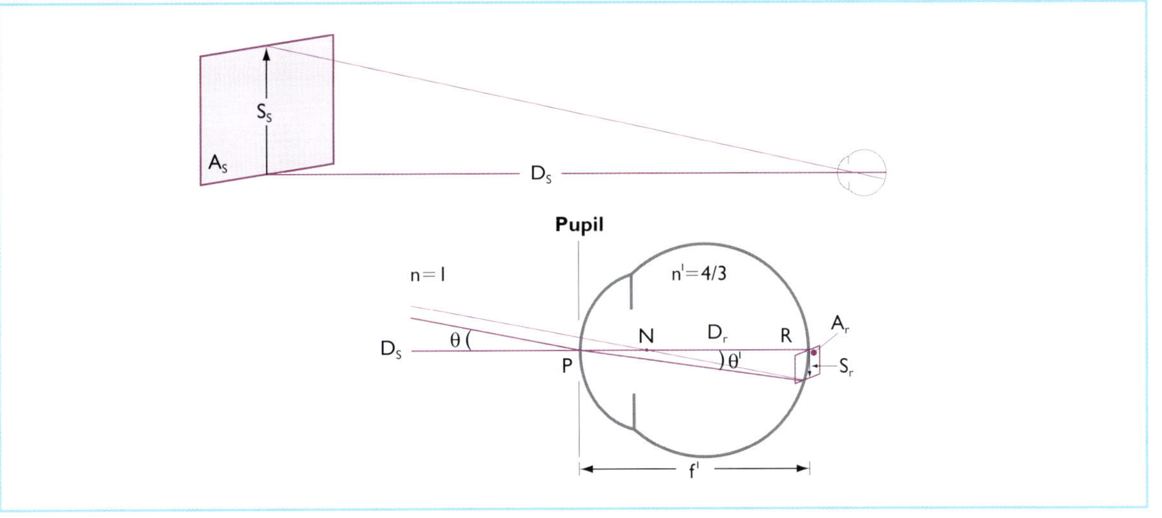

Figure 2.43 **The geometry of the reduced schematic eye (Elmsley, 1952) used to predict the dimensions of the retinal image. The upper figure shows the object space including the area, A_s, height, S_s, and distance, D_s, of the object being viewed. The lower half of the figure is an expanded view of the image space showing the area, A_r, height, S_r, and distance, D_r, of the image being formed. *P* is the point at which the optical axis intersects the cornea, the only refracting element in the reduced eye. Rays incident on *P* at an angle θ with respect to the optical axis will be bent towards the optical axis making a reduced angle θ' that can be calculated from Snell's Law and the refractive indices *n* and n'. *N* is the nodal point through which a ray passes unbent. f' is the focal length of the model eye.**

which implies that 1° of visual angle corresponds to about 0.291 mm on the retina, or that one minute of arc corresponds to 4.85 μm.

Consider the second ray from the object point that is coincident with a normal to the refracting surface. This ray will not be bent at all and will intersect the optic axis at point N. Point N is called the nodal point of the eye. The ray continues through N, intersecting the retina at the same point as the first ray. Rays that pass through N have the valuable property that angles inside and outside the eye are equal. This allows us an alternative and simpler way to compute the size of the retinal image, by using similar right triangles. In the reduced eye, the distance between N and the retina, which is sometimes called the posterior nodal distance, D_r, is 16.67 mm. The posterior nodal distance, incidentally, is the posterior focal length of a schematic eye that consists of a thin lens and equal refractive indices inside and outside the eye. In this case,

$$S_s/D_s = S_r/D_r$$

In terms of area, if we let A_s be the area of the surface, S_s^2 and A_r be the area of the retinal image, S_r^2, we can write

$$A_s/D_s^2 = A_r/D_r^2$$

This expression simply says that the solid angles with respect to the nodal point outside and inside the eye are equal.

2.8.4.2 Computing retinal photon flux irradiance

We are now in a position to compute the retinal photon flux irradiance for a monochromatic stimulus. Typically we might be given the luminance or radiance of the stimulus. If we are given luminance, then we must first convert to radiometric units which we can do by

$$L_e = L_v/K_m V(\lambda)$$

If we are given the radiance of the stimulus or after we have converted luminance to radiance, the next step is to convert to photon flux radiance by

$$L_p = 5.0341 \times 10^{15}\, \lambda L_e$$

Given the photon flux radiance of the surface, we can compute the photon flux in the pupil by

$$P_p = L_p A_s A_p / D_s^2$$

This expression tells us the number of photons/s arriving at the pupil from the source. Next, we need to compute how these photons will be distributed on the retina. We can calculate the area of the retinal image using a rearranged version of one of the equations developed above for the simplified schematic eye.

$$A_r = D_r^2 A_s / D_s^2$$

Knowing both the photon flux radiance and the area of the retinal image we can then calculate photon flux irradiance from

$$E_p = TP_p / A_r = TL_p A_p / D_r^2$$

The expression for photon flux irradiance on the right is calculated by substituting for P_p and A_r and taking into account light losses in the optical media by including its transmittance, T.

We can now calculate the photon flux arriving at any area of the retina by

$$P_p = E_p A_r$$

where Ar is the area of interest. For example, photon flux for a particular stimulus could be calculated by setting A_r equal to the stimulus area. The number of photons/s arriving at a single photoreceptor can be estimated by setting A_r equal to the area of the photoreceptor aperture. Examples, which are explained in section 2.2.4 can be found in Table 2.2.

2.9 APPENDIX B: GENERALIZED PUPIL FUNCTION AND IMAGE FORMATION

2.9.1 QUANTITATIVE DESCRIPTION OF THE GENERALIZED PUPIL FUNCTION

The optics of the eye can be evaluated by determining what happens to a planar wave front as it passes through the optics to the retina. In an aberrated eye, the light waves passing through different parts of the pupil will be delayed by different amounts resulting in an imperfect retinal image. A map of the amount that light is delayed as it passes through the pupil is known as the wave aberration. The generalized pupil function is an extension of the wave aberration that takes into account not only the delays introduced by the eye's optics but also their transmittance. If the generalized pupil function is known, it becomes possible to calculate the point spread function, which is a complete description of image quality.

The generalized pupil function is:

$$P(\eta,\xi) = P_0(\eta,\xi) \cdot \exp\left(i\frac{2\pi}{\lambda}W(\eta,\xi)\right)$$

where (η,ξ) are 2-d spatial coordinates in the entrance pupil and $W(\eta,\xi)$ is the eye's wave aberration, which describes errors in the delay of light at each location in the pupil. $P_0(\eta,\xi)$ is the amplitude transmittance across the eye's optics, the truncating effect of the iris being the most important. The variation in the absorption of the cornea and lens across the pupil is small enough in the normal eye that it can usually be ignored. However, because of the antenna properties of cones, the quantum efficiency of the retina depends on the entry point of light in the pupil. Though this effect, known as the Stiles–Crawford effect (see section 2.5.4.1), is caused by the optics of the retina, it is equivalent to reducing the amplitude transmittance towards the perimeter of the entrance pupil. Therefore, the generalized pupil function for the eye includes the directional sensitivity of the retina in $P_0(\eta,\xi)$.

The PSF is the squared modulus of the Fourier transform of the generalized pupil function. That is,

$$PSF(x, y) = |\Im(P(\lambda d\eta, \lambda d\xi))|^2$$

where the Fourier transform is given by

$$\Im(f(\eta, \xi)) = \iint f(\eta, \xi) \cdot exp[+i2\pi(x\eta + y\xi)]d\eta d\xi$$

2.9.2 COMPUTING RETINAL IMAGES FOR ARBITRARY OBJECTS

The retinal image for an arbitrary object, as illustrated in Figure 2.14, can be computed either in the spatial domain or the frequency domain. In the spatial domain, the intensity distribution of the image, $I(x,y)$, is the convolution of the PSF with the intensity distribution of the object, $O(x,y)$. That is,

$$I(x,y) = PSF(x, y) \otimes O(x/M, y/M)$$

where M is the magnification between the object and image planes.

The convolution of two functions $f(x,y)$ and $g(x,y)$ is

$$f(x, y) \otimes g(x, y) = \iint f(x, y) \cdot g(r - x, s - y)dxdy.$$

In practice, the computation of the retinal image is more efficient in the spatial frequency domain. In that case, the intensity distribution of the object. $O(x, y)$, is Fourier transformed to provide the object Fourier spectrum, $o(f_x, f_y)$. That is,

$$o(f_x, f_y) = \Im(O(x, y))$$

The object Fourier spectrum is then multiplied by the optical transfer function (OTF) of the eye to give the image Fourier spectrum:

$$i(f_x, f_y) = OTF(f_x, f_y) \cdot o(Mf_x, Mf_y)$$

By taking the inverse Fourier transform of the image spectrum, one obtains the retinal image.

$$I(x, y) = \Im^{-1}(i(f_x, f_y))$$

The OTF is the autocorrelation of the generalized pupil function. Alternatively, the OTF can be computed by Fourier transforming the PSF. The OTF is complex, consisting of two parts, a modulation transfer function (MTF) and a phase transfer function (PTF). The MTF indicates how faithfully the contrast of individual spatial frequency components of the object is transferred to the image. The PTF indicates how individual spatial frequency components of the object have been translated in the retinal image.

For the diffraction-limited eye, optical performance can be characterized by the modulation transfer function (MTF) alone since diffraction produces no phase error. In this case, the MTF is

$$D(s,s_0) = \frac{2}{\pi}\left[\cos^{-1}\left(\frac{s}{s_0}\right) - \left(\frac{s}{s_0}\right)\sqrt{1-\left(\frac{s}{s_0}\right)^2}\right]$$

$$\text{for } s < s_0$$

where s is spatial frequency in cycles/degree, and s_0 is the incoherent cut-off frequency for a diffraction-limited imaging system with a circular pupil. The incoherent cut-off frequency is the spatial frequency above which the optical transfer function is zero. In radians, the incoherent optical cutoff is

$$s_0 = a/\lambda$$

where a is the diameter of the pupil and λ is the wavelength of light.

ACKNOWLEDGMENTS

The authors wish to thank Joe Carroll, David Brainard, Larry Thibos, and Walt Makous for their comments on the manuscript and Antonio Guirao, Heidi Hofer, and Geun-Young Yoon for their assistance. We acknowledge financial support from the National Eye Institute.

REFERENCES

Abadi, R.V. and Cox, M.J. (1992) The distribution of macular pigment in human albinos. *Invest Ophthalmol Vis Sci*, 33, 494–7.

Abramov, I. and Gordon, J. (1977) Color vision in the peripheral retina. I. Spectral sensitivity. *J Opt Soc Am*, 67, 195–202.

Adams, D.L., Horton, J.C. (2002) Shadows cast by retinal blood vessels mapped in primary visual cortex. *Science*, 298(5593): 572–6.

Ahnelt, P.K., Kolb, H., and Pflug, R. (1987) Identification of a subtype of cone photoreceptor, likely to be blue sensitive, in the human retina. *J Comp Neurol*, 255, 18–34.

Alpern, M. (1986) The Stiles–Crawford effect of the second kind (SCII): a review. *Perception*, 15, 785–99.

Anderson, S.J. and Hess, R.F. (1990) Post-receptoral undersampling in normal human peripheral vision. *Vision Res*, 30, 1507–15.

Applegate, R.A. and Lakshminarayanan, V. (1993) Parametric representation of Stiles–Crawford functions: normal variation of peak location and directionality. *J Opt Soc Am A*, 10, 1611–23.

Artal, P., Derrington, A.M., and Colombo, E. (1995) Refraction, aliasing, and the absence of motion reversals in peripheral vision. *Vision Res*, 35, 939–47.

Artal, P., Marcos, S., Navarro, R., and Williams, D.R. (1995) Odd aberrations and double-pass measurements of retinal image quality. *J Opt Soc Am A*, 12, 195–201.

Atchison, D.A., Joblin, A., and Smith, G. (1998) Influence of Stiles–Crawford effect apodization on spatial visual performance. *J Opt Soc Am A*, 15, 2545–51.

Barlow, H.N. (1977) Retinal factors in human vision limited by noise. In H.N. Barlow and P. (eds), *Photoreception in Vertebrates*. London: Academic Press.

Baylor, D.A., Nunn, B.J., and Schnapf, J.L. (1984) The photocurrent, noise, and spectral sensitivity of rods of the monkey *Macaca fascicularis*. *J Physiol (Lond)*, 357, 575–607.

Baylor, D.A., Nunn, B.J., and Schnapf, J.L. (1987) Spectral sensitivity of cones of the monkey *Macaca fascicularis*. *J Physiol (Lond)*, 390, 145–60.

Bergmann, C. (1858) Anatomisches und Physiologisches uber die Netzhaut des Auges. Zeitschrift fur ration. *Medicin*, 2, 83–108. [Translated by D'Zmura, M. (1996) Bergmann on visual resolution. *Perception*, 25, 1223–34.]

Bird, A.C. and Weale, R.A. (1974) On the retinal vasculature of the human fovea. *Exp Eye Res*, 19, 409–17.

Boettner, E.A. and Wolter, J.R. (1962) Transmission of the ocular media. *Invest Ophthalmol Vis Sci*, 1, 776–83.

Bone, R.A., Landrum, J.T., and Tarsis, S.L. (1985) Preliminary identification of the human macular pigment. *Vision Res*, 25, 1531–5.

Bowmaker, J.K. and Dartnall, H.J. (1980) Visual pigments of rods and cones in a human retina. *J Physiol (Lond)*, 298, 501–11.

Boyd, R.W. (1983) *Radiometry and the Detection of Optical Radiation*. New York: John Wiley.

Bradley, A., Zhang, X.X., and Thibos, L.N. (1991) Achromatizing the human eye. *Optom Vis Sci*, 68, 608–16.

Brainard, D.H. and Williams, D.R. (1993) Spatial reconstruction of signals from short-wavelength cones. *Vision Res*, 33, 105–16.

Brainard, D.H., Roorda, A., Yamauchi, Y., Calderone, J.B., Metha, A., Neitz, M., Neitz. J., Williams, D.R., and Jacobs, G.H. (2000) Functional consequences of the relative numbers of L and M cones. *J Opt Soc Am A*, 17, 607–14.

Brewster, D. (1832) On the undulations excited in the retina by the action of luminous points and lines, *London and Edinburgh Philosoph Mag and J Sci*, pp. 1–169.

Brindley, G.S. (1953) The effects on colour vision of adaptation to very bright lights. *J Physiol (Lond)*, 122, 332–50.

Bumsted, K.M., Jasoni, C.L., and Hendrickson, A.E. (1996) Developmental appearance of the monkey cone mosaic detected by opsin mRNA and protein expression. *Invest Ophthalmol Vis Sci*, 37, S149.

Burns, S.A. and Elsner, A.E. (1985) Color matching at high illuminances: the color-match-area effect and photopigment bleaching. *J Opt Soc Am A*, 2, 698–704.

Burns, S.A., Wu, S., He. J.C., and Elsner, A.E. (1997) Variations in photoreceptor directionally across the central retina. *J Opt Soc Am A*, 14, 2033–40.

Burton, G.W. and Ingold, K.U. (1984) Beta-carotene: an unusual type of lipid antioxidant. *Science*, 224, 569–73.

Byram, G.M. (1944) The physical and photochemical basis of visual resolving power. Part II. Visual acuity and the photochemistry of the retina. *J Opt Soc Am*, 34, 718–38.

Campbell, F.W. and Green, D.G. (1965) Optical and retinal factors affecting visual resolution. *J Physiol (Lond)*, 181, 576–93.

Campbell, F.W. and Gubisch, R.W. (1967) The effect of chromatic aberration on visual acuity. *J Physiol (Lond)*, 192, 345–58.

Carroll, J., Neitz, J., and Neitz, M. (2002) Estimates of L:M cone ratio from ERG flicker photometry and genetics. *J Vision*, 2, 531–42.

Charman, W.N. (1995) Optics of the eye. In Michael Bass (ed.), *Handbook of Optics*. New York: McGraw-Hill, pp. 24.3–24.54.

Chen, B. and Makous, W. (1989) Light capture by human cones. *J Physiol (Lond)*, 414, 89–109.

Chen, B., Makous, W., and Williams, D.R. (1993) Serial spatial filters in vision. *Vision Res*, 33, 413–27.

Cicerone, C.M. and Nerger, J.L. (1989) The relative numbers of long-wavelength-sensitive to middle-wavelength-sensitive cones in the human fovea centralis. *Vision Res*, 29, 115–28.

Cooper, G.F. and Robson, J.G. (1969) The yellow colour of the lens of man and other primates. *J Physiol (Lond)*, 203, 411–17.

Cornsweet, T.N. and Crane, H.D. (1973) Accurate two-dimensional eye tracker using first and fourth Purkinje images. *J Opt Soc Am*, 63, 921–8.

Curcio, C.A. and Allen, K.A. (1990) Topography of ganglion cells in human retina. *J Comp Neurol*, 300, 5–25.

Curcio, C.A., Allen, K.A., Sloan, K.R., Lerea, C.L., Hurley, J.B., Klock, I.B., and Milam, A.H. (1991) Distribution and morphology of human cone photoreceptors stained with anti-blue opsin. *J Comp Neurol*, 312, 610–24.

Curcio, C.A., Sloan, K.R., Kalina, R.E., and Hendrickson, A.E. (1990) Human photoreceptor topography. *J Comp Neurol*, 292, 497–523.

Dartnall, H.J. (1968) Quantum efficiency of rhodopsin bleaching. *Vision Res*, 8, 339–58.

Dartnall, H.J., Bowmaker, J.K., and Mollon, J.D. (1983) Human visual pigments: microspectrophotometric results from the eyes of seven persons. *Proc R Soc Lond B Biol Sci*, 220, 115–30.

Deeb, S.S., Diller, L.C., Williams, D.R., and Dacey, D.M. (2000) Interindividual and topographical variation of L:M cone rations in monkey retinas. *J Opt Soc Am A*, 17, 538–44.

de Monasterio, F.M., Schein, S.J., and McCrane, E.P. (1981) Staining of blue-sensitive cones of the macaque retina by a fluorescent dye. *Science*, 213, 1278–81.

de Monasterio, F.M., McCrane, E.P., Newlander, J.K., and Schein, S.J. (1985) Density profile of blue-sensitive cones along the horizontal meridian of macaque retina. *Invest Ophthalmol Vis Sci*, 26, 289–302.

Dolin, P.J. (1994) Ultraviolet radiation and cataract: a review of the epidemiological evidence. *Br J Ophthalmol*, 78, 478–82.

Einthoven, W. (1885) Stereoskopie durch farbendifferenz. *Albrecht von Graefes Archiv fur Ophthalmologie*, 31, 211–38.

Elmsley, H.H. (1952) *Visual Optics*, 5th edn, Vol. 1. London: Butterworths.

Enoch, J.M. and Lakshminarayanan, V. (1991) Retinal fibre optics. In J. Cronly-Dillon (ed.), *Vision and Visual Dysfunction*, Vol. I. Boca Raton: CRC Press, pp. 280–309.

Enoch, J.M. and Stiles, W.S. (1961) The colour change of monochromatic light with retinal angle of incidence. *Optica Acta*, 8, 329–58.

Erb, M.B. and Dallenbach, K.M. (1939) 'Subjective' colors from line patterns. *Am J Psych*, 52, 227.

Field, D.J. (1987) Relations between the statistics of natural images and the response properties of cortical cells. *J Opt Soc Am A*, 4, 2379–94.

Galvin, S.J. and Williams, D.R. (1992) No aliasing at edges in normal viewing. *Vision Res*, 32, 2251–9.

Geisler, W.S. (1989) Sequential ideal-observer analysis of visual discriminations. *Psychol Rev*, 96, 267–314.

Geller, A.M., Sieving, P.A., and Green, D.G. (1992) Effect on grating identification of sampling with degenerate arrays. *J Opt Soc Am A*, 9, 472–7.

Goodman, J.W. (1996) *Introduction to Fourier Optics*. New York: McGraw-Hill.

Grassman, H.G. (1853) Zur theorie der farbenmischung. *Annalen der Physik und Chemie*, 89, 69–84.

Haegerstrom-Portnoy, G. (1988) Short-wavelength-sensitive-cone sensitivity loss with aging: a protective role for macular pigment? *J Opt Soc Am A*, 5, 2140–4.

Hagstrom, S.A., Neitz, J., and Neitz, M. (1997) Ratio of M/L pigment gene expression decreases with retinal eccentricity. In C.R. Cavonious (ed.), *Colour Vision Deficiencies XIII*. Dordrecht: Kluwer Academic, pp. 59–66.

Hagstrom, S.A., Neitz, J., and Neitz, M. (2000) Cone pigment gene expression in individual photoreceptors and the chromatic topography of the retina. *J Opt Soc Am A*, 17, 527–37.

Hallett, P.E. (1987) Quantum efficiency of dark-adapted human vision. *J Opt Soc Am A*, 4, 2330–5.

Ham, W.T., Jr, Mueller H.A., Ruffolo, J.J., Jr, Guerry, D. 3d, and Guerry, R.K. (1982) Action spectrum for retinal injury from near-ultraviolet radiation in the aphakic monkey. *Am J Ophthalmol*, 93, 299–306.

Hansen, G. (1946) The influence of the Stiles–Crawford effect on measurements with the Pulfrich photometer. *J Opt Soc Am*, 36, 321–5.

He, J.C., Marcos, S., and Burns, S.A. (1999) Comparison of cone directionality determined by psychophysical and reflectometric techniques. *J Opt Soc Am A*, 16, 2363–9.

Hecht, S., Shlaer, S., and Pirenne, M.H. (1942) Energy, quanta, and vision. *J Gen Physiol*, 25: 819–40.

Helmholtz, H. (1896) *Helmholtz's Treatise on Physiological Optics* (translated from the 3rd German edn, edited by J.P.C. Southall), 3rd edn (1962). New York: Dover.

Hendrickson, A.E. and Yuodelis, C. (1984) The morphological development of the human fovea. *Ophthalmology*, 91, 603–12.

Holmgren, F. (1884) Uber den Farbensinn. *Compte rendu du congrès international de science et medecine* (Vol 1: Physiology). Copenhagen, pp. 80–98.

Hsu, A., Smith, R.G., Buchsbaum, G., and Sterling, P. (2000) Cost of cone coupling to trichromacy in primate fovea. *J Opt Soc Am A*, 17, 635–40.

Jacobs, G.H. and Deegan, J.F. 2nd (1997) Spectral sensitivity of macaque monkeys measured with ERG flicker photometry. *Vis Neurosci*, 14, 921–8.

Jacobs, G.H. and Neitz, J. (1993) Electrophysiological estimates of individual variation in the L/M cone ratio. In B. Drum (ed.), *Colour Vision Deficiencies XI*. Dordrecht: Kluwer Academic, pp. 107–12.

Jennings, J.A. and Charman, W.N. (1981) Off-axis image quality in the human eye. *Vision Res* 21, 445–55.

Jordan, G., Mollon, J.D. (1993) The Nagel anomaloscope and seasonal variation of colour vision. *Nature*, J363(6429): 546–9.

Judd, D.B. (1951) Report of the U.S. Secretariat Committee on Colorimetry and Artificial Daylight, CIE Proceedings, Vol. 1, Part 7, p. 11 (Stockholm 1951). Paris, Bureau Central de la CIE.

Kraft, J.M. and Werner, J.S. (1999) Aging and the saturation of colors. 2. Scaling of color appearance. *J Opt Soc Am A*, 16, 231–5.

Krantz, D.H. (1975) Color measurement and color theory: I. Representation theorem for Grassman structures. *J Math Psychol*, 12, 283–303.

Krauskopf, J. (1978) On identifying detectors. In J.C. Armington, J. Krauskopf, and B.R. Wooten (eds), *Visual Psychophysics and Physiology*. New York: Academic Press, pp. 283–95.

Laties, A.M. and Enoch, J.M. (1971) An analysis of retinal receptor orientation. I. Angular relationship of neighboring photoreceptors. *Invest Ophthalmol*, 10, 69–77.

Legge, G.E., Mullen, K.T., Woo G.C., and Campbell, F.W. (1987) Tolerance to visual defocus. *J Opt Soc Am A*, 4, 851–63.

Liang, J. and Williams, D.R. (1997) Aberrations and retinal image quality of the normal human eye. *J Opt Soc Am A*, 14, 2873–83.

Liang, J., Williams, D.R., and Miller, D.T. (1997) Supernormal vision and high resolution imaging through adaptive optics. *J Opt Soc Am A*, 14, 2884–92.

Luckiesh, M. and Moss, F.K. (1933) A demonstrational test of vision. *Am J Psych*, 45, 135.

McLellan, J.S., Marcos, S., Prieto, P.M., Burns, S.A. (2002) Imperfect optics may be the eye's defence against chromatic blur. *Nature*, 417(6885): 174–6.

MacLeod, D.I.A. (1985) Receptoral restraints on color vision. In D. Ottoson and S. Zeki (eds), *Central and Peripheral Mechanisms of Colour Vision*. London: Macmillan, pp. 103–16.

MacLeod, D.I. and Webster, M.A. (1988) Direct psychophysical estimates of the cone-pigment absorption spectra. *J Opt Soc Am A*, 5, 1736–43.

MacLeod, D.I.A., Williams, D.R., and Makous, W. (1992) A visual nonlinearity fed by single cones. *Vision Res*, 32, 347–63.

Makous, W. (1997) Fourier models and loci of adaptation. *J Opt Soc Am A*, 14, 2323–45.

Makous, W. (1998) Optics. In R.H.S. Carpenter and J.G. Robson (eds), *Vision Research: a Practical Guide to Laboratory Methods*. Oxford: Oxford University Press, pp. 1–49.

Marcos, S., Burns, S.A., Moreno-Barriusop, E., Navarro, R. (1999) A new approach to the study of ocular chromatic aberrations. *Vision Res*, 39(26): 4309–23.

Miller, W.H. and Bernard, G.D. (1983) Averaging over the foveal receptor aperture curtails aliasing. *Vision Res*, 23, 1365–9.

Mino, M. and Okano, Y. (1971) Improvement in the OTF of a defocussed optical system through the use of shaded apertures. *Applied Optics*, 10, 2219–25.

Miyahara, E., Pokorny, J., Smith, V.C., Baron, R., and Baron, E. (1998) Color vision in two observers with highly biased LWS/MWS cone ratios. *Vision Res*, 38, 601–12.

Mollon, J.D. (1982) Color vision. *Ann Rev Psychol*, 33, 41–85.

Mollon, J.D. and Bowmaker, J.K. (1992) The spatial arrangement of cones in the primate fovea. *Nature*, 360, 677–9.

Navarro, R., Artal, P., and Williams, D.R. (1993) Modulation transfer of the human eye as a function of retinal eccentricity. *J Opt Soc Am A*, 10, 201–12.

Neitz, J., Carroll, J., Yamauchi, Y., Neitz, M., Williams, D.R. (2002) Color perception is mediated by a plastic neural mechanism that remains adjustable in adults. *Neuron*, 35, 783–92.

Nussbaum, J.J., Pruett, R.C., and Delori, F.C. (1981) Historic perspectives. Macular yellow pigment. The first 200 years. *Retina*, 1, 296–310.

Osterberg, G.A. (1935) Topography of the layer of rods and cones in the human retina. *Acta Ophthalmol*, 6 (Suppl. 13), 1–102.

Packer, O., Hendrickson, A.E., and Curcio, C.A. (1989) Photoreceptor topography of the retina in the adult pigtail macaque (*Macaca nemestrina*). *J Comp Neurol*, 288, 165–83.

Packer, O.S., Williams, D.R., and Bensinger, D.G. (1996) Photopigment transmittance imaging of the primate photoreceptor mosaic. *J Neurosci*, 16, 2251–60.

Pelli, D.G. (1990) The quantum efficiency of vision. In C. Blakemore (ed.), *Vision: Coding and Efficiency*. Cambridge: Cambridge University Press, pp. 3–24.

Pettersen, D.P. and Middleton, D. (1962) Sampling and reconstruction of wave number limited functions in N-dimensional euclidean space. *Information and Control*, 5, 279–323.

Piotrowski, L.N. and Campbell, F.W. (1982) A demonstration of the visual importance and flexibility of spatial-frequency amplitude and phase. *Perception*, 11, 337–46.

Pirenne, M.H. (1962) Absolute thresholds and quantum effects. In H. Davson (ed.), *The Eye*, Vol. 2. New York: Academic Press, pp. 123–40.

Pokorny, J. and Smith, V.C. (1977) Evaluation of single pigment shift model of anomalous trichromacy. *J Opt Soc Am*, 67, 1196–209.

Pokorny, J., Smith, V.C., and Lutze, M. (1987) Aging of the human lens. *Applied Optics*, 26, 1437–40.

Polyak, S.L. (1957) *The Vertebrate Visual System*. Chicago: University of Chicago Press.

Pulos, E. (1989) Changes in rod sensitivity through adulthood. *Invest Ophthalmol Vis Sci*, 30, 1738–42.

Reading, V.M. and Weale, R.A. (1974) Macular pigment and chromatic aberration. *J Opt Soc Am*, 64, 231–4.

Rodieck, R.W. (1973) *The Vertebrate Retina; Principles of Structure and Function*. San Francisco, Freeman.

Roorda, A., Metha, A.B., Lennie, P., and Williams, D.R. (2001) Packing arrangement of the three cone classes in primate retina. *Vision Res*, 41, 1291–306.

Roorda, A. and Williams, D.R. (1999) The arrangement of the three cone classes in the living human eye. *Nature*, 397, 520–2.

Roorda, A., Williams, D.R. (2002) Optical fiber properties of individual human cones. *J Vision*, 2, 404–12.

Ruddock, K.H. (1972) Light transmission through the ocular media and its significance for psychophysical investigation. In D. Jameson and L.M. Hurvich (eds), *Handbook of Sensory Physiology*, Vol. VII/4. New York: Springer-Verlag, pp. 455–69.

Rushton, W.A.H. and Baker, H.D. (1964) Red/green sensitivity in normal vision. *Vision Res*, 4, 75–85.

Rushton, W.A.H. (1965) Stray light and the measurement of mixed pigments in the retina. *J Physiol (Lond)*, 176, 46–55.

Rynders, M.C., Lidkea, B.A., Chisholm, W.J., and Thibos, L.N. (1995) Statistical distribution of foveal transverse chromatic aberration, pupil centration, and angle psi in a population of young adult eyes. *J Opt Soc Am A*, 12, 2348–57.

Safir, A., Hyams, L., and Philpot, J. (1970) Movement of the Stiles–Crawford effect. *Invest Ophthalmol*, 9, 820–5.

Schefrin, B.E. and Werner, J.S. (1990) Loci of spectral unique hues throughout the life span. *J Opt Soc Am A*, 7, 305–11.

Sekiguchi, N., Williams, D.R., and Brainard, D.H. (1993a) Aberration-free measurements of the visibility of isoluminant gratings. *J Opt Soc Am A*, 10, 2105–17.

Sekiguchi, N., Williams, D.R., and Brainard, D.H. (1993b) Efficiency in detection of isoluminant and isochromatic interference fringes. *J Opt Soc Am A*, 10, 2118–33.

Shannon, C.E. (1949) Communication in the presence of noise. *Proc IRE*, 37, 10.

Sharpe, L.T. (1990) The light-adaptation of the human rod visual system. In R.F. Hess, L.T. Sharpe, and K. Nordby (eds), *Night Vision: Basic, Clinical and Applied Aspects*. Cambridge: Cambridge University Press, p. 9.

Shevell, S.K. and Burroughs, T.J. (1988) Light spread and scatter from some common adapting stimuli: computations based on the point-source light profile. *Vision Res*, 28, 605–9.

Skinner, B.F. (1932) A paradoxical color effect. *J Gen Psychol*, 7, 481.

Smith, R.A. and Cass, P.F. (1987) Aliasing in parafovea with incoherent light. *J Opt Soc Am A*, 4, 1530–4.

Snodderly, D.M., Brown, P.K., Delori, F.C., and Auran, J.D. (1984a) The macular pigment. I. Absorbance spectra, localization, and discrimination from other yellow pigments in primate retinas. *Invest Ophthalmol Vis Sci*, 25, 660–73.

Snodderly, D.M., Auran, J.D., and Delori, F.C. (1984b) The macular pigment. II. Spatial distribution in primate retinas. *Invest Ophthalmol Vis Sci*, 25, 674–85.

Snodderly, D.M., Weinhaus, R.S., and Choi, J.C. (1992) Neural-vascular relationships in central retina of macaque monkeys (*Macaca fascicularis*). *J Neurosci*, 12, 1169–93.

Snodderly, D.M. (1995) Evidence for protection against age-related macular degeneration by carotenoids and antioxidant vitamins. *Am J Clin Nutr*, 62(6 Suppl), 1448S–61S.

Snyder, A.W. and Hall, P.A. (1969) Unification of electromagnetic effects in human retinal receptors with three pigment colour vision. *Nature*, 223, 526–8.

Snyder, A.W. and Pask, C. (1973a) The Stiles–Crawford effect – explanation and consequences. *Vision Res*, 13, 1115–37.

Snyder, A.W. and Pask, C. (1973b) Letter: Waveguide modes and light absorption in photoreceptors. *Vision Res*, 13, 2605–8.

Snyder, A.W., Bossomaier, T.R., and Hughes, A. (1986) Optical image quality and the cone mosaic. *Science*, 231, 499–501.

Sperling, H.G., Johnson, C., and Harwerth, R.S. (1980) Differential spectral photic damage to primate cones. *Vision Res*, 20, 1117–25.

Stromeyer, C.F. 3rd, Kronauer, R.E., and Madsen, J.C. (1978) Apparent saturation of blue-sensitive cones occurs at a color-opponent stage. *Science*, 202, 217–19.

Starr, S.J. (1977) Effect of wavelength and luminance on the Stiles–Crawford effect in dichromats. PhD dissertation, University of Chicago, Chicago, IL.

Stiles, W.S. (1937) The luminous efficiency of monochromatic rays entering the eye pupil at different points and a new colour effect. *Proc R Soc Lond B Biol Sci*, 123, 90–118.

Stiles, W.S. (1939) The directional sensitivity of the retina and the spectral sensitivities of the rods and cones. *Proc R Soc Lond B Biol Sci*, 127, 64–105.

Stiles, W.S. and Burch, J.M. (1959) National Physical Laboratory colour-matching investigation: final report. *Optica Acta*, 6, 1–26.

Stiles, W.S. and Crawford, B.H. (1933) The luminous efficiency of rays entering the eye pupil at different points. *Proc R Soc Lond B Biol Sci*, 112, 428–50.

Sykes, S.M., Robison, W.G. Jr, Waxler, M., and Kuwabara, T. (1981) Damage to the monkey retina by broad-spectrum fluorescent light. *Invest Ophthalmol Vis Sci*, 20, 425–34.

Thibos, L.N. (1987) Calculation of the influence of lateral chromatic aberration on image quality across the visual field. *J Opt Soc Am A*, 4, 1673–80.

Thibos, L.N., Bradley, A., Still, D.L., Zhang, X., and Howarth, P.A. (1990) Theory and measurement of ocular chromatic aberration. *Vision Res*, 30, 33–49.

Thibos, L.N., Still, D.L., and Bradley, A. (1996) Characterization of spatial aliasing and contrast sensitivity in peripheral vision. *Vision Res*, 36, 249–58.

Thibos, L.N., Walsh, D.J., and Cheney, F.E. (1987) Vision beyond the resolution limit: aliasing in the periphery. *Vision Res*, 27, 2193–7.

Toraldo di Francia, G. (1949) The radiation pattern of retinal receptors. *Proc R Soc (Lond) Ser B*, 62, 461–2.

van Blokland, G.J. and van Norren, D. (1986) Intensity and polarization of light scattered at small angles from the human fovea. *Vision Res*, 26, 485–94.

van de Kraats, J., Berendschot, T.T., and van Norren, D. (1996) The pathways of light measured in fundus reflectometry. *Vision Res*, 36, 2229–47.

van Kampen, E.J. and Zijlstra, W.G. (1983) Spectrophotometry of hemoglobin and hemoglobin derivatives. *Adv Clin Chem*, 23, 199–257.

van Norren, D. and Vos, J.J. (1974) Spectral transmission of the human ocular media. *Vision Res,* 14, 1237–44.

van Norren, D. and Tiemeijer, L.F. (1986) Spectral reflectance of the human eye. *Vision Res,* 26, 313–20.

Vimal, R.L., Pokorny, J., Smith, V.C., and Shevell, S.K. (1989) Foveal cone thresholds. *Vision Res,* 29, 61–78.

Vos, J.J. (1963) Contribution of the fundus oculi to entoptic scatter. *J Opt Soc Am,* 53, 1449.

Walls, G.L. (1963) *The Vertebrate Eye and Its Adaptive Radiation.* New York: Hafner.

Weale, R.A. (1953) Spectral sensitivity and wavelength discrimination of the peripheral retina. *J Physiol (Lond),* 121, 170–90.

Weale, R.A. (1954) Light absorption by the lens of the human eye. *Optica Acta,* 1, 107–10.

Weale, R.A. (1981) On the problem of retinal directional sensitivity. *Proc R Soc Lond B Biol Sci,* 212, 113–30.

Webster, M.A. and MacLeod, D.I. (1988) Factors underlying individual differences in the color matches of normal observers. *J Opt Soc Am A,* 5, 1722–35.

Werner, J.S., Donnelly, S.K., and Kliegl, R. (1987) Aging and human macular pigment density. *Vision Res,* 27, 257–68.

Werner, J.S. and Schefrin, B.E. (1993) Loci of achromatic points throughout the life span. *J Opt Soc Am A,* 10, 1509–16.

Werner, J.S. and Steele, V.G. (1988) Sensitivity of human foveal color mechanisms throughout the life span. *J Opt Soc Am A,* 5, 2122–30.

Werner, J.S., Steele, V.G., and Pfoff, D.S. (1989) Loss of human photoreceptor sensitivity associated with chronic exposure to ultraviolet radiation. *Ophthalmology,* 96, 1552–8.

Westheimer, G. and Liang, J. (1995) Influence of ocular light scatter on the eye's optical performance. *J Opt Soc Am A,* 12, 1417–24.

Wikler, K.C. and Rakic, P. (1990) Distribution of photoreceptor subtypes in the retina of diurnal and nocturnal primates. *J Neurosci,* 10, 3390–401.

Wijngaard, W. (1974) Some normal modes of an infinite hexagonal array of identical circular dielectric rods. *J Opt Soc Am,* 64, 1136–44.

Williams, D.R. (1985) Aliasing in human foveal vision. *Vision Res,* 25, 195–205.

Williams, D.R. (1988) Topography of the foveal cone mosaic in the living human eye. *Vision Res,* 28, 433–54.

Williams, D.R. (1990) The invisible cone mosaic. In: *Advances in Photoreception: Proceedings of a Symposium on Frontiers of Visual Science.* Washington, DC: National Academy Press, pp. 135–48.

Williams, D.R. and Collier, R. (1983) Consequences of spatial sampling by a human photoreceptor mosaic. *Science,* 221, 385–7.

Williams, D.R., MacLeod, D.I., and Hayhoe, M.M. (1981) Punctate sensitivity of the blue-sensitive mechanism. *Vision Res,* 21, 1357–75.

Williams, D.R., Sekiguchi, N., and Brainard, D. (1993) Color, contrast sensitivity, and the cone mosaic. *Proc Natl Acad Sci U S A,* 90, 9770–7.

Williams, D.R., Sekiguchi, N., Haake, W., Brainard, D., and Packer, O. (1991) The cost of trichromacy for spatial vision. In A. Valberg and B.B. Lee (eds), *From Pigments to Perception.* New York: Plenum, pp. 11–22.

Williams, D.R., Artal, P., Navarro, R., McMahon, M.J., and Brainard, D.H. (1996) Off-axis optical quality and retinal sampling in the human eye. *Vision Res* 36, 1103–4.

Wooten, B.R. and Geri, G.A. (1987) Psychophysical determination of intraocular light scatter as a function of wavelength. *Vision Res,* 27 (8), 1291–8.

Wright, W.D. (1928–29) A re-determination of the mixture curves of the spectrum. *Trans Opt Soc,* 31, 201.

Wyszecki, G. and Stiles, W.S. (1980) High-level trichromatic color matching and the pigment-bleaching hypothesis. *Vision Res,* 20, 23–37.

Wyszecki, G. and Stiles, W.S. (1982) *Color Science: Concepts and Methods, Quantitative Data and Formulae,* 2nd edn. Wiley: New York.

Yamaguchi, T., Motulsky, A.G., and Deeb, S.S. (1997) Visual pigment gene structure and expression in the human retinae. *Hum Mol Genet,* 6, 981–90.

Yellott, J.I. (1982) Spectral analysis of spatial sampling by photoreceptors: topological disorder prevents aliasing. *Vision Res,* 22, 1205–10.

Yellott, J.I. (1983) Spectral consequences of photoreceptor sampling in the rhesus retina. *Science,* 221, 382–5.

Yoon, G.Y. and Williams, D.R. (2002) Visual performance after correcting the monochromatic and chromatic aberrations of the eye. *J Opt Soc Am A,* 19, 266–75.

Zhang, X.X., Ye, M., Bradley, A., and Thibos, L.N. (1999) Apodization by the Stiles–Crawford effect moderates the visual impact of retinal image defocus. *J Opt Soc Am A,* 16, 812–20.

3 Color Matching and Color Discrimination

Vivianne C. Smith and Joel Pokorny

Departments of Ophthalmology & Visual Science and Psychology, University of Chicago, 940 East Fifty-Seventh Street, Chicago, IL 60637, USA

CHAPTER CONTENTS

The Science of Color
ISBN 0–444–512–519

3.1 INTRODUCTION

The purpose of this chapter is to summarize the data of color matching, detection of spectral lights, and discrimination of lights on the basis of differences in chromaticity. Matching, detection, and discrimination are all tasks in which the spectral content of the lights is an important parameter. The tasks involve either identity matching or detection of a just noticeable difference. Data are expressed in physical units. The color appearance at the identity match or at the just noticeable difference is irrelevant and rarely noted. Although color names are often used to refer to lights as a shortcut form of expression (e.g. red light for a 660 nm spectral light or white light for a continuous spectral power distribution), we have tried to avoid such terminology in this chapter.

The data of matching, detection, and discrimination have been modeled successfully by considering early retinal processing. All the phenomena described in this chapter can be modeled by the activity of parvocellular (PC-), koniocellular (KC-) and magnocellular (MC-) pathways (see Chapter 6). Some readers may find it helpful to read Chapter 6 concurrently with this chapter.

We will concentrate primarily on the classical studies in the literature. These studies have involved small (1° or 2°) or moderate (10°) sized foveally fixated, circular stimuli. Luminance levels of matching and discrimination stimuli are usually at low to medium photopic levels, with retinal illuminations of 5–1000 trolands (td). In detection studies, large concentric backgrounds are often employed and light levels may extend to levels where substantial photopigment bleaching occurs.

3.2 COLOR MIXTURE

A human observer looking at a colored object has no way of knowing from its appearance the spectral composition of the physical stimulus. Colorimetry provides a system of color measurement and specification based upon the concept of equivalent-appearing stimuli. In a color match, two fields of differing spectral radiation appear identical. The match represents a unique neural state in which neural signals generated by the fields are identical.

3.2.1 PRINCIPLES AND PROCEDURES

Metamers: Metameric lights are lights that though of dissimilar spectral radiation are seen as the same by the observer. In a prototypical color-matching experiment using additive lights, the metamers are presented in a bipartite field. For 2° foveal fields, metamers have three important properties that allow treatment of color mixture as a linear system (Grassmann, 1853):

1. The additive property. When a radiation is identically added to both sides of a color mixture field, the metamerism is unchanged.
2. The scalar property. When both sides of the color mixture field are changed in radiance by the same proportion, the metamerism is unchanged.
3. The associative property. A metameric mixture may be substituted for a light without changing the metameric property of the color fields.

According to Grassmann's laws, a color match is invariant under a variety of experimental conditions that may alter the appearance of the matching fields. Metameric matches will hold with the addition of a chromatic surround or following pre-exposure to a moderately bright chromatic field.

Trichromacy: A fundamental property of normal human color vision is the existence of color matches of lights that differ in spectral composition. It is possible to find a metamer for any light (spectral power distribution) by variation of the energies of three fixed lights, which are called primaries. The terms trichromat and trichromacy refer to this property of human color vision. There is wide freedom in the choice of primaries. A formal requirement is that one primary cannot be metameric to a mixture of the other two. In practice, it is desirable that the primaries be spectrally separated as much as possible and that the matching field is at a mid-photopic level. The choice of primaries is dictated largely by experimental convenience. Primaries may or may not themselves be spectral. However, in the development of a colorimetric system, the test lights should be spectral or near-spectral in order to derive the largest color gamut.

It has become customary to present the results of color mixture experiments as color equations. Suppose we have three primaries, $\mathbf{P}_1$, $\mathbf{P}_2$, $\mathbf{P}_3$ and a test light, S, arranged in a bipartite field. We find that a mixture of S and $\mathbf{P}_3$ appears identical to a mixture of $\mathbf{P}_1$ and $\mathbf{P}_2$, when the radiant energies of S, $\mathbf{P}_1$, $\mathbf{P}_2$, $\mathbf{P}_3$ are P_S, $P_{S,1}$, $P_{S,2}$ and $P_{S,3}$ respectively. This is written:

$$P_S S \oplus P_{S,3}\mathbf{P}_3 \equiv P_{S,1}\mathbf{P}_1 \oplus P_{S,2}\mathbf{P}_2 \qquad (3.1)$$

where '$\equiv$' means visually identical and '$\oplus$' means physical mixture. The quantities $P_{S,1}$, $P_{S,2}$ and $P_{S,3}$ are called the tristimulus values. Their subscripts identify the test light (S) and the primaries (1, 2 or 3). Using Grassmann's law we treat this mixture equation as an algebraic equation and express the match in terms only of S:

$$P_S S = P_{S,1}\mathbf{P}_1 + P_{S,2}\mathbf{P}_2 - P_{S,3}\mathbf{P}_3 \qquad (3.2)$$

where the minus sign reflects the fact that in the color match, the primary $\mathbf{P}_3$ actually was added to the test light. Given a set of primaries, ($\mathbf{P}_1$, $\mathbf{P}_2$, $\mathbf{P}_3$), a color match can be made to all lights, of any spectral power distribution. When the test light is a narrow spectral band, one of the primaries is always either negative; i.e. physically superimposed with the spectral test light to match the remaining two primaries, or zero. When the test light has a broad spectral power distribution, the three primaries may all be positive.

As a consequence of Grassmann's law, the match to a broad spectral power distribution can be considered as the sum of constituent narrow-band spectral matches. Consider a distribution of unit energy at every spectral wavelength (the equal energy spectrum, abbreviated EES). According to the law of additivity, the color match to this distribution is considered as the sum of the matches to unit energies of the spectral wavelengths.

$$P_{EES}EES = [\Sigma(P_\lambda)]\ EES = [\Sigma(P_{\lambda,1})]\ \mathbf{P}_1 + [\Sigma(P_{\lambda,2})]\ \mathbf{P}_2 + [\Sigma(P_{\lambda,3})]\ \mathbf{P}_3 \qquad (3.3)$$

Data of color matching: Early measurements of color matching are reviewed by Bouma (1947) and Le Grand (1968). The data on which 2° colorimetry was formulated were those of Wright (1929, 1946) and Guild (1931). Stiles (1955) has discussed this work and presented modern data for both 2° and 10° fields. Here we describe Wright's experiment and how the colorimetric observer was formulated.

Wright used a technique known as maximum saturation matching. The primaries and the spectral test lights are arranged pairwise in a bipartite field so that a mixture of the spectral test light and one primary are matched to a mixture of the two other primaries. The spectral primaries were at 650 nm ($\mathbf{P}_1$), 530 nm ($\mathbf{P}_2$), and 460 nm ($\mathbf{P}_3$). The spectral test wavelengths varied in 10 or 20 nm steps between 410 and 700 nm. For each test wavelength, a color match was obtained and the amount of each primary was measured and expressed as an equation. Every spectral wavelength could be specified in terms of the three primaries, with one of the three being negative or zero. Wright also made a match to his instrument broadband (white) source, which was filtered tungsten with a color temperature of 4800 K. This source was essentially equivalent to one adopted formally by the CIE and termed Standard Illuminant B.[1]

3.2.2 REPRESENTATION OF COLOR MATCHING DATA

The quantities of the test wavelengths are customarily referred to an equal energy spectrum. There are several conventions to represent the unit of measurement for the primaries (Wright, 1946; Stiles, 1955; Stiles and Burch, 1959; Le Grand, 1968). It is convenient for the purpose of discussion to redefine the tristimulus values $P_{S,1}$, $P_{S,2}$, and $P_{S,3}$ of equations 3.1–3.2, using new terms, $C_{S,1}$, $C_{S,2}$, and $C_{S,3}$:

$$C_{S,i} = P_{S,i}/e_i \qquad (3.4)$$

where $P_{S,i}$ is the radiant flux of primary (i) specified relative to a radiant unit, e_i. If the three radiant units are equivalent and unity, the data will be expressed in watts, as implied in equations 3.1–3.3. In practice, however, other normalizations are used. In energy units, the short-wavelength $\mathbf{C}_1$ primary amount is much higher than the others. In representing color mixture data, it was considered desirable that the amounts of the primaries have similar scales. Recalculating a new normalization simply requires weighting all the values of C_i. Suppose e'_i is the new primary unit:

$$P_{S,i} = C_{S,i}\, e'_i = C_{S,i}\, e_i \tag{3.5}$$
$$C_{S,I} = C_{S,i}\, e_i / e'_i \tag{3.6}$$

Chromaticity diagrams: The data of a color matching experiment can be expressed in terms of vectors in a three-dimensional space (Schrödinger, 1920). The tristimulus values, $C_{1,1}$, $C_{2,2}$, and $C_{3,3}$, at the three primaries form unit vectors. A resultant vector represents the location of a mixture of the three primaries. According to the Grassmann laws, the scaling of the unit vectors is arbitrary; if the radiance were doubled, the entire diagram would be expanded but would maintain its shape. A two-dimensional unit plane can be defined in the space where the sum of the tristimulus values is unity. The relative positions of the resultant vectors are preserved in such a plane. The tristimulus values are converted into a form where the sum of the three always equals unity. For a test color S:

$$c_{S,1} = C_{S,1}/[C_{S,1} + C_{S,2} + C_{S,3}], \tag{3.7}$$
$$c_{S,2} = C_{S,2}/[C_{S,1} + C_{S,2} + C_{S,3}] \tag{3.8}$$
$$c_{S,3} = C_{S,3}/[C_{S,1} + C_{S,2} + C_{S,3}]. \tag{3.9}$$

The quantities $c_{S,i}$ are termed chromaticity coordinates (trichromatic coefficients in the older literature). The unit plane for Wright's data is plotted in Cartesian coordinates in Figure 3.1. The horseshoe shape shows the location of the spectral test wavelengths and the head of vector B represents the location of Wright's instrument white (Standard Illuminant B).

The chromaticity diagram is a two-dimensional representation of the results of a color mixture experiment. Figure 3.2 shows Wright's data replotted in a chromaticity diagram where c_1 is plotted against c_2 on Cartesian axes. The coordinates for $\mathbf{P}_1$, $\mathbf{P}_2$, and $\mathbf{P}_3$ form a right-angled triangle. Points that fall outside this triangle represent the negative values of the spectral tristimulus values. The values for the spectral wavelengths again demonstrate a characteristic horseshoe-shaped curve; this is called the spectrum locus. Standard Illuminant B appears near the center of the right-angled triangle as point S_B.

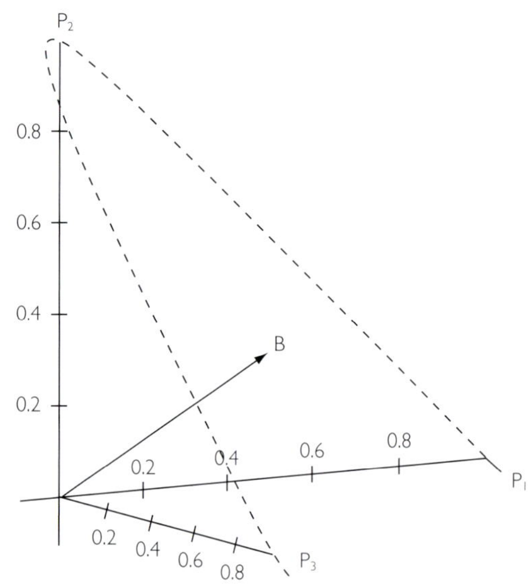

Figure 3.1 **Representation of Wright's color matching data in a three-dimensional space. The three primaries $\mathbf{P}_1$, $\mathbf{P}_2$, $\mathbf{P}_3$ form the axes. Wright's chromaticity coordinates for the spectral test lights are shown plotted in the unit plane. The arrowhead represents the vector for source B.**

WDW normalization: W.D. Wright performed his experiment using a method of normalization now termed WDW normalization. This normalization is a practical choice, because it ensures that the tristimulus values will have rather similar weights, but does not require the experimenter to have an absolute calibration of the radiant energies of the primaries and test lights. There is additionally a theoretical significance to data expressed in this normalization.

In WDW normalization, two test wavelengths, the first intermediate between $\mathbf{P}_1$ and $\mathbf{P}_2$ and the second intermediate between $\mathbf{P}_2$ and $\mathbf{P}_3$, are chosen as normalizing wavelengths. Wright used 582.5 nm and 494 nm. The energy units are chosen so that the amount C_1 of the $\mathbf{P}_1$ primary is set equal to the amount C_2 of the $\mathbf{P}_2$ primary at the match to the first normalizing wavelength and the amount C_3 of the $\mathbf{P}_3$ primary is set equal to the amount C_2 of the $\mathbf{P}_2$ primary at the match

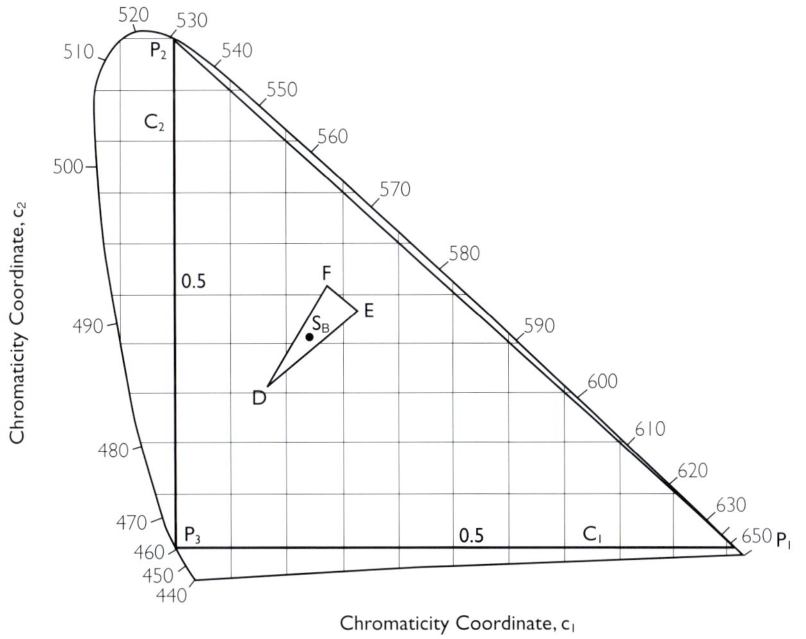

Figure 3.2 The chromaticity diagram calculated for Wright's data with WDW normalization and C_2 plotted versus C_1. The coordinates for S_B represent the position of the average match to Standard Illuminant B made by 36 observers, at coordinates (0.243, 0.410). The triangle DEF shows the spread of the individual white matches. (From Y. Le Grand, *Light, Colour, and Vision*, translated by R.W.G. Hunt, J.W.T. Walsh, and F.R.W. Hunt, Dover Publications, New York, 1957; reprinted with permission.)

to the second normalizing wavelength. In Figure 3.2, the spectrum locus is the averaged data of 10 observers. The coordinates for S_B represent the position of the average match to the instrument white made by 36 observers, at coordinates (0.243, 0.410). The triangle DEF shows the spread of the individual white matches. Figure 3.3 shows the chromaticity coordinates for the spectrum for Wright's observers plotted as a function of wavelength. The solid line shows the average data for 10 observers and the dashed lines show the matches of extreme observers. The interobserver variability is partitioned among the spectral wavelengths and the white point.

The importance of the WDW normalization is that it separates interobserver variance caused by receptor variation from interobserver variance caused by prereceptoral variation. It may be shown algebraically that in the WDW system, interobserver variation in the chromaticity coordinates for the spectrum greater than experimental error can be attributed to interobserver differences in the spectral absorption characteristics of the visual photoreceptors. Individual variation in the distribution of the coefficients for the white point greater than experimental error must be attributed to variation in prereceptoral filters, e.g. the lens and macular pigment (Wright, 1946; Wyszecki and Stiles, 1982) (see Chapter 2).

Photometry and colorimetry: The discussion until now has assumed that the primary units are specified in radiant energy. However, that is not how colorimetry developed. Historically, the radiant energy levels were not available in the early studies of Wright and Guild. Wright circumvented this problem by use of the WDW normalization and he expressed his data in chromaticity coordinates.

Equation (3.4) can also be expressed in luminous quantities, F:

$$F_{\lambda 1} = K_m V_{\lambda 1} P_\lambda \qquad (3.10)$$

where K_m is the constant relating lumens to watts (683 lumens/watt) and V_λ is the spectral

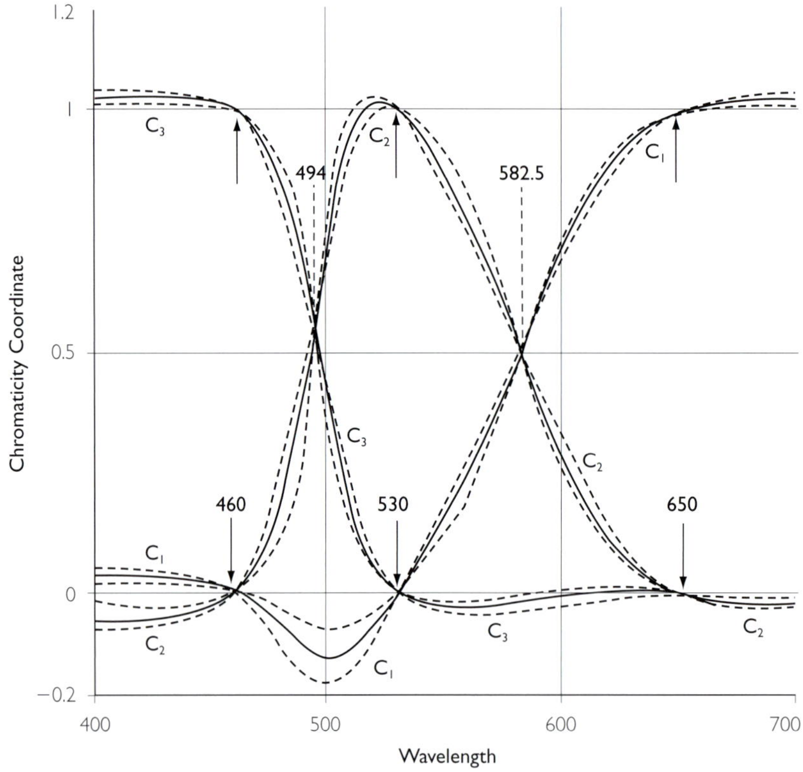

Figure 3.3 Wright's chromaticity coordinates plotted as a function of wavelength with WDW normalization. The solid line represents the average of 10 observers; the dashed lines show the matches of extreme observers. (From Y. Le Grand, *Light, Colour and Vision*, translated by R.W.G. Hunt, J.W.T. Walsh, and F.R.W. Hunt, Dover Publications, New York, 1957; reprinted with permission.)

luminous efficiency of the human eye. The V_λ had been adopted as a standard by the CIE in 1924 (CIE, 1926), just a few years before Wright's experiments. Equation (3.4) can thus be rewritten:

$$C_{\lambda,i} = F_{\lambda,i}/l_i \qquad (3.11)$$

where $F_{\lambda,i}$ is the luminous flux of primary light, (i) specified relative to its luminous unit, l_i. Wright measured the luminous units for the primaries using heterochromatic flicker photometry. The measured values were adjusted to predict the chromaticity coefficients of Standard Illuminant B, consistent with the V_λ curve. The relative luminance of the $\mathbf{P}_1$, $\mathbf{P}_2$, and $\mathbf{P}_3$ primaries was calculated to be in the ratio of 0.65:1:0.044.

The colorimetric match is a statement of identity of appearance. At the match, the luminous fluxes must also be equivalent. Therefore for any test light S, of luminous flux F_S:

$$F_S = F_{S1} + F_{S2} + F_{S3} = l_1C_{S1} + l_2C_{S2} + l_3C_{S3} \qquad (3.12)$$

For the spectral test lights referred to, an equal energy spectrum, F_λ is proportional to V_λ. Further, the luminous unit, l_λ for a spectral test light, C_λ of luminous flux F_λ can be defined:

$$l_\lambda = F_\lambda/C_\lambda = (l_1C_{\lambda,1} + l_2C_{\lambda,2} + l_3C_{\lambda,3})/(C_{\lambda,1} + C_{\lambda,2} + C_{\lambda,3}) \qquad (3.13)$$

$$= l_1c_{\lambda,1} + l_2c_{\lambda,2} + l_3c_{\lambda,3} \qquad (3.14)$$

If the spectral chromaticity coordinates and the luminous units, l_i, of the primaries are known, the spectral tristimulus values can be derived from the equations above:

$$C_{\lambda,i}(\lambda) = c_{\lambda,i}V(\lambda)/(l_1c_{\lambda,1} + l_2c_{\lambda,2} + l_3c_{\lambda,3}) \qquad (3.15)$$

The data for Figure 3.1 were derived in this manner from Wright's tabulation of the chromaticity coefficients and the values of the relative luminous units given above. In modern terminology, for a set of three primaries, identified as $\mathbf{P}_1$, $\mathbf{P}_2$, $\mathbf{P}_3$, the tristimulus values are identified as $P_{\lambda,1}$, $P_{\lambda,2}$, and $P_{\lambda,3}$, and the chromaticity coordinates are $p_{\lambda,1}$, $p_{\lambda,2}$, and $p_{\lambda,3}$. The tristimulus values for an arbitrary light, S, are $P_{S,1}$, $P_{S,2}$, and $P_{S,3}$.

Linear transformations of color matching data: Grassmann's (1853) observation that color mixture data show the associative property allows expression of a set of data in sets of primaries other than those used in a particular experiment. This can be noted intuitively since any test wavelength is a linear combination of a given primary set ($\mathbf{P}_1$, $\mathbf{P}_2$, $\mathbf{P}_3$). These primaries can themselves be considered as a linear sum of some other primary set ($\mathbf{Q}_1$, $\mathbf{Q}_2$, $\mathbf{Q}_3$). The equations are more economically set up in matrix notation.

A transformation from one set of primaries ($\mathbf{P}_1$, $\mathbf{P}_2$, $\mathbf{P}_3$) to another set ($\mathbf{Q}_1$, $\mathbf{Q}_2$, $\mathbf{Q}_3$) is specified by a general homogeneous linear transformation. The rules for choosing the new primaries ensure that the matrix A relating ($\mathbf{P}_1$, $\mathbf{P}_2$, $\mathbf{P}_3$) to ($\mathbf{Q}_1$, $\mathbf{Q}_2$, $\mathbf{Q}_3$) has an inverse (i.e. the determinant of A $\neq$ zero). A test color in the original primary set can be described in terms of either primary set. In particular, a given test color S with tristimulus values $P_{S,i}$ in Primary set ($\mathbf{Q}_1$, $\mathbf{Q}_2$, $\mathbf{Q}_3$):

$$\begin{matrix} P_{S,1} \\ P_{S,2} \\ P_{S,3} \end{matrix} = \begin{bmatrix} a_{11} & a_{12} & a_{13} \\ a_{21} & a_{22} & a_{23} \\ a_{31} & a_{32} & a_{33} \end{bmatrix} \begin{bmatrix} \mathbf{Q}_{S,1} \\ \mathbf{Q}_{S,2} \\ \mathbf{Q}_{S,3} \end{bmatrix} \tag{3.16}$$

has tristimulus values $Q_{S,i}$ in Primary set ($\mathbf{P}_1$, $\mathbf{P}_2$, $\mathbf{P}_3$):

$$\begin{matrix} Q_{S,1} \\ Q_{S,2} \\ Q_{S,3} \end{matrix} = \begin{bmatrix} b_{11} & b_{12} & b_{13} \\ b_{21} & b_{22} & b_{23} \\ b_{31} & b_{32} & b_{33} \end{bmatrix} \begin{bmatrix} \mathbf{P}_{S,1} \\ \mathbf{P}_{S,2} \\ \mathbf{P}_{S,3} \end{bmatrix} \tag{3.17}$$

where matrix B is the inverse of matrix A. In particular, if the tristimulus values at the new primary set ($\mathbf{Q}_1$, $\mathbf{Q}_2$, $\mathbf{Q}_3$) are known in the original set ($\mathbf{P}_1$, $\mathbf{P}_2$, $\mathbf{P}_3$), the matrix A can be written explicitly:

$$\begin{bmatrix} a_{11} & a_{12} & a_{13} \\ a_{21} & a_{22} & a_{23} \\ a_{31} & a_{32} & a_{33} \end{bmatrix} = \begin{bmatrix} {}^{P}\mathbf{Q}_{1,1} & {}^{P}\mathbf{Q}_{2,1} & {}^{P}\mathbf{Q}_{3,1} \\ {}^{P}\mathbf{Q}_{1,2} & {}^{P}\mathbf{Q}_{2,2} & {}^{P}\mathbf{Q}_{3,2} \\ {}^{P}\mathbf{Q}_{1,3} & {}^{P}\mathbf{Q}_{2,3} & {}^{P}\mathbf{Q}_{3,3} \end{bmatrix} \tag{3.18}$$

where ${}^{P}\mathbf{Q}_{1,1}$, ${}^{P}\mathbf{Q}_{1,2}$, and ${}^{P}\mathbf{Q}_{1,3}$ are the tristimulus values of primary $\mathbf{Q}_1$, ${}^{P}\mathbf{Q}_{2,1}$, ${}^{P}\mathbf{Q}_{2,2}$, and ${}^{P}\mathbf{Q}_{2,3}$ are the tristimulus values of primary $\mathbf{Q}_2$, and ${}^{P}\mathbf{Q}_{3,1}$, ${}^{P}\mathbf{Q}_{3,2}$, and ${}^{P}\mathbf{Q}_{3,3}$ are the tristimulus values of primary $\mathbf{Q}_3$ in the $\mathbf{P}_1$, $\mathbf{P}_2$, $\mathbf{P}_3$ primary set. These assignments uniquely determine the transformation. However, the data will be normalized to the energy units of the spectral matches. To obtain the same normalization as the original $\mathbf{P}_1$, $\mathbf{P}_2$, $\mathbf{P}_3$ primary set, a diagonal matrix containing the inverse of the energy units, e_i is used to multiply matrix B.

The properties of a homogeneous linear transformation (also called an affine transformation) include: straight lines remain straight after transformation; parallel lines remain parallel; and plane surfaces remain plane surfaces.

Transformations may also be made directly between chromaticity coefficients. If matrix B is known, the chromaticity coordinates, q_1 and q_2, are given by:

$$q_1 = b11p_1 + b12p_2 + b13p_3/[(b11 + b12 + b13)p_1 + (b12 + b22 + b23)p_2 + (b31 + b32 + b33)p_3] \tag{3.19}$$

$$q_2 = b21p_1 + b22p_2 + b23p_3/[(b11 + b12 + b13)p_1 + (b12 + b22 + b23)p_2 + (b31 + b32 + b33)p_3] \tag{3.20}$$

The transformation of chromaticity coefficients is projective rather than linear. Straight lines remain straight, but parallel lines need not remain parallel.

The subset of physically realizable lights may be thought of as only a small portion of a chromaticity space. The possibility exists of defining new primaries determined by locations in chromaticity space that lie outside the spectrum locus. In this case, the tristimulus values are not known. A transformation matrix, B′ is determined, except for an arbitrary scaling factor, by four unique loci in the chromaticity space, the three new primary coordinates and a fourth locus, usually the equal energy spectrum. These coordinates provide coefficients for three sets of simultaneous equations, one for each new primary, which are solved to yield the elements of matrix B′.

Primary transformations have been used for widely diverse purposes, including: comparison of data sets; derivation of an all-positive (imaginary) primary system (Judd, 1930); derivation of color planes in which equal vector lengths represent equal steps in discriminability (Judd, 1935; Galbraith and Marshall, 1985); derivation of a coordinate system in which the primaries represent the cone spectral sensitivities (König and Dieterici, 1893; Vos and Walraven, 1971; Smith and Pokorny, 1975; Stockman *et al.*, 1993; Stockman and Sharpe, 2000); and derivation of a coordinate system in which the primaries represent physiologically relevant opponent channel sensitivities (Schrödinger, 1925; Judd, 1951a).

3.2.3 CIE STANDARD COLORIMETRIC OBSERVERS

The industrial importance of trichromacy is in prediction of visual equivalency of a wide array of spectral power distributions. The colorimetric data provide a numerical specification at unit wavelength steps from which can be calculated tristimulus values for any spectral power distribution. The CIE in 1931 defined a standard observer for colorimetry, based on 2° color matching. The 2° observer is recommended for fields up to 4°. A 10° observer was defined in 1964 (CIE, 1964). The characteristics of the large-field observer are recommended for visual stimuli whose extent exceeds 4°, but should only be used at high photopic illuminances. Revision and evaluation of the standard observers remains a current interest of the CIE.

The 2° observer: The 1931 CIE standard observer for colorimetry incorporates both colorimetric and photometric behavior. The basic data were averaged chromaticity coefficients of Wright (1929) and Guild (1931). These were expressed in Wright's primaries and normalized to Standard Illuminant B. The luminous units of the primaries were adjusted to be consistent with the location of Standard Illuminant B and with the luminosity of the 1924 CIE standard observer for photometry.

Two equivalent statements of the color-matching behavior of the 1931 CIE standard observer were embodied in the (**R,G,B**) and (**X,Y,Z**) systems of units. The (**R,G,B**) system represented a first step in which spectral primaries were retained but all the negative values were in the $G(\lambda)$. Normalization was to the equal energy spectrum. An important consideration was that, following transform of the chromaticity coordinates, color matching functions using equation (3.15) were determined by incorporating $V(\lambda)$, the luminous efficiency function of the 1924 Standard observer for photometry. The 1924 CIE photometric observer was based on an entirely different set of observations than the color matching. The accuracy of the 1931 CIE colorimetric observer is thus dependent both on the accuracy of the Wright and Guild color matching data and on the accuracy of the 1924 CIE spectral luminous efficiency function. Stiles presented color matching data based on absolute radiometric calibration. His calculated chromaticity coefficients were very close to those of Wright and Guild.

The (**X,Y,Z**) system is an all-positive system derived by a linear transformation of the (**R,G,B**) system. An all-positive system means that the primaries enclose the spectrum locus; the primaries are not realizable lights and are sometimes called 'imaginary' primaries. The transformation was defined so that the color matching function, Y_λ was equivalent to $V(\lambda)$, the CIE photopic luminous efficiency function for the standard observer. Therefore, the **X** and **Z** primaries have zero luminance. In color space the line of zero luminance is called the alychne (Schrödinger, 1920). Given that the luminous units of the (**R,G,B**) system are in the ratio 1:4.5907:0.0601, the equation for the alychne obeys:

$$r + 4.5901g + 0.0601b = 0 \tag{3.21}$$

The **X** and **Y** primaries were placed on a line connecting the color matches made above 550 nm. This means that **Z** has no contribution to color matching at long wavelengths. The **Y** and **Z** primaries were placed on a line tangent to the spectrum locus at 504 nm. This choice was to minimize the area between the unit triangle and the spectrum locus. The intersections of the three lines determine the chromaticity coordinates (r, g) of the new primaries. Normalization was to the equal-energy white. The (**X,Y,Z**) system is specified by a set of color matching functions, X_λ, Y_λ, and Z_λ shown in Figure 3.4 and a chromaticity diagram, x_λ, y_λ shown in Figure 3.5.

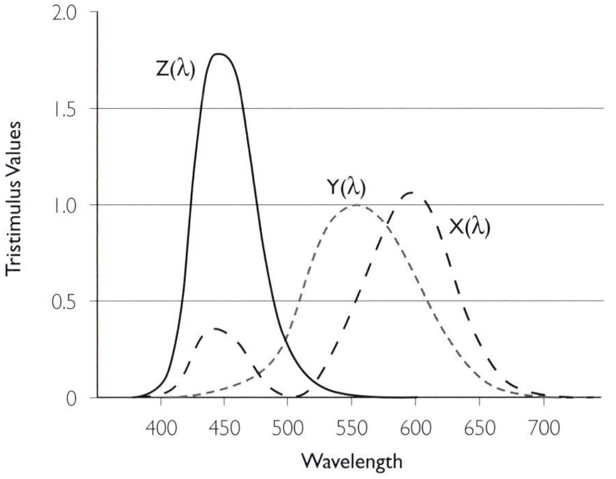

Figure 3.4 **CIE 1931 color matching functions. Spectral tristimulus values of constant radiance stimuli for different wavelengths. The three functions of wavelength define the color-matching properties of the CIE 1931 standard colorimetric observer. (Plotted from Table 3.1.)**

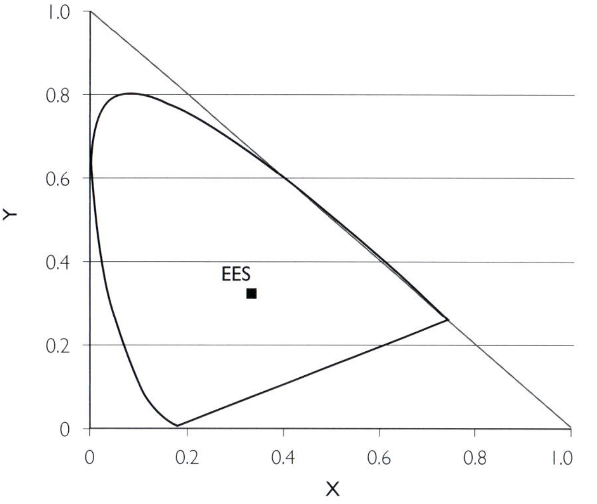

Figure 3.5 **CIE 1931 chromaticity diagram. CIE 1931 (x,y)-chromaticity diagram. (Plotted from Table 3.1.)**

The (**X,Y,Z**) system is widely used for color specification in industry. Table 3.1 shows color matching functions and chromaticity coordinates at 10 nm intervals.

The Judd (1951) modified 2° observer (Judd 1951b): After the acceptance of the 1931 CIE observer, problems were noted in the estimates of continuous spectral power distributions. The difficulties were ascribed to underestimation of luminosity at short wavelengths in the 1924 CIE photometric observer. Judd proposed a revision of the 1931 CIE colorimetric observer, with a modification of the Y_λ function below 460 nm and a slight modification of the chromaticity coordinates. The Judd revised colorimetric observer gave new functions, $X_{J,\lambda}$, $Y_{J,\lambda}$, and $Z_{J,\lambda}$ in the short wavelength region. The Judd revised colorimetric observer did not replace the CIE 2° observer, which remains widely used in industry. However, the Judd revised colorimetric observer is frequently used in color vision theory. Smith, Pokorny, and Zaidi (1983) observed that the Judd revised colorimetric observer is characterized by less lens and more prereceptoral macular pigment absorption than is the CIE 2° observer. Table 3.2 shows color matching functions and chromaticity coordinates at 10 nm intervals for the Judd (1951) revised observer.

In 1988, the CIE recommended a supplementary observer for photometry, termed V_M (λ). This observer differs from the Judd revised $y_{J\lambda}$ below 410 nm. The further revision to give V_M (λ) was originally proposed by Vos (1978), who also provided tabulations for an amended colorimetric observer.

The 10° observer: The 1964 CIE large-field standard observer for colorimetry was based on color matching data from the laboratories of Stiles and Burch (1959) and Speranskaya (1959, 1961). Since cone-dependent color matching functions were desired, the experimenters were concerned to avoid rod intrusion (changes in color matches caused by rod activity). Stiles and Burch (1959) maintained high photopic luminance of the matching fields. Multiple primary sets were used to minimize rod contamination of the color matches. Finally, Stiles and Burch (1959) made mathematical corrections to the data using a theoretical expectation of the nature of rod intrusion (see also Wyszecki and Stiles, 1982; Shapiro *et al.*, 1994).

The CIE transformed the data into an all-positive system with properties similar to those of the 1931 (**X,Y,Z**) system. The 1964 10° standard observer is specified by a set of color matching functions, $X_{10}(\lambda)$ $Y_{10}(\lambda)$, and $Z_{10}(\lambda)$ and a chromaticity diagram, $x_{10}(\lambda)$, $y_{10}(\lambda)$. The $Y_{10}(\lambda)$ represents the relative spectral luminous

Table 3.1 Color matching functions and chromaticity coordinates for the CIE (1931) Standard colorimetric observer

Wavelength	X	Y	Z	x	y
380	0.0014	0	0.0065	0.1772	0.0000
390	0.0042	0.0001	0.0201	0.1721	0.0041
400	0.0143	0.0004	0.0679	0.1731	0.0048
410	0.0435	0.0012	0.2074	0.1726	0.0048
420	0.1344	0.0040	0.6456	0.1714	0.0051
430	0.2839	0.0116	1.3856	0.1689	0.0069
440	0.3483	0.0230	1.7471	0.1644	0.0109
450	0.3362	0.0380	1.7721	0.1566	0.0177
460	0.2908	0.0600	1.6692	0.1440	0.0297
470	0.1954	0.0910	1.2876	0.1241	0.0578
480	0.0956	0.1390	0.813	0.0913	0.1327
490	0.032	0.2080	0.4652	0.0454	0.2950
500	0.0049	0.3230	0.272	0.0082	0.5384
510	0.0093	0.5030	0.1582	0.0139	0.7502
520	0.0633	0.7100	0.0782	0.0743	0.8338
530	0.1655	0.8620	0.0422	0.1547	0.8058
540	0.2904	0.9540	0.0203	0.2296	0.7543
550	0.4334	0.9950	0.0087	0.3016	0.6924
560	0.5945	0.9950	0.0039	0.3731	0.6245
570	0.7621	0.9520	0.0021	0.4441	0.5547
580	0.9163	0.8700	0.0017	0.5125	0.4866
590	1.0263	0.7570	0.0011	0.5752	0.4242
600	1.0622	0.6310	0.0008	0.6270	0.3725
610	1.0026	0.5030	0.0003	0.6658	0.3340
620	0.8544	0.3810	0.0002	0.6915	0.3084
630	0.6424	0.2650	0	0.7080	0.2920
640	0.4479	0.1750	0	0.7191	0.2809
650	0.2835	0.1070	0	0.7260	0.2740
660	0.1649	0.0610	0	0.7300	0.2700
670	0.0874	0.0320	0	0.7320	0.2680
680	0.0468	0.0170	0	0.7335	0.2665
690	0.0227	0.0082	0	0.7346	0.2654
700	0.0114	0.0041	0	0.7347	0.2653
710	0.0058	0.0021	0	0.7347	0.2653
720	0.0029	0.0010	0	0.7347	0.2653
730	0.0014	0.0005	0	0.7347	0.2653
740	0.0007	0.0003	0	0.7347	0.2653
750	0.0003	0.0001	0	0.7347	0.2653
760	0.0002	0.0001	0	0.7347	0.2653
770	0.0001	0	0	0.7347	0.2653
780	0	0	0	0.7347	0.2653

efficiency function of the 10° standard observer, although it has never been accepted as a standard for photometry. Since the data are representative of matches made by an observer without rod function, 10° matches made by color normal observers with other primaries and luminances need not in general correspond to the 10° CIE Standard observer.

Properties of the chromaticity diagram: In the all-positive (**X,Y,Z**) system, an isosceles right triangle completely encloses the experimentally determined chromaticity diagram (Figure 3.5). The abscissa ($y = 0$) is the alychne. The spectrum locus forms its characteristic horseshoe shape. A line connects the coordinates for 380 nm and 700 nm and represents mixtures formed by the extreme short wavelength and the extreme long wavelength lights.

Chromaticity coordinates (x, y) may be calculated for light of any spectral power distribution. The tristimulus values of Q are given by:

Table 3.2 Color matching functions and chromaticity coordinates for the Judd (1951) Revised colorimetric observer. Values are tabulated at 10 nm intervals between 380 nm and 780 nm

Wavelength	X	Y	Z	x	y
380	0.0045	0.0004	0.0224	0.1648	0.0147
390	0.0201	0.0015	0.0925	0.1762	0.0131
400	0.0611	0.0045	0.2799	0.1768	0.0130
410	0.1267	0.0093	0.5835	0.1761	0.0129
420	0.2285	0.0175	1.0622	0.1747	0.0134
430	0.3081	0.0273	1.4526	0.1723	0.0153
440	0.3312	0.0379	1.6064	0.1677	0.0192
450	0.2888	0.0468	1.4717	0.1598	0.0259
460	0.2323	0.0600	1.2880	0.1470	0.0380
470	0.1745	0.0910	1.1133	0.1266	0.0660
480	0.092	0.1390	0.7552	0.0933	0.1409
490	0.0318	0.2080	0.4461	0.0464	0.3033
500	0.0048	0.3230	0.2644	0.0081	0.5454
510	0.0093	0.5030	0.1541	0.0140	0.7548
520	0.0636	0.7100	0.0763	0.0748	0.8354
530	0.1668	0.8620	0.0412	0.1559	0.8056
540	0.2926	0.9540	0.0200	0.2310	0.7532
550	0.4364	0.9950	0.0088	0.3030	0.6909
560	0.597	0.9950	0.0039	0.3741	0.6235
570	0.7642	0.9520	0.0020	0.4448	0.5541
580	0.9159	0.8700	0.0016	0.5124	0.4867
590	1.0225	0.7570	0.0011	0.5742	0.4251
600	1.0544	0.6310	0.0007	0.6253	0.3742
610	0.9922	0.5030	0.0003	0.6635	0.3363
620	0.8432	0.3810	0.0002	0.6887	0.3112
630	0.6327	0.2650	0.0001	0.7047	0.2952
640	0.4404	0.1750	0	0.7156	0.2844
650	0.2787	0.1070	0	0.7226	0.2774
660	0.1619	0.0610	0	0.7263	0.2737
670	0.0858	0.0320	0	0.7284	0.2716
680	0.0459	0.0170	0	0.7297	0.2703
690	0.0222	0.0082	0	0.7303	0.2697
700	0.0114	0.0041	0	0.7347	0.2653
710	0.0058	0.0021	0	0.7347	0.2653
720	0.0029	0.0010	0	0.7347	0.2653
730	0.0014	0.0005	0	0.7347	0.2653
740	0.0007	0.0003	0	0.7347	0.2653
750	0.0003	0.0001	0	0.7347	0.2653
760	0.0002	0.0001	0	0.7347	0.2653
770	0.0001	0	0	0.7347	0.2653
780	0	0	0	0.7347	0.2653

$$\begin{bmatrix} X_Q \\ Y_Q \\ Z_Q \end{bmatrix} \begin{matrix} = \\ = \\ = \end{matrix} \begin{bmatrix} K\,\Sigma\, P(\lambda) \\ K\,\Sigma\, P(\lambda) \\ K\,\Sigma\, P(\lambda) \end{bmatrix} \begin{bmatrix} X(\lambda), \\ Y(\lambda), \\ Z(\lambda), \end{bmatrix} \qquad \begin{matrix} (3.22) \\ (3.23) \\ (3.24) \end{matrix}$$

where K is a constant and $P(\lambda)$ is the spectral power distribution. The chromaticity coordinates of Q are given by:

$$x_Q = X_Q/(X_Q + Y_Q + Z_Q), \qquad (3.25)$$
$$y_Q = Y_Q/(X_Q + Y_Q + Z_Q). \qquad (3.26)$$

Useful relations to transfer among the tristimulus values and the chromaticity coordinates are:

$$X_Q = (x_Q/y_Q)Y_Q \qquad (3.27)$$
$$Z_Q = (z_Q/y_Q)\ Y_Q = ((1 - x_Q - y_Q)/y_Q)Y_Q \qquad (3.28)$$

In equations 3.22–3.24, K is a normalizing constant that disappears from the chromaticity coordinates. In the definition of the 1924 CIE standard observer for photometry, K is identified with k_m the conversion factor for lumens/watt. The value Y_Q can thus be expressed in lumens. The spectral power distribution Q is completely specified colorimetrically by its tristimulus values, X_Q, Y_Q, Z_Q, or alternatively by its chromaticity coordinates and luminance, x_Q, y_Q, Y_Q.

Representation of papers or filters in the x,y chromaticity diagram: There is an alternative way to consider K that is useful for specification of transmitting filters or reflective surfaces, such as papers. In this case, the colorimetric properties of the filter or paper under the illuminant are important but the absolute radiance level of the source is irrelevant. Suppose there is a pigment sample of spectral reflectance $\rho(\lambda)$ or a filter of spectral transmission $\tau(\lambda)$ viewed under an illumination, H of spectral distribution $H(\lambda)$. Equations 3.22–3.24 are rewritten to incorporate the spectral properties of the sample, S. For a pigment sample:

$$X_S = K \sum_\lambda \rho(\lambda)H(\lambda)\, X(\lambda), \tag{3.29}$$

$$Y_S = K \sum_\lambda \rho(\lambda)H(\lambda)\, Y(\lambda), \tag{3.30}$$

$$Z_S = K \sum_\lambda \rho(\lambda)H(\lambda)\, Z(\lambda). \tag{3.31}$$

With K set at $100/\sum_\lambda H(\lambda)Y(\lambda)$, Y_S has the value of $100[\sum_\lambda \rho(\lambda)H(\lambda)Y(\lambda)]/[\sum_\lambda H(\lambda)Y(\lambda)]$. If the object is a perfectly diffusing surface, with $\rho(\lambda) = 1.0$ for all wavelengths, or a perfectly transmitting object, with $\tau(\lambda) = 1.0$ for all wavelengths, Y has the value 100. Thus, Y may be interpreted as the percentage luminous reflectance or percentage luminous transmittance of the sample. Calculation of the percentage luminous reflectance or transmittance is ratified only for the 1931 CIE colorimetric standard observer (Wyszecki and Stiles, 1982). Figure 3.6 shows the necessary calculations for a Wratten gelatin (No. 78) and CIE Standard Illuminant A[1].

A sample whose chromaticity coordinates are known may be specified by its dominant wavelength, λ_d, and its excitation purity, p_e, (Figure 3.6) for a specified CIE Illuminant. The dominant wavelength of sample S for Standard Illuminant A is the wavelength occurring at the intersection of the spectrum locus and a line extending from the locus of A through Q. If Q occurs in a region of the diagram for which the line extending from A to Q has no intersection with the spectrum locus, then the complementary wavelength may be used and should be noted by $-\lambda_d$ or λ_c. The excitation purity is the ratio of the distance from A to Q and the distance from A to λ_d:

$$p_e = (x_Q - x_A)/(x_d - x_A) = (y_Q - y_A)/(y_d - y_A) \tag{3.32}$$

In the case of a light whose dominant wavelength is $-\lambda_d$, the intersection with the line joining 380 nm and 700 nm is used. Excitation purity is zero when A and Q coincide and unity when Q and λ_d coincide. Both dominant wavelength and excitation purity may be estimated graphically. Precise computational methods for calculation of dominant wavelength are detailed by Wyszecki and Stiles (1982). The specification of dominant wavelength and excitation purity is widely used by manufacturers of colored filters.

Primary transformations using the CIE observers: Primary transformations using one of the CIE observers are simple because the tristimulus values (X,Y,Z) may be calculated for any choice of three lights. As an example of a problem applicable to visual science, consider the use of a color monitor system. The primaries are the three phosphors. All lights that can be produced on the monitor are combinations of possible light outputs of the three phosphors. Calibration of the relative spectral power distribution will yield the chromaticity coordinates (x_i, y_i) and calibration of the maximal luminance will yield $Y_{max,i}$ for phosphor (i). The luminance for phosphor (i) to light S is described by

$$Y_{S,i} = p_{S,i}\, Y_{max,i} \tag{3.33}$$

where $p_{S,i}$ is the proportion of maximal phosphor output for phosphor (i). Further, the CIE tristimulus values for light S can be calculated from $Y_{S,1}$, $Y_{S,2}$, and $Y_{S,3}$:

$$\begin{aligned} X_S &= X_{S,1} + X_{S,2} + X_{S,3} \\ &= (x_1/y_1)Y_{S,1} + (x_2/y_2)Y_{S,2} \\ &\quad + (x_3/y_3)Y_{S,3} \end{aligned} \tag{3.34}$$

$$Y_S = Y_{S,1} + Y_{S,2} + Y_{S,3} \tag{3.35}$$

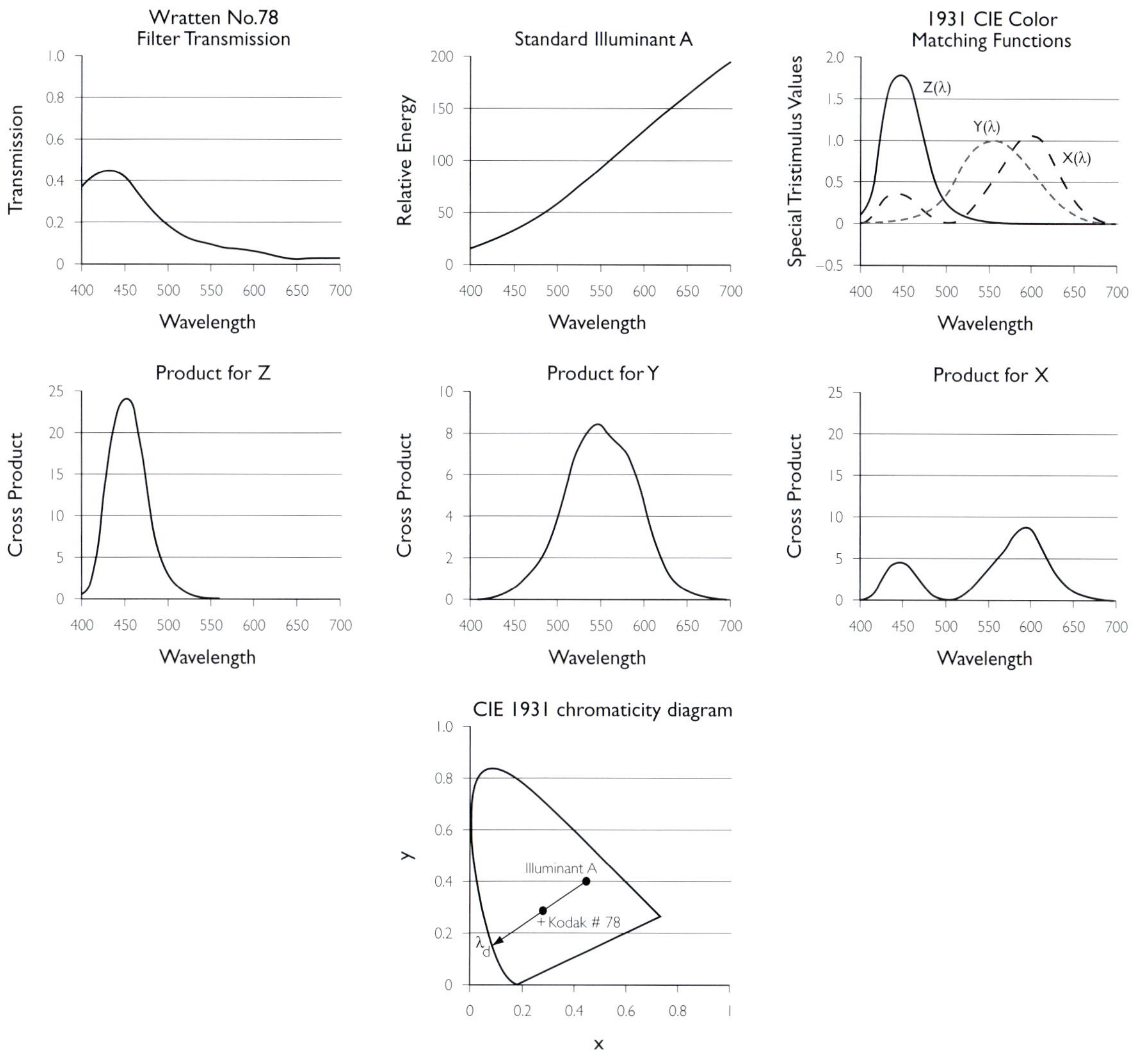

Figure 3.6 Calculation of tristimulus values and chromaticity coordinates for Wratten filter (No. 78) viewed under CIE Standard Illuminant A. The upper three panels show the transmission for the filter, the relative energy output for Standard Illuminant A and the 1931 CIE color matching functions. The middle three panels show the cross products of the filter transmission, CIE Standard Illuminant A, and the color matching functions. The lower panel shows the chromaticity diagram with the chromaticity coordinates of CIE standard illuminant A and the filter-illuminant combination. The line extending from CIE standard illuminant A, through the chromaticity coordinates of the filter-illuminant combination to the spectrum locus gives the dominant wavelength of 482 nm. The excitation purity is 0.45 and the luminous transmittance is 8.8%.

$$\begin{aligned} Z_S &= Z_{S,1} + Z_{S,2} + Z_{S,3} \\ &= (z_1/y_1)Y_{S,1} + (z_2/y_2)Y_{S,2} \\ &\quad + (z_3/y_3)Y_{S,3} \end{aligned} \qquad (3.36)$$

This can be written in matrix form as:

$$\begin{bmatrix} X_S \\ Y_S \\ Z_S \end{bmatrix} \begin{matrix} = \\ = \\ = \end{matrix} \begin{bmatrix} x_1/y_1 & x_2/y_2 & x_3/y_3 \\ 1 & 1 & 1 \\ z_1/y_1 & z_2/y_2 & z_3/y_3 \end{bmatrix} \begin{bmatrix} Y_{S,1} \\ Y_{S,2} \\ Y_{S,3} \end{bmatrix} \qquad (3.37)$$

where $Y_{S,i}$ is given by equation (3.33). It is seen that matrix A contains only the chromaticity coefficients which are a characteristic of the phosphors. The inverse matrix gives the luminances of the phosphors required to produce a desired chromaticity and luminance specified in CIE coordinates.

3.2.4 EXPERIMENTAL VARIABLES

The Wright (1929) and Guild (1931) data were based on a 2° field viewed with foveal fixation. The method was maximum saturation matching in which the test light and one primary were matched to the remaining primaries in a bipartite field. The effects of procedure, field size, retinal illuminance, and fixation are important in color matching experiments and are detailed below.

Maxwell matching: In Maxwell matching, the spectral light plus a broadband light (such as the EES) are presented in one hemifield and compared to the three primaries presented in the other hemifield (Crawford, 1965). There are subtle differences in the color matching functions derived from the two methodologies which have eluded explanation (Zaidi, 1986). Stiles and Burch (1955) observed that the precision of color matches in the short wavelength region of the spectrum was improved by superimposing a mid-spectrum light on both fields.

Effect of field size: Color matches depend on the field of view; for example, color matching functions based on a 1.5° field (Fridrikh, 1957) show systematic differences from the 2° data (Pokorny *et al.*, 1976). A match for a 2° field will not hold for a larger or smaller field. There is a continuous change in the amounts of the primaries required for the color match as field size is increased (Pokorny and Smith, 1976).

For certain color stimuli in a 10° colorimetric field, a color inhomogeneity may appear at the area of fixation. This appears as an ill-defined ellipse with major axis horizontal, extending 1° or 2°, and is called the Maxwell spot. The spot follows fixation and is best observed by switching rapidly from viewing one half of the bipartite field to the other. In 10° trichromatic matching, the observer must ignore the Maxwell spot (e.g. Stiles and Burch, 1959). Alternatively an annular field may be used (e.g. Speranskaya, 1959, 1961). The Maxwell spot is usually attributed to higher density of macular pigment in the central 1–2° of the fovea. Trezona (1970) advanced an alternate hypothesis that the Maxwell spot might be a rod contrast color. This conclusion was based on her studies of 10° color matching using a tetrachromatic technique. A fourth primary was added to the mixture field to allow the observer to balance the rods in a dark-adapted state. By repeating the matching procedure in light- and dark-adapted states, a match is eventually obtained that holds in both light- and dark-adapted states. This 'tetrachromatic' match does not show a Maxwell spot. Palmer (1981) analyzed Trezona's paradigm and showed that her stimulus situation also reduced the differential effect of macular pigment in the two halves of the bipartite field.

When the color mixture field is reduced below 30' of arc, there is a severe loss of discrimination. With stable fixation, if the field subtends 15' or 20' and is viewed either foveally or at 20' or 40' from the fovea, the normal trichromatic observer becomes dichromatic, requiring only two primaries for full spectrum color matching (Thomson and Wright, 1947). The color matches resemble those of the stationary congenital color defect, tritanopia (see section 3.5).

Effect of retinal illuminance: The scalar property states that metamers hold for all levels of retinal illumination; however, the range for which the 2° trichromatic metamers hold is limited to about 1–8000 td. Chromatic discrimination is optimal in a similar range of retinal illuminance. When the retinal illuminance exceeds 5000–10 000 td, lights that were metamers are no longer perceived as such (Brindley, 1953; Terstiege, 1967; Alpern, 1979; Wyszecki and Stiles, 1980). For example, in the match of 589 nm to a mixture of 545 nm and 670 nm primaries, a greater proportion of the 670 nm primary is required as retinal illuminance increases above 8000 td. The retinal illuminance at which the metamers break down is a level at which photopigment is significantly depleted by bleaching. While the change in match is a failure of the scalar property, the matches remain trichromatic. The effect and its explanation are described further in section 3.2.5.

With reduction in retinal illuminance, color matches continue to hold as low as 1 td. One effect of reduction in retinal illuminance is discrimination loss, similar to small-field tritanopia (Grigorovici and Aricescu-Savopol, 1958). With further reduction in luminance, rod intrusion becomes evident (Richards and Luria, 1964). Whether this is due to rod function in a foveal 2°

area or to changes in fixation with decreases in luminance is unknown. Estévez (1979) suggested that the Wright (1929), Guild (1931), and Stiles (1955) 2° data have a small rod contribution. Pokorny and Smith (1981) and Pokorny, Smith, and Went (1981) noted rod contribution in some color-defective individuals for 50 td fields as small as 1°. Rod intrusion is more easily seen in the color-defective observer whose cone-dominated color vision is compromised.

Peripheral color matching: Color matching may also be performed using the parafoveal or peripheral retina. With the dark-adapted eye and a scotopic illuminance, the normal observer is monochromatic over most of the spectrum, using the rod mechanism for color matching. At mesopic and photopic levels, parafoveal and peripheral color matching is trichromatic. Color matching data that allow the description of peripheral color matches in terms of foveal color vision have been described by Moreland and Cruz (1959) using an asymmetric matching procedure. For a spectral test field of $40' \times 80'$ viewed by the periphery and a $40' \times 80'$ mixture field viewed by the fovea with WDW normalization (section 3.2.2 above) at the foveal match, Moreland and Cruz determined the proportions of foveal primaries necessary to match various peripherally viewed stimuli. The chromaticity coefficients were all inside rather than on the spectrum locus for Wright's 2° foveal data, indicating that a spectral radiation of fixed size viewed in the peripheral retina is desaturated in appearance compared with its appearance at the fovea. Abramov, Gordon, and Chan (1991) have emphasized that a peripheral stimulus must be larger than a foveal stimulus in order to appear colored (see section 4.2.1 in Chapter 4). Stabell and Stabell (1976) used the Moreland and Cruz paradigm to evaluate rod contribution to color matching by taking measurements during the cone-plateau period following intense light adaptation and noted that rod participation produces changes in all three chromaticity coordinates.

3.2.5 INTERPRETATION OF COLOR MATCHING

It was acknowledged by Young (1802) that every spectral wavelength is not recognized independently in the visual system. He proposed three physiological mechanisms or fundamentals that are differentially sensitive in the visible spectrum. In principal, the limitation of trichromacy could occur at any stage in the visual system (Brindley, 1970). Brindley proposed that foveal trichromacy is photopigment-limited. However, with a larger matching field or with parafoveal viewing, a fourth photoreceptor type, the rod, becomes active. Color matching remains trichromatic but does not obey Grassmann's laws. In this case, trichromatic color matching is neurally limited (Smith and Pokorny, 1977).

The quantal hypothesis: Brindley formalized the biological interpretation of color matching with his proposal that 2° foveal color matching is achieved when the quantal catch rate is equivalent for each active photopigment (Brindley, 1970). Since three sets of cone photopigments are active in the normal 2° fovea, color matching is trichromatic and photopigment-limited. Thus, foveal color matching can be considered a powerful tool in understanding human color vision, since the appropriate linear transform will reveal the effective absorption spectra of the cone visual photopigments. At the same time, color matching is a limited tool in understanding human color vision since it can give us no information on the subsequent neural transformations performed by the retina and visual cortex.

The spectral sensitivity of the fundamentals must be a linear transform of the color matching functions. However, since there are infinitely many possible linear transformations of color matching functions, external criteria are needed to guide and limit the transformation. The classic assumption, made by König was that congenital color-defectives (section 3.5) represented reduction forms of normal color vision. An early set of fundamentals, which relied on color matching data from congenital color-defective observers was published by König and Dieterici (1886, 1893). Fundamentals that rely on properties of color-defective vision are called König fundamentals.

Cone fundamentals: König hypothesized that the dichromatic forms of color defect represent reduced forms of normal color vision. Modern fundamentals are based on the König hypothesis

(Vos and Walraven, 1971; Smith and Pokorny, 1975; Stockman *et al.*, 1993; Stockman and Sharpe, 2000). We term the fundamentals S_λ, M_λ, and L_λ to indicate that these fundamentals explicitly represent the energy-based, corneal spectral sensitivities of the short-wavelength (SWS), middle-wavelength (MWS), and long-wavelength (LWS) sensitive cones respectively.

Vos and Walraven (1971) suggested that the Judd (1951) revised observer should be used to derive fundamentals. They further postulated that the three fundamentals should add to make the Judd (1951) luminous efficiency function, $y_{J,\lambda}$. Smith and Pokorny (1975) suggested that the luminous efficiency function should be determined only by $L(\lambda)$ and $M(\lambda)$, giving the property that the relative height of $S(\lambda)$ is undetermined. Their values for $L(\lambda)$ and $M(\lambda)$ differ only at short wavelengths from Vos and Walraven. Since the protanopic and deuteranopic copunctal points fall on the inverse diagonal of the spectrum locus in the chromaticity diagram, both transformations equate $S(\lambda)$ with $Z(\lambda)$. The Smith and Pokorny (1975) transformation equations, with $S(\lambda)/Y_j(\lambda)$ scaled to have a height of unity at 400 nm, are:[2]

$$L_\lambda = 0.15516\ X_{J,\lambda} + 0.54307\ Y_{J,\lambda}\ 0.03287\ Z_{J,\lambda} \quad (3.38)$$

$$M_\lambda = -0.15516\ X_{J,\lambda} + 0.45692\ Y_{J,\lambda} + 0.03287\ Z_{J,\lambda} \quad (3.39)$$

$$S_\lambda = 0.01608\ Z_{J,\lambda} \quad (3.40)$$

According to the requirement for the transformation:

$$Y_{J,\lambda} = L_{,\lambda+}\ M_\lambda \quad (3.41)$$

Table 3.3 shows the Smith and Pokorny fundamentals as calculated from equations 3.38–3.40.

Table 3.3 Color matching functions and chromaticity coordinates for the Smith and Pokorny fundamentals. Values are tabulated at 10 nm intervals between 400 nm and 700 nm

Wavelength	L	M	S	V_λ	l	s
400	0.0027	0.0018	0.0045	0.0045	0.6055	1.0002
410	0.0055	0.0038	0.0094	0.0093	0.5948	1.0089
420	0.0100	0.0075	0.0171	0.0175	0.5741	0.9760
430	0.0149	0.0124	0.0234	0.0273	0.5453	0.8556
440	0.0192	0.0187	0.0258	0.0379	0.5059	0.6816
450	0.0219	0.0249	0.0237	0.0468	0.4670	0.5057
460	0.0263	0.0337	0.0207	0.0600	0.4383	0.3452
470	0.0399	0.0511	0.0179	0.0910	0.4385	0.1967
480	0.0649	0.0741	0.0121	0.1390	0.4672	0.0874
490	0.1032	0.1048	0.0072	0.2080	0.4963	0.0345
500	0.1675	0.1555	0.0043	0.3230	0.5185	0.0132
510	0.2695	0.2335	0.0025	0.5030	0.5359	0.0049
520	0.3929	0.3171	0.0012	0.7100	0.5534	0.0017
530	0.4927	0.3693	0.0007	0.8620	0.5715	0.0008
540	0.5628	0.3912	0.0003	0.9540	0.5900	0.0003
550	0.6078	0.3872	0.0001	0.9950	0.6108	0.0001
560	0.6329	0.3621	0.0001	0.9950	0.6360	0.0001
570	0.6355	0.3165	0.0000	0.9520	0.6676	0.0000
580	0.6145	0.2555	0.0000	0.8700	0.7064	0.0000
590	0.5697	0.1873	0.0000	0.7570	0.7526	0.0000
600	0.5063	0.1247	0.0000	0.6310	0.8023	0.0000
610	0.4271	0.0759	0.0000	0.5030	0.8491	0.0000
620	0.3377	0.0433	0.0000	0.3810	0.8865	0.0000
630	0.2421	0.0229	0.0000	0.2650	0.9135	0.0000
640	0.1634	0.0116	0.0000	0.1750	0.9336	0.0000
650	0.1014	0.0056	0.0000	0.1070	0.9472	0.0000
660	0.0582	0.0028	0.0000	0.0610	0.9549	0.0000
670	0.0307	0.0013	0.0000	0.0320	0.9591	0.0000
680	0.0164	0.0006	0.0000	0.0170	0.9620	0.0000
690	0.0079	0.0003	0.0000	0.0082	0.9632	0.0000
700	0.0040	0.0001	0.0000	0.0041	0.9745	0.0000

The height of the LWS fundamental at its λ_{max} is 0.6373; that for the MWS fundamental at its λ_{max} is 0.3924. Figure 3.7 shows the Smith and Pokorny fundamentals, renormalized to their peak and plotted on a logarithmic axis.

A recent development is the use of the Stiles and Burch (1955, 1959) data to derive König fundamentals, e.g. (Estévez, 1979; Stockman *et al.*, 1993; Stockman and Sharpe, 2000). The goal of these attempts was to avoid the criticism that the CIE and Judd standard observers represent an amalgam of colorimetric and photometric data obtained from different individuals. A new difficulty is introduced. The Stiles and Burch pilot data do not incorporate luminosity, since the matching functions were obtained with direct energy calibrations of the primaries and test wavelengths. However, it is now considered useful for physiological fundamentals to incorporate luminosity. While the Y of the CIE 10° XYZ Standard Observer can be used to represent the relative luminous efficiency function, there are no measured dichromatic copunctal points for 10° fields (see section 3.5).

Physiologically based chromaticity diagram:

A physiologically based chromaticity space was suggested as early as Maxwell (1860). He postulated an isosceles triangle with the cone fundamentals at each corner. Although inherently attractive, the Maxwell triangle is difficult to use.

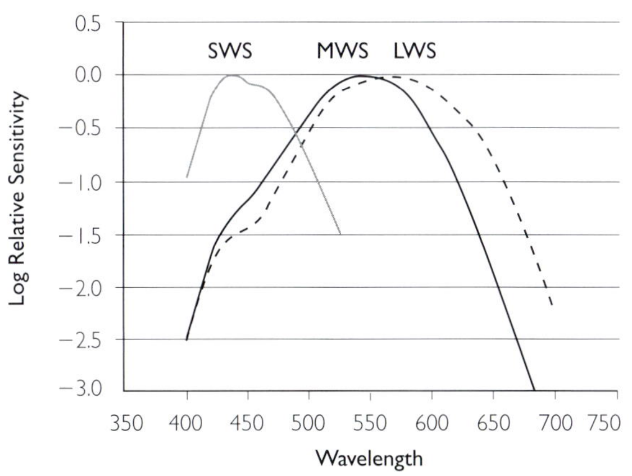

Figure 3.7 **Relative spectral sensitivity of the cone visual photopigments as proposed by Smith and Pokorny (1975). The curves are normalized to their own maxima.**

MacLeod and Boynton (1979) suggested that a useful and easily used chromaticity chart would be a constant luminance plane in which the cone spectral sensitivities formed rectangular axes. This is essentially the chromaticity diagram formed by the Smith and Pokorny fundamentals with the value of S_λ/Y_λ arbitrarily placed at unity at its peak.

$$l_\lambda = L_\lambda/(L_\lambda + M_\lambda) \tag{3.42}$$

$$m_\lambda = M_\lambda/(L_\lambda + M_\lambda) \tag{3.43}$$

$$s_\lambda = S_\lambda/(L_\lambda + M_\lambda) \tag{3.44}$$

This cone-based diagram includes the specific assumption that s_λ does not contribute to luminance. Figure 3.8 shows the cone-based diagram with s_λ plotted against l_λ. In the cone-based diagram the horizontal axis represents the exchange of LWS and MWS cone excitation at equiluminance, i.e. an increase in LWS cone excitation is offset by a decrease in MWS cone excitation but the sum is unity. The vertical axis represents variation in SWS cone excitation at a constant retinal illuminance. The protan

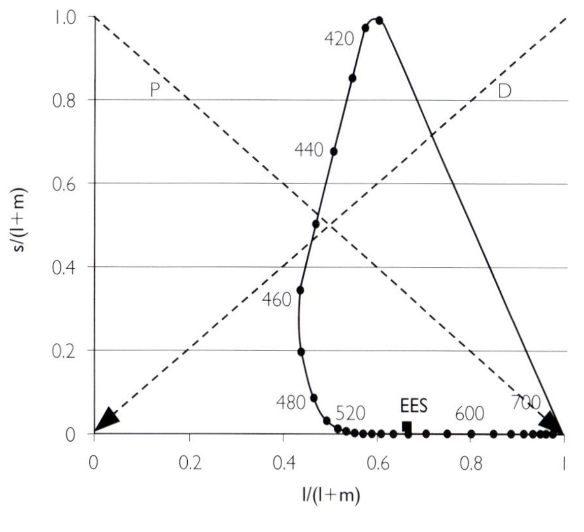

Figure 3.8 **MacLeod–Boynton (1979) diagram. Chromaticity diagram representing relative cone excitation. The relative SWS cone excitation s/(l+m) is plotted against l/(l+m), the proportion of LWS cone stimulation from equiluminant stimuli. The isochromatic lines for protanopes P and deuteranopes D converge at l=1 (point representing LWS) and m=1 (point representing MWS), respectively. Tritanopic isochromatic lines plot as parallel lines orthogonal to the ordinate.**

copunctal point is at coordinate (0,1); the deutan copunctal point is at (0,0). Tritan confusions are represented by a set of parallel, vertical lines. Although it is customary to refer to the MacLeod–Boynton diagram as a cone excitation diagram, it should be emphasized that the cone excitations are not equivalent to quantal excitation of the cones (see below).

Rod excitation relative to photopic luminance may be incorporated in the cone excitation diagram as a third dimension, by plotting $\mathbf{V}_{J\lambda}/V_{\lambda}$ on the z axis (Pokorny and Smith, 1986). For chromaticities produced by three physical primaries, rod confusion lines for a fixed scotopic luminance will be sets of parallel lines in the equiluminance plane (Shapiro *et al.*, 1996). The angles of these lines will be determined by the particular choice of primaries.

Cone trolands: Boynton and Kambe (1980) proposed the definition of a new unit, the cone troland. Following their suggestion, we can define the L, M, and S cone trolands at wavelength, λ as:

$$L_{\lambda}td = (I)\ L_{\lambda}/\mathbf{V}_{J\lambda} \quad (3.45)$$
$$M_{\lambda}td = (I)\ M_{\lambda}/\mathbf{V}_{J\lambda} \quad (3.46)$$
$$S_{\lambda}td = (I)\ S_{\lambda}\ 1.6064/\mathbf{V}_{J\lambda} = (I)\ Z_{\lambda}/\mathbf{V}_{J\lambda} \quad (3.47)$$

where I is the retinal illuminance in trolands, L_{λ}, M_{λ}, and S_{λ} are the Smith and Pokorny cone fundamentals, and $\mathbf{V}_{J\lambda}$ is the spectral luminous efficiency of the Judd (1951) observer. The SWS fundamental is renormalized to be equivalent to the Z_{λ} of the Judd observer (the normalization is arbitrary in the Smith and Pokorny fundamentals and was set for convenience in the MacLeod–Boynton diagram).

The cone troland has two important properties. First, cone trolands are proportional to the quantal excitation rate of the photoreceptors. Quanta are related to trolands at wavelength λ by the formula:

$$Q_{\lambda} = I/\ \mathbf{V}_{J\lambda}(10^7/8)(\lambda/555) \quad (3.48)$$

where Q_{λ} is the number of trolands, and the other symbols are described above. The quantal excitation rate for a given photoreceptor is proportional to the number of quanta multiplied by the relative absorption spectrum of the photoreceptor. For the LWS cone:

$$L_{Q,\lambda} = Q_{\lambda}(,L\lambda/L_{max})(\lambda_{Q,L}/\lambda) \quad (3.49)$$

L/L_{max} represents the relative spectral sensitivity of the photoreceptor and $(\lambda_{Q,L}/\lambda)$ converts from the energy base of the fundamental to the quantal base of an absorption spectrum. The term $(\lambda_{Q,L})$ is the wavelength at which the LWS absorption spectrum has its peak absorption. The peak of the absorption spectrum is shifted to shorter wavelength than the peak of the fundamental. When equations 3.48 and 3.49 are combined for each cone type:

$$L_{Q,\lambda} = L_{td,\lambda}/L_{max}(10^7/8)\ (\lambda_{Q,L}/555) \quad (3.50)$$
$$M_{Q,\lambda} = Q_{\lambda}M_{\lambda}/M_{max})\ (\lambda_{Q,M}/\lambda)$$
$$= M_{ts,\lambda}/M_{max}(10^7/8)\ (\lambda_{Q,M}/555) \quad (3.51)$$
$$S_{Q,\lambda} = Q_{\lambda}S_{\lambda}/S_{max}\ (\lambda_{Q,S}/\lambda)$$
$$= S_{td,\lambda}/Z_{max}(10^7/8)\ (\lambda_{Q,S}/555) \quad (3.52)$$

Thus for a given cone type, the quantal excitation at any wavelength is proportional to the cone trolands weighted by a constant.

Second, colorimetric calculations are easily made using the cone troland space (Smith and Pokorny, 1996). A light, Q specified by the Judd revised observer as x_{JQ}, y_{JQ}, Y_{JQ}, has a unique specification in the cone space given by l_Q, z_Q, Y_{JQ}. The tristimulus values, L_Q, $Y_{J,Q}$, Z_Q are calculated in the same way as for $X_{J,Q}$, $Y_{J,Q}$, and $Z_{J,Q}$. Expression in other primary systems follows the usual rules (for example, to transform between cone trolands and the phosphors of a color monitor). The equations (3.38–3.40) can be rewritten:

$$\begin{bmatrix} L_Q \\ Y_{JQ} \\ S_Q \end{bmatrix} \begin{matrix} = \\ = \\ = \end{matrix} \begin{bmatrix} l_1/y_{J1} & l_2/y_{J2} & l_3/y_{J3} \\ 1 & 1 & 1 \\ s_1/y_{J1} & s2/y_{J2} & s_3/y_{J3} \end{bmatrix} \begin{bmatrix} Y_{JQ,1} \\ Y_{JQ,2} \\ Y_{JQ,3} \end{bmatrix} \quad (3.53)$$

where the terms l, y_{Ji}, z_{Ji} represent the specification in chromaticity coordinates for phosphor (i) and $Y_{J,Q,j}$ represents the luminance of light Q for phosphor (i).

3.2.6 SOURCES OF INDIVIDUAL DIFFERENCES IN COLOR MATCHING

The parameter variables that may modify color matching data were discussed in section 3.2.4. These included the field size, the luminance level, the choice of primaries, and the method. Here we discuss the physiological mechanisms that may play a role in modifying matches for an individual or that may play a role in explaining inter-individual differences in matching. Since color matches are a linear transform of photopigment spectral sensitivity, factors that modify the spectral sensitivity can modify color matches. These factors include individual variation in photopigment spectra, variation in optical density of the photopigments, photoreceptor optics, and pre-retinal filters.

Variation in photopigment spectra: Modern molecular biology has defined the protein structure of the genes coding the photopigment opsins. To date there is at least one well-documented polymorphism of the L photopigment opsin (either the amino acid serine or alanine at position 180 on the L- opsin gene; Neitz *et al.*, 1991; Merbs and Nathans, 1992) which changes the peak wavelength of the absorption spectrum by a small amount (~3–5 nm). Sanocki, Shevell, and Winderickx (1994), using a technique which eliminates in large part inter-observer differences in prereceptoral filtering and photopigment optical density, show reliable small differences in color matching in the red–green spectral region for observers having the two different alleles. The same allele pattern also is present for the M-cone photopigment but at a low frequency and it is probable that there are other polymorphisms capable of modifying extinction spectra by small spectral shifts. There is now accumulating evidence that individuals with normal color vision exhibit small variation in the absorption spectra of the photopigments in their L and M cones.

An estimate of the extreme values that photopigment variation and optical density might assume in the normal population may be obtained by theoretically manipulating these variables and establishing the extreme values that fall within the intra-observer variability of color matching data. If WDW normalization (Wright, 1946; Wyszecki and Stiles, 1982) is used for both data and the synthesized CMFs, the effects of individual differences in prereceptoral filtering are eliminated. The choices of primaries and normalizing wavelengths are unimportant as long as the same are used for both the data and the synthesized CMFs. Smith, Pokorny, and Starr (1976) performed such an analysis for the Stiles and Burch (1955) 2° color matching data and a set of theoretical spectra based in large part on a transformation of the Judd (1951) color matching functions. The analysis can define the potential extreme limits of normal variation but cannot specify which variable or combination of the variables is responsible for the normal variation. Calculated variation in the S, M, and L cone spectral positions indicated the data variability was dominated by the theoretical L and M cone spectral shifts; S cone shifts had relatively little effect. Wavelength shifts in a range from −4 to +2 nm in the M cone spectrum and −3 to +7 nm in the L cone spectrum predicted WDW unit coordinates that fell within the extremes of the Stiles data.

Effective optical density of the photopigments: Light must be absorbed in the photopigments to be seen. The concentration of the pigment and the length of the light path affect an absorption spectrum. As light traverses a greater concentration of pigment, more light is absorbed and the extinction spectrum broadens. The rule governing absorption follows Beer's law. In the case of a visual photopigment, expressed in decadic base:

$$A = (1 - 10^{-\varepsilon_\lambda cl}) \qquad (3.54)$$

where A is the fraction absorbed, ε_λ is the decadic extinction coefficient, c refers to the concentration and l to the pathlength. The extinction coefficient, ε_λ, is a wavelength-dependent function that is characteristic of the photopigment. For visual photopigments, concentration and pathlength can be grouped as a single factor, the effective optical density of the photopigment.

A graphical sketch to demonstrate how the absorption spectrum broadens as the effective optical density increases is shown in Figure 3.9. The insert in the top panel schematically illustrates a path through a beaker of the rod photopigment rhodopsin. The curves show the calculated effective fractional absorbance at each successive layer of pigment. Light reaching each successive layer is the product of the incoming

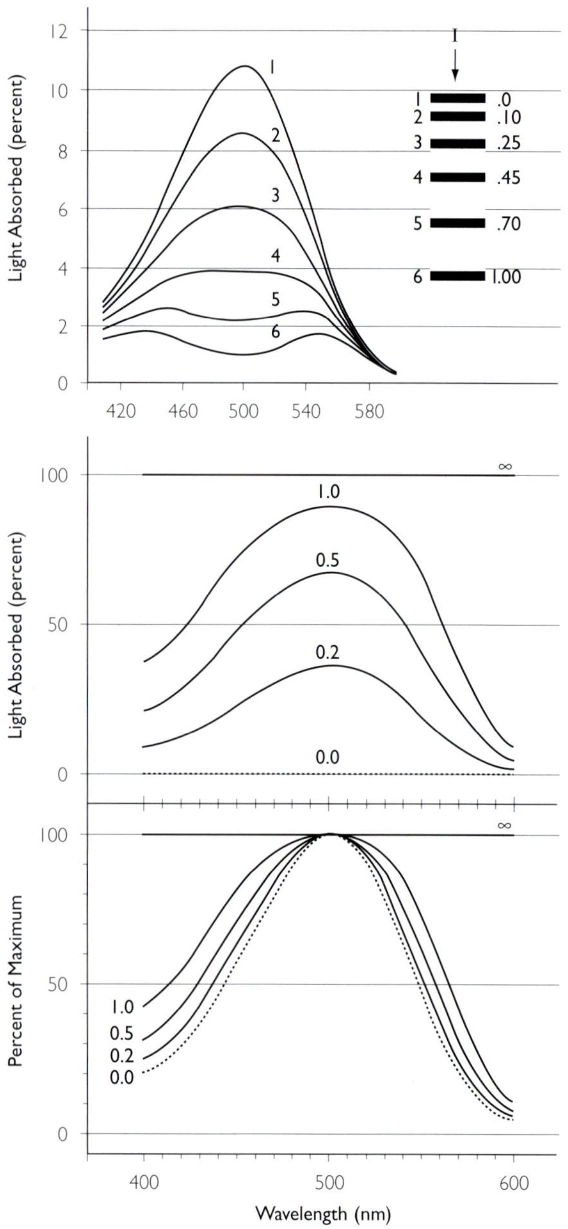

Figure 3.9 Effect of optical density on spectral sensitivity. (The top panel is from Goldstein and Williams, 1966; the bottom two panels are from Dartnall, 1962.)

light and the transmission of the layers that precede them. At the initial layer (1), the absorption resembles that of the extinction spectrum. At the final layer (6), most of the absorption is taking place in the tails of the extinction spectrum. The absorptance spectrum is the sum of the absorbances of all layers. The middle panel shows the fractional absorption spectrum, calculated for different optical densities of pigment. The lower panel shows the relative fractional absorption.

The analysis proposed by Smith, Pokorny and Starr can also be applied to variation in optical density. Calculated variation in photopigment optical densities could also predict the variability of the Stiles and Burch data. In this analysis a higher optical density was required for the L cone photopigment, a result found for all published comparisons of L and M cone optical density (Miller, 1972; Smith and Pokorny, 1973; Bowmaker *et al.*, 1978; Wyszecki and Stiles, 1980; Burns and Elsner, 1993). An optical density range of 0.15 to 0.45 for the M cone spectrum and 0.25 to 0.55 for the L cone spectrum predicted WDW unit coordinates that fell within the extremes of the Stiles (1955) data. The estimated standard deviation was 0.05.

Cone photoreceptors vary in length, with retinal position being longest in the center of the fovea (Polyak, 1957). Field size is an important variable in matching which may be attributed partially to changes in the effective optical density of photopigments. Pokorny, Smith and Starr (1976) extended their analysis to the difference of the Stiles (1955) 2° and the Stiles and Burch (1959) 10° data. The differences between the mean 2° and 10° data could be explained by a reduction in optical density of 0.10–0.15. Pokorny, Smith and Starr also calculated the theoretically acceptable range of optical densities of the L and M cone photopigments for data collected with a small field at several eccentricities. Thomson and Wright (1947) obtained small field tritanopic data from W.D. Wright's eye with a 15' field fixated directly or placed at eccentricities of 20' and 40' from fixation. There have been a number of experimental verifications of the change in color matches with field size (Horner and Purslow, 1947; Pokorny and Smith, 1976; Burns and Elsner, 1985; Eisner *et al.*, 1987; Swanson and Fish, 1996). These studies are all consistent with the interpretation that the effective optical densities of the photopigments decrease as field sizes increase. Figure 3.10 shows the estimated L cone optical density as a function of field size from a number of studies.

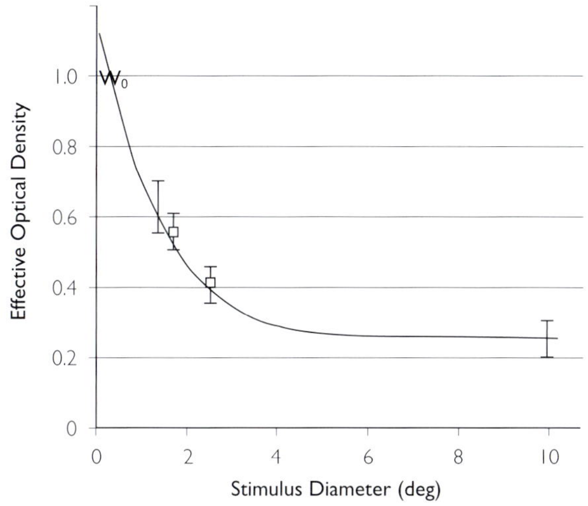

Figure 3.10 **Optical density of the L cones as a function of field size. (From Pokorny *et al.*, 1976.)**

Pre-retinal filters: The other major sources of variation in color matching are pre-retinal filters, namely the lens and macular pigment density. Figure 3.11 shows the density spectra for an average lens of a 32-year-old observer and the average macular pigment for a 2° field. These both show substantial variation in the population.

There is significant inter-individual variation in lens transmission and also a substantial change with age. Van Norren and Vos (1974) calculated from Crawford's (1949) scotopic spectral sensitivity data that individual variation in ocular absorption for a group of 50 young observers (17–30 year) is about ±25% of the average absorption at short wavelengths. Adult lens transmission has been characterized as having two components, T_{L1} and T_{L2} with T_{L1} varying with age (Tan, 1971; Pokorny *et al.*, 1987). An algorithm that allows calculation of an average lens transmission between the ages of 20 and 60 years is:

$$T_L = T_{L1}\,[1 + 0.02(A - 32)] + T_{L2} \qquad (3.55)$$

where T_L, T_{L1}, and T_{L2} represent the spectral lens densities tabulated in Table 3.4 and A is the chronological age. Beyond the age of 60, there is an acceleration in decrease in lens (Pokorny *et al.*, 1987). This acceleration is characteristic of a population average but was not observed in studies where observers were screened so as to eliminate those with incipient cataracts (Weale, 1988; Moreland *et al.*, 1991).

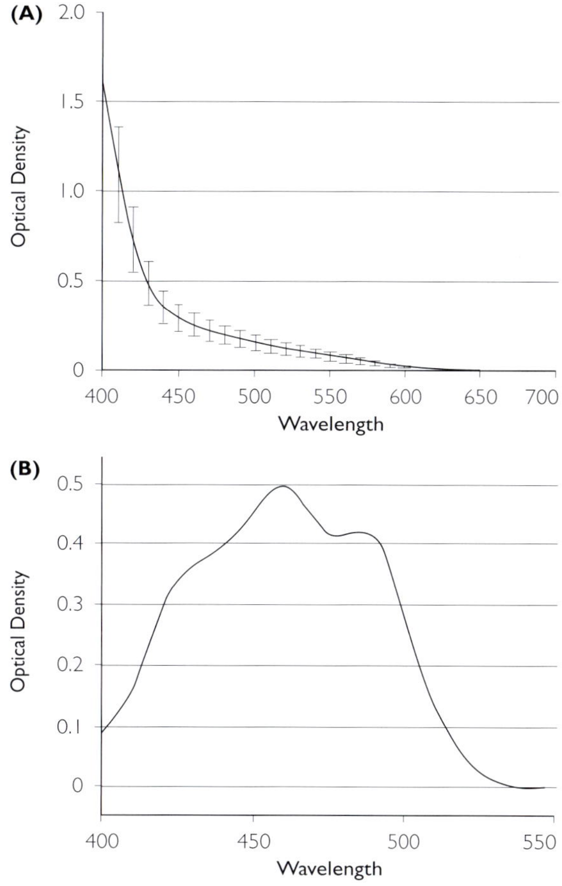

Figure 3.11 **(A) The optical density of the lens (van Norren and Vos, 1974) and (B) the macular pigment (Wyszecki and Stiles, 1982).**

The macular region of the human retina contains a non-photolabile pigment that selectively filters light arriving at the receptors. Entopic viewing of Maxwell's spot (section 3.2.4) is interpreted as a visualization of the spatial distribution of macular pigment (Palmer, 1978). For many observers Maxwell's spot is seen to be darkest in the center of the fovea but for others there is considerable spatial structure (Miles, 1954).

Studies of the optical density of the macular pigment have used widely different methodologies. Since macular pigment varies with field position (see below), it is necessary when evaluating literature reports to take into account the field size employed in the various studies. Perhaps the most striking feature of the literature reports

Table 3.4 Tabulation of the Optical Density of the Total Lens Transmission Function T_L for an Average 32-year-old Observer and Separation of T_L into Components: T_{L1} Represents Portion Affected by Aging after age 20, and T_{L2} Represents Portion Stable after age 20.* (After Pokorny, Smith and Lutze, 1987)

Wavelength	Optical Density			Wavelength	Optical Density		
nm	T_L	T_{L1}	T_{L2}	nm	T_L	T_{L1}	T_{L2}
400	1.933	0.600	1.333	530	0.120	0.120	–
410	1.280	0.510	0.770	540	0.107	0.107	–
420	0.787	0.433	0.354	550	0.093	0.093	–
430	0.493	0.377	0.116	560	0.080	0.080	–
440	0.360	0.327	0.033	570	0.067	0.067	–
450	0.300	0.295	0.005	580	0.053	0.053	–
460	0.267	0.267	–	590	0.040	0.040	–
470	0.233	0.233	–	600	0.033	0.033	–
480	0.207	0.207	–	610	0.027	0.027	–
490	0.187	0.187	–	620	0.020	0.020	–
500	0.167	0.167	–	630	0.013	0.013	–
510	0.147	0.147	–	640	0.007	0.007	–
520	0.133	0.133	–	650	0.000	0.000	–

*The optical density of the lens of an average observer between the ages of 20 and 60 years old may be estimated by

$$T_L = T_{L1}\,[1 + 0.02(A-32)] + T_{L2}.$$

For an average observer over the age of 60

$$T_L = T_{L1}\,[1.56 + 0.0667(A-60)] + T_{L2},$$

where A is the observer's age.

T_L is the van Norren and Vos (1974) tabulation of lens density scaled by 1.333 to represent a 32-year-old observer (the average age of the Stiles and Burch observers) with a small pupil (<3mm). To estimate the lens density function for a completely open pupil (>7mm), multiply the tabulated values by 0.86.

For the Wyszecki and Stiles (1982) lens density function, the following values may be substituted:

Wavelength	Optical Density		
nm	T_L	T_{L1}	T_{L2}
400	1.600	0.600	1.000
410	1.093	0.510	0.583
420	0.733	0.433	0.300

is the marked individual variation in macular pigment; for a 2° field size, individuals may vary from 0.0 to >1.0 optical density at 460 nm, the wavelength of peak absorption (Vos, 1972; Pease *et al.*, 1987; Werner *et al.*, 1987).

Psychophysically measured density of the macular pigment decreases with increase in field size. Estimates from literature reviews of the average macular pigment optical density for a 2° field vary from 0.35 (Vos, 1972) to 0.50 (Wyszecki and Stiles, 1982). Stiles (1955) reported that the 10° colorimetric data are characterized by macular pigment densities of about 0.25 times the 2° optical density. Four studies have attempted to characterize the retinal distribution of macular pigment by comparison of data taken for a small field at a number of retinal eccentricities (Ruddock, 1963; Stabell and Stabell, 1980; Viénot, 1983; Hammond *et al.*, 1997). These data may be characterized with an exponential decrease in macular pigment optical density with retinal eccentricity (Moreland and Bhatt, 1984; Hammond *et al.*, 1997).

3.3 CHROMATIC DETECTION

Detection refers to the ability to recognize a change in light level. The threshold for detection can be measured in the fully dark-adapted eye (absolute threshold) or on a background (increment threshold). The threshold represents some criterion change presumably correlated with a change in a neural response from its steady-state adapting level. It is possible to specify absolute threshold in terms of the number of quanta needed for detection. The increment threshold is usually expressed either as the increment or change in quanta, ΔQ, from the background level or as the contrast ratio of the increment to the background, $\Delta Q/Q$. Increment thresholds may equally well be expressed in quantal, radiance or luminance units.

Sensitivity is inversely related to detection; it is the reciprocal of the quanta at the detection threshold. The human visual system maintains an approximately even state of contrast sensitivity over a billion-fold range of light levels. Detection thresholds can be measured over this entire range of illumination. In the mid-periphery of the dark-adapted eye, where the visual system is most sensitive, the absolute detection threshold requires only a few quanta. The visual system continues to maintain sensitivity even at steady-state background levels of $10^{11.5}$ quanta (about 20 000 td at 555 nm). At this quantal excitation level, there is a 50% depletion of the MWS and LWS cone photopigments. At such levels, an increment of many millions of quanta is needed to detect a change from the steady excitation level.

Part of the sensitivity range of the human visual system is obtained by the duplex nature of the retina. There are two sub-systems each with an operating range over a million-fold, that show overlapping ranges of sensitivity. One receptor system, the rods, constitutes a high sensitivity, low visual acuity, color-blind system. The other system, the cones, represents a high threshold, high visual acuity, color system. There are a variety of sources which treat the topics of detection and sensitivity more fully (Cornsweet, 1970; Barlow, 1972; Hood and Finkelstein, 1986). Here we briefly review some explanatory concepts in detection and review chromatic detection data aimed at isolating cone mechanisms and/or postreceptoral channels.

3.3.1 THRESHOLD-VERSUS-RADIANCE (TVR) FUNCTIONS

Detection thresholds can be measured as a small, brief increment, ΔR on a larger steady background of radiance R. At each background level, the observer first adapts to the background. If the test and background are foveally fixated and the spectral distribution is uniform, detection will be mediated by cone mechanisms. The data may be expressed in several different metrics. The detection threshold can be plotted as the log ΔR versus log R and the function is called a threshold-versus-radiance (TVR) function. Alternately, the data may be expressed in units of retinal illuminance and the function is called a threshold-versus-illuminance (TVI) function. Data may also be specified in quanta/deg^2/sec. The TVR function shows a characteristic shape. At low radiances, detection threshold is unchanged from the absolute threshold on a zero background. As the background is increased, threshold starts to increase and reaches a limiting $\Delta R/R$ slope of unity. At this limiting slope, sensitivity is said to be in the Weber region; threshold is a constant percentage of the background, or a constant contrast.

3.3.2 EXPLANATORY CONCEPTS IN DETECTION

In the psychophysical literature, there have been three important explanatory concepts in describing the TVR function. These are adaptation, saturation, and noise.

3.3.2.1 Adaptation

Adaptation refers to mechanisms that expand the dynamic range of response of the system as a whole. Any given retinal element has a limited response range of perhaps 400-fold. Thus, without adaptation, as light level increases the range available for greater stimulation decreases. Following adaptation, a neural element may maintain this 400-fold response range for a wide range of background light levels. The literature distinguishes two major sub-types of adaptation. Subtractive adaptation resets the steady-state signal without affecting the response to a stimulus pulse. Multiplicative adaptation scales both the responses to the steady-state and to a stimulus pulse. Multiplicative adaptational mechanisms are sometimes called gain controls.

Multiplicative adaptation has many sources. The reflex response of the closing of the pupil in bright illumination is a source of multiplicative adaptation in the natural environment. Pupil constriction reduces the amount of retinal illumination from both a steady-state background and from a light increment. Pupil constriction allows a 16-fold increase in the total operating range of the visual system, under conditions of natural viewing and thus plays a relatively minor role in adaptation in the natural environment. In threshold experiments, the effective pupil is often held constant by use of an artificial pupil (Troland, 1915; Pokorny and Smith, 1997) allowing the study of neural adaptational mechanisms. An artificial pupil is an aperture smaller that the natural pupil which the observer looks through. An alternate technique sometimes used in Maxwellian view systems places a limiting aperture in a plane conjugate to the natural pupil.

Photopigment depletion is another source of multiplicative adaptation. Breakdown and regeneration of photopigment are reciprocal processes. At low illuminations, regeneration works to maintain a full complement of photopigment. At high illuminations, the visual photopigment is depleted (sometimes termed bleaching). In steady illumination, there is no net effect. For a first order kinetic process (Rushton, 1972) the amount of photopigment depleted (1−p) is given by:

$$(1-p) = I/(I + I_o) \qquad (3.56)$$

where p is the amount of photopigment available, I is the retinal illuminance and I_o is a constant, the illumination at which 50% of the photopigment is depleted. For cone photopigments at their λ_{max}, the value of I_o is $10^{11.5}$ quanta (about 20 000 td at 555 nm). At levels above 20 000 td, there is sufficient depletion that only a lower percent of the incident background quanta are absorbed. If the system is responsive at low bleaching levels, it will remain responsive at higher levels since further increases in incident background quanta will be offset by the reduced probability of absorption. This mechanism of adaptation usually plays only a small role in the natural environment, however, snow fields and sunlit beaches may provide sufficient illumination to allow substantial bleaching.

The most important sources of multiplicative adaptation occur neurally. Recordings from primate horizontal cells, second-order neurons in the retina show adaptation over a wide range of light levels (Smith *et al.*, 2001) though the extent of adaptation is not as great as found later in the retina (Lee *et al.*, 1990), or psychophysically.

It is common to lump sources of multiplicative adaptation in a single term. At a computational level, multiplicative adaptation is a scalar less than one that modifies the adapted response, R_A to both the background, Q_A and the increment, ΔQ. The response to the background is given by:

$$R_A = Q_A/(1 + kQ_A) \qquad (3.57)$$

where k is an adaptation constant. Provided that the threshold increment does not perturb the adaptation level, the increment threshold is described by the equation:

$$\Delta Q = (Q_{th})\,(1 + kQ_A) \qquad (3.58)$$

where (Q_{th}) is the absolute threshold, determined by criterion, noise, and/or quantal requirements. The adaptation constant, k, is the reciprocal of the quanta at which threshold is raised two-fold. On a double logarithmic scale, the limiting slope is unity, as demanded in the Weber region. This equation describes the data of TVR functions obtained for the cone mechanisms on large steady backgrounds. The function is sketched in Figure 3.12.

Subtractive adaptation is considered to remove part of the adapting background (Geisler, 1981; Adelson, 1982; Hayhoe *et al.*, 1987). When subtractive adaptation is added to

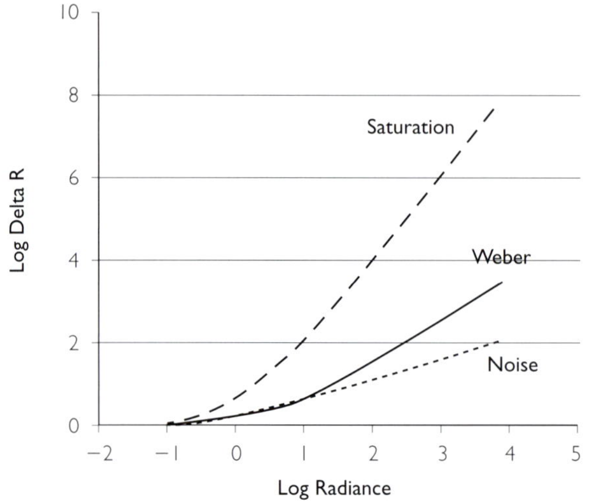

Figure 3.12 The increment threshold functions predicted by three types of detection mechanism, a saturation function, adaptation following Weber's law, and a noise mechanism.

a process already controlled by multiplicative adaptation, the effect is to shift the TVR function on the horizontal axis.

3.3.2.2 Saturation

Any given neural element has a limited response range of perhaps 400-fold. The response of a non-adapting retinal element initially increases with the incident quanta, but with diminishing slope. At a high level above threshold, the response is constant and is said to have saturated. In vision, the saturating response, R is usually described by a Naka–Rushton equation:

$$R = R_{max}\,(Q)/(Q + Q_{sat}) \qquad (3.59)$$

where R_{max} is the maximal response, Q is the incident quanta and Q_{sat} is the semi-saturation, or number of quanta at which the response is half the maximum value. It is clear from equation (3.60) that sensitivity is greatest at low light levels, and that at high light levels where the response has saturated, a detectable increment in response will not be measurable. The equation for detection for a saturating system obeying the Naka–Rushton equation is:

$$\Delta R = (\delta/R_{max})\,(Q + Q_{sat})^2/(Q_{sat} - (\delta/R_{max})\,(Q + Q_{sat})) \qquad (3.60)$$

where δ is the criterion, R_{max} is the maximal response, Q is the incident quanta and Q_{sat} is the semi-saturation, or number of quanta at which the response is half the maximum value. Normally the term (δ/R_{max}) is very small. At absolute threshold, where Q is zero:

$$\Delta R \sim (\delta/R_{max})\,(Q_{sat}) \qquad (3.61)$$

At higher quantal excitation levels where $Q >> Q_{sat}$:

$$\Delta R \sim (\delta/R_{max})\,(Q^2) \qquad (3.62)$$

This equation then describes a function that has a slope of two, steeper than the limiting slope of the Weber function. For some values of δ, R_{max} and Q_{sat}, the denominator of equation 3.60 becomes negative, implying that negative light is required at threshold. It is at this point that the system is said to have saturated. Equation 3.60 is sketched in Figure 3.12.

Saturation can be found in cone-mediated TVR functions under special conditions of measurement. Protocols that reveal saturation include pulsed backgrounds (King-Smith and Webb, 1974; Shevell, 1977; Stockman *et al.*, 1993) and the probe-flash technique (Hayhoe *et al.*, 1987; Hood, 1998). A large steady background controls the overall state of adaptation. An adapting pulse of a second or so, called the flash is superimposed on the background, and a brief test pulse, the probe is superimposed on the adapting flash. The probe may be presented at any time interval during the flash presentation. If the probe is presented in the middle of the flash duration, threshold follows a Weber function, indicative of neural adaptation to the flash. If the probe is presented at flash onset, threshold is elevated above the Weber function demonstrating a slope of two before saturation, indicative of a saturating process. The probe-flash technique has been used to delineate a different time course for subtractive and multiplicative adaptation (Geisler, 1981; Hayhoe *et al.*, 1987).

Mechanisms of neural adaptation: The neural multiplication and neural subtractive adaptation inferred from the data described above has computational importance. Another approach is to ask what kind of neural mechanism might exist. Neural mechanisms may be feed-forward or feed-backward. Historically, feed-forward is considered unsatisfying since it must be subject to saturation.

In **subtractive feedback**, a portion, k of the signal is subtracted from the signal. In the steady state subtractive feedback is described as

$$R = Q - (kR) \qquad (3.63)$$

$$R = Q/(1+k) \qquad (3.64)$$

Subtractive feedback acts to shift the start of a saturating mechanism to a higher radiance level. Models of subtractive feedback may postulate that the feedback is developed slowly in time compared with the signal. Slow subtractive feedback shows pronounced overshoots following a rapid increase in radiance level.

In **divisive feedback** the signal is divided by a portion of the signal. In the steady state response is given by:

$$R = Q/(1+kR) \tag{3.65}$$
$$R = -\tfrac{1}{2}k + [(1+4kQ)/4k^2]^{0.5} \tag{3.66}$$

In divisive feedback, the response increases as the square root of the signal; i.e. only part of the signal is removed by the adapting mechanism. Subtractive feedback acts to shift a saturating mechanism by the square root of the steady-state radiance.

Combined neural mechanisms: The subtractive and divisive feedbacks described above do not produce Weber behavior. There is interest in the literature as to how Weber behavior may be produced. One possibility, as proposed by Koenderink, van de Grind, and Bouman (1970) was to weight a subtractive feedback pathway with a feed-forward signal that represented the average radiance over time.

3.3.2.3 Noise

An important concept in detection is that the signal may be noisy. There are two consequences of the noise concept in visual thresholds. First, noise affects the slope of the psychometric function and, second, a noise-limited process affects the slope of the TVR function. The applicability of the noise concept at absolute threshold followed the recognition that the statistics of light emission in a brief pulse follow a Poisson process. The introduction of the noise concept in visual processing occurred at a time when engineers were developing methods to assess signal transmission in electronic transmission, i.e. signal detection theory. A detection event then requires that the response to a signal on a noisy background be some criterion amount larger than the noise level alone. If the noise is Poisson-limited, its variance is given by the mean. Suppose threshold is defined at 55% correct detection, i.e., detection occurs at one standard deviation above the noise. The increment threshold is defined as:

$$\Delta R = (Q^{0.5}) \tag{3.67}$$

In the classic paper of Hecht, Shlaer, and Pirenne (1942), the slope of the psychometric function at rod absolute threshold was related to the uncertainty in the number of quanta delivered per light pulse. An important and undisputed conclusion from this study was that a single quantum is sufficient to excite a photoreceptor. However, the study also suggested that on average five to eight absorptions were required for detection on 55% of the trials. Thus detection is limited not by absorption but by some neural criterion. Barlow (1956) introduced the idea that the photoreceptor responses might themselves be noisy in the absence of stimulation. This idea is sometimes called 'equivalent noise,' EN. Equation (3.60) can be rewritten:

$$\Delta R = (EN + Q)^{0.5} \tag{3.68}$$

In the absence of a real background, absolute threshold will be limited by the equivalent noise. Once the background noise exceeds the neural noise, detection will be limited by the background noise. The limiting slope of a noise-limited TVR function is 0.5 (see Figure 3.12).

The noise concept has been most important at absolute threshold. As the steady-state light level increases, multiplicative adaptation processes take over and detection is in the Weber region. Provided the multiplicative adaptation process follows the source of the noise, it will reduce the effect of both the average background and its variance. Thus, the level of stimulus noise or early neural noise will approach a constant value once gain mechanisms are active. It is also recognized that threshold may be limited by late neural noise that follows gain mechanisms. There are data that suggest that the intrinsic noise of spike generation at the retinal ganglion cell is constant at different superthreshold illuminations (Troy and Robson, 1992; Troy and Lee, 1994).

There are conditions for which cone-mediated detection obeys equation (3.68) (Barlow, 1957; Bouman and Koenderink, 1972). The conditions to obtain noise-limited detection in cones involve the use of very small test and adaptation fields. These conditions probably restrict the role of neural adaptation.

3.3.3 DETECTION ON SPECTRAL BACKGROUNDS

The TVR function for foveally fixated achromatic targets measured with large steady backgrounds and small test stimuli follows the form of equation (3.58). However, when chromatic backgrounds and tests are used, multiple branches or partial components of multiple TVR functions can be measured depending on the choice of test and background wavelengths. Further, the spectral sensitivity of the detection mechanisms varies, depending on the background wavelength. These results were attributed to multiple underlying cone mechanisms (i.e. a photoreceptor and its adaptation mechanism). An early goal of these studies was to separate and measure the spectral sensitivity of the cone mechanisms with the view that they would reveal the underlying visual photopigments.

One important pre-theoretical concept was that a spectral background might exert a differential effect on the three classes of cones. The differential spectral sensitivity of the cone photopigments might be exploited to allow isolation of each cone mechanism by an appropriate choice of background wavelength e.g. Wald (1964). This idea in turn originated in the photochemical studies of extracted pigments (Dartnall, 1957). It was recognized that the constituents of extracted photopigment mixtures could be studied by partial bleaching, i.e. by bleaching with a spectral wavelength that exploited the differential transmissivity of the pigment mixture. In human psychophysics, it became clear that this exploitation could be achieved at levels below photopigment depletion. These data suggested that the neural adaptation mechanisms of the cone mechanisms were equivalently independent. The major development of the relation between cone-mediated TVR functions and the underlying cone mechanisms was performed by Stiles (1959, 1978).

3.3.3.1 Displacement laws

When TVR functions are measured using monochromatic lights for test and background stimulus, there are two important laws which govern the placement of the TVR function on the horizontal or vertical axis. Consider a single mechanism consisting of a photopigment with neural elements that show multiplicative adaptation, giving a classical TVR function. From equation (3.58), we see that two independent factors govern the TVR function. The term Qth for absolute threshold determines the vertical intercept and the term k for adaptation determines the transition to the Weber region.

The vertical displacement law (test wavelength variation): Suppose test and background are chosen near the peak absorption of the photopigment. At absolute threshold, the mechanism is at its most sensitive, since the chosen wavelength allows the highest probability of absorption. If the test wavelength is now changed, the absolute threshold will be higher, since absolute threshold is determined partially by the reciprocal absorptivity of the underlying photopigment (Chapter 2). The transition to the Weber region, however, is determined by the relative absorptivity of the photopigment at the adapting background that remains unchanged. The TVR functions for different test wavelengths will be displaced vertically, but will make their transition into the Weber region at the same background radiance. The vertical displacement law states that variation in test wavelength can only affect the vertical position of the TVR function for a single mechanism.

The horizontal displacement law (background wavelength variation): In comparison, consider variation in the background wavelength, leaving the test wavelength fixed near the peak absorption of the photopigment. The value of absolute threshold is not affected by the choice of background wavelength. However, the effectiveness of the background, Q_A is determined by the absorption probability of the photopigment. The transition to the Weber region occurs at higher radiances for background wavelengths other than at the peak absorptivity of the photopigment. The TVR functions will be displaced horizontally on the radiance axis but will share the same vertical position since they are pinned at absolute threshold. The horizontal displacement law states that variation in background wavelength can only affect the horizontal position of the TVR function for a single mechanism.

It is clear that the spectral sensitivity of a single mechanism can be assessed in two different ways. Spectral sensitivity can be assessed by using a background of fixed wavelength and a test stimulus of varying wavelength. The background radiance is fixed and test radiance is varied to achieve increment threshold. This is called a test sensitivity function. Alternatively, spectral sensitivity can be assessed by using a test stimulus of fixed wavelength and a background stimulus of varying wavelength. The radiance of the background is varied to achieve a 10-fold rise in test wavelength threshold above absolute threshold. This spectral sensitivity function is called a field sensitivity function. The two methods each have advantages and disadvantages. The test sensitivity method is more straightforward, and requires minimal data collection (one threshold per test wavelength). Test sensitivity has seen the greater use (Wald, 1964; Eisner and MacLeod, 1981; Yeh *et al.*, 1989). Its disadvantage is that the human cone mechanisms are highly overlapping, while the success of the technique depends on a large differential sensitivity between constituent mechanisms. It is virtually impossible to choose a background wavelength that will yield test spectral sensitivity for the entire spectrum for a given cone mechanism. The field sensitivity method is more data-intensive; a TVR function must be measured at each background wavelength. The overlap of the human cone spectral sensitivities may result in overlap of the TVR functions. Thus, a value for the spectral sensitivity at 10× absolute threshold may in some cases depend on extrapolation of a fitted TVR function rather than a direct measurement.

The π mechanisms: If the cones have independent adaptation pathways, then the displacement laws will hold for each independent mechanism. Additionally, provided the adaptation mechanism is such as to generate a TVR function showing Weber's law, then the spectral sensitivity of the underlying mechanism may be inferred even if only a small segment of the TVR function is measurable. It is also possible to test the independence of the adapting mechanisms, by superimposing backgrounds that are mixtures of component wavelengths. Stiles developed the rationale of the displacement laws and the field sensitivity technique. Stiles used a consistent experimental paradigm. The background was 10° and the test was a 1° by 1° square pulsed for 100–200 msec. Stiles obtained a number of functions of differing spectral sensitivity, associated with different combinations of test and field wavelength. He termed these π mechanisms (Figure 3.13). These were subsequently replicated and subjected to tests of independence (Pugh and Kirk, 1986).

π 1,2,3: The first three Stiles π mechanisms are associated with the SWS cone mechanism. The π 2 mechanism is the most sensitive mechanism, obtained at absolute threshold. The π 2 mechanism occurs variably among observers, and thus has not been the subject of extensive analysis. The π 1 mechanism is obtained at low to moderate adapting levels. The π 3 mechanism is obtained when adaptation fields are close to bleaching levels for the LWS and MWS cones. One difficulty in obtaining the π 1 and the π 3 mechanisms is that even with a 435 nm test flash near the peak of the SWS cone spectral sensitivity, an auxiliary long wavelength conditioning field is needed to suppress the other cone types. The finding of multiple mechanisms for SWS cone function was disappointing in that it revealed a failure to isolate a unitary mechanism that could be associated with a presumed SWS cone photopigment. Further, the long wavelength sensitivity slopes of the π 1, the π 2, and the π 3 mechanisms were not consistent with typical absorption functions for photopigments. These findings led Stiles to realize that his techniques did not reveal a unitary adapting

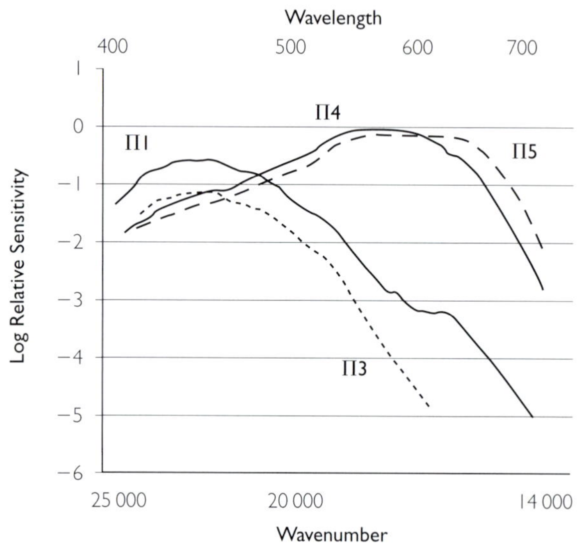

Figure 3.13 **Stiles field mechanisms. Log relative quantal field sensitivities of the π mechanisms plotted as a function of wavenumber.**

mechanism. Subsequent studies provided further indication that the π 1 to π 3 are not consistent with unitary adapting mechanisms (Pugh, 1976; Mollon and Polden, 1977; Pugh and Mollon, 1979). In particular, there were failures of additivity when the adapting field was composed of short wavelength and long wavelength components. When the background was composed of low luminance short wavelength and long wavelength components, threshold was raised more than predicted from the additivity of the component fields (Pugh, 1976). When the background was composed of a high luminance short wavelength and lower luminance long wavelength components, threshold was raised less than predicted from the additivity of the component fields. Another irregularity of the π 1 to π 3 mechanisms was called the 'limited conditioning effect.' As a long wavelength background was raised, threshold for a 435 nm test flash rose for about 0.7–0.8 log unit, and then stabilized, i.e. showed no further effect of an increase in the adapting background. The threshold started to increase again only when the background reached a level capable of bleaching the LWS and MWS cones. The final abnormality of the π 1 mechanism was one of temporal adaptation and termed 'transient tritanopia.' Following extinction of a long wavelength background, threshold for a short wavelength test flash first rose precipitously and then recovered very slowly. In comparison following extinction of a short wavelength background that caused the same steady threshold increment, sensitivity fell rapidly. A model of the π 1 and π 3 pathways was suggested by Pugh and Mollon (1979) in which the SWS cone was subject to two independent sources of adaptation. Adaptation could occur both in the SWS cone and at a later 'second' site where there was spectral opponency between SWS cones and summed activity of LWS and MWS cones (see Chapter 6 on spectral opponency in the retina). The failure of the independence tests for π 1 was attributed to independence of first site and second site adaptation. The limited conditioning effect of long wavelength adapting fields was attributed to stabilization of the steady-state response at the second site at bleaching levels of the LWS and MWS cones. Transient tritanopia was attributed to the adaptational properties of the second site. In modern models of adaptational mechanisms, the gain controls are carried forward to subsequent sites. An early stage of multiplicative adaptation serves to stabilize the later opponent sites and thus the first and second sites cannot be truly independent. The adaptational abnormalities of the π 1 mechanism are not predicted if the SWS cone shows Weber adaptation preceding the second site. The Pugh and Mollon model can be rephrased if we consider that the SWS cone pathway is subject only to partial adaptation at the first site. There is adaptation at the second site that acts to subtract most of the opponent signal.

π 4 and π 5: The remaining Stiles π mechanisms are associated with detection mediated primarily by MWS and LWS cones. These mechanisms obey the displacement laws and fulfil many criteria for unitary mechanisms. The mechanism Stiles termed π 4 has often been associated with the MWS photopigment and to a lesser extent π 5 has been associated with the LWS photopigment. Nonetheless, other evidence suggested that π 4 and π 5 did not represent photopigment sensitivities. This evidence came from many sources: The π 4 and π 5 were broader than the spectral sensitivities of X-chromosome linked dichromats believed to have only one of these mechanisms (Boynton, 1963). The π 4 and π 5 mechanisms showed unexpected interactions that were not consistent with unitary mechanisms (Boynton, Ikeda and Stiles, 1964). If the parameters of the test size and duration are changed, the spectral sensitivities of the isolated mechanisms do not necessarily agree with those of the π 4 and π 5 mechanisms (Ingling and Martinez, 1981; Stockman and Mollon, 1986). Finally, test sensitivity measurements yield narrower functions than the classical Stiles field mechanisms (Wald, 1964; Eisner and MacLeod, 1981; Yeh *et al.*, 1989; Stockman *et al.*, 1993).

Today it is conceded that the π mechanisms do not represent isolated cone spectral sensitivities. With the acceptance of the parallel pathway description of the retina (Chapter 6), it is recognized that the choice of spatio-temporal parameters will favor detection either in PC- or in MC-pathways. Thus, obedience of the displacement laws may represent isolation of a higher order neural mechanism by choice of the spatio-temporal presentation, rather than isolation of a single photoreceptor by adaptation. The spatio-temporal parameters of the stimulus will determine the relative sensitivities of the MC- and PC-pathway channels. If these sensitivities are similar, probability summation among pathways should be considered. The choice of a 100–200 msec square-wave pulse is one that favors both MC- and PC-pathway channels. In comparison, a brief 5 msec pulse would favor the MC-pathway while a 1 second gaussian-shaped pulse would favor the PC-pathway.

3.3.4 INCREMENT DETECTION ON WHITE

With a white-adapting field, a test sensitivity function may be obtained as a function of test wavelength for a large, long test pulse. This function shows three peaks, separated by two notches (Sperling and Harwerth, 1971). There is a prominent peak near 450 nm with a notch near 500 nm. There are peaks at 540 and 600 nm, separated by a notch near 570 nm. The prominence of the peaks depends on the spatio-temporal characteristics of the test stimulus and the size and luminance of the background (Figure 3.14). The most prominent peaks are obtained when the background is a pedestal spatially coextensive with the test (Nacer *et al.*, 1989) and when the test is of long duration (King-Smith and Carden, 1976).

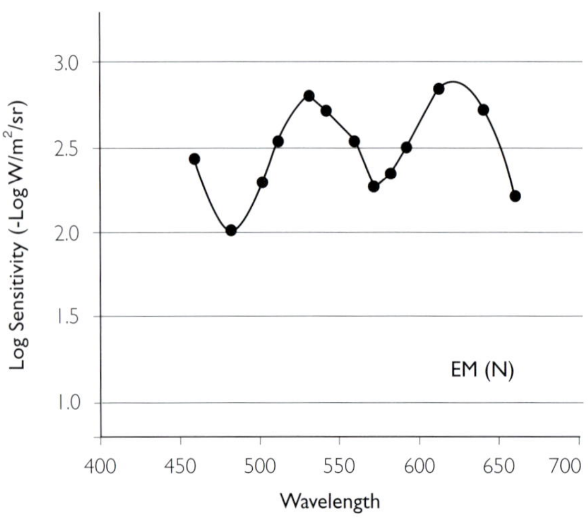

Figure 3.14 Increment threshold spectral sensitivity function for 2° test stimuli presented on a coextensive 4600 K, 800 td pedestal within a larger 200 td surround. (Data replotted from Figure 6 of Miyahara *et al.*, 1996.)

Interpretation: The characteristic lobes and notches of the increment spectral sensitivity on a white background are usually interpreted as reflecting spectrally opponent processing (see Chapter 6). Detection in the spectrally opponent channels is most comparable to KC-pathway 'blue-on,' and PC-pathway 'green-on' and 'red-on' responses (Sperling and Harwerth, 1971; Thornton and Pugh, 1983). The channels are weighted and fit to the data. This approach does not specify adaptation in a mechanistic form, but the weights serve this purpose. An alternative interpretation is in terms of psychophysically specified achromatic and chromatic visual pathways (King-Smith and Carden, 1976). The white background is considered a powerful adapting stimulus for the achromatic but not the two chromatic pathways. The lobes reflect weighted chromatic opponent activity; the notches represent weighted achromatic activity. This approach also does not specify adaptation in a mechanistic form.

3.4 CHROMATIC DISCRIMINATION

Discrimination refers to the ability to detect a difference between two lights that differ on some physical continuum. In studies of chromatic discrimination, the lights may differ in wavelength, in colorimetric purity, or in chromaticity, but do not differ in luminance. The threshold represents some criterion change presumably correlated with a difference in a neural response to the two lights. Thresholds may be expressed in wavelength steps or in chromaticity steps. A modern approach that attempts to relate detection and discrimination uses cone troland units (defined in section 3.2), which allows comparison of detection and discrimination in terms of quantal excitation of the receptors. If a surround is present and discrimination is measured from the surround chromaticity, the threshold may conceptually be considered as a detection, and related to the detection experiments described in section 3.3. In modern studies of chromatic discrimination, the test chromaticity may differ from the surround chromaticity.

3.4.1 HISTORICAL APPROACHES

Wavelength discrimination: Wavelength discrimination refers to the ability of an observer to detect chromatic differences along the spectrum locus. In the classical wavelength discrimination experiment, the observer views a bipartite field, one half filled with light of a standard wavelength and the other with light of a comparison wavelength. Both standard and comparison fields are narrow spectral bands of light that are varied in spectral composition and radiance.

A common procedure is the step-by-step method in which both fields are initially of identical spectral composition and radiance (isomeric fields). The wavelength of the comparison field is changed in small steps (one nanometer or less) and the observer adjusts the radiance of the comparison field following each change to seek a match. Discrimination threshold is reached when the observer reports that the fields do not appear identical regardless of the radiance of the comparison field. The wavelength discrimination step is expressed in terms of the difference in wavelength, $\Delta\lambda$, between the standard and comparison fields. The procedure is repeated for a series of standard wavelengths throughout the visible spectrum. Data are reported either as the $\Delta\lambda$ in one direction, for example scaling toward longer wavelengths, or as the average of $\Delta\lambda$ for comparison lights scaled in both directions.

In an alternative technique, the standard deviation of a repeated series of color matches is taken as being proportional to the discrimination step. In this procedure, the two fields are initially different in wavelength. The observer adjusts the wavelength and radiance of the comparison field until it appears to be the same as the standard. The procedure is repeated many times, in order to determine the standard deviation of the comparison field settings. In terms of experimental convenience, the step-by-step method is more rapid but it requires absolute calibration of wavelength for both the standard and the comparison fields. The standard deviation procedure is time-consuming but may be more accurate as it shows less dependence on criterion changes of the observer. This technique also bridges measurements of color matching and color discrimination. The standard deviation of a set of color matches can be used as an index of color discrimination.

Figure 3.15 compares wavelength discrimination data from several laboratories. MacAdam's (1942) standard deviation data appear to be approximately one-fifth the discrimination thresholds measured by step-by-step procedures. The peaks and valleys vary somewhat among the different authors. A similar variation occurs among the functions measured in different individuals.

Colorimetric purity discrimination: Colorimetric purity discrimination typically refers to measurements of the least colorimetric purity, p_c, the minimum amount of spectral light that allows a mixture of a spectral light and white to be distinguished from white.

$$p_c = L_\lambda/(L_w + L_\lambda) \qquad (3.69)$$

where L_λ is the luminance of the spectral color and Lw is the luminance of the white. Figure 3.16(A) shows the data expressed as the reciprocal (p_c) of least colorimetric purity as a function of retinal illuminance. The results show a minimum in the 570–580 nm region, and best discrimination at the spectral extremes.

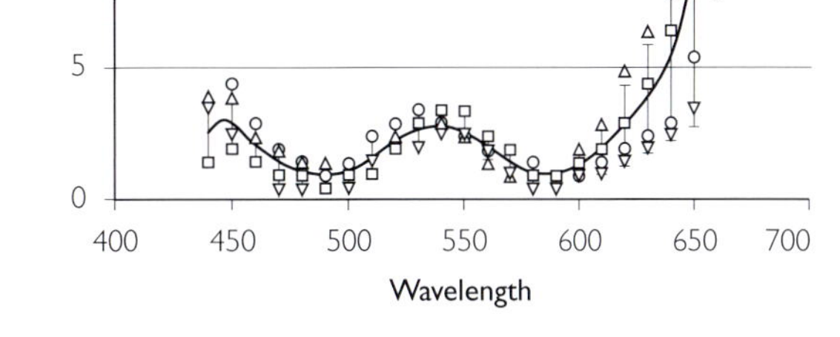

Figure 3.15 Wavelength discrimination plotted as a function of wavelength. The symbols show data from four observers (Pokorny and Smith, 1970). The solid line is the average.

Colorimetric purity of a sample, S, denoted by its chromaticity coefficients (x_S, y_S) in the CIE diagram is related to excitation purity, pe (section 3.2) by:

$$p_c = (y_\lambda / y_S) p_e \tag{3.70}$$

where y_λ is the chromaticity coefficient of the dominant wavelength of sample S and y_S is the chromaticity coefficient of the sample.

If colorimetric purity discrimination is measured as the first step from the spectrum (i.e. least amount of white added to a spectral light), the results in the literature are rather variable but show a much flatter function than when colorimetric purity is measured as the first step from white (Jones and Lowry, 1926; Martin *et al.*, 1933; Wright and Pitt, 1937; Kaiser *et al.*, 1976). Yeh, Smith, and Pokorny (1993) reexamined this question carefully and found the shape of the first step from the spectrum function to be highly retinal illuminance dependent with flatter functions at higher light levels (Figure 3.16B).

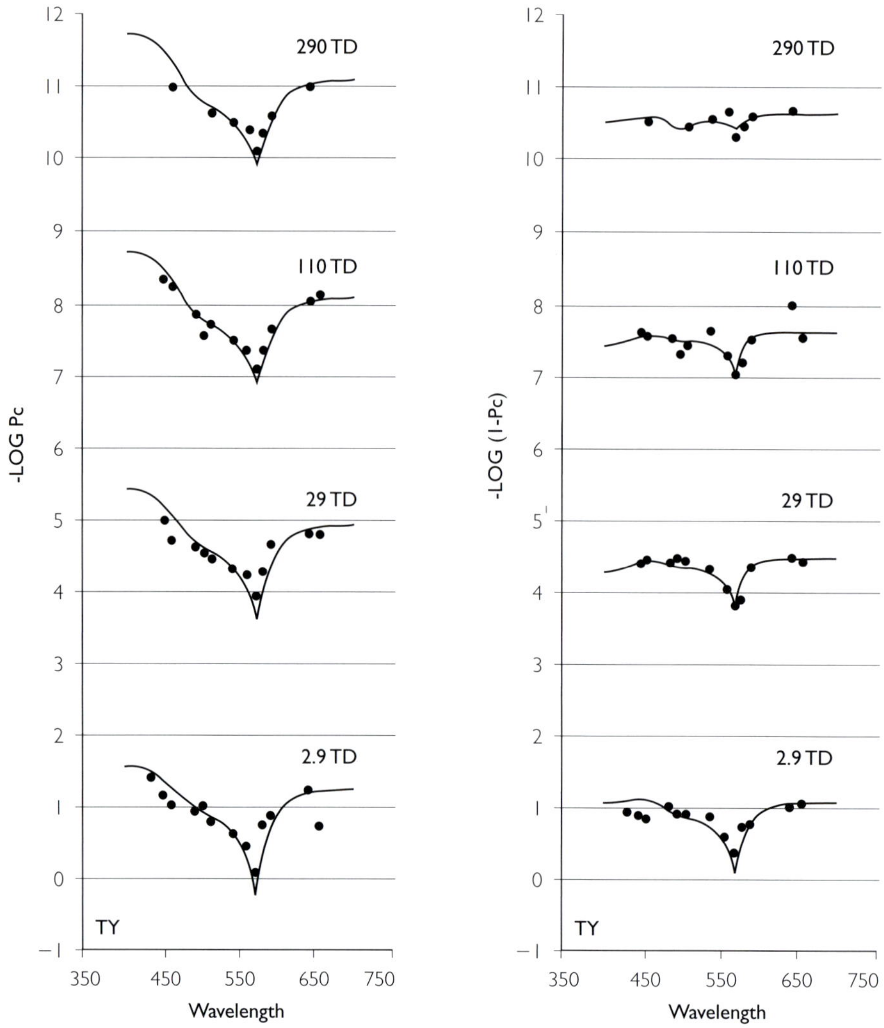

Figure 3.16 Colorimetric purity discrimination plotted as a function of wavelength. Left panel shows colorimetric purity thresholds measured from white and right panel shows colorimetric purity thresholds measured from the spectrum. Data for the higher luminance levels are successively scaled vertically by 3 log units. Data are shown for one observer, data of four other observers showed closely similar trends. (From Yeh *et al.*, 1993.)

MacAdam ellipses: Wavelength and colorimetric purity discrimination represent two special cases of chromaticity discrimination: discriminations along the spectrum locus and discrimination along axes between white and the spectrum locus. It is possible to sample chromatic discrimination systematically starting at an arbitrary chromaticity (e.g. Wright, 1941). The data are represented in the 1931 CIE chromaticity diagram (MacAdam, 1942; Brown and MacAdam, 1949; Wyszecki and Fielder, 1971). MacAdam used the standard deviation of color matches to represent chromaticity discrimination. For a number of different points in chromaticity space, MacAdam derived a series of discrimination ellipses, which represent the discriminable distance for a number of directions from each point. MacAdam ellipses represent data from a single observer. Figure 3.17 shows MacAdam's data plotted in the 1931 chromaticity diagram with each of the ellipses representing ten times the measured standard deviations.

In the equiluminant plane, discriminations are based solely on chromaticity differences. It is also possible to evaluate the joint effects of chromaticity and luminance in determining discrimination steps (Brown and MacAdam, 1949; Noorlander *et al.*, 1980). These data also describe ellipsoids in a three-dimensional chromaticity and luminance space (Poirson and Wandell, 1990).

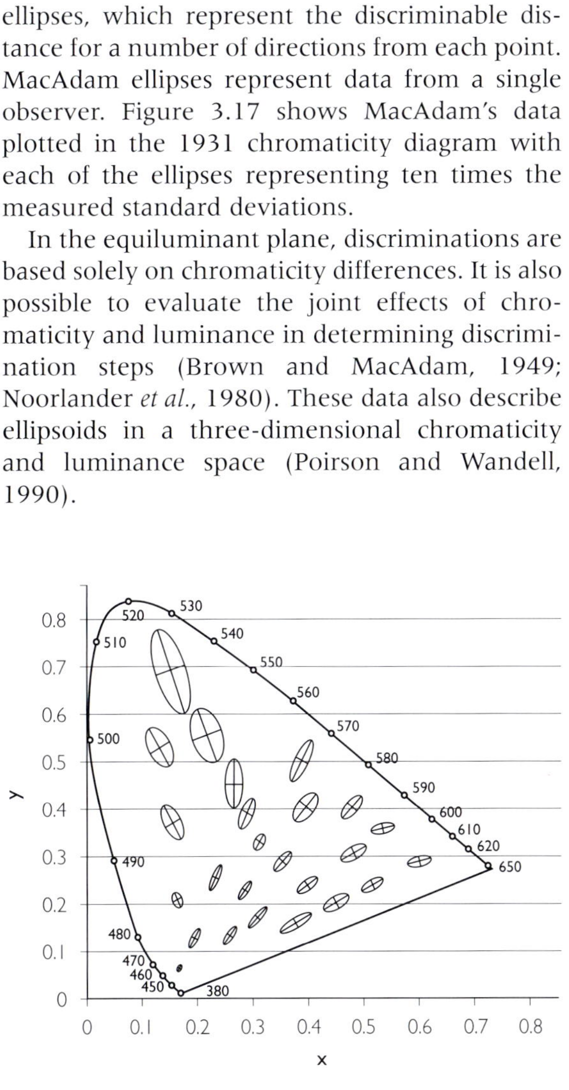

Figure 3.17 **The MacAdam ellipses plotted in the CIE chromaticity diagram. (From MacAdam, 1942.)**

Watson (1911) and Tyndall (1933) investigated the effects of adding white light to discrimination fields composed of spectral lights. For wavelengths greater than 490 nm, the discrimination step is increased with increases in the white light content. Tyndall extended these observations into the short wavelength region of the spectrum and found rather striking results. For 455 nm fields, discrimination improved with the addition of white light. Discrimination improved and was optimal when the white light was four to ten times higher in luminance than the spectral discrimination lights. This improvement has been termed the Tyndall effect. Polden and Mollon (1980) coined the term 'combinative euchromatopsia' to describe the enhanced sensitivity to hue differences.

3.4.2 EXPERIMENTAL VARIABLES

The effects of the luminance level, spatial structure, temporal presentation and retinal position are important in chromatic discrimination. The effect of surrounds is considered separately in section 3.4.4.

Effect of field size: Chromatic discrimination improves when the field size is increased from 2° to 10° by a factor of about two (Brown, 1952; Wyszecki and Stiles, 1982). The improvement is independent of the sampling direction in chromaticity space. Chromatic discrimination deteriorates when the field size is reduced below 1° (Pokorny and Smith, 1976). Chromatic discriminations are possible for bipartite fields as small as 3' (MacAdam, 1959). Steady fixation of small fields (20' or less) leads to a deterioration of discrimination mediated by the SWS cones (small field tritanopia, König, 1894; Thomson and Wright, 1947). The small field tritanopic effect also occurs with steady fixation of parafoveal fields (Hartridge, 1945; Thomson and Wright, 1947) and is reduced or eliminated by employing a scanning or glance technique (Bedford and Wyszecki, 1958b; McCree, 1960).

Effect of retinal illuminance: Discrimination functions show little change over a range of retinal illuminance of 100–3500 troland (Bedford and Wyszecki, 1958a; Cornu and Harlay, 1969). However, discrimination deteriorates at low levels of retinal illuminance. The effect is particularly marked for discriminations based upon SWS cones (Brown, 1951; Verriest *et al.*, 1963; Knoblauch *et al.*, 1987). There is a strong interaction between field size and luminance; the deterioration of SWS cone discrimination is more pronounced with the joint reduction of field size and luminance (Farnsworth, 1955; Clarke, 1967; Yonemura and Kasuya, 1969).

The gap effect: Discrimination is also affected by the presence of a separation between two halves of a bipartite field (Sharpe and Wyszecki, 1976; Boynton *et al.*, 1977). The effect of introducing a gap is not the same for different types of discriminations. Luminance discrimination is best when the two half fields are precisely juxtaposed. Chromatic discrimination for red–green discriminations is unimpaired by a gap and discriminations based on differential SWS cone excitations improve.

Temporal presentation: Wavelength discrimination improves with increasing exposure duration but there is little agreement in the literature as to the optimal exposure (Farnsworth, 1961; Siegel, 1965; Regan and Tyler, 1971; Hita *et al.*, 1982). Discrimination deteriorates if stimuli are presented successively rather than simultaneously (Uchikawa and Ikeda, 1981; Uchikawa, 1983; Sachtler and Zaidi, 1992; Jin and Shevell, 1996).

Retinal location: Peripheral fixation of the fields results in a marked reduction of discrimination, particularly in the 490–530 nm (Moreland, 1972). Rods have been implicated as the source of degradation of discrimination (Lythgoe, 1931; Stabell and Stabell, 1977; Stabell and Stabell, 1982).

Temporal and spatial contrast sensitivity: A number of studies have measured the contrast sensitivity function for equiluminous chromatic alternation in space (van der Horst *et al.*,1967; Hilz and Cavonius, 1970), time (de Lange, 1958; Kelly and van Norren, 1977; Wisowaty, 1981; Swanson *et al.*, 1987), and joint variation of space and time (van der Horst and Bouman, 1969; Noorlander *et al.*, 1981). The studies report that equiluminous chromatic modulation showed a low pass function with poor sensitivity to high spatial or temporal frequencies.

Assessment of the spatial contrast sensitivity for equiluminant stimuli is technically demanding due to the presence of chromatic aberration in the eye. Chromatic aberration can introduce unwanted luminance information in the nominally equiluminous grating. Since the data reveal that a pure color grating has low contrast sensitivity, chromatic aberration must be carefully minimized (Mullen, 1985) or eliminated (Sekiguchi *et al.*, 1993).

A number of techniques have been used to assess the temporal and spatial characteristics of isolated receptor mechanisms. In general, the LWS and MWS mechanism have similar spatial (Brindley, 1954; Green, 1968; Cavonius and Estévez, 1975) and temporal properties (Brindley *et al.*, 1966; Green, 1969; Estévez and Cavonius, 1975). The SWS mechanism exhibits lower spatial (Stiles, 1949; Brindley, 1954; Green, 1968) and temporal (Brindley *et al.*, 1966; Green, 1969; Kelly, 1974; Wisowaty and Boynton, 1980) resolution.

3.4.3 MODERN APPROACH TO CHROMATICITY DISCRIMINATION

The Boynton and Kambe experiment: Boynton and Kambe (1980) performed a systematic sampling of chromaticity space in a constant luminance plane. Their study showed notable differences from the earlier studies. One major difference was that discrimination was measured along theoretically critical axes in the equiluminant plane which correspond to the axes of the MacLeod–Boynton chromaticity space (section 3.2.5). One set of axes maintained a constant amount of SWS cone stimulation, $s/(l+m)$ and discrimination was measured for test chromaticities varying in their ratios of LWS to MWS cone stimulation, $l/(l+m)$. A second set of axes maintained a constant LWS to MWS cone stimulation $l/(l+m)$ and discrimination was evaluated for test chromaticities varying in SWS cone excitation, $s/(l+m)$. The $l/(l+m)$ cone discriminations showed a minimum. The minimum occurred near a value of 0.667 for $l/(l+m)$ which is comparable to data obtained with a surround chromaticity at the equal energy spectrum (see section 3.4.4). The $l/(l+m)$ discriminations were primarily independent of the level of s/(l+m), although there appeared a small contribution of SWS cone activity at high s/(l+m) levels. On the S cone axis, discrimination was dependent on s/(l+m) at the test chromaticity. Further, s/(l+m) axis discriminations were affected only by the level of s/(l+m) and were independent of the l/(l+m) component of the stimulus. Subsequently, Krauskopf, Williams and Healy (1982) confirmed the independence of the l/(l+m) and s/(l+m) lines in an experiment using chromatic adaptation. They found highly selective chromatic effects with an adaptation field that was modulated in a l/(l+m) direction. The l/(l+m) discrimination was impaired by previous adaptation to a l/(l+m) stimulus, but discrimination along the s/(l+m) line was unaffected. Conversely, adaptation on a s/(l+m) affected s/(l+m) discrimination but not l/(l+m) discriminations. Luminance modulation had little effect on chromatic thresholds. Chromatic modulation had little effect on luminance thresholds.

The Boynton and Kambe data when expressed in chromaticity showed general agreement with MacAdam's (1942) ellipses. The Boynton and Kambe experiment was designed to yield high criterion color-difference steps. The observer was required to identify the color direction at threshold. Boynton and Kambe's discrimination steps are equivalent to approximately 13 of MacAdam's standard deviations.

A second major advance in the Boynton and Kambe formulation lies in the ability to relate discrimination data to detection by use of the cone troland. Boynton and Kambe showed that at 115 td optimal discrimination on the l/(l+m) axis required an increase of one L td (accompanied by a decrease of one M td). In comparison, optimal discrimination on the s/(l+m) axis required an increase of eight S td.

3.4.4 THE EFFECT OF SURROUNDS

Surrounds are important since they control the state of adaptation, as was clear from detection experiments. In early studies it was established that chromatic discrimination is best when the test chromaticity is at or near the chromaticity of the surround (Brown, 1952; Hurvich and Jameson, 1961; Pointer, 1974; Loomis and Berger, 1979). Modern studies, assessing discrimination on LWS, MWS cone, and on SWS cone excitation axes have confirmed and extended this finding (Krauskopf *et al.*, 1982; Zaidi *et al.*, 1992; Miyahara *et al.*, 1993; Smith *et al.*, 2000). The data show that l/(l+m) cone discriminations show a symmetrical V shape with minimum near the l/(l+m) chromaticity of the surround (Figure 3.18). Chromatic discrimination data obtained with no surround show a shallower V shape whose minimum coincides with that obtained when the surround chromaticity is that of the equal energy spectrum (Boynton and Kambe, 1980; Yeh *et al.*, 1993). Discriminations on the s/(l+m) axis also show a V shape with a minimum near the s/(l+m) cone chromaticity of the surround. The V is not symmetrical (Zaidi *et al.*, 1992; Miyahara *et al.*, 1993), rising more sharply when the s/(l+m) level of the test chromaticity is higher than that of the surround (Figure 3.19).

3.4.5 INTERPRETATION

An interpretation of chromatic discrimination data at equiluminance can be viewed in terms of spectral signals generated in the PC-pathway. A PC-pathway retinal ganglion cell has a steady resting level to a steady EES adapting field of 100–1000 trolands. If the field luminance or

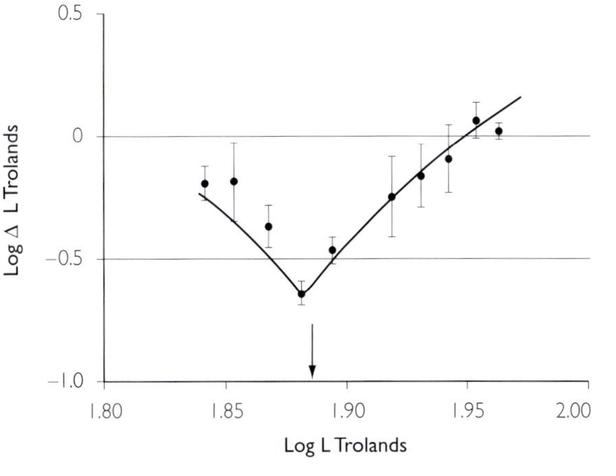

Figure 3.18 Chromatic discrimination in the equiluminant plane for lights varying only in their l/(l+m) content. The observer is adapted to the equal energy spectrum. The data are expressed in L tds (see section 3.1) with log ΔL plotted vs. log L at the starting chromaticity. (From unpublished data of the authors.)

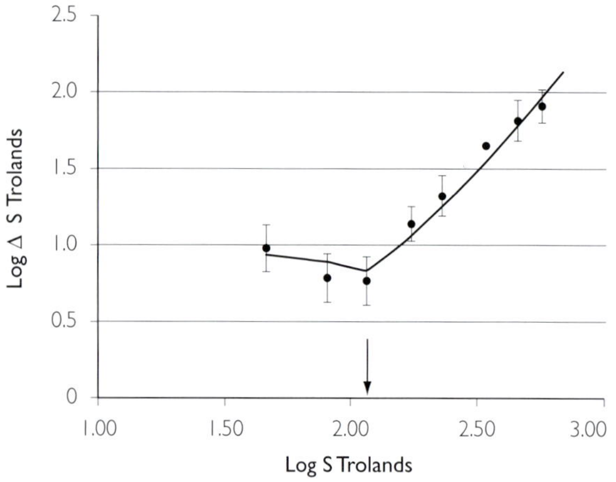

Figure 3.19 Chromatic discrimination in the equiluminant plane for lights varying only in their s/(l+m) content. The observer is adapted to the equal energy spectrum. The data are expressed in S tds (see section 3.1) with log ΔS plotted vs. log S at the starting chromaticity. (From unpublished data of the authors.)

chromaticity is changed, there is a return to near the resting level. This is indicative of almost complete adaptation to both chromaticity and luminance, occurring before or at the generation of the PC-pathway retinal ganglion cell signal. This adaptation could be either multiplicative or subtractive, as discussed in section 3.3. If a brief chromatic pulse is presented, the cell responds, showing a Naka–Rushton saturation function (Figure 3.12 in section 3.3) as the pulse is increased from the adaptation state. The V-shapes of chromatic discrimination can be viewed as characteristic of saturation functions following an earlier stage of neural adaptation (Zaidi *et al.*, 1992). At the point of the V, discrimination is assessed at the adapting chromaticity. These discriminations can also be considered as detections (section 3.3). The decrease in discrimination ability at low light levels is consistent with the idea that the neural adaptation becomes effective only above 1–10 trolands in the P pathway.

3.5 CONGENITAL COLOR DEFECT

Congenital color defects represent a hereditary, stationary condition in which there is an abnormality of color matching and/or color discrimination. Other visual function, including visual acuity, is normal. Such defects represent only a subset of the classification of human color defect which includes color vision problems accompanying hereditary and acquired eye disorders (Pokorny *et al.*, 1979). Congenital color defects have fascinated visual science since their discovery at the end of the eighteenth century. The fascination lies in the idea that color defects represent 'mistakes' of nature that can help elucidate the mechanisms of normal color vision. Today it is recognized that congenital color defects arise because of point mutations, rearrangements, and deletions of the opsin genes that determine the structure and function of the cone visual photopigments.

Congenital color defects may be classified on two dimensions: a qualitative dimension which states how color vision is affected and a quantitative dimension which describes the extent of discrimination loss. There are three major qualitative categories of defect, termed protan, deutan, and tritan.[3] The most common congenital defects are the protan and deutan defects. These defects show X-chromosome-linked inheritance and occur in 8% of the European male and 0.4% of the European female population (4–5% of the total European white population). The incidence in the United States is considered to be higher (Paulson, 1973). The tritan defect is rarer, occurring equally in both sexes in about 1 in 15 000 to 1 in 50 000 (0.002–0.007%) of the European population. The tritan defect has autosomal dominant inheritance. The inheritance, incidence, and classification of these defects are summarized in Table 3.5.

3.5.1 THE PROTAN AND DEUTAN DEFECTS

There are two qualitatively different forms of X-chromosome linked congenital defect. Protan observers show spectral sensitivity with long wavelength luminosity loss. Deutan observers show spectral sensitivity in the normal range at long wavelengths. The protan and deutan defects include a dichromatic form called protanopia and deuteranopia respectively. In the dichromatic defect, the affected observer requires only two primaries for full spectrum color matching. Protanopia and deuteranopia

Table 3.5 The inheritance, incidence and classification of congenital color vision defects

Type	Inheritance	Incidence	Classification
Protan and Deutan	X-chromosome linked recessive	8–10%(males) <1%(females)	
Protanopia		1%(males)	Dichromatic
Deuteranopia		1%(males)	Dichromatic
Protanomaly		1%(males)	Trichromatic
Deuteranomaly		5%(males)	Trichromatic
Tritan defect	Autosomal dominant	0.002–0.007	Dichromatic and Trichromatic

have traditionally been regarded as a 'reduction' form of color vision (von Kries, 1897). The dichromat was considered to lack function of one of the normal color fundamentals. The spectral sensitivity of protanopes and deuteranopes is shown in Figure 3.20. There are also trichromatic forms called protanomalous trichromacy (protanomaly) or deuteranomalous trichromacy (deuteranomaly). The color matches of protanomalous and deuteranomalous trichromats differ from each other and from those of normal trichromats. Anomalous trichromacy was historically regarded as an 'alteration' system (von Kries, 1897), but modern interpretation is in terms of inheritance of polymorphic forms of either the LWS (deuteranomalous) or the MWS (protanomalous) cone photopigments (see section 3.2.6).

The severity in discrimination loss of the protan and deutan defects varies considerably. The dichromatic form is more severe than the trichromatic form. It should be noted that variation is minimal within a family pedigree, i.e. both the qualitative and the quantitative extent of the defect are inherited. Color confusions and spectral sensitivity of protanopes and protanomalous trichromats or of deuteranopes and deuteranomalous trichromats are qualitatively similar, justifying the inclusive terms 'protan' and 'deutan' (Farnsworth, 1947). These similarities also allow the design of rapid screening tests for X-chromosome linked defects.

Full-spectrum colorimetry, spectral sensitivity, and wavelength and colorimetric purity discrimination functions for a limited number of observers have been described in the literature (Pokorny *et al.*, 1979). Some major features of protan and deutan color defects are summarized in Table 3.6.

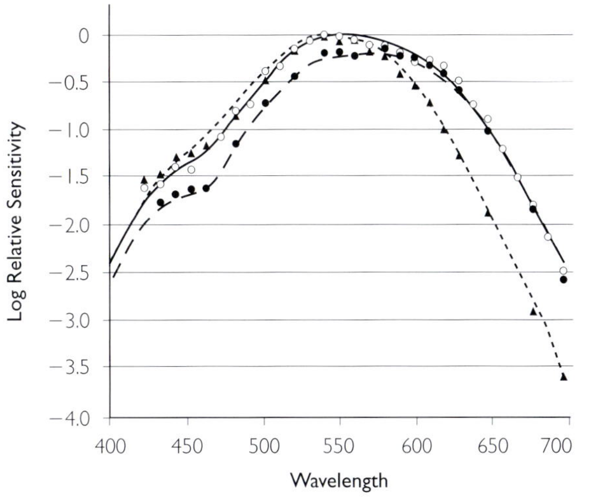

Figure 3.20 Dichromatic spectral sensitivity data. The symbols show the threshold data of Hsia and Graham. The solid lines represent the Smith and Pokorny (1975) fundamentals of Figure 3.7, adjusted vertically by eye to pass near the data.

The assumption that protanopes and deuteranopes lack one of the normal fundamentals allows the dichromatic color matches to be represented in the normal chromaticity diagram. The dichromatic color matches are normalized in the same manner as the normal matches. The dichromatic chromaticity coordinates fall on a line joining the two primaries. The chromaticity coordinates are joined to the corresponding test wavelength, forming a confusion line. The data reveal axes of discrimination loss characteristic of the type of defect. In the Judd revised chromaticity diagram, the confusion lines converge at a point, called the copunctal point (Figure 3.21). The copunctal point is considered the locus of the 'missing fundamental.' It is these copunctal points that form the new primaries in

Table 3.6 Major features of congenital color vision defects

Characteristic	Normal	Protan	Deutan	Tritan
Number of primaries used in color mixture	3	2(P) 3(PA)	2(D) 3(DA)	2 or 3
Neutral point (dichromats only)		494 nm	499 nm	570 nm
Copunctal point (dichromats only)		$X_p = 0.7635$ $Y_p = 0.2365$	$X_d = 1.4000$ $Y_d = -0.400$	$X_t = 0.1748$ $Y_t = 0.0000$
λ_{max} of luminosity	555 nm	540 nm	560 nm	555 nm
Minimum delta λ (best wavelength discrimination)	590 nm	490 nm	495 nm	590 nm
Minimum Pc (worst purity discrimination)	570 nm	494 nm	499 nm	570 nm

transforming from the Judd color matching functions to a set of König fundamentals (see section 3.2.5). One confusion line passes from the chromaticity coordinates through the equal energy spectrum to the spectrum locus. The spectral wavelength at the intersection is called the neutral point.

The X-chromosome linked defects are diagnosed and classified using a specialized color match, the Rayleigh equation. The Rayleigh equation presents a match of a 589 nm spectral test light to a mixture of two spectral primaries, 545 nm and 670 nm. Since the primaries fall near the linear portion of the long wavelength spectrum locus, a third primary is unnecessary. An anomaloscope is used to measure the Rayleigh match; the instrument is designed so that the mixture field has fixed energy levels, only the proportion of 545 nm:670 nm lights is varied. The 589 nm test is variable in luminance. For some primary ratios, the trichromatic observer can adjust the 589 nm test field and obtain a match. Protanopic and deuteranopic observers can match all the primary ratios with suitable adjustment of the 589 nm test luminance. Normal, protanomalous and deuteranomalous trichromats use very different 545 nm:670 nm primary ratios in their matches, thus allowing classification with high specificity. The accepted classification of X-chromosome linked defects, based on Rayleigh matching with a 2° field of low photopic luminance is shown in Table 3.5. This classification has been extended (Franceschetti, 1928) and replicated in large-scale studies (Schmidt, 1955; Helve, 1972). It is important to recognize that change in the parameters of study (e.g. test field size, primaries, etc.) will not yield the same classification. For example, few dichromats will accept the full range of primary ratio with an 8° test field. Most would then be classified as anomalous trichromats. Screening tests based upon discrimination rather than color matching do not permit conclusive classification of color defect nor usually do they indicate the severity of discrimination loss.

The genetic study of the protan and deutan defects has revealed point mutations (single nucleotide changes) or deletions within the opsin genes on the X chromosome. The opsins for normal MWS and LWS photopigments lie in a tandem array on the X chromosome. There may be multiple copies of these genes and the factors controlling their expression are not yet delineated. The nucleotide sequences of the MWS and LWS opsin genes are very similar. Only a few nucleotide changes differentiate whether the absorption spectrum will be that of an LWS or MWS photopigment. Some variation in these nucleotides (polymorphism) occurs naturally in the color-normal population. The protan and deutan defects are correlated with

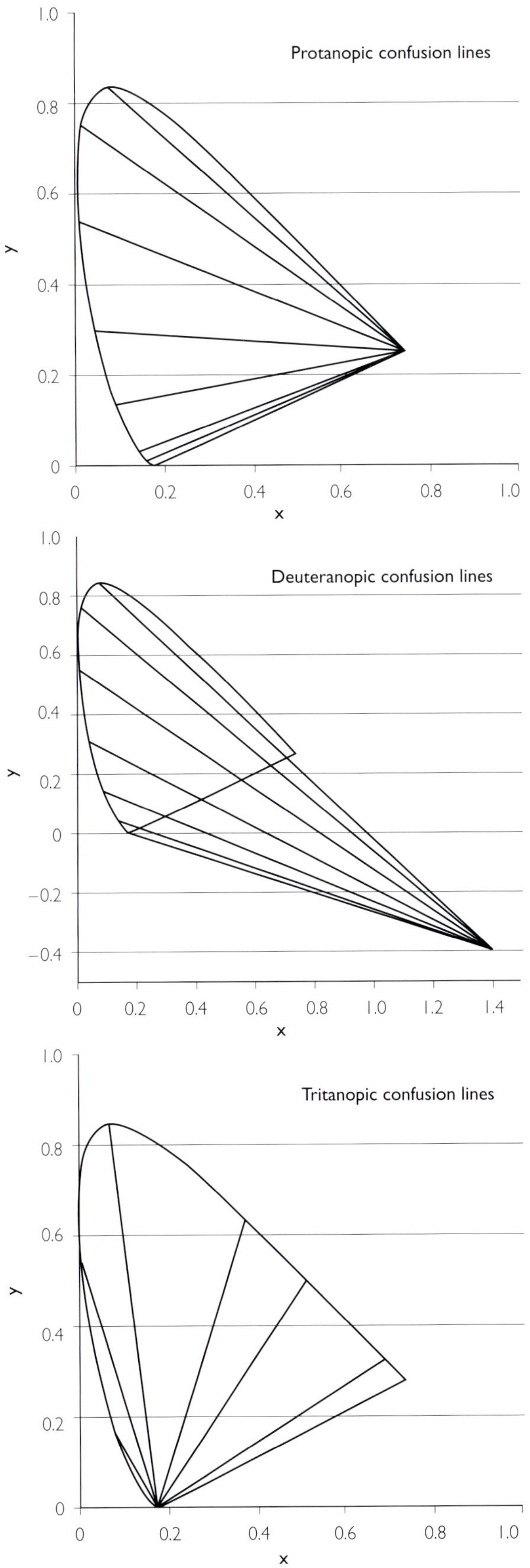

more pronounced alterations or with deletions of the opsin genes on the X-chromosome. The qualitative classification is well correlated with the type of gene alteration. The quantitative classification is less well correlated with the gene array. The correlation of genotype and phenotype remains an area of concentrated research.

3.5.2 TRITAN DEFECTS

The tritan defect is characterized by a lack of function of the mechanism that allows normals to discriminate colors that differ by the amount of short-wavelength light they contain. Discriminations dependent on LWS and MWS cone function are normal. Tritans show discrimination loss for SWS-cone mediated discrimination but do not show a specific alteration in color matching that would implicate variation in the absorption spectrum of the SWS photopigment. Some characteristics of tritan color deficiency are summarized in Table 3.6.

There is considerable variability in chromatic discrimination both within and between family pedigrees with tritan defect. Classification by color matching is less clear-cut. Some tritans make dichromatic color matches, but the majority do not. Discrimination improves with increase in field size (Pokorny *et al.*, 1981). Wright (1952) used a 1.2° field to classify and define tritanopia. For dichromatic tritans, the color matches can be treated as for protanopes and deuteranopes. The characteristic confusion axes for tritan defect are shown in Figure 3.21. There is no analog of anomalous trichromacy in autosomal dominant tritan defect size (Pokorny *et al.*, 1981).

The genetic study of the tritan defect has revealed point mutations (single nucleotide changes) or deletions within an opsin gene on the 7th chromosome ascribed to the SWS photopigment. The type of mutation is consistent within a pedigree of tritan defect.

Figure 3.21 Dichromatic confusion lines plotted on the Judd revised chromaticity diagram. The upper panel shows protanopic confusion lines, the middle panel shows deuteranopic confusion lines and the lower panel shows tritanopic confusion lines. (Copunctal points from Smith and Pokorny, 1975).

ACKNOWLEDGMENT

Preparation work for this chapter was supported in part by NIH Grant EY00901.

NOTES

1 The CIE has recommended standard sources for use in colorimetric specification. See Wyszecki and Stiles (1982) for further information. Those mentioned in this chapter include Standard Illuminants A, B, and C. CIE Standard Illuminant A is an incandescent tungsten filament lamp operated at a color temperature of approximately 2854 K. CIE Standard Illuminant B approximates noon sunlight, with a correlated color temperature of approximately 4870 K. CIE Standard Illuminant C approximates an overcast skylight, with a correlated color temperature of approximately 6740 K (Wyszecki and Stiles, 1982).

2 Differences in these equations from those in Smith and Pokorny (1975) result from rounding errors in the original calculation. Dr. Yasuhiso Nakano kindly noted and corrected them.

3 In the older literature, these defects were termed 'red-blind,' 'green-blind,' and 'blue-blind.' These terms, implying failure to perceive whole domains of color percepts, were dropped for the more agnostic terms now used. Nonetheless, color terms such as 'red–green defect' for the protan and deutan defects and 'blue–yellow defect' for the tritan defect remain common. Most protans and deutans recognize a wide variety of colors in the real world.

REFERENCES

Abramov, I., Gordon, J., and Chan, H. (1991) Color appearance in the peripheral retina: effects of stimulus size. *Journal of the Optical Society of America A*, 8, 404–14.

Adelson, E.H. (1982) Saturation and adaptation of the rod system. *Vision Research*, 22, 1299–312.

Alpern, M. (1979) Lack of uniformity in colour matching. *Journal of Physiology (London)*, 288, 85–105.

Barlow, H.B. (1956) Retinal noise and absolute threshold. *Journal of the Optical Society of America*, 46, 634–9.

Barlow, H.B. (1957) Increment thresholds at low intensities considered as signal/noise discrimination. *Journal of Physiology*, 136, 469–88.

Barlow, H.B. (1972) Dark and light adaptation: psychophysics. In D. Jameson and L.M. Hurvich (eds), *Handbook of Sensory Physiology, Visual Psychophysics* (Vol. VII/4). Berlin: Springer-Verlag, pp. 1–28.

Bedford, R.E. and Wyszecki, G.W. (1958a) Luminosity functions for various field sizes and levels of retinal illuminance. *Journal of the Optical Society of America*, 48, 406–11.

Bedford, R.E. and Wyszecki, G.W. (1958b) Wavelength discrimination for point sources. *Journal of the Optical Society of America*, 48, 129–35.

Bouma, P.J. (1947) *Physical Aspects of Colour*. Eindhoven: N.V. Philips Gloeilampenfabrieken.

Bouman, M.A. and Koenderink, J.J. (1972) Psychophysical basis of coincidence mechanisms in the human visual system. *Ergebnisse der Physiolgie*, 65, 126–72.

Bowmaker, J.K., Dartnall, H.J.A., Lythgoe, J.N., and Mollon, J.D. (1978) The visual pigments of rods and cones in the rhesus monkey, *Macaca mulatta*. *Journal of Physiology (London)*, 274, 329–48.

Boynton, R.M. (1963) Contributions of threshold measurements to color-discrimination theory. *Journal of the Optical Society of America*, 53, 165–78.

Boynton, R.M., Hayhoe, M.M., and MacLeod, D.I.A. (1977) The gap effect: chromatic and achromatic visual discrimination as affected by field separation. *Optica Acta*, 24, 159–77.

Boynton, R.M., Ikeda, M., and Stiles, W.S. (1964) Interactions among chromatic mechanisms as inferred from positive and negative increment thresholds. *Vision Research*, 4, 87.

Boynton, R.M. and Kambe, N. (1980) Chromatic difference steps of moderate size measured along theoretically critical axes. *Color Research and Application*, 5, 13–23.

Brindley, G.S. (1953) The effects on colour vision of adaptation to very bright lights. *Journal of Physiology (London)*, 122, 332–50.

Brindley, G.S. (1954) The summation areas of human colour-receptive mechanisms at increment threshold. *Journal of Physiology (London)*, 124, 400–8.

Brindley, G.S. (1970) *Physiology of the Retina and the Visual Pathway*, 2nd edn. Baltimore, MD: Williams and Wilkins.

Brindley, G.S., du Croz, J.J., and Rushton, W.A.H. (1966) The flicker fusion frequency of the blue-sensitive mechanism of colour vision. *Journal of Physiology (London)*, 183, 497–500.

Brown, W.R.J. (1951) The influence of luminance level on visual sensitivity to color differences. *Journal of the Optical Society of America*, 41, 684–8.

Brown, W.R.J. (1952) The effect of field size and chromatic surroundings on color discrimination. *Journal of the Optical Society of America*, 42, 837–44.

Brown, W.R.J. and MacAdam, D.L. (1949) Visual sensitivities to combined chromaticity and luminance differences. *Journal of the Optical Society of America*, 39, 808–34.

Burns, S. and Elsner, A. (1985) Color matching at high illuminances: the color-match-area-effect and photopigment bleaching. *Journal of the Optical Society of America A*, 2, 698–704.

Burns, S.A. and Elsner, A.E. (1993) Color matching at high illuminances: photopigment optical density and pupil entry. *Journal of the Optical Society of America A*, 10, 221–30.

Cavonius, C.R. and Estévez, O. (1975) Sensitivity of human color mechanisms to gratings and flicker. *Journal of the Optical Society of America*, 65, 966–8.

CIE (1926) *Proceedings*, 1924, (pp. 1–232). Cambridge: Cambridge University Press.

CIE (1964) *Proceedings*, 1963 (Vienna Session), Vol. B. (Committee Report E–1.4.1), Paris, Bureau Central de la CIE, pp. 209–20.

Clarke, F.J.J. (1967) Colour measurement in industry. The effect of field–element size on chromaticity discrimination. Paper presented at the Proceedings of a Symposium on Colour Measurement in Industry, London.

Cornsweet, T.N. (1970) *Visual Perception*. New York: Academic Press.

Cornu, L. and Harlay, F. (1969) Modifications de la discrimination chromatique en fonction de l'eclairement. *Vision Research*, 9, 1273–87.

Crawford, B.H. (1949) The scotopic visibility function. *Proceedings of the Physical Society, B*, 62, 321–34.

Crawford, B.H. (1965) Colour matching and adaptation. *Vision Research*, 5, 71–8.

Dartnall, H.J.A. (1957) *The Visual Pigments*. London: Methuen and Company.

Dartnall, H.J.A. (1962) Extraction, measurement, and analysis of visual photopigment. In H. Davson (ed.), *The Eye*, Vol. 2. New York: Academic Press.

de Lange, H. (1958) Research into the dynamic nature of the human fovea–cortex systems with intermittent and modulated light. *Journal of the Optical Society of America*, 48, 779–89.

Eisner, A., Fleming, S.A., Klein, M.L., and Mouldin, W.M. (1987) Sensitivities in older eyes with good acuity: Cross-sectional norms. *Investigative Ophthalmology and Visual Science*, 28, 1824–31.

Eisner, A. and MacLeod, D.I.A. (1981) Flicker photometric study of chromatic adaptation: selective suppression of cone inputs by colored backgrounds. *Journal of the Optical Society of America*, 71, 705–18.

Estévez, O. (1979) On the fundamental data base of normal and dichromatic vision. Doctoral Dissertation (Vol. 17). Amsterdam: Krips Repro Meppel.

Estévez, O. and Cavonius, C.R. (1975) Flicker sensitivity of the human red and green color mechanisms. *Vision Research*, 15, 879–81.

Farnsworth, D. (1947) *The Farnsworth Dichotomous Test for Color Blindness – Panel D–15*. New York: Psychological Corporation.

Farnsworth, D. (1955) Tritanomalous vision as a threshold function. *Die Farbe*, 4, 185–97.

Farnsworth, D. (1961) A temporal factor in colour discrimination. *NPL Symposium No. 8, Visual Problems of Colour* (Vol. 2). New York: Chemical Publishing Co., pp. 65–78

Franceschetti, A. (1928) Die Bedeutung der Einstellungsbreite am Anomaloskop fur die Diagnose der eizelnen Typen der Farbensinnstorungen nebst Bemerkungen uber ihre Vererbungsmodus. *Schweizerische Medizinische Wochenschrift*, 52, 1273–8.

Fridrikh, L. (1957) Colour-combination curves for normal trichromats determined by direct energy measurements. *Biophysics* [translation of *Biofizika*], 2, 129–32.

Galbraith, W. and Marshall, P.N. (1985) A survey of transforms of the CIE 1931 chromaticity diagram with some new non-linear transforms and histological illustrations of their utility. *Acta Histochemica*, 77, 79–100.

Geisler, W.S. (1981) Effects of bleaching and backgrounds on the flash response of the cone system. *Journal of Physiology (London)*, 312, 413–34.

Goldstein, E.B. and Williams, T.P. (1966) Calculated effects of 'screening pigments', *Vision Research*, 6, 39–50.

Grassmann, H. (1853) Zur Theorie der Farbenmischung. *Annalen der Physik (Leipzig)*, 89, 60–84. [English trans. *Philosophical Magazine (London)*, 1854, 7: 254–64.]

Green, D.G. (1968) The contrast sensitivity of the colour mechanisms of the human eye. *Journal of Physiology (London)*, 196, 415–29.

Green, D.G. (1969) Sinusoidal flicker characteristics of the color-sensitive mechanisms of the eye. *Vision Research*, 9, 591–601.

Grigorovici, R. and Aricescu-Savopol, I. (1958) Luminosity and chromaticity in the mesopic range. *Journal of the Optical Society of America*, 48, 891–8.

Guild, J. (1931) The colorimetric properties of the spectrum. *Philosophical Transactions of the Royal Society London A*, 230, 149–87.

Hammond, B.R., Wooten, B.R., and Snodderly, D.M. (1997) Individual variations in the spatial profile of human macular pigment. *Journal of Optical Society of America, A*, 14, 1187–96.

Hartridge, H. (1945) The change from trichromatic to dichromatic vision in the human retina. *Nature*, 155, 657–62.

Hayhoe, M., Benimoff, N.I., and Hood, D.C. (1987) The time-course of multiplicative and subtractive adaptation processes. *Vision Research*, 27, 1981–96.

Hecht, S., Shlaer, S., and Pirenne, M.H. (1942) Energy, quanta and vision. *Journal of General Physiology*, 224, 665–99.

Helve, J. (1972) A comparative study of several diagnostic tests of colour vision used for measuring types and degrees of congenital red–green defects. *Acta Ophthalmologica Supplement*, 115, 1–64.

Hilz, R. and Cavonius, C.R. (1970) Wavelength discrimination measured with square-wave gratings. *Journal of the Optical Society of America*, 60, 273–7.

Hita, E., Romero, J., Jimenez del Barco, L., and Martinez, R. (1982) Temporal aspects of color discrimination. *Journal of the Optical Society of America*, 72, 578–82.

Hood, D.C. (1998) Lower-level visual processing and models of light adaptation. *Annual Review of Psychology*, 49, 503–35.

Hood, D.C. and Finkelstein, M.A. (1986) Sensitivity to light. In K.R. Boff, L. Kaufman, and J.P. Thomas (eds), *Handbook of Perception and Human Performance, Vol I: Sensory Processes and Perception*. New York: John Wiley and Sons, pp. 5-1–5-66.

Horner, R.G. and Purslow, E.T. (1947) Dependence of anomaloscope matches on viewing distance or field size. *Nature*, 160, 23–4.

Hurvich, L.M. and Jameson, D. (1961) Opponent chromatic induction and wavelength discrimination. In R. Jung and H. Kornhuber (eds), *The Visual System: Neurophysiology and Psychophysics*. Berlin: Springer, pp. 144–52.

Ingling, C.R. and Martinez, E. (1981) Stiles' Π 5 mechanism: failure to show univariance is caused by opponent–channel input. *Journal of the Optical Society of America*, 71, 1134–7.

Jin, E.W. and Shevell, S.K. (1996) Color memory and color constancy. *Journal of the Optical Society of America A*, 13, 1981–91.

Jones, L.A. and Lowry, E.M. (1926) Retinal sensibility to saturation differences. *Journal of the Optical Society of America*, 13, 25–34.

Judd, D.B. (1930) Reduction of data on mixture of color stimuli. *Journal of Research National Bureau of Standards (USA)*, 4, 515–48.

Judd, D.B. (1935) A Maxwell triangle yielding uniform chromaticity scales. *Journal of the Optical Society of America*, 25, 24–35.

Judd, D.B. (1951a) Basic correlates of the visual stimulus. In S.S. Stevens (ed.), *Handbook of Experimental Psychology*. New York: Wiley, pp. 811–67.

Judd, D.B. (1951b) Colorimetry and artificial daylight. In Technical Committee No. 7 Report of Secretariat United States Commission, International Commission on Illumination, Twelfth Session, Stockholm, pp. 1–60.

Kaiser, P.K., Comerford, J.P., and Bodinger, D.M. (1976) Saturation of spectral lights. *Journal of the Optical Society of America*, 66, 818–26.

Kelly, D.H. (1974) Spatio-temporal frequency characteristics of color-vision mechanisms. *Journal of the Optical Society of America*, 64, 983–90.

Kelly, D.H. and van Norren, D. (1977) Two-band model of heterochromatic flicker. *Journal of the Optical Society of America*, 67, 1081–91.

King-Smith, P.E. and Carden, D. (1976) Luminance and opponent-color contributions to visual detection and adaptation and to temporal and spatial integration. *Journal of the Optical Society of America*, 66, 709–17.

King-Smith, P.E. and Webb, J.R. (1974) The use of photopic saturation in determining the fundamental spectral sensitivity curves. *Vision Research*, 14, 421–9.

Knoblauch, K., Saunders, F., Kusuda, M., Hynes, R., Podgor, M., Higgens, K.E., and deMosasterio, M. (1987) Age and illuminance effects in the Farnsworth–Munsell 100-hue test. *Applied Optics*, 26, 1441–8.

Koenderink, J.J., van de Grind, W.A., and Bouman, M.A. (1970) Models of retinal signal processing at high luminances. *Kybernetik*, 6, 227–37.

König, A. (1894) Uber den menschlichen Sehpurpur und seine Bedeutung fur das Sehen. *Akademie der Wissenschaften Berlin, Sitzungsberichte*, pp. 577–98.

König, A. and Dieterici, C. (1886) Die Grundempfindungen und ihre Intensitats–Vertheilung im Spectrum. *Akademie der Wissenschaften Berlin, Sitzungsberichte, Pt.2*, pp. 805–29.

König, A. and Dieterici, C. (1893) Die Grundempfindungen in normalen und anomalen Farben Systemen und ihre Intensitats-Verthielung im Spectrum. *Zeitschrift für Psychologie und Physiologie der Sinnesorgane*, 4, 241–347.

Krauskopf, J., Williams, D.R., and Heeley, D.W. (1982) Cardinal directions of color space. *Vision Research*, 22, 1123–31.

Le Grand, Y. (1968) *Light, Colour and Vision*, 2nd edn. London: Chapman and Hall, pp. 1–564.

Lee, B.B., Pokorny, J., Smith, V.C., Martin, P.R., and Valberg, A. (1990) Luminance and chromatic modulation sensitivity of macaque ganglion cells and human observers. *Journal of the Optical Society of America A*, 7, 2223–36.

Loomis, J.M. and Berger, T. (1979) Effects of chromatic adaptation on color discrimination and color appearance. *Vision Research*, 19, 891–901.

Lythgoe, R. (1931) Dark-adaptation and the peripheral colour sensations of normal subjects. *British Journal of Ophthalmology*, 15, 193–210.

MacAdam, D.L. (1942) Visual sensitivities to color differences in daylight. *Journal of the Optical Society of America*, 32, 247–74.

MacAdam, D.L. (1959) Small-field chromaticity discrimination. *Journal of the Optical Society of America*, 49, 1143–6.

MacLeod, D.I.A. and Boynton, R.M. (1979) Chromaticity diagram showing cone excitation by stimuli of equal luminance. *Journal of the Optical Society of America*, 69, 1183–5.

Martin, L.C., Warburton, F.L., and Morgan, W.J. (1933) The determination of the sensitiveness of the eye to differences in the saturation of colours. *Great Britain Medical Research Council*, 188, 5–42.

Maxwell, J.C. (1860) On the theory of compound colors and relations of the colors of the spectrum. *Philosophical Transactions*, 150, 57–84. [Reprinted with commentary by Qasim Zaidi in: *Color Research and Application*, 1993, 18, 270–87.]

McCree, K.J. (1960) Small-field tritanopia and the effects of voluntary fixation. *Optica Acta*, 7, 317–23.

Merbs, S.L. and Nathans, J. (1992) Absorption spectra of human cone pigments. *Nature*, 356, 433–5.

Miles, W.R. (1954) Comparison of the functional and structural areas in human fovea. I. Method of entoptic plotting. *Journal of Neurophysiology*, 17, 22–38.

Miller, S.S. (1972) Psychophysical estimates of visual pigment densities in red–green dichromats. *Journal of Physiology (London)*, 223, 89–107.

Miyahara, E., Pokorny, J., and Smith, V.C. (1996) Increment threshold and purity discrimination spectral sensitivities of X-chromosome-linked color defective observers. *Vision Research*, 36, 1597–613.

Miyahara, E., Smith, V.C., and Pokorny, J. (1993) How surrounds affect chromaticity discrimination. *Journal of the Optical Society of America A*, 10, 545–53.

Mollon, J.D. and Polden, P.G. (1977) An anomaly in the response of the eye to light of short wavelengths. *Philosophical Transactions of the Royal Society of London – Series B: Biological Sciences*, 278, 207–40.

Moreland, J.D. (1972) Peripheral Colour Vision. In D. Jameson and L.M. Hurvich (eds), *Handbook of Sensory Physiology, Visual Psychophysics*, Vol. VII/4. Berlin: Springer-Verlag, pp. 517–36.

Moreland, J.D. and Bhatt, P. (1984) Retinal distribution of macular pigment. *Documenta Ophthalmologica Proceedings Series*, 39, 127–32.

Moreland, J.D. and Cruz, A. (1959) Colour perception with the peripheral retina. *Optica Acta*, 6, 117–51.

Moreland, J.D., Torczynski, E., and Tripathi, R. (1991) Rayleigh and Moreland matches in the ageing eye. *Documenta Ophthalmologica Proceedings Series*, 54, 347–52.

Mullen, K.T. (1985) The contrast sensitivity of human colour vision to red–green and blue–yellow chromatic gratings. *Journal of Physiology (London)*, 359, 381–400.

Nacer, A., Murray, I.J., and Carden, D. (1989) Interactions between luminance mechanisms and colour opponency. In C.M. Dickinson and I.J. Murray (eds), *Seeing Contour and Colour*. Oxford: Pergamon Press, pp. 357–60.

Neitz, M., Neitz, J., and Jacobs, G.H. (1991) Spectral tuning of pigments underlying red–green color vision. *Science*, 252, 971–3.

Noorlander, C., Heuts, M.J.G., and Koenderink, J.J. (1980) Influence of the target size on the detection threshold for luminance and chromaticity contrast. *Journal of the Optical Society of America*, 70, 1116–21.

Noorlander, C., Heuts, M.J.G., and Koenderink, J.J. (1981) Sensitivity to spatiotemporal combined luminance and chromaticity contrast. *Journal of the Optical Society of America*, 71, 453–9.

Palmer, D.A. (1978) Maxwell spot and additivity in tetrachromatic matches. *Journal of the Optical Society of America*, 68, 1501–5.

Palmer, D.A. (1981) Nonadditivity in color matches with four instrumental primaries. *Journal of the Optical Society of America*, 71, 966–9.

Paulson, H.M. (1973) Comparison of color vision tests used by the Armed Forces. *Color Vision*. National Academy of Sciences.

Pease, P.L., Adams, A.J., and Nuccio, E. (1987) Optical density of human macular pigment. *Vision Research*, 27, 705–10.

Pointer, M.R. (1974) Color discrimination as a function of observer adaptation. *Journal of the Optical Society of America*, 64, 750–9.

Poirson, A.B. and Wandell, B.A. (1990) The ellipsoidal representation of spectral sensitivity. *Vision Research*, 30, 647–52.

Pokorny, J. and Smith, V.C. (1970) Wavelength discrimination in the presence of added chromatic fields. *Journal of the Optical Society of America*, 69, 562–9.

Pokorny, J. and Smith, V. C. (1976) Effect of field size on red–green color mixture equations. *Journal of the Optical Society of America*, 66, 705–8.

Pokorny, J. and Smith, V.C. (1981) A variant of red–green color defect. *Vision Research*, 21, 311–17.

Pokorny, J. and Smith, V.C. (1986) Colorimetry and Color Discrimination. In K.R. Boff, L. Kaufman, and J P. Thomas (eds), *Handbook of Perception and Human Performance, Vol I: Sensory Processes and Perception*. New York: John Wiley and Sons, pp. 8-1–8-51.

Pokorny, J. and Smith, V.C. (1997) How much light reaches the retina? In C.R. Cavonius (ed.), *Colour Vision Deficiencies XIII. Documenta Ophthalmologica Proceedings Series*, 59, 491–511.

Pokorny, J., Smith, V. C., and Lutze, M. (1987) Aging of the human lens. *Applied Optics*, 26, 1437–40.

Pokorny, J., Smith, V.C., and Starr, S.J. (1976) Variability of color mixture data – II. The effect of viewing field size on the unit coordinates. *Vision Research*, 16, 1095–8.

Pokorny, J., Smith, V.C., Verriest, G., and Pinckers, A.J.L.G. (eds) (1979) *Congenital and Acquired Color Vision Defects*. New York: Grune and Stratton.

Pokorny, J., Smith, V.C., and Went, L.N. (1981) Color matching in autosomal dominant tritan defect. *Journal of the Optical Society of America*, 71, 1327–34.

Polden, P.G. and Mollon, J.D. (1980) Reversed effects of adapting stimuli on visual sensitivity. *Proceedings of the Royal Society of London Series B*, 210, 235–72.

Polyak, S.L. (1957) *The Vertebrate Visual System*. Chicago: University of Chicago Press.

Pugh, E.N. (1976) The nature of the π-1 colour mechanism of W.S. Stiles. *Journal of Physiology (London)*, 257, 713–47.

Pugh, E.N.J. and Kirk, D.B. (1986) The pi mechanisms of WS Stiles: an historical review. [Review]. *Perception*, 15, 705–28.

Pugh, E.N.J. and Mollon, J.D. (1979) A theory of the π-1 and π-3 color mechanisms of Stiles. *Vision Research*, 19, 293–312.

Regan, D. and Tyler, C.W. (1971) Temporal summation and its limit for wavelength changes: an analog of Bloch's Law for color vision. *Journal of the Optical Society of America*, 61, 1414–21.

Richards, W. and Luria, S.M. (1964) Color-mixture functions at low luminance levels. *Vision Research*, 4, 281–313.

Ruddock, K.H. (1963) Evidence for macular pigmentation from colour matching data. *Vision Research*, 3, 417–29.

Rushton, W.A.H. (1972) Visual pigments in man. In H.J.A. Dartnall (ed.), *Handbook of Sensory Physiology*, Vol. VII/I. Berlin: Springer, pp. 364–94.

Sachtler, W.L. and Zaidi, Q. (1992) Chromatic and luminance signals in visual memory. *Journal of the Optical Society of America A*, 9, 877–94.

Sanocki, E., Shevell, S.K., and Winderickx, J. (1994) Serine/Alanine amino acid polymorphism of the

L-cone photopigment assessed by dual Rayleigh-type color matches. *Vision Research*, 34, 377–82.

Schmidt, I. (1955) Some problems related to testing color vision with the Nagel anomaloscope. *Journal of the Optical Society of America*, 45, 514–22.

Schrödinger, E. (1920) Grundlinien einer Theorie der Farbenmetrik im Tagessehen. *Annalen der Physik (Leipzig)*, 63, 134–82. English translation in D.L. MacAdam (ed.), *Sources of Color Science*. Cambridge, MA: The MIT Press, 1970.

Schrödinger, E. (1925) Ueber das Verhaltnis der Vierfarben- zur Dreifarbentheorie. *Sitzungsberichte der Mathematisch–naturwissenschaftlichen Klasse der Kaiserlichen Akademie der Wissenschaften Wien, 134, Abt. IIa*, 471–90. [Commentary by Qasim Zaidi and National Translation Center translation 'On the relationship of four-color theory to three-color theory', *Color Research and Application*, 1994, 19, 37–47.]

Sekiguchi, N., Williams, D.R., and Brainard, D.H. (1993) Aberration-free measurements of the visibility of isoluminant gratings. *Journal of the Optical Society of America A*, 10, 2105–17.

Shapiro, A.G., Pokorny, J., and Smith, V.C. (1994) Rod contribution to large field color-matching. *Color Research and Application*, 19, 236–45.

Shapiro, A.G., Pokorny, J., and Smith, V.C. (1996) Cone-rod receptor spaces, with illustrations that use CRT phosphor and light-emitting-diode spectra. *Journal of the Optical Society of America A*, 13, 2319–28.

Sharpe, L.T. and Wyszecki, G. (1976) Proximity factor in color-difference evaluations. *Journal of the Optical Society of America*, 66, 40–9.

Shevell, S.K. (1977) Saturation in human cones. *Vision Research*, 17, 427–34.

Siegel, M.H. (1965) Color discrimination as a function of exposure time. *Journal of the Optical Society of America*, 55, 566–8.

Smith, V. and Pokorny, J. (1973) Psychophysical estimates of optical density in human cones. *Vision Research*, 13, 1099–202.

Smith, V.C. and Pokorny, J. (1975) Spectral sensitivity of the foveal cone photopigments between 400 and 500 nm. *Vision Research*, 15, 161–71.

Smith, V.C. and Pokorny, J. (1977) Large-field trichromacy in protanopes and deuteranopes. *Journal of the Optical Society of America*, 67, 213–20.

Smith, V.C. and Pokorny, J. (1996) The design and use of a cone chromaticity space. *Color Research and Application*, 21, 375–83.

Smith, V.C., Pokorny, J., Lee, B.B., and Dacey, D.M. (2001) Primate Horizontal Cell Dynamics: An Analysis of Sensitivity Regulation in the Outer Retina. *Journal of Neurophysiology*, 85, 545–58.

Smith, V.C., Pokorny, J., and Starr, S.J. (1976) Variability of color mixture data – I. Interobserver variability in the unit coordinates. *Vision Research*, 16, 1087–94.

Smith, V.C., Pokorny, J., and Sun, H. (2000) Chromatic contrast discrimination: Data and prediction for stimuli varying in L and M cone excitation. *Color Research and Application*, 25, 105–15.

Smith, V.C., Pokorny, J., and Zaidi, Q. (1983) How do sets of color-matching functions differ? In J.D. Mollon and L.T. Sharpe (eds), *Colour Vision: Physiology and Psychophysics*. London: Academic Press, pp. 93–105.

Speranskaya, N.I. (1959) Determination of spectrum color coordinates for twenty-seven normal observers. *Optics and Spectroscopy*, 7, 424–8.

Speranskaya, N.I. (1961) Methods of determination of the co-ordinates of spectrum colours. *NPL Symposium No. 8, Visual Problems of Colour* (Vol. 1). New York: Chemical Publishing Co., pp. 319–25.

Sperling, H.G. and Harwerth, R.S. (1971) Red–green cone interaction in the increment-threshold spectral sensitivity of primates. *Science*, 172, 180–4.

Stabell, B. and Stabell, U. (1976) Rod and cone contributions to peripheral colour vision. *Vision Research*, 16, 1099–104.

Stabell, U. and Stabell, B. (1977) Wavelength discrimination of peripheral cones and its change with rod intrusion. *Vision Research*, 17, 423–6.

Stabell, U. and Stabell, B. (1980) Variation in density of macular pigmentation and in short-wave cone sensitivity with eccentricity. *Journal of the Optical Society of America*, 70, 706–11.

Stabell, U. and Stabell, B. (1982) Color vision in the peripheral retina under photopic conditions. *Vision Research*, 22, 839–44.

Stiles, W.S. (1949) Increment thresholds and the mechanisms of colour vision. *Documenta Ophthalmologica*, 3, 138–63.

Stiles, W.S. (1955) 18th Thomas Young Oration. The basic data of colour-matching. *The Yearbook of the Physical Society*, pp. 44–65.

Stiles, W.S. (1959) Color vision: The approach through increment threshold sensitivity. *Proceedings National Academy of Sciences USA*, 45, 100–14.

Stiles, W.S. (1978) *Mechanisms of Colour Vision*. London: Academic Press.

Stiles, W.S. and Burch, J.M. (1955) Interim report to the Commission Internationale de l'Eclairage, Zurich, 1955, on the National Physical Laboratory's investigation of colour-matching. *Optica Acta*, 2, 168–81.

Stiles, W.S. and Burch, J.M. (1959) NPL colour-matching investigation: final report. *Optica Acta*, 6, 1–26.

Stockman, A., MacLeod, D.M., and Johnson, N.E. (1993) Spectral sensitivities of the human cones. *Journal of the Optical Society of America*, 10, 2491–521.

Stockman, A., MacLeod, D.M., and Vivien, J.A. (1993) Isolation of the middle- and long-wavelength sensitive cones in normal trichromats. *Journal of the Optical Society of America*, 10, 2471–90.

Stockman, A. and Mollon, J. (1986) The spectral sensitivities of the middle- and long-wavelength cones: an extension of the two-colour threshold technique of W.S. Stiles. *Perception*, 15, 729–54.

Stockman, A. and Sharpe, L.T. (2000) The spectral sensitivities of the middle- and long-wavelength-sensitive cones derived from measurements in observers of known genotype. *Vision Research*, 40, 1711–37.

Swanson, W.H. and Fish, G.E. (1996) Age-related changes in the color-match-area effect. *Vision Research*, 36, 2079–85.

Swanson, W.H., Ueno, T., Smith, V.C., and Pokorny, J. (1987) Temporal modulation sensitivity and pulse detection thresholds for chromatic and luminance perturbations. *Journal of the Optical Society of America A*, 4, 1992–2005.

Tan, K.E.W.P. (1971) *Vision in the Ultraviolet*. Utrecht: Drukkerij Elinkwijk.

Terstiege, H. (1967) Untersuchungen zum Persistenz- und Koeffizientensatz. *Die Farbe*, 16, 1–120.

Thomson, L.C. and Wright, W.D. (1947) The colour sensitivity of the retina within the central fovea of man. *Journal of Physiology (London)*, 105, 316–31.

Thornton, J.E. and Pugh, E.N.J. (1983) Red/green color opponency at detection threshold. *Science*, 219, 191–3.

Trezona, P.W. (1970) Rod participation in the 'blue' mechanism and its effect on colour matching. *Vision Research*, 10, 317–32.

Troland, L.T. (1915) The theory and practise of the artificial pupil. *Psychological Review*, 22, 167–76.

Troy, J.B. and Lee, B.B. (1994) Steady discharges of macaque retinal ganglion cells. *Visual Neuroscience*, 11, 111–18.

Troy, J.B. and Robson, J.G. (1992) Steady discharges of X and Y retinal ganglion cells of cat under photopic illuminance. *Visual Neuroscience*, 9, 535–53.

Tyndall, E.P.T. (1933) Chromaticity sensibility to wave-length difference as a function of purity. *Journal of the Optical Society of America*, 23, 15–24.

Uchikawa, K. (1983) Purity discrimination: successive vs simultaneous comparison method. *Vision Research*, 23, 53–8.

Uchikawa, K. and Ikeda, M. (1981) Temporal deterioration of wavelength discrimination with successive comparison method. *Vision Research*, 21, 591–5.

van der Horst, G.J.C. and Bouman, M.A. (1969) Spatiotemporal chromaticity discrimination. *Journal of the Optical Society of America*, 59, 1482–8.

van der Horst, G.J.C., de Weert, C.M.M., and Bouman, M.A. (1967) Transfer of spatial chromaticity contrast at threshold in the human eye. *Journal of the Optical Society of America*, 57, 1260–7.

van Norren, D. and Vos, J.J. (1974) Spectral transmission of the human ocular media. *Vision Research*, 14, 1237–44.

Verriest, G., Buyssens, A., and Vanderdonck, R. (1963) Etude quantitative de l'effet qu'exerce sur les resultats de quelques tests de la discrimination chromatique une diminution non selective du niveau d'un eclairage. *Revue d'Optique*, 3, 105–19.

Viénot, F. (1983) Can variation in macular pigment account for the variation of colour matches with retinal position? In J.D. Mollon and L.T. Sharpe (eds), *Colour Vision*. New York: Academic Press, pp. 107–16.

von Kries, J. (1897) Uber Farbensysteme. *Zeitschrift für Psychologie Physiologie Sinnesorg*, 13, 241–324.

Vos, J.J. (1972) Literature review of human macular absorption in the visible and its consequences for the cone receptor primaries (2F1972–17). TNO Report, Institute for Perception, Soesterberg The Netherlands.

Vos, J.J. (1978) Colorimetric and photometric properties of a 2° fundamental observer. *Color Research and Application*, 3, 125–8.

Vos, J.J. and Walraven, P.L. (1971) On the derivation of the foveal receptor primaries. *Vision Research*, 11, 799–818.

Wald, G. (1964) The receptors of human color vision. *Science*, 145, 1007.

Watson, W. (1911) Note on the sensibility of the eye to variations of wave-length. *Proceedings of the Royal Society (London)*, B84, 118–21.

Weale, R.A. (1988) Age and the transmittance of the human crystalline lens. *Journal of Physiology (London)*, 395, 577–87.

Werner, J.S., Donnelly, S.K., and Kliegl, R. (1987) Aging and human macular pigment density. *Vision Research*, 27, 257–68.

Wisowaty, J.J. (1981) Estimates for the temporal response characteristics of chromatic pathways. *Journal of the Optical Society of America*, 71, 970–7.

Wisowaty, J.J. and Boynton, R.M. (1980) Temporal modulation sensitivity of the blue mechanism: measurements made without chromatic adaptation. *Vision Research*, 20, 895–909.

Wright, W.D. (1929) A re-determination of the trichromatic coefficients of the spectral colours. *Transactions of the Optical Society*, 30, 141–64.

Wright, W.D. (1941) The sensitivity of the eye to small colour differences. *Proceedings of the Physical Society (London)*, 53, 93–112.

Wright, W.D. (1946) *Researches on Normal and Defective Colour Vision*. London: Henry Kimpton.

Wright, W.D. (1952) The characteristics of tritanopia. *Journal of the Optical Society of America*, 42, 509–20.

Wright, W.D. and Pitt, F.H.G. (1937) The saturation-discrimination of two trichromats. *Proceedings of the Physical Society (London)*, 49, 329–31.

Wyszecki, G. and Fielder, G.H. (1971) New color-matching ellipses. *Journal of the Optical Society of America*, 61, 1135–52.

Wyszecki, G. and Stiles, W.S. (1980) High-level trichromatic color matching and the pigment-bleaching hypothesis. *Vision Research*, 20, 23–37.

Wyszecki, G. and Stiles, W.S. (1982) *Color Science – Concepts and Methods, Quantitative Data and Formulae*, 2nd edn. New York: John Wiley and Sons.

Yeh, T., Pokorny, J., and Smith, V.C. (1993) Chromatic discrimination with variation in chromaticity and luminance: data and theory. *Vision Research*, 33, 1835–45.

Yeh, T., Smith, V.C., and Pokorny, J. (1989) The effect of background luminance on cone sensitivity functions. *Investigative Ophthalmology and Visual Science*, 30, 2077–86.

Yeh, T., Smith, V. C., and Pokorny, J. (1993) Colorimetric purity discrimination: data and theory. *Vision Research*, 33, 1847–57.

Yonemura, G.T. and Kasuya, M. (1969) Color discrimination under reduced angular subtense and luminance. *Journal of the Optical Society of America*, 59, 131–5.

Young, T. (1802) On the theory of light and colours. *Philisophical Transactions (London)*, 92, 12–48.

Zaidi, Q. (1986) Adaptation and color matching. *Vision Research*, 26, 1925–38.

Zaidi, Q., Shapiro, A., and Hood, D. (1992) The effect of adaptation on the differential sensitivity of the S-cone color system. *Vision Research*, 32, 1297–318.

4 Color Appearance

Steven K. Shevell

Departments of Psychology and Ophthalmology & Visual Science,
University of Chicago, 940 East Fifty-seventh Street,
Chicago, IL 60637, USA

CHAPTER CONTENTS

The Science of Color
ISBN 0–444–512–519

4.1 INTRODUCTION

4.1.1 LIGHT, COLOR, AND NEURONS

When speaking of *color* in ordinary conversation we usually mean the aspect of visual experience that goes beyond perceived intensity (dim to bright). A light, a surface or an object appears a particular shade of blue or orange. Acronyms are learned by children in school for the colors we perceive when light is refracted by a prism or is seen in a rainbow: ROY G BIV (red–orange–yellow–green–blue–indigo–violet). A first course in physics describes light as the part of the electromagnetic spectrum from 400 to 700 nm. The shortest wavelengths appear violet, the longest appear red; from 400–700 nm the colors change continuously according to ROY G BIV in reverse order. A tempting conclusion is that the colors we see are explained by the color in each wavelength of light. That conclusion, however, would be wrong.

Color appearance is a mental phenomenon, not a physical one. No wavelength of light is endowed with a color. For example, 700 nm is perceived as red only because that wavelength selectively and unequally stimulates the eye's several types of photoreceptors, which transduce physical light to physiological neural responses. *Red* is a human experience resulting from subsequent neural events in the retina and brain. There is no red in a 700 nm light, just as there is no pain in the hooves of a kicking horse. We experience red or pain when an external physical stimulus – a 700 nm light or a hoof – excites a human sensory system.

Two observations demonstrate the dissociation between color appearance and the wavelengths of light that reach the eye. First, examine the three rings in the top row of Figure 4.1. All three rings are physically identical; that is, they reflect the same light to the eye. The rings differ in their appearance because color perception is affected by the lights in the surrounding regions. Similarly, the three rings in the second row are all identical but vary in appearance with the surrounding light. This is an example of chromatic induction (section 4.3.3): a surrounding region alters the perceived color of the light entering the eye (Chevreul, 1839).

Another demonstration of color as a mental construction, not a property of light, is the appearance of Figure 4.1 under much reduced illumination. Find a room with a light fixture

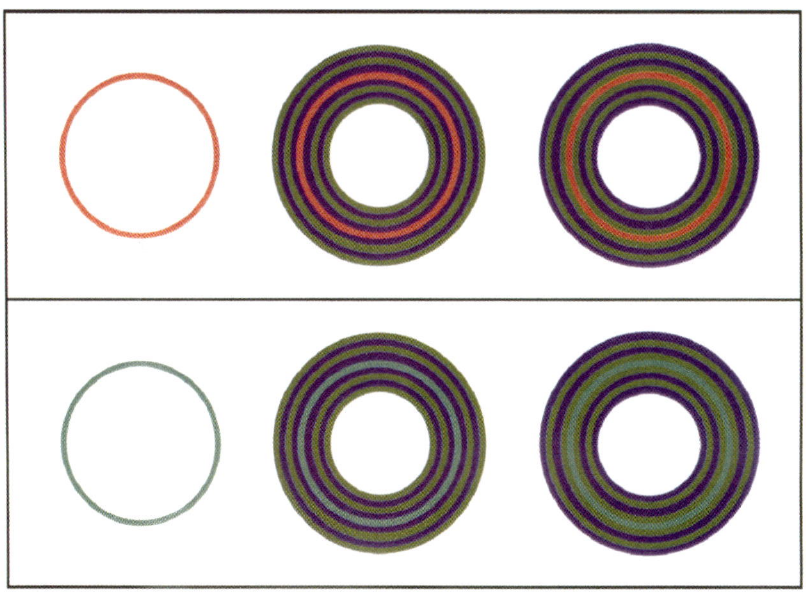

Figure 4.1 **The three rings in the top row are physically identical but appear to be different in color because of surrounding light. Similarly, the three rings in the bottom row are the same physically. These are examples of chromatic induction.**

controlled by a dimmer switch. The room should be completely dark when the light is off. Examine the colors in Figure 4.1 with the room light at its maximum and then slowly dim it. The color in the figure will disappear when the room is nearly dark. The regions that appeared red, green or blue will be seen as shades of gray. This change in color appearance is caused by a transition from cones, the photoreceptors used in normal viewing, to rods. Rods are much more sensitive than cones and thus useful for night vision but they produce neural signals that encode only intensity (dim to bright), not color. Color is a mental experience that depends on neural codes from receptors, not on the wavelength of light stimulating the receptors, so rod vision is colorless.

In general, the color appearance of an object is not related in a simple way to the properties of the object alone. Perceived color can depend on the source of light illuminating the object, the spectrally selective reflectance of that light by the object, other objects in view, and the current state of the neural pathways of eye and brain that mediate visual experience. Of these, only the spectral reflectance is a property of the object.

4.1.2 COLOR APPEARANCE VERSUS MATCHING OR DISCRIMINATION

The technical definition of color vision is based on discrimination (Chapter 3) rather than appearance: color vision is the ability to distinguish two lights regardless of their radiances. A light that appears red will not be perceived as identical to a light that appears green no matter what the level of the second light. Color matching and discrimination are of fundamental importance for determining the limits of the human visual system, for diagnosing color vision abnormalities, and for revealing properties of photoreceptors and neural pathways. Matching and discrimination, however, do not depend on appearance. An observer can judge whether two lights appear identical (a match) or are distinguishable (a discrimination) without considering *how* they appear. As aptly put by Brian Wandell, an author of Chapter 8, color matching and discrimination measure what we cannot see. The colors we actually perceive are the province of color appearance.

4.1.3 UNRELATED AND RELATED COLORS

A single light viewed in isolation has three perceptual dimensions of appearance: hue, saturation, and brightness (Figure 4.2). Hue is the aspect of the percept that differentiates it from white. ROY G BIV is a set of hue names. Saturation is the degree to which the percept is different from white. For example, powder blue is less saturated than royal blue, and pink is less saturated than red. Brightness is the dimension of perceived overall level, ranging from dim to dazzling. The percepts of single isolated lights are called *unrelated colors*.

We seldom see a single light when outside the laboratory. The visual stimulus is normally a mosaic of different patches due to light reflected from many objects in view. The percept of a light viewed within the context of at least one other light is called a *related color*. Some colors (e.g., red, blue, orange) may be perceived as related or as unrelated colors but others, such as brown, maroon, and gray, exist as only related colors. The three dimensions of hue, saturation, and brightness are insufficient to describe the appearance of all related colors.

In natural viewing, color is usually perceived as a property of an object that has other perceptual attributes, such as size, shape, and location. An object in view is visible because it reflects light from an external illuminant such as the sun or a lamp. A color perceived to belong to an object is said to be in the *object mode* of appearance. Object mode is used in a minority of studies of color vision, despite its ecological validity. The alternatives to object mode are *surface mode*, in which the color is perceived to belong to a surface that diffusely reflects illuminating light (for example, a painted wall or a sheet of paper), or *illuminant mode*, in which the color appears to be from an emitting light source (for example, traffic signals or Christmas-tree bulbs). Most color research is conducted in surface mode or illuminant mode. The mode is determined by the observer's impression of the stimulus, not by the physical stimulus itself. A video display, which emits light, can generate under appropriate conditions stimuli perceived in surface mode or in object mode. Object and surface mode apply only to related colors.

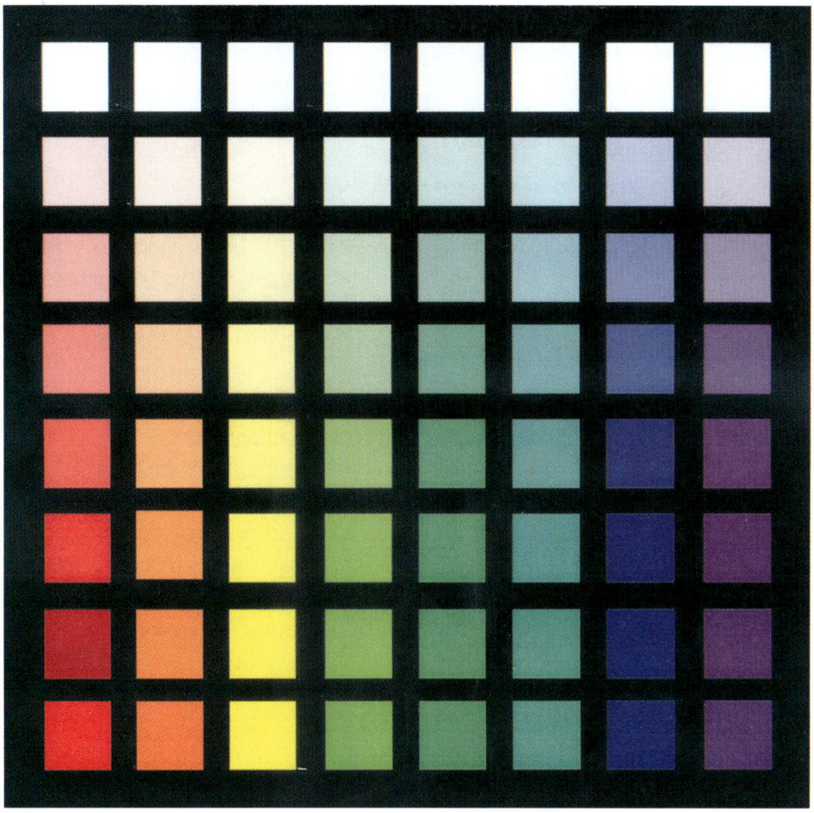

Figure 4.2 **Colors that vary in saturation (within each column) or hue (within each row, except the top one).**

Unrelated colors are perceived in illuminant mode.

4.2 UNRELATED COLORS

4.2.1 MONOCHROMATIC SPECTRAL LIGHTS

Hue: Lights of a single wavelength, called monochromatic lights, have a characteristic hue and saturation when viewed in isolation (the percept of brightness varies with the radiance of the light). Typical descriptions of hue are violet for 400–450 nm; blue near 470 nm; blue–green for 480–495 nm; green near 500 nm; yellow–green for 520–560 nm; yellow near 580 nm; orange for 600–630 nm; and red for 640–700 nm. These wavelength ranges should be considered a rough guide to the color names assigned to monochromatic lights. Wavelength discrimination is much finer than these ranges (Chapter 3).

In general, the exact hue of a particular wavelength of light cannot be specified. Differences among color-normal individuals would permit at best typical or average descriptions. For example, the wavelength that appears pure green (no hint of blueness or yellowness) varies among observers in a range from 495 to 530 nm or higher (Jordan and Mollon, 1995; Rubin, 1961). Furthermore, the hue of a given wavelength changes with light level. The change in hue with retinal illumination, called the *Bezold–Brücke hue shift,* is quantified in Figure 4.3 for a modest change of light level (Purdy, 1931b). Hue matches between two adjacent half-fields were measured with one half-field maintained at 100 td and the other at 1000 td (about the level of reading light). The wavelength of the dimmer field was varied until the two half-fields were judged to be the same hue. If there were no hue shift, all of the points would fall at zero. The measurements at 600 nm and above, however, show the match occurred with the dimmer field

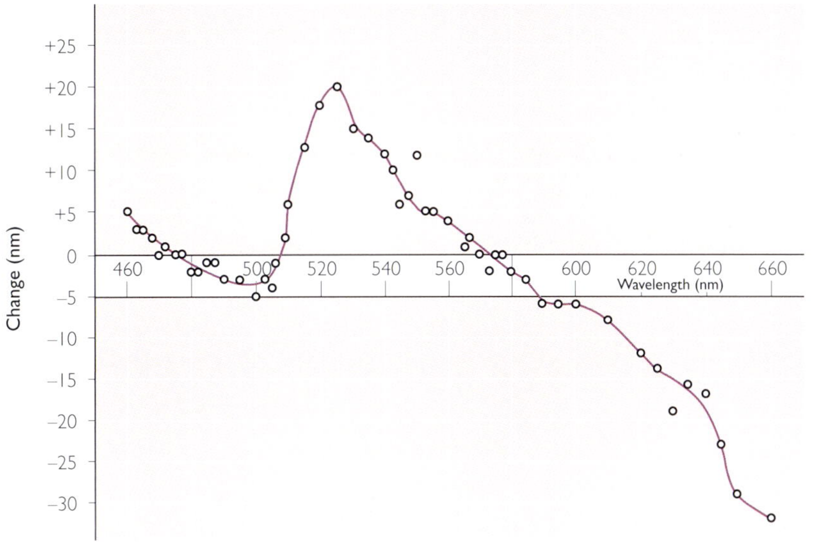

Figure 4.3 **The shift in hue with light level (Bezold-Brücke hue shift). Plotted points show the difference in wavelength required for a match in hue, when two fields differ in light level by a factor of 10. (From Purdy, 1931b, reproduced from the *American Journal of Psychology*. Copyright 1931 by the Board of Trustees of the University of Illinois. Used with the permission of the University of Illinois Press.)**

at a shorter wavelength than the more intense field. This implies a light of fixed wavelength shifts toward yellow at the higher level. At middle wavelengths a match resulted with the dimmer field set at a longer wavelength than the more intense field (also a shift toward yellow at the higher level).

The unique hues: ROY G BIV does not, of course, exhaust the names we use to describe colors. Many other terms are common (e.g., pink, turquoise, chartreuse), and compound descriptions provide a limitless color vocabulary (e.g., royal blue, lime green, fire-engine red, Kodak yellow). The *Color Name Dictionary* gives the meaning of 7500 color names (Kelly and Judd, 1955). A fundamental property of color appearance, however, is the minimal set of hues, called *unique hues*, that alone or in combination can describe all hue percepts. By definition, unique hues cannot be described by any other unique-hue name(s) (Wyszecki and Stiles, 1982). Orange, for example, is yellowish red so is not a candidate for this minimal set.

The unique hues are red, green, yellow, and blue. Each unique hue refers to the perceptual experience of that hue alone. Unique yellow is pure yellow with no hint of red (approaching orange) or green (approaching lime green), and similarly for the other unique hues. The hue of every monochromatic light in the visible spectrum can be described as red, green, yellow or blue, or by one of the four combinations yellow–red, blue–red, yellow–green, or blue–green. None of the unique hues (red, green, yellow or blue) can be described by the other three hues alone or in combination.

Saturation: Saturation is the perceived difference between a color and white. The saturation of all monochromatic lights is not equal. There is no reason to expect a 450 nm light and a 580 nm light to be perceived as equally different from white, and indeed they are not so judged. Long-wavelength lights and short-wavelength lights are perceived as more saturated than wavelengths near 580 nm. The relation between perceived saturation and wavelength is shown in Figure 4.4 for lights of equal luminance. The upper panel shows average ratings of briefly presented monochromatic stimuli viewed under neutral (tungsten) adaptation. Each wavelength was rated on an 11-point scale from 0 to 10, defined respectively as a complete lack of any chromatic content and a complete lack of any achromatic content (Jacobs, 1967). The lower panel shows a similar pattern of results for brief flashes presented in an otherwise dark field

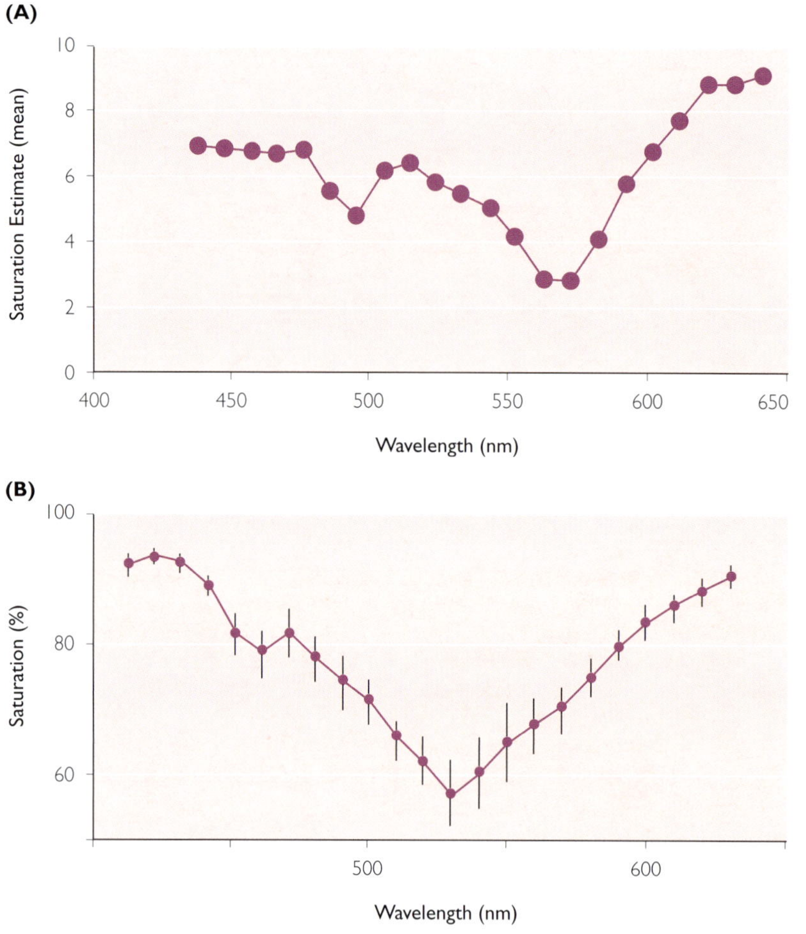

Figure 4.4 **Perceived saturation as a function of wavelength. (A) Rating on 0–10 scale where 10 is most saturated (average data replotted from Jacobs, 1967). (B) Judged percentage of chromatic content. (From Gordon and Abramov, 1988. Copyright © 1988 John Wiley & Sons, Inc., reproduced by permission.)**

(Gordon and Abramov, 1988). The measure is the judged percentage of overall chromatic content (as opposed to achromatic content – 0% is a purely achromatic percept). Differences in saturation among monochromatic lights imply that excitation purity (section 3.2.3) is not an index of saturation, as all monochromatic lights have equal purity (1.0).

Saturation, like hue, cannot be specified precisely as a function of wavelength because saturation depends strongly on the level of light. Monochromatic lights appear achromatic near (photopic) detection threshold, except for long-wavelengths, which appear reddish. The *photochromatic interval* is the difference between the energy of a light at absolute threshold and the least energy perceived to have a chromatic appearance. Thresholds for detecting light and for perceiving color are shown in Figure 4.5 as a function of wavelength. The photochromatic interval depends strongly on wavelength, ranging from about 10 times absolute threshold near 580 nm to virtually zero at long wavelengths (Graham and Hsia, 1969). Above the threshold level for seeing color, saturation increases with radiance until reaching a maximum at an intermediate light level (Purdy, 1931a). Saturation then decreases gradually as radiance is raised further. Some wavelengths appear nearly achromatic at very high light levels.

Brightness, luminance, and radiance: Brightness of an unrelated color is the perceived level of light emitted by the source. Brightness is

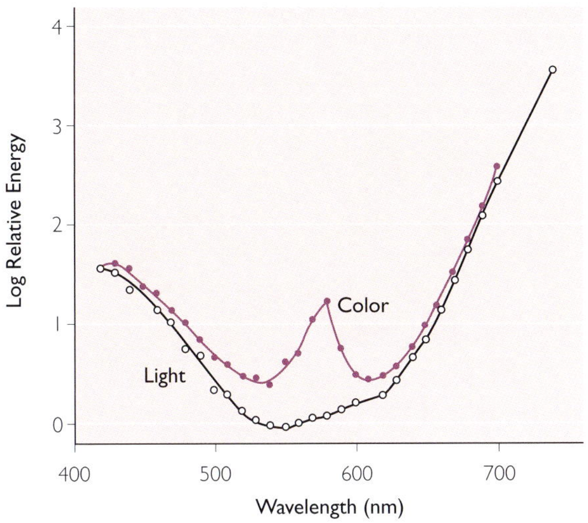

Figure 4.5 The photochromatic interval as a function of wavelength. (From Graham and Hsia, 1969, Fig. 5. Copyright © Optical Society of America, reproduced with permission.)

not linearly related to radiance, an energy-based unit, even for a light of fixed wavelength. The relation between brightness (ψ_{Br}) and stimulus radiance (x) at wavelength λ is approximately a power function with exponent 0.33 (Stevens and Stevens, 1963): $\psi_{Br} = a_{\lambda}x^{0.33}$, where a_{λ} is a proportionality constant that depends on wavelength. Values of a_{λ} do not merely relate energy to the luminous efficiency of photopic vision (section 2.8.2); if they did, the equation for brightness could be rewritten in terms of stimulus luminance (L) rather than radiance, $\psi_{Br} = aL^{0.33}$, which would imply lights of different wavelength but equal luminance would appear equally bright. It is well known, however, that they do not. Perceptual measurements of monochromatic lights show that short-wavelengths, which appear violet, are brightest, followed by long wavelengths, which appear red, and wavelengths that appear blue–green or green (480–510 nm). The least bright wavelength is near 580 nm, which appears yellow. The distinction between brightness and luminance is shown in Figure 4.6, which compares luminance efficiency and brightness efficiency as a function of wavelength (upper panel). The difference between the two spectral efficiency functions is plotted in the lower panel. If lights of equal luminance were equally bright, all values in the lower panel would fall on the horizontal line at

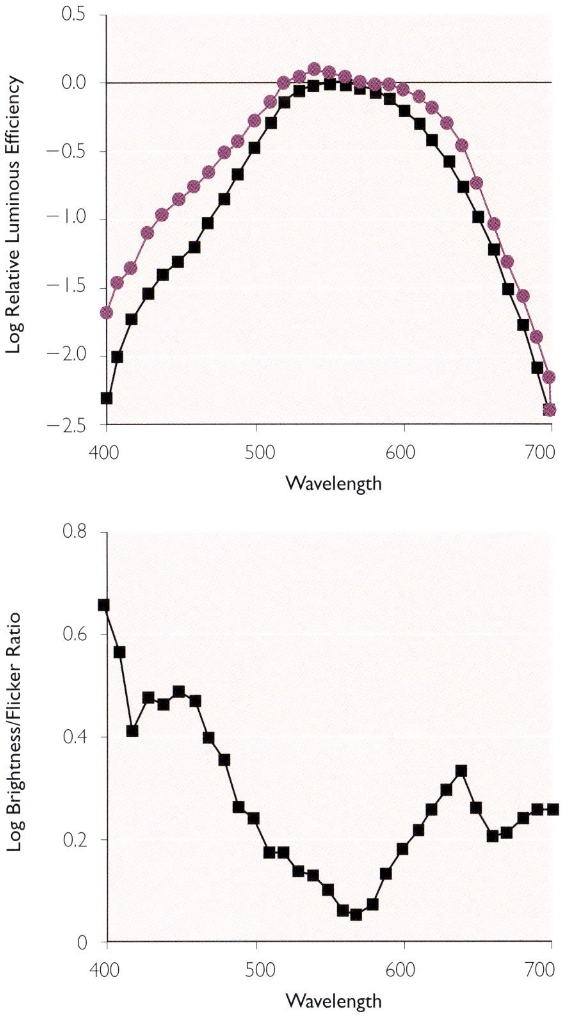

Figure 4.6 (A) Luminous efficiency (squares) versus brightness efficiency (circles), as a function of wavelength. (B) The difference between brightness and luminous efficiency spectra. (From Pokorny *et al.*, 1991, reproduced by permission of Macmillan Publishers Ltd.)

zero. Deviations from zero show the enhanced brightness perceived at short and at long wavelengths.

Color naming: In most studies of color vision a physical stimulus is varied until the observer achieves a perceptual criterion. The change of hue with light level (Figure 4.3), for example, is measured by varying the wavelength of a light at one level until its hue is identical to that of a fixed wavelength at a different level. The photochromatic interval is determined from the lowest radiance of a spectral light perceived to have a chromatic appearance (Figure 4.5). In these and many other procedures an observer judges whether a physical stimulus satisfies a perceptual criterion (e.g., no difference in hue between two lights, no difference in brightness between two lights, no chromatic content), but not *what* is perceived. Color naming, on the other hand, seeks a direct report of the hue or hues evoked by a stimulus.

An implicit difficulty with color naming is quantifying the responses. The vocabulary for color is immense and in most cases imprecise. A solution is provided by the unique hues: red, green, yellow, and blue. By definition, they form a minimal set of hues that alone or in combination can describe the hue of every spectral light. One variant of color naming permits an observer to assign one or two unique-hue names to a percept. If two names are used, one must be designated the predominant hue (Boynton and Gordon, 1965). An arbitrary scoring rule assigns a value of 2 to the predominant hue and 1 to the other hue; a score of 3 is given when a stimulus is described with a single hue name. The hue names assigned in this way to monochromatic lights from 440 to 660 nm at 100 td are summarized in the upper panel of Figure 4.7. The values plotted at each wavelength are the accumulated scores from 25 stimulus repetitions (thus the theoretical maximum on the ordinate is 75). These results suggest how hue varies with wavelength.

In another variant of color naming, called *hue estimation*, the observer describes color sensation by assigning percentages to the hue names red, green, yellow, and blue, such that the sum adds to 100% (e.g. 70% green, 30% yellow). The percentages assigned to equiluminant monochromatic lights at 100 td are shown in the lower panel of Figure 4.7.

Color-naming measurements have been found to be reliable both within and across observers. Boynton and Gordon (1965) noted differences among observers in absolute value but typically not in the shapes of functions. An advantage of color naming is that the observer views only the stimulus being judged, unlike hue- or brightness-matching procedures (as in Figures 4.3 and 4.6) that rely on abstracting a single perceptual attribute from two obviously distinguishable stimuli. Color naming also eliminates potential effects of adaptation or induction caused by a comparison field simultaneously in view.

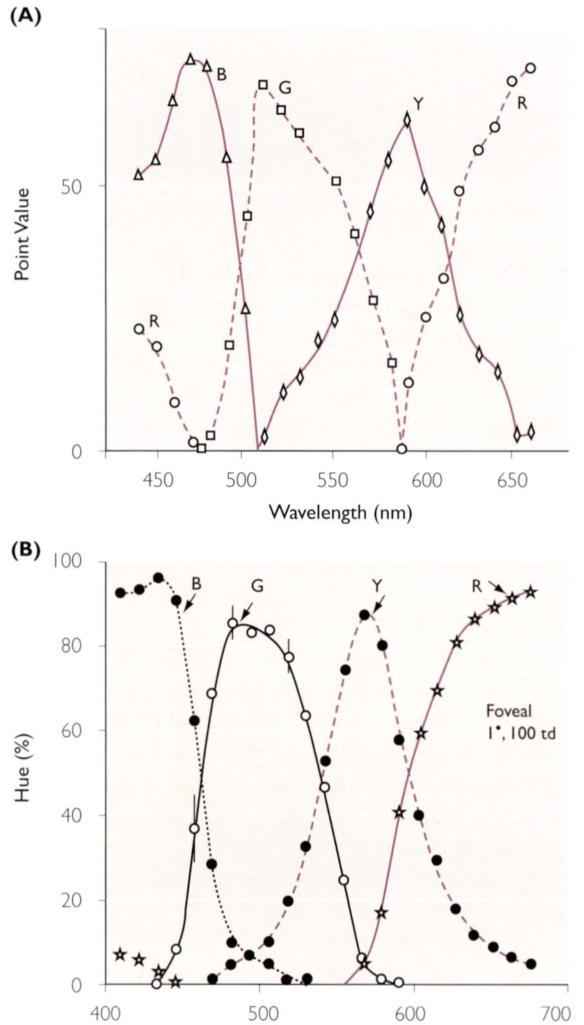

Figure 4.7 **(A) Hue names given to monochromatic lights (maximum value for each hue is 75; from Boynton and Gordon, 1965, Fig. 3a. © Copyright Optical Society of America, reproduced with permission). (B) Percentages of each hue assigned to monochromatic lights. (From Gordon and Abramov, 1988. Copyright © 1988 John Wiley & Sons, Inc., reproduced by permission.)**

Retinal location and size of stimulus: The hue and saturation of a light depend on the part of retina illuminated. Color matches between a foveal comparison field and a spectral light of the same size in peripheral retina show that stimuli in the periphery appear less saturated. Saturation falls progressively as the stimulus is located farther from the fovea (Moreland and

Cruz, 1959). Similar results are found for judgments of chromatic content of a 1° field, out to 40° nasally or temporally (Abramov *et al.*, 1991). Saturation of peripheral stimuli increases with field size. Hue also is affected by peripheral versus foveal stimulation (Stabell and Stabell, 1982).

Perceptual map of colors derived from similarity judgments: A different approach to inferring the perceptual space of color appearance relies on observers' judgments of similarity. No specification of color is required. An observer assesses only the similarity of a pair of colors. In a typical study, the observer examines all pairs of several different stimuli. For example, in an experiment with 14 monochromatic lights there are 91 possible pairs of lights. Each pair is presented in turn. The subject's task is to evaluate the similarity of each pair of colors, typically using an ordinal rating scale with, say, 1 as most similar and 25 as least similar. The perceptual space of colors is inferred using a multidimensional scaling model that finds coordinates on two or more dimensions for each of the 14 lights. The coordinates are chosen to be in accord with the similarity judgments, assuming lights closer to each other in the coordinate space are judged as more similar. The ordering of the distances between all pairs of lights in the space, from shortest to longest, seldom corresponds exactly to the ordering of judged similarity of all pairs of stimuli. For example, 14 stimuli in a two-dimensional space have 28 coordinates to be estimated by the model while a perfect fit to the data requires a match to an ordering of 91 distances between pairs. Multidimensional-scaling procedures seek to optimize the correspondence between the ordering of the pairs' distances in the derived perceptual space and the ordering of the pairwise similarity judgments.

A perceptual color space determined from multidimensional scaling is shown in Figure 4.8 for 14 narrow-band lights with peak wavelengths from 434 and 674 nm (Shepard, 1962). The space is derived from a similarity measure for each pair of wavelengths (Ekman, 1954), which is the only information about the stimuli required for multidimensional scaling. The 14 stimuli fall in an approximately circular pattern from shortest to longest wavelength (the curve through the points and the hue names do not come from scaling but were added by Shepard to aid interpretation). Note that (Euclidean) distances between points within a coordinate space are invariant with rotation so, in general, substantive interpretation of the horizontal and vertical axes is inappropriate unless special scaling models or metrics are used (Schiffman *et al.*, 1981).

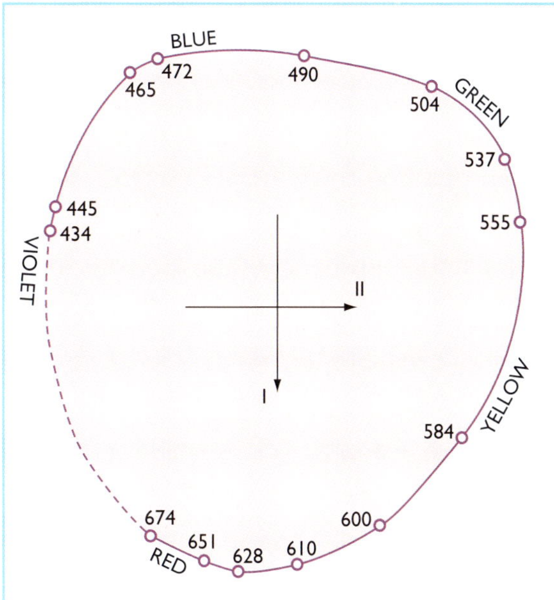

Figure 4.8 Perceptual color space derived from similarity measures for pairs of wavelengths, using multidimensional scaling. (From Shepard, 1962, reproduced by permission of the author and *Psychometrika*.)

4.2.2 MIXTURES OF SPECTRAL LIGHTS

Appearance of mixtures: Nearly all lights that we see include more than one wavelength. Even most laboratory stimuli labeled 'monochromatic' are really a narrow range of the visible spectrum composed of at least several adjacent wavelengths. The distinction between a single wavelength and a mixture of several adjacent wavelengths normally is inconsequential for color appearance. Mixtures of more separated wavelengths, on the other hand, greatly expand our range of color percepts. The fundamental achromatic percept of white, for example, is not experienced with any monochromatic light; and purple, which is a different color than violet, results from mixing short-wavelength and long-wavelength lights. If restricted to only monochromatic lights, we could perceive fewer than 200 different colors (Chapter 3); with mixtures of monochromatic lights, the number of distinguishable unrelated colors[1] is more than 5000.

The complete set of unrelated colors that can be perceived with mixtures is represented schematically on a CIE chromaticity diagram (section. 3.2.3) that shows the approximate percept of the mixture represented by each chromaticity coordinate (Figure 4.9). The colors of monochromatic lights are around the 'horseshoe,' from 380 nm at lower left to 700 nm at lower right. The straight line at the bottom of the horseshoe joins the two points representing 380 and 700 nm; these mixtures are perceived as purples. The points in the interior of the horseshoe represent all possible light mixtures. White is the percept of a mixture that combines every wavelength in the visible spectrum at equal energy. This mixture is represented by CIE coordinate (x,y) = (0.33,0.33).

Spectral complements: A mixture of all wavelengths at equal energy appears white, but not all percepts of white are due to this mixture. Other light mixtures with chromaticity coordinate (0.33,0.33) are perceptually indistinguishable (section 3.2). A mixture of two monochromatic lights with chromaticity coordinate (0.33,0.33) defines a pair of *complementary colors*. The complement of wavelength λ_1 is the

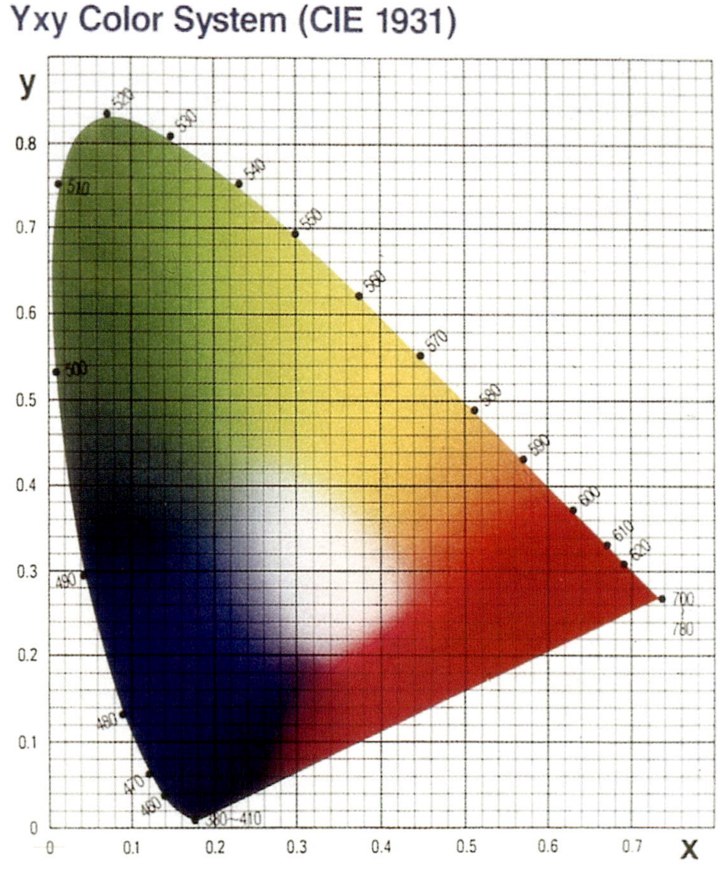

Figure 4.9 **Approximate rendition of the perceived color of isolated lights at given CIE x,y chromaticities. (Courtesy of Minolta Corporation.)**

wavelength λ_2 that can be added to λ_1, in an appropriate amount, to give a percept identical to that of equal-energy white.

The concept of complementary colors can be extended also to other 'whites,' for example to the spectral distribution of CIE Standard Illuminant A or of Illuminant D_{65} with, respectively, chromaticity coordinates (0.45,0.41) or (0.31,0.33). The wavelengths of a complementary pair depend on the specific achromatic stimulus chosen as the reference 'white.' For example, the complement of 460 nm is 580 nm with Illuminant A as 'white' but 570 nm with Illuminant D_{65}.

With D_{65} as 'white,' wavelengths from 400 to 493 nm and from 567 to 700 nm have monochromatic complements (Wyszecki and Stiles, 1982). Wavelengths from 494 to 566 nm must be combined with at least two other wavelengths (for example, 400 and 700 nm) to achieve the reference achromatic percept. The dozens of different complementary-wavelength pairs, all of which result in the same indistinguishable white percept, are a further example of the dissociation between wavelengths of light stimulating photoreceptors and the color appearance we experience.

Abney effect: Most of the mixtures in Figure 4.9 can be considered an additive combination of light represented by coordinate (0.33,0.33), which appears white, and a monochromatic light.[2] As saturation is the perceived difference between a color and white, one might expect that adding a light at (0.33,0.33) to a monochromatic stimulus would only desaturate the percept of the monochromatic light; that is, the monochromatic light alone as well as mixtures that are monochromatic plus equal-energy white in proportions 90%/10%, 50%/50% or 10%/90% would have the same hue but different saturations. This, however, is not the case (Abney, 1910), which serves to point out that metrics derived from color matching, such as the CIE X,Y,Z system, should not be used as scales of color appearance (see Chapter 5). Adding a light that appears white causes a shift toward redness if the monochromatic light alone appears orange or blue, or toward less yellowness if the monochromatic light alone appears green (Newhall *et al.*, 1943; Burns *et al.*, 1984). These hue shifts are depicted in the CIE chromaticity diagram by curved loci representing stimuli of constant hue (section 5.2.1.6).

Failure of brightness additivity: The distinction between stimulus luminance (section 2.8.2) and brightness was discussed in section 4.2.1 with respect to monochromatic lights, where it was pointed out that lights of equal luminance but different wavelength are not equally bright. Luminance is additive by definition, so combining a light of wavelength λ_1 at luminance L_1 with a light of wavelength λ_2 at luminance L_2 yields a physical light mixture $\lambda_1 \oplus \lambda_2$ of luminance L_1+L_2 (note the distinction between physical admixture of light and algebraic addition, indicated respectively by the symbols $\oplus$ and $+$). More generally, additivity implies that the luminance of any spectral power distribution, SPD(λ), can be calculated by summing the luminance of each component wavelength: $\int_\lambda \mathrm{SPD}(\lambda)V(\lambda)d\lambda$, where $V(\lambda)$ is the luminous efficiency function (section 2.8.2) The *brightness* of the admixture of $\lambda_1 \oplus \lambda_2$ or of SPD(λ), however, cannot be determined by adding the brightnesses of the components.

Violations of brightness additivity may occur as brightness enhancement or inhibition. In brightness enhancement, an additive mixture of, say, monochromatic lights $\lambda_1 \oplus \lambda_2$ appears brighter than the sum of the brightness of λ_1 viewed alone plus the brightness of λ_2 viewed alone. For example, define one unit of 422 nm light as the luminance that matches the brightness of a fixed achromatic standard. Similarly, define one unit of 521 nm light as its luminance that matches the same brightness standard. Then mix the 422 and 521 nm lights, with the luminance of 521 nm at half of its matching level (that is, at 0.5 unit). The mixture field and the fixed standard will match in brightness with 421 nm at about 0.35 unit, well below the 0.5 value specified by brightness additivity. In brightness inhibition, the brightness of a mixture is less than the sum of the brightnesses of the components viewed alone. For example, a mixture of 0.5 unit of 521 nm and about 0.9 unit of 647 nm will match the brightness standard. Brightness matches using other wavelengths in an admixture with 0.5 unit of 521 nm are plotted in Figure 4.10 (Guth *et al.*, 1969). These results should be considered average values as

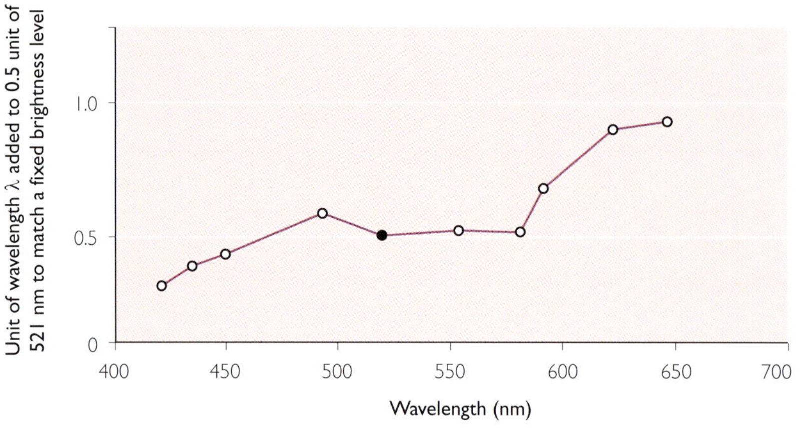

Figure 4.10 Measurements showing failure of brightness additivity. (Plot modified from Wyszecki and Stiles, 1982, based on data from Guth *et al.*, 1969; reproduced with permission.)

differences among individuals are substantial. The magnitude of additivity failure is little affected by the level of the standard light.

4.2.3 OPPONENT HUE CANCELLATION

The four unique hues (section 4.2.1) can be combined theoretically into six possible pairs yet we experience only four of them. Yellow–red (orange) and blue–red (violet) are common, as are yellow–green (lime green) and blue–green (turquoise). No hue, however, is perceived as red–green or as yellow–blue. This observation is the basis of *opponent-colors theory* (Hering, 1920), which posits two bipolar perceptual hue dimensions: red(+)/green(−) and yellow(+)/blue(−). The assignment of red and yellow to positive values is arbitrary but now conventional (Jameson and Hurvich, 1955). Every hue can be described by two values, one on each dimension. Orange, for example, has a positive value on both dimensions. A null (zero) value on one dimension implies a unique hue on the other; a null value on both dimensions represents an achromatic (white) percept.

Perceptual opponency of red/green and of yellow/blue forms the conceptual basis for quantifying the redness, greenness, yellowness, and blueness of monochromatic lights. In a classic study, Jameson and Hurvich (1955) reasoned that the amount of redness in a monochromatic light can be measured by combining it with a second light that appears green when viewed alone. The level of the second light is adjusted until an observer judges the appearance of the mixture to be neither reddish nor greenish (that is, yellow, blue or achromatic). Such percepts are called *red–green equilibrium colors*. This measurement of judged hue is repeated with wavelengths from throughout the visible spectrum whose appearance has a reddish component (violet, orange, red). The redness of each monochromatic light is quantified by the magnitude of the 'green' addend required for red–green equilibrium.

Not all wavelengths appear reddish. Those that do not, appear greenish, or are pure (unique) yellow or blue. Greenness is measured using a red-appearing addend, the level of which is adjusted until the mixture is in red–green equilibrium. The level of the addend quantifies greenness. Every monochromatic light can be brought to red–green equilibrium by adding some amount of either a green-appearing or a red-appearing light. The amount of addend may be zero, in which case the wavelength appears unique yellow or blue. The magnitude of redness or of greenness measured in this way is plotted as a function of wavelength in Figure 4.11 (solid symbols). By convention, redness has positive values and greenness has negative values. Yellowness or blueness of each wavelength is measured similarly using, respectively, blue-appearing or yellow-appearing addends adjusted in level so an observer perceives a color that is pure red, pure green or achromatic (the *yellow–*

blue equilibrium colors). These measurements also are shown in Figure 4.11 (open symbols), using the convention of positive values for yellowness.

The outcome measure from the hue-cancellation experiment is labeled 'chromatic response' (Figure 4.11). This value incorporates several assumptions. First, a unit is needed for the green-appearing light used to cancel redness, and for the red-appearing light used to cancel greenness. These units are determined using an admixture of the green-appearing and red-appearing addend lights. Their relative contributions to the mixture are adjusted so the appearance is a red–green equilibrium color. The energies of the lights at this point are defined as equal units of redness and of greenness. The units for yellowness and for blueness are defined in a similar manner, using an admixture of the blue-appearing and yellow-appearing addends perceived to be in yellow-blue equilibrium. Second, the height of the red–green function must be scaled relative to the height of the yellow–blue curve. The heights are set by finding those wavelengths perceived to have two hues in equal amounts (e.g., an orange judged to have equal redness and yellowness). A plot comparing redness, greenness, yellowness, and blueness, as in Figure 4.11, must incorporate some set of normalizing assumptions of this nature.

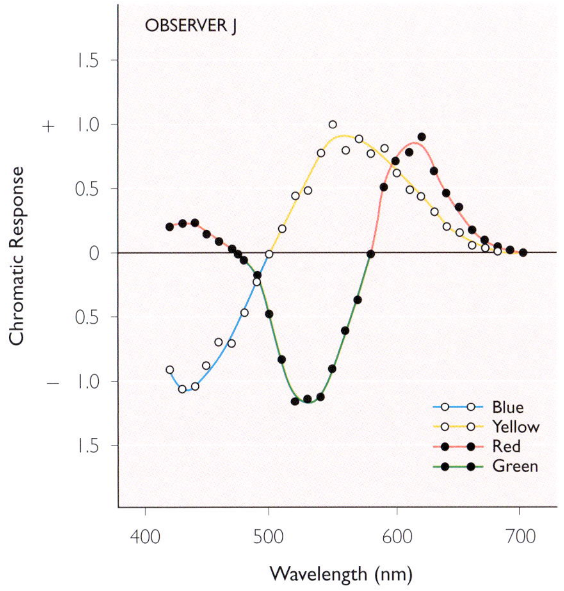

Figure 4.11 Redness, greenness, yellowness, and blueness as a function of wavelength, inferred from hue-cancellation measurements. (From Jameson and Hurvich, 1955, Fig. 5. © Copyright Optical Society of America, reproduced with permission.)

The generality of the results in Figure 4.11 requires two further assumptions (Krantz, 1975). First, while the chromatic responses are shown for spectral lights of equal radiance, which is an energy-based unit, the actual measurements were made with lights of equal luminance (10 mL). Values in the plot are calculated by assuming the scaling factor applied at each test wavelength, to convert from equal luminance to equal radiance, applies also to the canceling addend. For example, if the measured level of canceling light is t for test-wavelength λ at 10 mL, and the scaling factor required for equal radiance is α_λ, then the level of canceling light for equal radiance is assumed to be $\alpha_\lambda t$. Second, the generality of Figure 4.11 depends on independence from the particular canceling addends used by Jameson and Hurvich in their experiments. Both of these empirical properties are implied if the red/green and yellow/blue chromatic responses are linear transformations of the cones' spectral sensitivities (or, equivalently, of the CIE X,Y,Z color matching functions):

$$(\text{red/green})_\lambda = c_{11}S_\lambda + c_{12}M_\lambda + c_{13}L_\lambda,$$
$$(\text{yellow/blue})_\lambda = c_{21}S_\lambda + c_{22}M_\lambda + c_{23}L_\lambda,$$

where S_λ, M_λ, and L_λ are the S-, M-, and L-cone fundamentals (section 3.2.5), and constants c_{ij} are weights, some with negative values.

Linearity implies that a light in red/green (or yellow/blue) equilibrium remains so at all stimulus levels (Krantz, 1975). A special case is the monochromatic wavelengths perceived as unique hues. Linearity requires these wavelengths to remain constant regardless of radiance level. In general, however, hue depends on light level (section 4.2.1); the exceptions are the three wavelengths where there is no (zero) shift (see Figure 4.3). If the chromatic responses are linear then the wavelengths perceived as unique hues, determined from color-appearance judgments, must be the three wavelengths with no shift, determined from hue matching. Measurements show this is the case. Unique blue, green, and yellow are perceived near 478 nm, 500 nm, and 578 nm, respectively. Further, the wavelengths of these unique hues are virtually constant over a 100-fold change of light levels (Larimer *et al.*, 1974, 1975). This is consistent with linearity.

No monochromatic wavelength appears unique red. The longest wavelengths in the visible spectrum appear slightly yellowish red. A mixture of long- and short-wavelength lights, therefore, is required to perceive unique red. A mixture that appears unique red at one light level appears bluish-red at higher levels (Larimer *et al.*, 1975). This implies yellow/blue, the chromatic response in equilibrium at unique red, is not linear.

Linearity implies further that an additive mixture of lights must be perceived as a red/green (yellow/blue) equilibrium color if each of the components in the mixture is in red/green (yellow/blue) equilibrium (Krantz, 1975). For example, any mixture of the wavelengths that appear unique blue and unique yellow (478 and 578 nm, respectively) should be in red/green equilibrium. This means the line in chromaticity space joining the points representing 478 and 578 nm should define a set of mixture lights in red/green equilibrium; similarly, the line joining the points for unique green (500 nm) and for extra-spectral unique red should represent light mixtures in yellow/blue equilibrium (black lines in left panels of Figure 4.12). While initial measurements using mixtures were consistent with linearity (Larimer *et al.*, 1975), more recent studies reveal linearity failures. Some mixtures of the wavelength appearing unique yellow and the wavelength appearing unique blue result in a desaturated reddish-blue percept, not a red/green equilibrium color (Burns *et al.*, 1984). In general, the set of light mixtures found to be in red/green equilibrium is not represented by a straight line in the chromaticity diagram (black line in top right panel of Figure 4.12; note curvature toward the left) though linearity can be a reasonable approximation for mixtures from 'white' to the long-wave spectral locus. Deviations from linearity are more severe for light mixtures in yellow/blue equilibrium (black line in bottom right panel of Figure 4.12). In general, the chromatic response functions in Figure 4.11 should not be considered entirely independent of light level or of the particular green-appearing, red-appearing, blue-appearing, and yellow-appearing lights used to cancel, respectively, redness, greenness, yellowness, and blueness.

4.3 RELATED COLORS

Unrelated colors are useful stimuli in the laboratory for studying the perceptual dimensions of color, and for measuring the relations between the physical features of a stimulus and color appearance. In the natural world, however, a single isolated light is rare. The colors experienced in daily life are related colors, in which one color is perceived in the presence of others.

4.3.1 HUE, CHROMA, AND LIGHTNESS

Hue, saturation, and brightness provide a complete description of an unrelated color. Additional perceptual dimensions apply to related colors. These dimensions characterize a percept *in relation* to other color percepts. Lightness is the perceived level of emitted light relative to light from a region that appears white. In natural viewing, lightness is usually more salient than brightness, which is the perceived overall level of emitted light (section 4.2.1). The difference between brightness and lightness can be appreciated by standing outside on a sunny day. When one puts on sunglasses, the entire scene appears less bright but each part of the scene has about the same lightness. For an achromatic percept, brightness varies from very dim to dazzling, while lightness varies from black to gray to white (Judd, 1940).

Saturation and chroma are perceptual dimensions that also are distinguished by whether the attribute depends on another percept. Saturation (section 4.2.1) is the perceived difference between a color and white, regardless of lightness (or brightness). Chroma, as a relative value, is the perceived difference between a color and an achromatic percept of the same lightness. Chroma, therefore, depends on a reference color that varies according to the lightness of the stimulus under consideration. The reference color is often a gray; in natural scenes, it may not be present for simultaneous viewing. Examples of colors that vary in chroma are shown in Figure 5.1. While the lightness of a patch within a scene is often apparent to a naive observer, chroma usually is not (Wyszecki, 1986).

The distinction between chroma and saturation is illustrated by a chromatic patch

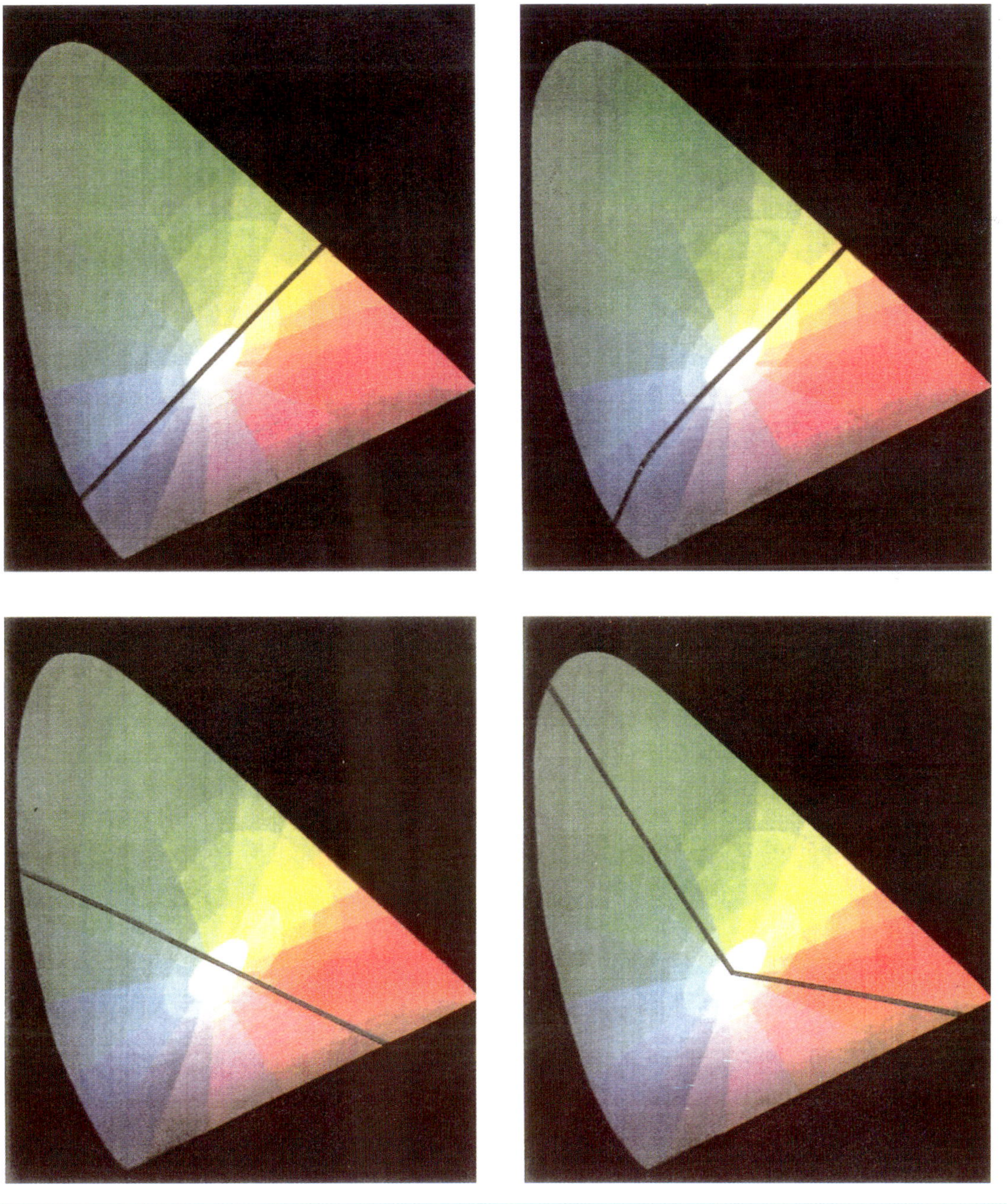

Figure 4.12 **The loci of equilibrium hues (red/green above, yellow/blue below). Left: Predicted loci assuming the red/green and yellow/blue chromatic responses are a linear transformation of the L, M and S cone spectral sensitivities. Right: Measurements of equilibrium hue loci (Burns *et al.*, 1984), which show deviations from linearity. (From Pokorny *et al.*, 1991, reproduced by permission of Macmillan Publishers Ltd.)**

surrounded by an achromatic (gray) region of the same lightness, all on a white background of greater lightness (Figure 4.13). Chroma is the perceived difference in color between the chromatic center and the immediate surround of comparable lightness. Saturation is the perceived difference in color between the chromatic center and the white background.

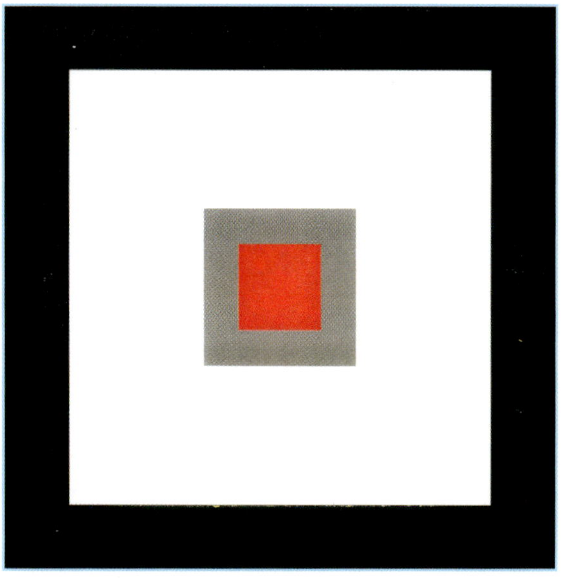

Figure 4.13 **The distinction between chroma and saturation. Chroma is the perceived difference between the chromatic center patch and the immediately surrounding gray of the same lightness. Saturation is the perceived difference between the chromatic patch and the white background.**

The conceptual meaning of chroma is well established but there is no universally accepted definition of the term. Color specification systems that include chroma, such as the Munsell color notation (Chapter 5), use a specific definition in accord with the conceptual meaning.

4.3.2 DARK COLORS

The distinction between brightness and lightness, above, points to a fundamental property of an isolated achromatic patch of light: an isolated patch can vary in brightness but not lightness because lightness, by definition, is perceived in relation to a second stimulus that appears white. If a single isolated patch cannot vary in lightness, which is the perceptual dimension ranging from black to white, then varying the radiance of an isolated achromatic patch should not alter its appearance along the black–white perceptual dimension. This is precisely what one observes. An isolated achromatic light of any radiance appears white, never gray or black. Reducing the luminance of the patch causes it to appear dimmer while still white. Stars that are barely visible in the night sky appear white.

The percepts of gray and black occur only as related colors, when a light is viewed simultaneously with other light of higher luminance. Gray and black are examples of dark colors, which in general are percepts that include a component of perceptual grayness or blackness. Chromatic dark colors include maroon, navy blue, and British racing green. Related colors significantly expand the range of colors that we can perceive, by introducing the dark-color percepts. The most significant addition is brown, which is experienced only as a related color (note that no area is brown in Figure 4.9). A patch of light that appears desaturated orange in isolation will appear brown when surrounded by achromatic light of significantly higher luminance.

The added perceptual experience that accompanies dark colors is called grayness (Evans, 1974). Consider a 700 nm light, which in isolation appears red. Surrounding the light by an achromatic field at 1000 times the 700 nm luminance causes the 700 nm light to appear black. Gradually raising the 700 nm luminance gives rise to a percept with some redness but an overall impression of dark red (reddish black). Further increasing 700 nm luminance adds redness and reduces grayness simultaneously; at some luminance of 700 nm the grayness in the percept is completely eliminated. The least luminance of the central patch without any grayness is called G_0. The G_0 luminance depends strongly on wavelength but generally is below the luminance of the surround (Evans, 1974).

Dark colors provide another demonstration of the dissociation between the physical wavelengths of light and color appearance. Dark colors are percepts that cannot be achieved with any single light alone.

4.3.3 CHROMATIC INDUCTION

Dark colors are an example of one light affecting the appearance of another. In general, the appearance of a given light will depend on other light(s) also in view. The change in appearance caused by introducing surrounding light is called chromatic induction, a term used here to include also induction from achromatic stimuli. Chromatic induction has been recognized as a property of human vision for more than 160 years. Chevreul (1839), as Director of Dyes for the Royal Manufactures at the Gobelins tapestry works in France, was charged with producing woolens of consistent color. He showed that a perceived difference in color between two identical but spatially separated samples of material was caused by the context of nearby regions within which each sample was viewed, not by a difference between the two woolen samples themselves.

Chromatic induction may result in chromatic contrast or chromatic assimilation. In chromatic contrast, the appearance of a light changes in a direction away from the color of the inducing light. For example, a patch that appears white when viewed alone becomes greenish when surrounded by a light that appears red. In chromatic assimilation, on the other hand, the appearance of a light shifts toward the color of the inducing light. The direction of chromatic induction, toward contrast or assimilation, depends on the properties of the stimuli, particularly their spatial frequencies.

Achromatic contrast: When stimuli are achromatic, introducing an inducing field can cause a light that appears white to become a brighter white, or to become gray or black. These are changes in brightness and/or lightness. When a patch is surrounded by light of somewhat lower luminance, the brightness of the patch is enhanced slightly compared to its brightness when viewed alone. As the luminance of the surround approaches and surpasses the luminance of the patch, the brightness of the patch falls rapidly. A surround at twice the luminance of the patch induces a dark color, so that no single light alone can match the appearance of the patch (Heinemann, 1955). Achromatic contrast is demonstrated by viewing an identical stripe within surrounds of various light levels, which range from well below that of the stripe to well above it (Figure 4.14).

Chromatic contrast: The perceived hue and saturation of a given light also depend on adjacent stimuli. In most stimulus configurations, a chromatic inducing field shifts the color of a patch away from the color of the inducing light. The specific change in color appearance depends on the chromaticities of both the inducing field and the patch, and on the spatial and temporal properties of the stimuli. Shifts in appearance can be substantial, as shown in Figure 4.15, which plots shifts in the perceptually matching chromaticity caused by introducing an inducing light that appears red, yellow, green or blue (Ware and Cowan, 1982). Results with each color of inducing stimulus are in a separate panel; the solid circle is the chromaticity of the inducing field, which was presented in repeated 18' wide stripes of a grating 2° wide by 1.5° high. The test color was presented between the inducing regions, in 6' wide stripes. The test and inducing lights were viewed by one eye while the observer matched the perceived color of the test-within-inducing-stripes by adjusting a trichromatic mixture presented to the other eye (haploscopic matching). The tail of each arrow is the chromaticity of the test light alone (no inducer); the head of the arrow is the matching chromaticity with the inducing field. In general, each inducing light shifts color appearance away

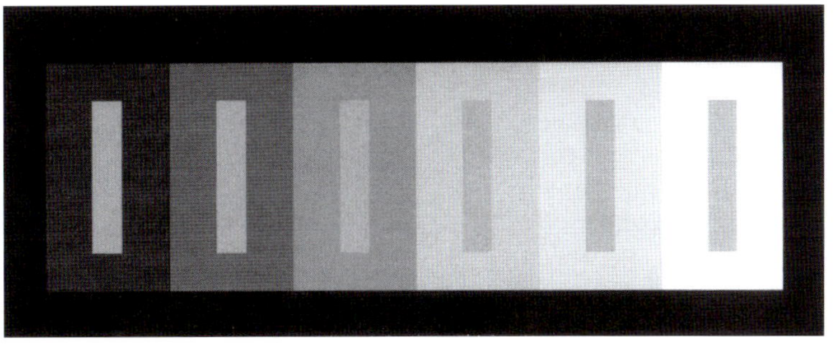

Figure 4.14 Example of achromatic contrast. All of the vertical stripes are physically identical but they appear different because of the light level in the surrounds.

from its chromaticity (arrows pointing away from solid circle in each panel). There are several exceptions, however, particularly with a short-wavelength 'blue' inducer (bottom panel) which shifts middle- and long-wavelength lights near the spectrum locus toward redness. Theories of chromatic induction are discussed in section 4.3.4.

Weaker contrast would be expected in natural viewing. The measurements in Figure 4.15 were made under conditions that optimize chromatic contrast: steady viewing, adaptation to the stimulus for more than a minute, similar luminances of the test and inducing lights, and with optical correction for chromatic aberration of the eye.

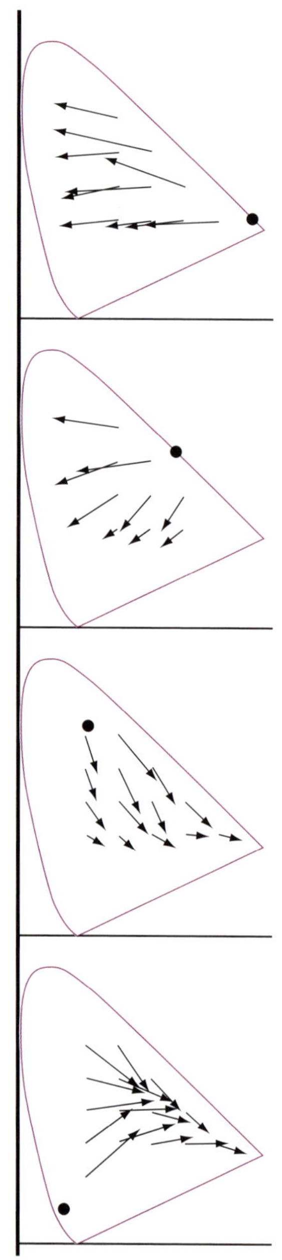

Figure 4.15 Shifts in color appearance caused by chromatic contrast (see text). (From Ware and Cowan, 1982, reproduced from *Vision Research* by permission of Elsevier Science.)

Achromatic and chromatic assimilation: Under some stimulus conditions, the appearance of a light shifts toward rather than away from the color of an inducing field. The phenomenon of assimilation was documented more than a century ago (von Bezold, 1876). We experience it when viewing a brick building: the perceived color of the brick depends on the color of the mortar. Achromatic assimilation is demonstrated in Figure 4.16, where two identical gray backgrounds have a superimposed grid of either black or white. The background with the black grid appears darker than the background with the white one. A step plate above and below the backgrounds allows them to be compared to the appearance of uniform bars. The upper background has a gray level near step 2 or 3 (counting steps from the left) while the lower one has an appearance near step 4 or 5.

Chromatic assimilation is shown in Figure 4.17. All three green regions (top half, center) are constructed from an identical uniform rectangle at the chromaticity of the uniform bar on the left; grids that appear yellow, red or blue are superimposed (the grids alone are shown on the right). Chromatic assimilation results in the three regions of different perceived color (top half, center). Assimilation from the same grids is shown below for an orange background.

Assimilation has been studied less thoroughly than contrast, despite its powerful influence on color appearance. In general, assimilation occurs with fields of relatively high spatial frequency. In studies with gratings composed of interleaved contiguous inducing and test stripes, there is a transition from assimilation to contrast when the stripes become wider than about 3–6 cycles per degree (Helson, 1963; Fach and Sharpe, 1986). This is a rough guide, however, because several factors affect the size of stimuli that result in

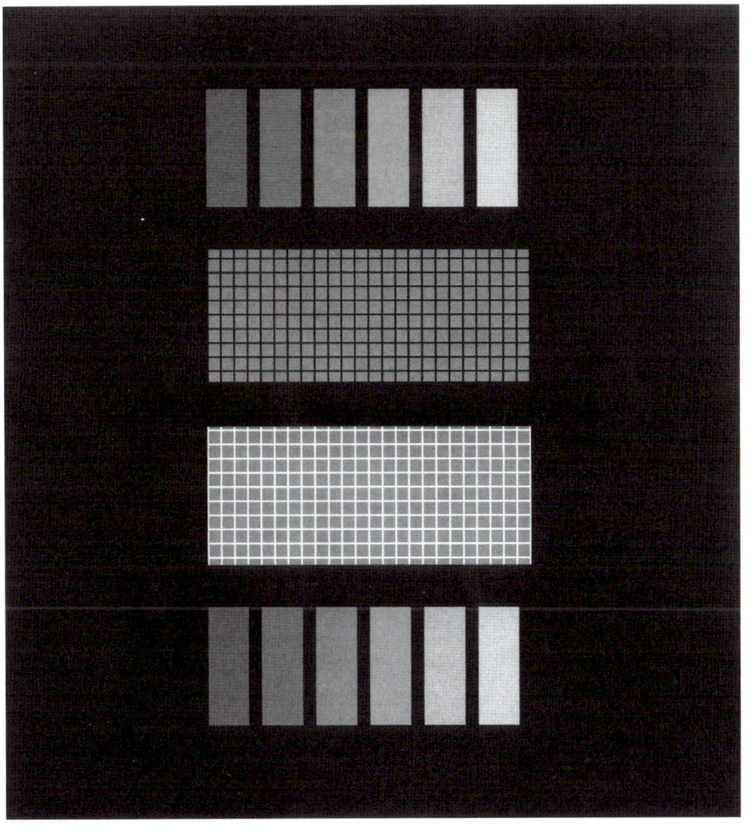

Figure 4.16 **Example of achromatic assimilation. All of the small squares are physically identical but they shift in appearance toward the appearance of the black or white overlaying grid.**

assimilation, and the degree of assimilation that occurs. These factors include the relative widths and chromaticities of the inducing and test stripes, and the background field on which the grating is viewed.

Assimilation is mediated by both optical and neural processes. Chromatic aberration and diffraction contribute to blurring of light on the retina, which is a factor in assimilation (Wandell, 1993; Marimont and Wandell, 1994). Ware and Cowan (1982), in their study of chromatic contrast, collected some additional data without the achromatizing lens that was used for the measurements shown in Figure 4.15. Removing the achromatizing lens substantially increased the blueness in the test field when the inducing field appeared blue. Optical factors, however, are unable to account completely for assimilation. Fach and Sharpe's (1986) measurements did not show greatest assimilation from short-wavelength light, which is the most defocused by chromatic aberration. Moreover, assimilation is observed in some experimental conditions with stimuli too large to be strongly affected by optical factors (Helson, 1963). Most investigators studying assimilation have concluded that a neural process also contributes to these changes in color appearance. This conclusion is qualitatively consistent with the neural point spread function derived for chromatic pathways (Sekiguchi *et al.*, 1993; Williams *et al.*, 1993).

4.3.4 CHROMATIC ADAPTATION TO SIMPLE FIELDS

In chromatic contrast and assimilation, the color appearance of a particular light depends on an adjacent light also in view. Contrast and assimilation are special cases of chromatic adaptation,

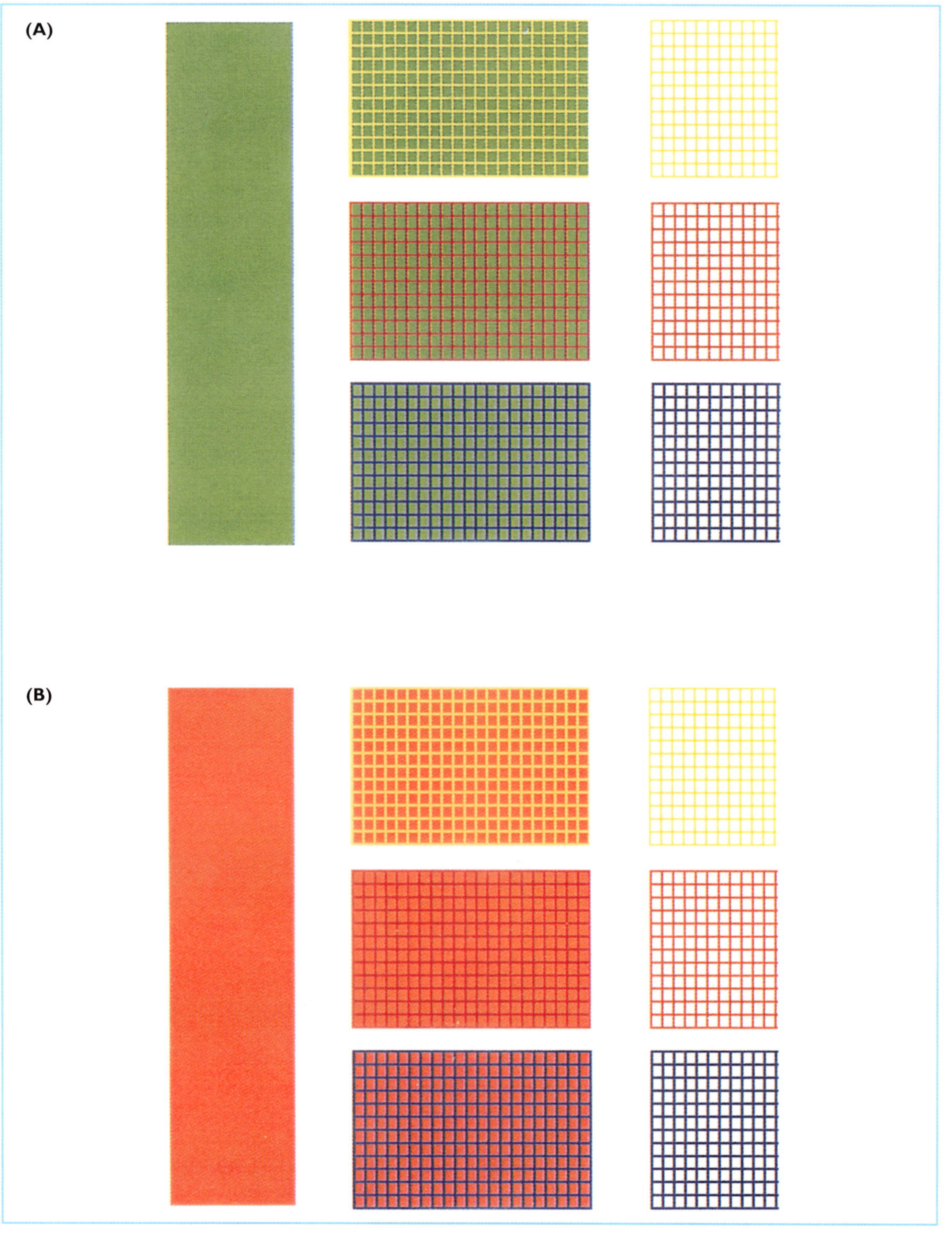

Figure 4.17 Examples of chromatic assimilation. (A) The three 'green' background regions in the center are physically identical, at the chromaticity of the uniform bar on the left. Overlaying grids that appear yellow, red or blue (shown alone on the right) shift the appearance of the 'green' background toward the appearance of the grids. (B) Assimilation from the same grids with a background that appears reddish-orange.

in which the neural response to a particular light is affected by other visual stimuli of arbitrary complexity and location in the visual field. The adapting stimulus may range from a large uniform field to a natural, variegated scene under some illumination, and may be viewed previously or simultaneously. Uniform adapting fields are considered here, together with basic theoretical issues concerning color appearance under chromatic adaptation. More complex fields are examined in the following section.

Chromatic adaptation has been studied using large uniform adapting lights on which a test field is superimposed. For example, a small test field that appears yellow when viewed alone can appear greenish when superimposed on a larger long-wavelength adapting field (Walraven, 1976; Shevell, 1978, 1982). Note that physical admixture of background and test light predicts the long-wavelength adapting field, which appears red, would shift the appearance of the superimposed test toward redness rather than greenness. Admixture of test and adapting light occurs at the photoreceptors but the light added by the adapting field can have surprisingly little effect on the appearance of a superimposed test. The shift toward greenness is accounted for by relative desensitization of L cones resulting from adaptation to long-wavelength light.

von Kries Coefficient Law: Receptoral sensitivity change is a classical explanation of color appearance under chromatic adaptation. According to the von Kries Coefficient Law, the neural response of each type of cone is attenuated by a gain factor that depends on the adapting light (von Kries, 1905). Several types of observations, however, are inconsistent with the Coefficient Law as a complete explanation of color appearance. First, consider two lights with spectral distributions $E_1(\lambda)$ and $E_2(\lambda)$, presented on patches of retina that are differentially adapted. The Coefficient Law implies that the two lights will have the same appearance when the response of each type of cone, L, M, and S, is the same for each of the lights. The condition for identical appearance is given by the three equalities

$$\begin{aligned}
\Sigma_\lambda\, [E_1(\lambda)\, a_{L1}\, q_L(\lambda)] &= \Sigma_\lambda\, [E_2(\lambda)\, a_{L2}\, q_L(\lambda)] \\
\Sigma_\lambda\, [E_1(\lambda)\, a_{M1}\, q_M(\lambda)] &= \Sigma_\lambda\, [E_2(\lambda)\, a_{M2}\, q_M(\lambda)] \\
\Sigma_\lambda\, [E_1(\lambda)\, a_{S1}\, q_S(\lambda)] &= \Sigma_\lambda\, [E_2(\lambda)\, a_{S2}\, q_S(\lambda)],
\end{aligned}$$

where $q_L(\lambda)$, $q_M(\lambda)$, and $q_S(\lambda)$ are the spectral sensitivities of each cone type and a_{ij} is the receptoral gain applied to cone-type i after adaptation to field j. The summation is over all wavelengths of light. These equations imply that if light $E_1(\lambda)$ matches light $E_2(\lambda)$ then changing the overall level of both lights by the same proportion, to $kE_1(\lambda)$ and $kE_2(\lambda)$, maintains their indistinguishable appearance (multiplying both sides of each equation by k does not upset the equalities). This prediction does not hold (Hurvich and Jameson, 1958; Jameson and Hurvich, 1959).

Additional evidence against simple receptoral sensitivity loss is apparent from a comparison of two types of measurements: color appearance and heterochromatic flicker photometry. If chromatic adaptation only alters receptoral sensitivity, then a given adapting field should have a corresponding effect on (i) the mixture ratio of 543⊕656 nm lights that appears equilibrium yellow and (ii) the ratio of 543 to 656 nm light that matches flicker photometrically. Monochromatic adapting fields in the range from 577 to 639 nm, however, alter the flicker match far more than the measurement for yellow, while recovery after adaptation is more rapid for flicker than for yellow (Ahn and MacLeod, 1993). This is inconsistent with chromatic adaptation causing only a selective sensitivity loss in receptoral signals that serve all later stages of vision.

The Coefficient Law fails to account also for the most simple case of chromatic adaptation: the change in appearance over time with extended viewing of a single light. Consider a 1° semi-circular monochromatic test field that can be varied between 558 and 630 nm, seen by the right eye. The appearance of a test wavelength in this range can be matched by a trichromatic mixture of 670 nm, 546 nm, and short-wavelength (broadband Wratten No. 47B) primaries presented to the left eye (haploscopic matching). The test wavelengths between 558 and 630 nm fall on the straight part of the spectrum locus in the chromaticity diagram, so they normally can be matched to a mixture of only 546⊕670 nm (no short-wavelength primary). This holds when the test and matching fields are presented for 1 second with an 11 second dark period between presentations, but fails when the test field (only) remains in view for 10 seconds of each 11 second intertrial interval (Vimal *et al.*, 1987). With self-adaptation during the intertrial interval, each monochromatic test light appears desaturated during the 1 second test presentation, compared to any mixture of 546⊕670 nm in the matching field; thus, some short-wavelength primary in the mixture is required for a match. The desaturated percept of these monochromatic lights after self-adaptation cannot be explained by the Coefficient Law because receptoral sensitivity loss could shift only the amounts of the 546 and 670 nm primaries required for the match.

Two-stage models: While the Coefficient Law fails to give a complete account of color perception under adaptation, many modern theories retain receptoral gain change as a first-stage process of adaptation. These theories include also a second stage of neural processing at which the responses of the L, M, and S cones are combined into a new trichromatic representation of color. The classical opponent-colors theory of Hurvich and Jameson (1957), for example, posits three second-stage opponent responses: red/green, yellow/blue, and white/black. Each opponent response is a weighted combination of signals from the L, M, and S cones (e.g., their red/green response is the difference between a redness signal, defined as a weighted sum of L and S cone excitations, and a greenness signal, defined as weighted M cone excitation). While the linear model of Hurvich and Jameson is not precisely correct for hue cancellation (section 4.2.3), many theories incorporate second-stage opponent responses defined as linear combinations of weighted first-stage receptor signals (Jameson and Hurvich, 1972; Shevell, 1978; Ware and Cowan, 1982; Guth, 1991; De Valois and De Valois, 1993; Poirson and Wandell, 1993). These theories can be only first-order approximations because they do not include known nonlinearities.

A broad class of these linear theories of chromatic adaptation can be characterized efficiently by considering multiplicative and/or additive processes of adaptation, occurring at the first (receptoral) stage and/or at a second (linear-opponent) stage. A general form for the response of one of the three trichromatic second-stage signals, R_n ($n = 1, 2, 3$), for a spectral distribution of light $E(\lambda)$ viewed under state of adaptation A, is

$$R_n[E(\lambda), A] = K_n(A) + \alpha_n(A) \{\Sigma_\lambda [E(\lambda) \{a_{S,n(A)}\, q_S(\lambda) + a_{M,n(A)}\, q_M(\lambda) + a_{L,n(A)}\, q_L(\lambda)\}] + k_{S,n(A)} + k_{M,n(A)} + k_{L,n(A)}\},$$

where $a_{i,n(A)}$ is the multiplicative gain for cone-type i feeding second-stage response n; $k_{i,n(A)}$ is an additive change in the response of cone-type i for response n; $\alpha_n(A)$ is the multiplicative gain applied to the second-stage signal n; and $K_n(A)$ is an additive shift in the second-stage signal n due to adaptation. Ware and Cowan (1982) used this framework to assess alternative theories for their measurements of chromatic induction (Figure 4.15). Their results were consistent only with theories that include a second-stage adapting effect (that is, $K_n(A) \neq 0$ and/or $\alpha_n(A) \neq 1$).

One model consistent with their analysis is the two-process theory of chromatic adaptation (Jameson and Hurvich, 1972; Shevell, 1978), which proposes that chromatic adaptation has two simultaneous influences on color appearance: receptoral gain changes, which are consistent with the Coefficient Law, and an additive shift at the second-stage opponent level. Under this model, the red/green chromatic response ($R_{r/g}$) for light $E(\lambda)$ under adaptation A is

$$R_{r/g}[E(\lambda), A] = K_{r/g}(A) + \Sigma_\lambda [E(\lambda) \{a_{S,r/g(A)}\, q_S(\lambda) + a_{M,r/g(A)}\, q_M(\lambda) + a_{L,r/g(A)}\, q_L(\lambda)\}]$$

where coefficients $a_{S,r/g(A)}$ and $a_{L,r/g(A)}$ are positive and coefficient $a_{M,r/g(A)}$ is negative. An implication of this theory is that mixtures of 540⊕660 nm lights that are red/green equilibrium colors (that is, neither the least reddish nor greenish in appearance; section 4.2.3) must follow a particular quantitative form, regardless of the adapting field A:

$$\Delta_{540} = [\Delta_{660} + f_{r/g(A)}]\, g_{r/g(A)},$$

where Δ_{540} and Δ_{660} are, respectively, the retinal illuminances of the 540 and 660 nm lights in the mixture judged in color; $g_{r/g(A)}$ is a parameter that depends on only the receptoral gains $a_{i,r/g(A)}$ and pre-receptoral filtering; and $f_{r/g(A)}$ includes the additive shift $K_{r/g}(A)$ due to adaptation.

This quantitative form implies that mixtures of 540⊕660 nm that appear neither reddish nor greenish must fall along a fixed template curve on a log-log plot of Δ_{540} light-level versus Δ_{660} light-level; the values of parameters $g_{r/g(A)}$ and $f_{r/g(A)}$ only shift the template parallel to the log coordinate axes (Shevell, 1978). The template fits experimental measurements well. Figure 4.18 shows measurements with long-wavelength adapting light at 10, 60 or 350 td. The linearity assumption implicit in the template is not problematic here because only 540 and 660 nm light is used. The same model accounts also for chromatic cancellation measurements with various spatial and temporal parameters and with adapting chromaticities from throughout color space (Shevell, 1982; Shevell and Humanski, 1988; Wei and Shevell, 1995).

Note that the formulation in terms of Δ_{540} and Δ_{660} includes only the light from the incremental test, not the adapting light on which the test is superimposed. The receptors stimulated by the test also absorb adapting light but the adapting light does not contribute directly to the appearance of a test when the test is distinguished from the adapting field in time, as a brief pulse, or in space, as a region smaller than the adapting area. Under some conditions, in fact, the added light from the adapting field may have a negligible effect on color appearance (Walraven, 1976); more generally, the additive contribution to color appearance from adapting light is often far less than expected from physical admixture (Shevell, 1982; Wei and Shevell, 1995). This implies a neural process tends to discount adapting light absorbed by receptors that are also stimulated by the test.

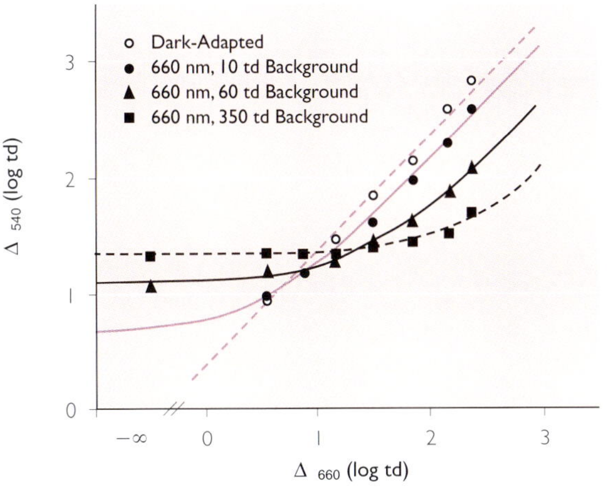

Figure 4.18 Mixtures of 540 and 660 nm light that appear neither reddish nor greenish, presented on a 660 nm background of 10, 60 or 350 trolands. Lines are fits of the template curve implied by the two-process theory. (From Shevell and Wesner, 1989.)

The two-process theory has been applied also to measurements of red/green equilibrium colors viewed within chromatic surrounds (Shevell, 1987; Shevell and Wesner, 1989). Chromatic surrounds alter receptoral gains $a_{i,n(A)}$, as do chromatic adapting fields, and can induce an additive shift $K_{r/g(A)}$ away from the appearance of the surround (for example a long-wavelength surround, which appears red, induces additive greenness).

Adapting to an illuminant: The human visual system, to a substantial degree, discounts the light illuminating objects so the objects appear about the same color under different spectral distributions of illumination (a full description of color constancy is in section 4.4.1). Chromatic adaptation to a uniform field of illuminating light has been studied in the context of adapting to, and thus discounting, the illuminant. Asymmetric color matches with the left (right) eye adapted to a uniform field of Illuminant A (Illuminant C) have been modeled within Ware and Cowan's general linear framework (Burnham *et al.*, 1957). Scaling methods also have been used in thorough studies of color perception following adaptation to different illuminants. A modified form of the Coefficient Law with nonlinear compression of the S-cone response (S^p) gives a fairly good account of these results (Bartleson, 1979).

4.3.5 CHROMATIC ADAPTATION TO COMPLEX FIELDS

Rich complex fields: Chromatic adaptation to rich complex fields is studied primarily with sets of chromatic surfaces viewed under different spectral illuminants. Chromatic adaptation in this case often is considered adaptation to the illuminant, though the separation of spectral illumination from spectral reflectance of the surfaces is frequently in the mind (or apparatus) of the experimenter, not in the stimulus entering the eye. This is particularly true of modern studies that use an emissive video display to simulate surfaces under a particular illuminant.

Models developed to explain adaptation to uniform fields (section 4.3.4) sometimes account well for the shifts in color appearance observed with a change in illumination. Adaptation to an array of 25 color surfaces, viewed under various (simulated) illuminants, gives color percepts consistent with the Coefficient Law (Brainard and Wandell, 1992; Bauml, 1995). In the simplest form of this model, a change in illumination alters the receptoral gain of each type of cone (L, M or S) in relation to the amount of light absorbed by only that cone-type; that is, the gain for each cone-type is independent of stimulation in the other types of cones. Failures of independence, however, have been found (Bauml, 1995) so, for example, S cone gain can depend on L and M stimulation while L cone gain can depend on S and M stimulation. These results corroborate a failure of independence found with uniform adapting fields (Cicerone *et al.*, 1975).

Many measurements using rich complex displays are described reasonably well by simple models, including the Coefficient Law for which specific violations are well known (section 4.3.4). The success of such models can provide useful first-order simplification. At the same time, the complexity of underlying mechanisms can be apparent in the way that parameters in the models depend on features of the adapting field. Measurements that are accounted for theoretically by gain controls applied to first-stage receptoral signals may, in fact, reflect higher visual processes that cause changes in color perception mimicked by receptoral gains. One example is contralateral (that is, opposite-eye) adaptation to a uniform chromatic field, which can cause multiplicative, gain-like changes in measurements of red/green equilibrium colors (Shevell and Humanski, 1984).

The correspondence between the measurements using complex displays and the predictions from models developed for uniform adapting fields would be expected if the adapting effect of a complex display were the same as the effect of some 'equivalent' uniform light. This is a fundamental issue considered below.

Modestly complex fields: One approach to understanding adaptation to complex fields is to examine the changes in appearance that result from modest modification of a uniform adapting field. A basic question is how the effect of adapting to two or more uniform regions viewed simultaneously, each one in a different part of the visual field, relates to the adapting effect of each uniform field presented alone. For example, a multi-light adapting field might be equivalent to a single uniform field at the spatial average of the lights. This would allow a complex stimulus to be reduced to a simple one by considering only physical lights. Alternatively, two or more lights in a complex field may establish a state of adaptation predicted from the adapting effect of each uniform light presented alone. This is an aggregation of neural processes of adaptation rather than of physical lights. A third alternative is that the state of adaptation established by a complex field cannot be specified from the adapting effect of each component light presented alone. This would follow if the state of adaptation depends, for example, on the range of chromaticities or the chromatic contrast within a complex field.

Consider changes in the color of a 1° test spot when it is superimposed on a uniform 3° monochromatic 540 nm adapting field. This is a simple adapting field; measurements of red/green equilibrium colors are consistent with the two-process theory. Now add broadband 'white' light in a 3–5° ring surrounding the 3° 540 nm field. Adding the remote achromatic ring shifts the appearance of the test toward greenness, toward the color of the 540 nm adapting field. This result shows attenuation of the neural effects of chromatic adaptation: compared to the 540 nm field alone, introducing the achromatic ring reduces receptoral gain changes and increases the influence of physical admixture from the 540 nm adapting light. Further, with 660 nm in place of 540 nm adapting light, introducing the same achromatic ring shifts color appearance toward redness, toward the color of the 660 nm adapting field (Wesner and Shevell, 1992). This shows that the remote achromatic ring is not directly influencing the color of the 1° test spot by either a physical or neural process, since the direction of color shift caused by introducing the ring depends on the wavelength of the adapting field (further, the 3–5° achromatic ring in an otherwise dark field causes a negligible change in color appearance of the test).

Chromatic adaptation to uniform long-wavelength light is attenuated also by small (2' diameter) achromatic 'dots' embedded very sparsely at random locations in the adapting field (Jenness and Shevell, 1995). Also, chromatic induction (section 4.3.3) is attenuated by spatial chromatic modulation in a region outside of a chromatic inducing surround (Shevell and Wei, 1998). Taken together, these observations show that the state of adaptation depends on the ensemble of lights that compose the complex adapting stimulus, not (i) on only the light near the boundary of a test field, (ii) on the space-average of light in the adapting field, or (iii) on a combination of effects determined from each element of the adapting stimulus presented alone (for example, not from the effect of the achromatic ring alone, which is nil, and a 3° monochromatic adapting field alone).

If a complex adapting field did establish the same state of adaptation as some 'equivalent' uniform field, then the contrast within the complex field would not be a critical factor mediating adaptation because, by definition, a uniform field has zero contrast. Adaptation specifically to contrast, however, does alter appearance. An achromatic demonstration is shown in Figure 4.19, in which the two circular regions are identical patterns of random texture elements at moderate contrast. The square regions surrounding each circle have the same space-averaged light level; the surround on the left is composed of high-contrast texture elements, and the surround on the right is a uniform field with no contrast within it. The contrast in the left square reduces the perceived contrast within the circle it surrounds, compared to the perceived contrast within the circle surrounded by the uniform field. Figure 4.19 is a static version of a rapidly changing dynamic display used by Chubb, Sperling, and Solomon (1989): a new random texture pattern in the center and surround was presented 60 times a second, so the time-averaged light level at every point was constant. Perceived contrast in the circle was measured with only a single circle-within-square (similar to the left half of Figure 4.19) using a cancellation procedure with slowly varying contrast in the surround. Their results showed that the magnitude of attenuation of perceived contrast within the circle follows the magnitude of contrast within the surround.

Figure 4.19 Demonstration of adaptation to achromatic contrast. The two circular regions are identical physically but the one on the left appears lower in contrast. The high-contrast texture elements in the left rectangle reduce perceived contrast within the circular region they surround. (Courtesy of Charles Chubb.)

Adaptation to an inhomogeneous surround has a specific effect also on the brightness of a uniform achromatic field, and on perceived chromatic contrast. The relation between the physical radiance and the perceived brightness of a uniform achromatic patch is affected by a surrounding achromatic inducing field (section 4.3.3). Brightness matches show that the quantitative relation measured with an inhomogeneous achromatic inducing surround is different from the relation found with *any* level of uniform surround (Schirillo and Shevell, 1996). Adaptation to contrast that is purely chromatic also affects appearance. Chromatic contrast within a surround attenuates perceived chromatic contrast within a central field (Singer and D'Zmura, 1994). Further, chromatic variation over time, rather than space, affects color perception according to the range of chromatic light presented, not just the time-averaged adapting light (Webster and Mollon, 1995). These findings show that a complex field can establish a state of adaptation not possible with a steady uniform adapting field.

Configurations of surfaces: A complex stimulus composed of many different regions at various lightnesses or chromaticities may be perceived as a collection of discrete lights or surfaces, or as an integrated pattern of related elements. Some patterns can even evoke the perception of a three-dimensional object. The perceptual interpretation of a complex stimulus depends on the spatial configuration of the regions. Most of the studies above used distinct regions designed to appear unrelated to each other, in order to avoid higher visual processes that mediate object perception. The perceived lightness and color of a given light, however, can vary according to the perceptual interpretation of the complete stimulus, which depends on the spatial arrangement of the various regions.

Perceptual organization affects lightness when a complex stimulus is interpreted to have subparts that are under distinct levels of illumination or that are viewed through unequal transmitting filters. The two arrowheads in the upper panel

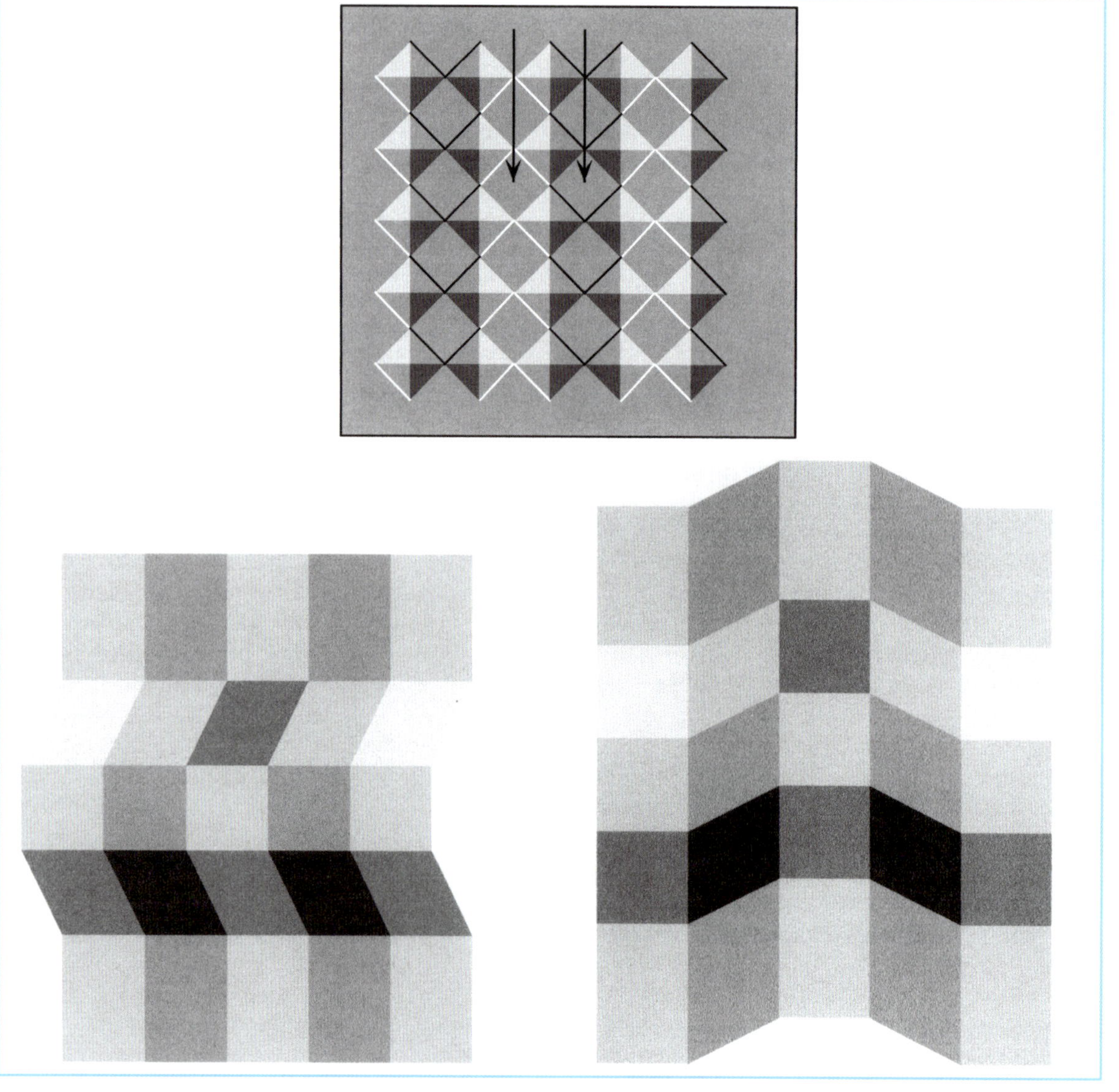

Figure 4.20 Demonstrations showing that perceptual organization alters appearance. (Above) The two arrowheads are in physically identical regions that appear quite different. (Below) In each figure, the middle vertical column contains two physically identical regions (the second and fourth ones from the top), which appear more different in the left figure than in the right one. See text for explanations. (Courtesy of Edward Adelson.)

of Figure 4.20 are located in diamonds that appear different in lightness: the diamond on the left is judged darker than the diamond on the right (Adelson, 1993). The two diamonds are actually identical with respect to the light reaching the eye, as can be seen by tracing each arrow from head to tail along a path of constant light level. Both arrows' tails are within the uniform background area. The difference in lightness can be accounted for by a perceived difference in the transmittance of filters inferred from the vertical strips. When the same amount of absolute light is detected in two strips with (inferred) filters of unequal transmittance, the region in the strip of weaker transmittance is perceived as lighter. The lightness percept discounts the loss of light due to the inferred filter absorption.

A similar effect on lightness is observed with a configuration of 25 regions arranged in a 5-row by 5-column display, perceived as a folded figure illuminated from the top of the page (Figure 4.20, lower left panel). In the middle vertical column, the second and fourth patches from the top deliver the same amount of light to the eye but the former appears darker. The inferred three-dimensional figure is consistent with illumination from the top, so the entire fourth row is perceived to be in shadow. The visual system compensates the weaker (inferred) illumination so a given level of light appears lighter in the fourth row than in the second row. When the same 25 regions are changed so as to alter the impression of shadow in the fourth row, the second and fourth patches in the middle column appear much more similar (Figure 4.20, lower right panel).

4.3.6 BASIC COLOR TERMS

An unlimited number of linguistic terms can be used to describe unrelated colors (section 4.2.1); the additional chromatic percepts that occur as only related colors expand these verbal descriptions. Despite this richness of color vocabulary, most modern languages have a small, predominant set of 11 color terms with comparable meanings. In English, these color terms are white, gray, black, red, green, blue, yellow, orange, purple, pink, and brown. The first three of these terms describe achromatic percepts; the next four are the unique-hue names (section 4.2.1), sometimes referred to as primary color terms; the last four are called secondary color terms because they can be described with a combination of the other seven terms. Berlin and Kay (1969), who studied the words used to describe color in many languages, called these 11 linguistic descriptions *basic color terms*.

Many nonbasic color terms are used commonly (for example beige, maroon, turquoise), and color names given by individuals can be idiosyncratic. How, then, can these 11 terms be considered a basic set? In addition to the cross-linguistic evidence (Berlin and Kay, 1969), laboratory measurements show the salience of the basic color terms with respect to the consistency and frequency with which they are used. When observers are asked to give monolexemic names (that is, names that are not compound terms such as dark green or reddish brown) to hundreds of uniform chromatic surfaces sampled broadly from color space, the basic color terms are used with better reliability when an individual names the same stimulus on more than one occasion, and with better consensus across different people, compared to nonbasic color names used by the same observers (Boynton and Olson, 1990). Further, an observer responds more quickly when he uses a basic color term than a nonbasic term. With respect to frequency of color term use, more than 7600 color-name responses were generated from hundreds of chromatic samples judged by many observers. One of the 11 basic color terms was the response on 67% of the trials; 71 different nonbasic terms were used on the other 33% of trials. The basic color terms clearly capture much of the linguistic description given to color appearance.

A controversial issue is whether the basic color terms reflect fundamental physiological responses that are common to all individuals with normal color vision (Ratliff, 1976; Boynton and Olson, 1990) or, alternatively, develop from cultural influences.

4.4 COLOR CONSTANCY

4.4.1 THE PHENOMENON OF COLOR CONSTANCY

Most objects we see are illuminated by a source of light, such as the sun, a light bulb, or a candle. Objects reflect light from the source, and some of this reflected light enters the eye (Figure 4.21). Our perception of objects depends on the light reflected from them. This light, however, is not a property of only the objects. The light entering the eye is determined by the spectral reflectance of the objects *and* the spectral power distribution of the illuminating light.

The light reflected from an object is an important factor in determining the object's color appearance. For example, a ping-pong ball that appears white in daylight appears violet with illumination from only, and thus reflection of only, short-wavelength light in an otherwise dark room, or red with illumination from only long-wavelength light. This page appears white under normal illumination because the paper reflects wavelengths throughout the visible spectrum in approximately equal amounts. The color figures in this book have regions that appear different in hue because the printer's ink reflects some wavelengths much more than others. A region that appears green, for example, is printed with ink that reflects middle wavelengths to a greater extent than other wavelengths.

A strict relation between the perceived color of an object and the light reflected from it does not hold, however, when the object is part of a complex scene, as noted in previous sections. A particularly clear demonstration is illustrated in Figure 4.22, from an experiment by McCann, McKee, and Taylor (1976). An observer viewed a complex patchwork of 17 colored papers (called a 'color Mondrian' because it resembles a painting by the Dutch artist Piet Mondrian). The colors in Figure 4.22 represent the papers as they appeared under normal illumination. The observer assessed the color of each patch by finding a matching colored paper in the *Munsell Book of Color* (1929), an atlas of color chips that spans a broad range of color percepts (see Munsell Color Order System, Chapter 5). The *Munsell Book of Color* was viewed with only the left eye and the Mondrian was viewed with only the right eye, so that retinal adaptation from viewing the Mondrian would not affect the matching color chosen from the book.

The Munsell book and the color Mondrian were illuminated by separate sources, each one a mixture of 450, 530, and 630 nm lights. The radiances of the three wavelengths illuminating the Munsell book were held fixed at levels giving a 'best' white (presumably close to a completely achromatic hue). The radiances of the three wavelengths illuminating the Mondrian were set initially to the same levels as used for the Munsell book. The observer easily found a colored paper in the book that matched each area in the Mondrian.

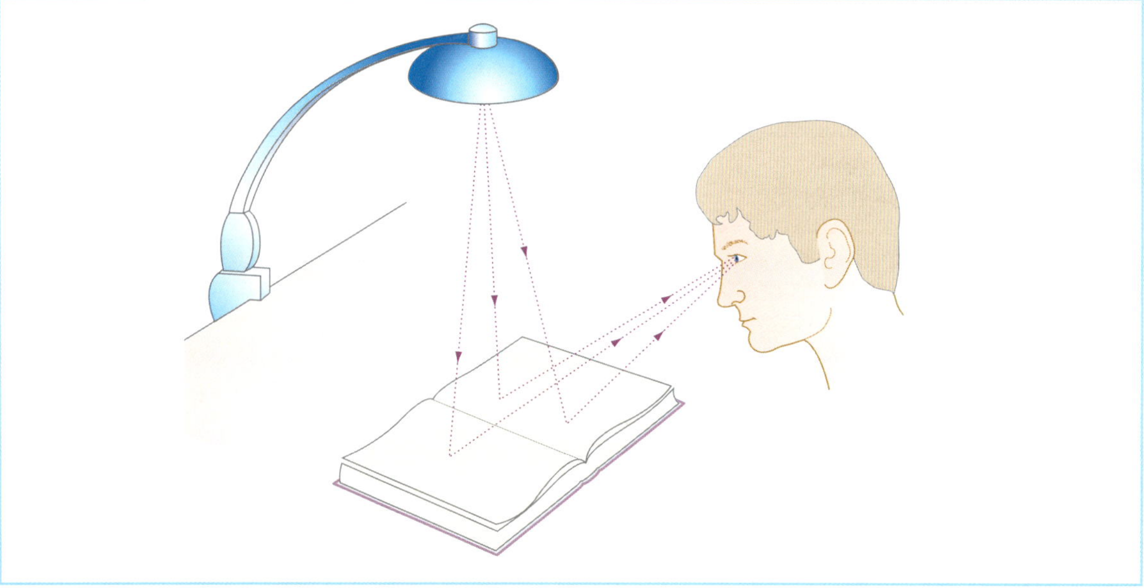

Figure 4.21 Light from most objects is reflected from a source of illumination, such as the lamp shown here. (Drawing courtesy of David Scott.)

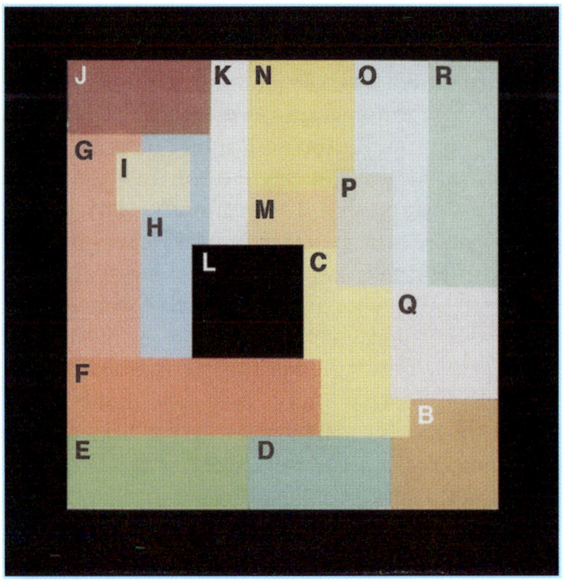

Figure 4.22 **The 'color Mondrian' used by McCann, McKee and Taylor (1976). See text for further detail.**

In the next part of the experiment, the light reflected from the neutral gray paper (area P) was measured spectroradiometrically, and then the illumination of *only* the Mondrian was changed so that the light reflected from the green paper (area R) was physically identical to the light previously reflected from the neutral gray (area P). If the primary determinant of a paper's color is the spectral power distribution of light reflected from it, the green paper under the new illuminant would appear the same as the gray paper under the initial illumination. Changing the illumination of the Mondrian, however, had little effect on the color appearance of the 17 papers. The perceived hue of the green paper was unchanged, even though it now reflected the same light as came previously from the neutral paper. Subsequently, the light illuminating the Mondrian was adjusted so a blue paper (area H), a red–purple paper (area G) or a yellow paper (area C) reflected the same light as the neutral gray paper under the initial illumination. Varying the illumination caused surprisingly little change in the appearance of the Mondrian. For example, area F always was judged red, area E green–yellow, and area O a blue (though sometimes a green–blue or a purple–blue). In general, the appearance of the 17 patches was not the color expected from the spectral distribution of light reflected from each paper.

Color constancy is the perceived stability of the color of objects or surfaces, despite changes in the light illuminating them. The color appearance of objects or surfaces can depend remarkably little on the illuminating light, as demonstrated in the Mondrian experiment, even though a change of illuminant alters the light absorbed by the photoreceptors that encode color.

The term constancy is slightly misleading because perfect constancy is not achieved in human color vision. The subtle variation of color in a painting of the sea can be inspiring at an outdoor exhibit but disappointingly drab in a living room illuminated by tungsten bulbs. Carved roast beef, cooked rare, looks less appetizing under fluorescent than tungsten illumination because the two sources of light differ in spectral emittance. The perceived colors of objects are not precisely stable when illumination is changed but human color percepts are much closer to constancy than to the color expected from the light reflected from the objects.

Color constancy in the classical sense refers to the stability of the color of objects under changes in illumination. A more modern interpretation extends constancy to the stability of color percepts also when the color of nearby objects is varied. The modern perspective is a theoretical ideal rather than a feature of human vision. The color of one object can affect the color of another, as in color contrast or assimilation (section 4.3.3).

4.4.2 HOW IS COLOR CONSTANCY POSSIBLE?

Color perception depends on the light absorbed by the three types of cones. This is obvious but at the same time paradoxical, because color constancy is the capability of the visual system to extract a stable color of an object *despite* changes in receptoral quantal absorptions caused by varying the illumination. The resolution of the paradox is that constancy depends on photoreceptor responses from more than one object.

Constancy is not achieved with only a single object, such as the isolated ping-pong ball.

Consider light reflected from the ball that includes only the wavelengths from 500–600 nm, all at the same energy. The visual system has no information to distinguish (a) a light of equal energy in only the spectral range 500–600 nm illuminating a ball that reflects all wavelengths nonselectively, from (b) a light of equal energy throughout the visible spectrum illuminating a ball that reflects equally but exclusively wavelengths from 500–600 nm (or an infinite number of other possible illuminants and reflectances that would produce the same light from the ping-pong ball).

An additional prerequisite for color constancy is an illuminant not restricted to a narrow part of the visible spectrum. In a demonstration 200 years ago to members of the Royal Academy of Sciences in Paris, Gaspard Monge showed color constancy is not achieved when only the long-wavelength light reflected from objects is allowed to enter the eye (Mollon, 1985). When an illuminant is monochromatic, the light reflected from objects in a complex scene varies only in level, not spectral composition. The pattern of receptoral quantal absorptions could be due to differences in the objects' spectral reflectances, or to differences in only the objects' overall level of reflectance (that is, all objects might reflect light spectrally nonselectively but vary in the fraction of incident light they reflect).

More recent studies confirm Monge's observation but show also that approximate constancy can be restored by adding only a few percent of broadband 'white' light to a strongly chromatic illuminant (Helson, 1938). Modern high-pressure sodium lamps, used to illuminate streets, take advantage of this fact. Sodium light alone, which is nearly monochromatic at 589 nm, gives roadways an eerie monochrome appearance. High pressure sodium lamps have an emission spectrum that includes small amounts of other wavelengths, which expand the range of perceived colors to a more normal gamut.

The ability of the visual system to maintain (nearly) stable colors of objects under changes in illumination is a form of visual adaptation. The visual system is adapting to the illumination. A modern approach to the problem of color constancy considers the biological information available to establish a state of adaptation that compensates for the illuminating light (Stiles, 1961; Maloney, 1985). With only one uniform object in view (for example, the ping-pong ball), the information carried by receptoral responses cannot separate information about the object from information that might mediate adaptation. With a narrow-band illuminant, differences among objects in spectral reflectance cannot be logically distinguished from differences that are not spectrally selective. More than one object must be illuminated by broadband (or more than one narrow-band) light in order that receptoral quantal absorptions may carry information useful for maintaining the stable color appearance of objects.

The visual system could, for example, adapt to the average of the light from the entire scene, as proposed by Helmholtz and several modern theorists. There is no guarantee, of course, that the average light reflected from the objects is an accurate measure of the illuminating light; in fact, there are common environments in which the average light reaching the eye is different from the illuminant (for example, a large lawn illuminated by sunlight). This is not, however, sufficient reason to reject the proposal. Whether or not the human visual system adapts to the average light, or to any other features of the scene, is an empirical question.

4.4.3 SPECTRAL ILLUMINATION, SPECTRAL REFLECTANCE, AND RECEPTORAL QUANTAL ABSORPTIONS

Color constancy in normal viewing is achieved effortlessly and with sufficient accuracy that one often fails to notice a change in illumination. An important question is whether a typical change in illumination alters receptoral quantal absorptions enough for easy detection. If not, then color constancy would be a simple consequence of failure to discriminate small differences in receptoral stimulation.

In fact, changes in receptoral stimulation due to varying illumination can be quite large. The amount of light absorbed by each of the three types of cone can be calculated directly from the spectral distribution of illuminating light $E(\lambda)$, the spectral reflectance of an object $R(\lambda)$, and the (corneal) spectral sensitivity of each cone type

$q_i(\lambda)$ (*i* denotes the cone type S, M or L). The amount of light at each wavelength reflected from the object is $E(\lambda)R(\lambda)$. The total number of quanta per second absorbed by each type of cone is $Q_i = \Sigma_\lambda[q_i(\lambda)E(\lambda)R(\lambda)]$. Restricting consideration to the visible spectrum from 400 to 700 nm, the total quantal absorptions Q_S, Q_M, and Q_L for the three cone types can be written in matrix form:

$$\begin{bmatrix} Q_S \\ Q_M \\ Q_L \end{bmatrix} = \begin{bmatrix} q_S(400)E(400) & q_S(401)E(401) & q_S(402)E(402) & \ldots & q_S(700)E(700) \\ q_M(400)E(400) & q_M(401)E(401) & q_M(402)E(402) & \ldots & q_M(700)E(700) \\ q_L(400)E(400) & q_L(401)E(401) & q_L(402)E(402) & \ldots & q_L(700)E(700) \end{bmatrix} \begin{bmatrix} R(400) \\ R(401) \\ R(402) \\ \cdot \\ \cdot \\ \cdot \\ R(700) \end{bmatrix}$$

The 3-row by 301-column matrix relating the spectral reflectances, $R(\lambda)$, to quantal absorptions, Q_i, has been called the lighting matrix to emphasize its dependence on the illuminant (Brainard and Wandell, 1986). Different objects illuminated by the same source of light can have different spectral reflectances $R(\lambda)$ but share the same lighting matrix.

Color papers that compose the Mondrian used by McCann, McKee, and Taylor (Figure 4.22) can demonstrate the changes in receptoral quantal absorptions due to a typical change of illumination. The spectral power distributions of two common illuminants are shown in the first column of Figure 4.23. These illuminants are designated CIE standard sources A and C. Illuminant A is an incandescent tungsten-filament lamp similar to an ordinary screw-in light bulb. Illuminant C has the approximate spectral distribution of overcast skylight. The change in illuminant from source A to source C, therefore, is similar to the difference between viewing the Mondrian indoors with illumination from a household lamp versus viewing it outdoors on an overcast day. Note that the spectral

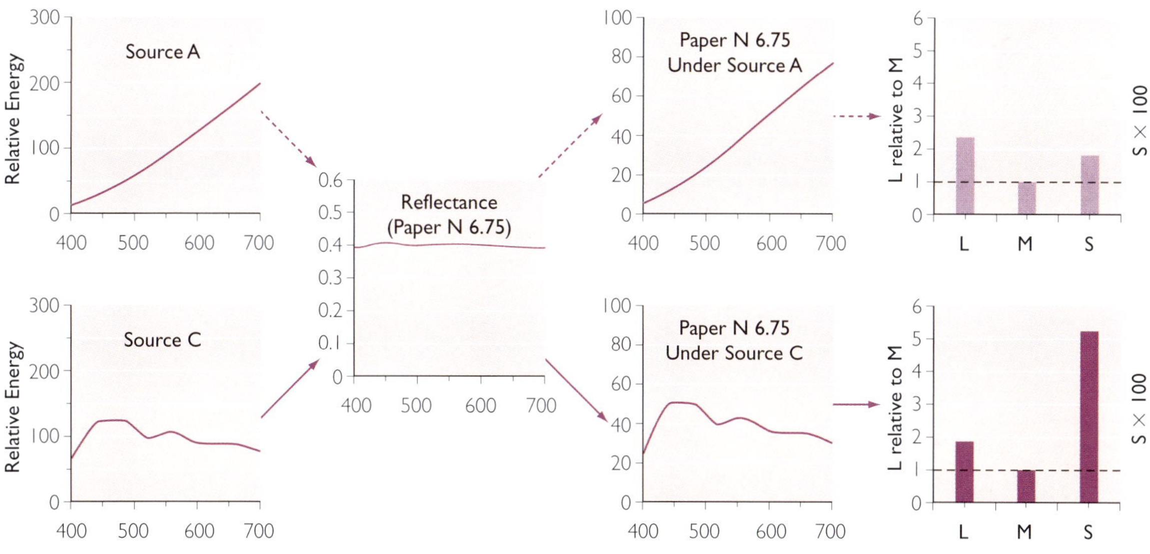

Figure 4.23 **The stimulation of L, M, and S cones from an illuminated paper. CIE standard sources A and C, with spectral distributions shown in the left column, illuminate Munsell paper N 6.75, with spectral reflectance shown in the second column. The spectral distribution of light from the paper under each source is shown in the third column. This results in the relative stimulation of L, M, and S cones shown in the last column (M normalized to 1.0).**

distributions of the illuminants are quite different. Source A has substantially less energy at short wavelengths than at long wavelengths, while source C is relatively flat but has somewhat more energy at short than at long wavelengths.

The reflectance spectrum of area P in Figure 4.22 is shown in the second column of Figure 4.23. Area P is constructed from Munsell paper N 6.75 which has nearly flat spectral reflectance.[3] The light reflected from this paper under source A or under source C is shown in separate panels in the third column. The L, M and S cone quantal absorptions for this paper under each illuminant are shown in the rightmost column. The L- and S-cone quantal absorptions are plotted relative to M-cone absorption, which is normalized to 1. The principle of univariance (see Chapter 1) implies that wavelengths of light are discriminated by relative stimulation of the L, M, and S cones. Relative stimulation of the three types of cone is seen directly by normalizing the M-cone absorption to 1. The change from source A to source C reduces relative L-cone quantal absorption by about 18% and raises relative S cone quantal absorption by nearly 200%. These are not marginal changes.

The spectral distributions of light reflected from four other regions in Figure 4.22 under Illuminant A or C are plotted in Figure 4.24. Areas F, N, E, and H are constructed from Munsell papers 5R 5/12, 5Y 7/8, 7.5GY 6/6, and 2.5PB 6/8, respectively. The lower panels show the relative stimulation of the cones under each illuminant. The magnitude of change in receptoral stimulation caused by changing from source A (lighter bars) to source C (darker bars) is qualitatively similar for all of the papers: a substantial drop in the relative stimulation of L cones and a large increase in the relative stimulation of S cones. This shows that color constancy is not a result of failing to detect small differences in receptoral stimulation.

A summary of the magnitude of effect due to changing illumination from source A to source C is plotted in Figure 4.25 for the five Munsell papers considered above. Relative L/(L+M) receptoral stimulation is plotted on the horizontal axis, and relative S cone stimulation is on the vertical axis (this is a MacLeod–Boynton diagram described in section 3.2.5). Note that the points for four of the five papers under source C (solid symbols) are outside the shaded region that includes the points for all five papers under source A. The difference in coordinates for the gray paper N 6.75 due to changing illuminants (dashed line) is larger than some of the differences

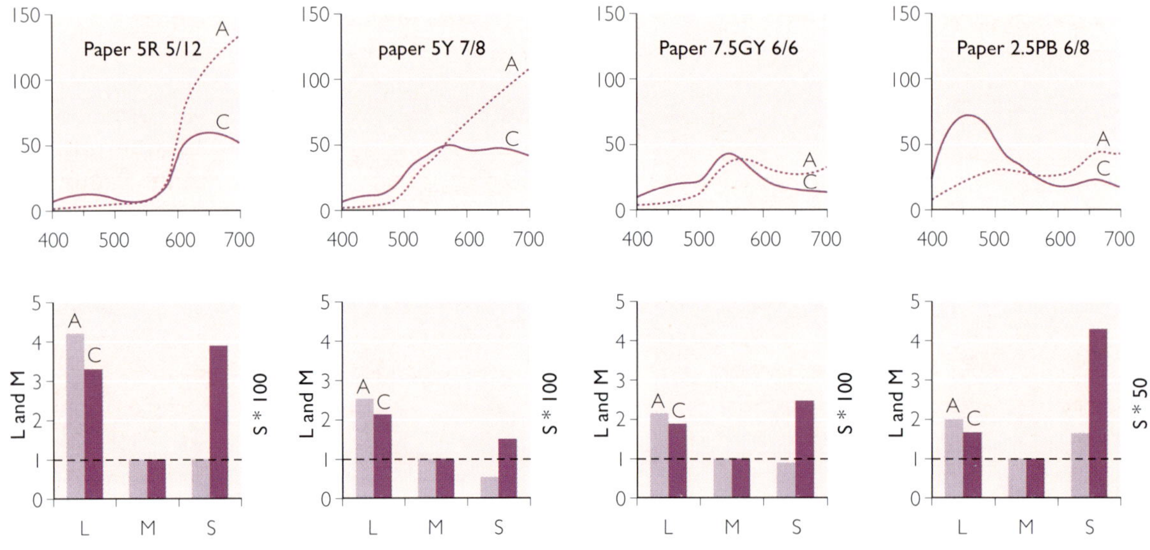

Figure 4.24 **(Above) The spectral distribution of light from four Munsell papers, 5R 5/12, 5Y 7/8, 7.5GY 6/6 and 2/5PB 6/8, under CIE standard sources A and C (dashed and solid lines, respectively). (Below) Relative stimulation of L, M, and S cones for the four Munsell papers, under each source of illumination (M normalized to 1.0).**

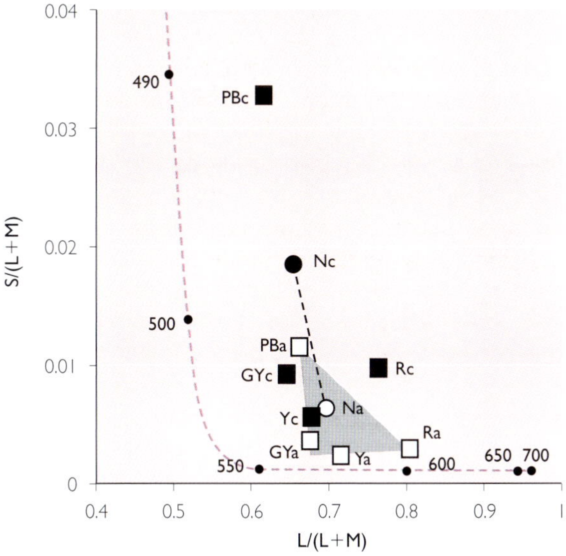

Figure 4.25 L, M, and S cone stimulation, plotted in the MacLeod–Boynton diagram, for five Munsell papers, under source A (open symbols) or source C (solid symbols). The shaded region includes all of the papers when illuminated by source A.

between paper N 6.75 under Illuminant A (open circle labeled Na) and the other papers also under Illuminant A (open squares). The difference in receptoral quantal absorptions for a single paper due to a change in illumination, therefore, can be comparable to the differences among clearly distinguishable, categorically different colors viewed under a single illuminant.

4.4.4 BASIC THEORETICAL ISSUES

Classical theories of color constancy focus on the mechanisms mediating the stable appearance of colored objects. Theories can be distinguished by the emphasis placed on peripheral sensory mechanisms versus central processes (including cognitive processes). Most theories include both retinal and cortical mechanisms.

Classical views assert that peripheral mechanisms by themselves are insufficient to account for constancy. Helmholtz (1866) proposed a learned, unconscious judgment process that somehow corrects for the illuminant. Hering (1920), who emphasized the importance of receptoral desensitization, retinal adaptation and even size of the pupil, included in his theory the memory of an object's color that is built up from seeing it on previous occasions. While many retinal mechanisms of chromatic adaptation now are well understood and no doubt affect color perception, modern research supports the classical position that retinal mechanisms are an incomplete explanation of color constancy (Arend and Reeves, 1986; Worthey and Brill, 1986; Cornelissen and Brenner, 1995).

There is clear evidence against the view that constancy is mediated entirely by an irreversible transformation of neural signals at a peripheral site. Consider two complex arrays of papers, each one like the color Mondrian, that are simulated on a computer-controlled video display. Each array of papers is illuminated by a different (simulated) light (the two illuminants are from the range bounded by the extremes of daylight). An experiment conducted by Arend and Reeves (1986) included two conditions that differed in only the instructions given to the observer: in the first condition the observer was asked to adjust a 'test' patch in one array to match the hue and saturation of a particular patch in the other array; in the second condition the subject was asked to adjust the test patch in one array to 'look as if it were cut from the same piece of paper' as a particular patch in the other array. Results from the two conditions were different. Moderately good color constancy was found with instructions to find a matching piece of paper (that is, a matching surface) but not with instructions to match hue and saturation. The two conditions were identical except for the instructions given to the observer, so the results argue strongly against an explanation of color constancy that relies on only automatic peripheral sensory mechanisms.

A pivotal element of many theories of constancy (and of color sensation; see next paragraph) is a 'white' or neutral point of a scene. In these theories, the neutral point serves as a reference standard, with discrepancies from it mediating the perceived colors of objects (Helson, 1938; Judd, 1940; Land and McCann, 1971). A theory of human perception must specify how the neutral point is determined from receptoral quantal absorptions or, if it depends on information other than light absorbed by photoreceptors (for example, prior knowledge about objects), how a particular object is awarded the status of the neutral one. Whether or not a neutral-appearing object is assumed to be identified in advance, these theories tend to be vague about the physiological mechanisms mediating constancy.

Proper theories of color constancy rely on only the information available to the nervous system. This distinguishes theories of constancy from theories that predict human color sensations under different types of illumination. The former address the visual processes that achieve the stable color appearance of objects; the latter concern the hue, saturation, and brightness of an object, given the spectral power distribution of the illuminant and the spectral reflectance of the object. Theories of color sensation take as given the physical properties of the illuminant and the objects, and specify the visual sensation (Helson, 1938; Judd, 1940). They examine how well, not *how*, the visual system maintains the color appearance of objects. Modern theories of constancy, on the other hand, take the receptoral quantal catches as given and specify the spectral reflectances of the objects. Experimental work on color sensation provides measurements useful for evaluating theories of constancy (in fact, if color sensations were predicted perfectly then theories of constancy could be tested with pencil and paper or a computer rather than with laboratory measurements of human percepts). Theories of color sensation, however, incorporate information other than receptoral quantal absorptions. They relate to constancy only to the extent that the information they require about a scene is recoverable from knowing the light absorbed by photoreceptors.

Recently, a computational approach to color constancy has stimulated theories that aim to reconstruct the spectral reflectances of objects from the number of quanta absorbed by each of the three types of cone. These theories exploit the information implicit in receptoral quantal absorptions, usually without considering the physiological mechanisms that might carry out the analog of the computations (see D'Zmura and Lennie, 1986, for a welcome exception). Photoreceptor quantal absorptions, however, carry insufficient information to specify exactly the illuminant and the objects' reflectances, so the information from receptors always is ambiguous about the spectral reflectances of objects. Computational theories of color constancy resolve the ambiguity with assumptions about the illuminant, the reflectances, and/or the human visual system.

4.4.5 AN ILLUMINANT WITH EXACTLY THREE MONOCHROMATIC COMPONENTS

Some theories of color constancy can be evaluated by examining the relation between spectral reflectance and quantal absorption. Consider again the von Kries Coefficient Law (section 4.3.4), which in this case holds that a change of illumination affects the gains of the three types of cones. The Coefficient Law does not predict perfect color constancy, as can be seen by considering the Mondrian experiment of McCann, McKee, and Taylor (Figure 4.22). The illuminant in the Mondrian experiment was restricted to three monochromatic lights, at 450, 530, and 630 nm, so the general lighting matrix with 301 columns (section 4.4.3) is reduced to only three columns:

$$\begin{bmatrix} Q_S \\ Q_M \\ Q_L \end{bmatrix} = \begin{bmatrix} q_S(450)E(450) & q_S(530)E(530) & q_S(630)E(630) \\ q_M(450)E(450) & q_M(530)E(530) & q_M(630)E(630) \\ q_L(450)E(450) & q_L(530)E(530) & q_L(630)E(630) \end{bmatrix} \begin{bmatrix} R(450) \\ R(530) \\ R(630) \end{bmatrix}.$$

The ratio of the quantal catch of the L cones under one illuminant (say E_1), $Q_{L|E1}$, to the quantal catch of the L cones under a second illuminant, $Q_{L|E2}$, is

$$\frac{Q_{L|E1}}{Q_{L|E2}} = \frac{q_L(450)E_1(450)R(450) + q_L(530)E_1(530)R(530) + q_L(630)E_1(630)R(630)}{q_L(450)E_2(450)R(450) + q_L(530)E_2(530)R(530) + q_L(630)E_2(630)R(630)}.$$

Similar equations can be written for the M and S cones. The Coefficient Law requires the value of $Q_{L|E1}/Q_{L|E2}$ to be the same for every object in the scene. This ratio is the sensitivity of the L cones under the first illuminant E_1 relative to their sensitivity under the second illuminant E_2. The equation for $Q_{L|E1}/Q_{L|E2}$, however, shows that the ratio is not the same for objects (or surfaces) with different spectral reflectances [R(450), R(530) and R(630)]. The same argument presents a problem for other theories that depend on only scaling the quantal catch of each type of cone (for example, a scaling factor that takes account of the quantal catch from a 'standard white' reference patch; Worthey and Brill, 1986).

Though the Coefficient Law does not predict perfect constancy, exact color constancy in the Mondrian experiment is possible with a standard reference patch of known reflectance and with an illuminant composed of the three monochromatic lights. The quantal absorptions for a reference standard with non-zero reflectances $R_{Std}(450)$, $R_{Std}(530)$, and $R_{Std}(630)$ are

$$\begin{bmatrix} Q_S \\ Q_M \\ Q_L \end{bmatrix} = \begin{bmatrix} q_S(450)R_{Std}(450) & q_S(530)R_{Std}(530) & q_S(630)R_{Std}(630) \\ q_M(450)R_{Std}(450) & q_M(530)R_{Std}(530) & q_M(630)R_{Std}(630) \\ q_L(450)R_{Std}(450) & q_L(530)R_{Std}(530) & q_L(630)R_{Std}(630) \end{bmatrix} \begin{bmatrix} E(450) \\ E(530) \\ E(630) \end{bmatrix}.$$

The known values of the reference-standard reflectances and of the spectral sensitivities of cones, $q_S(\lambda)$, $q_M(\lambda)$ and $q_L(\lambda)$, can be substituted in the matrix, and then the spectral power distribution, E(450), E(530), and E(630), found in terms of the quantal catches for the reference standard. Then, with the values of E(450), E(530), and E(630) determined, the reflectances R(450), R(530), and R(630) for any object can be found from the first matrix equation in this section (4.4.5) using the known values of $q_S(\lambda)$, $q_M(\lambda)$ and $q_L(\lambda)$, and the quantal catches Q_S, Q_M and Q_L for the object.

4.4.6 MODELING SPECTRAL REFLECTANCE AND ILLUMINATION (GENERAL CASES)

Color constancy would be achieved if the identical spectral reflectance of an object, $R(\lambda)$, could be calculated from the receptoral quantal catches Q_S, Q_M, and Q_L, given any spectral illuminant distribution $E(\lambda)$. Obviously it is not possible on mathematical grounds alone to invert the matrix equation in section 4.4.3 to solve for the 301 spectral reflectance values R(400), R(401), R(402), . . ., R(700) when only the three quantal absorptions, Q_S, Q_M, and Q_L, are known. Special forms of the matrix equation can be solved, however, by introducing assumptions about the spectra of the objects' reflectances and/or the illuminant. The specific choice of assumptions is what distinguishes some theories of constancy from each other.

Suppose, for example, all possible illuminants are some admixture of three known spectral power distributions, $e_1(\lambda)$, $e_2(\lambda)$, and $e_3(\lambda)$. The power of the illuminating light, $E(\lambda)$, is then a weighted sum of the three components: $a_1e_1(\lambda) + a_2e_2(\lambda) + a_3e_3(\lambda)$. The advantage of the weighted-sum approach is a simplification of the problem of color constancy. As in the Mondrian experiment, only three values are required to specify the illuminant: a_1, a_2, and a_3. Measurements of real illuminants suggest three values may be sufficient for many practical purposes. For example, any typical spectral distribution of daylight, which changes substantially with weather and over the course of a day, can be described accurately by a weighted sum of three specific spectral power distributions (Judd *et al.*, 1964).

Suppose further that the spectral reflectance of an object is some weighted sum of three known spectral reflectances, $r_1(\lambda)$, $r_2(\lambda)$, and $r_3(\lambda)$. The spectral reflectance of the object at every wavelength is then $b_1r_1(\lambda) + b_2r_2(\lambda) + b_3r_3(\lambda)$. This, too, is a fairly reasonable assumption because most spectral reflectances found in natural scenes can be described moderately well by a weighted sum of three components (Cohen, 1964). Color constancy would be achieved by determining b_1, b_2, and b_3.

Under these assumptions, the total number of quanta absorbed by the L cone, $Q_L = \Sigma_\lambda[q_L(\lambda)E(\lambda)R(\lambda)]$, is

$$Q_L = \Sigma_\lambda\{q_L(\lambda)\ [a_1e_1(\lambda) + a_2e_2(\lambda) + a_3e_3(\lambda)]\ [b_1r_1(\lambda) + b_2r_2(\lambda) + b_3r_3(\lambda)]\}.$$

Similar equations give Q_S and Q_M. Further, the L-cone quantal absorption for a standard reference patch of known reflectance $R_{Std}(\lambda)$ is

$$Q_L = \Sigma_\lambda\{q_L(\lambda)\ [a_1e_1(\lambda) + a_2e_2(\lambda) + a_3e_3(\lambda)]\ [R_{Std}(\lambda)]\ \}$$
$$= a_1[\Sigma_\lambda\{q_L(\lambda)e_1(\lambda)R_{Std}(\lambda)\}] + a_2[\Sigma_\lambda\{q_L(\lambda)e_2(\lambda)R_{Std}(\lambda)\}] + a_3[\Sigma_\lambda\{q_L(\lambda)e_3(\lambda)R_{Std}(\lambda)\}].$$

All of the terms within square brackets of the last equation have known values. Similar equations for Q_S and Q_M complete a set of three simultaneous equations which can be solved for the three unknown weights of the illuminant, a_1, a_2, and a_3. The standard reference patch thus provides the information necessary to find the illuminant: $E(\lambda) = a_1e_1(\lambda) + a_2e_2(\lambda) + a_3e_3(\lambda)$. With the illuminant $E(\lambda)$ known, the quantal catch of the L cones for a reflecting surface is

$$Q_L = \Sigma_\lambda\{q_L(\lambda)\ E(\lambda)\ [b_1r_1(\lambda) + b_2r_2(\lambda) + b_3r_3(\lambda)]\}$$
$$= b_1[\Sigma_\lambda\{q_L(\lambda)E(\lambda)r_1(\lambda)\}] + b_2[\Sigma_\lambda\{q_L(\lambda)E(\lambda)r_2(\lambda)\}] + b_3[\Sigma_\lambda\{q_L(\lambda)E(\lambda)r_3(\lambda)\}].$$

Again, all of the terms within square brackets of the final equation have known values. With similar equations for Q_S and Q_M, these three simultaneous equations can be solved for the three unknown parameters b_1, b_2, and b_3, which give the spectral reflectance of the object: $R(\lambda) = b_1r_1(\lambda) + b_2r_2(\lambda) + b_3r_3(\lambda)$.

Exact color constancy, therefore, is possible when (a) the illuminant is a weighted sum of three known spectral power distributions, (b) the reflectance of each object is a weighted sum of three known spectral reflectances, and (c) an object of known reflectance is identified as a reference standard (Sallstrom, 1973; Buchsbaum, 1980). No reference standard is required if, instead, one assumes the average spectral reflectance over all objects in the scene has a known distribution (for example, uniform spectral reflectance).

Alternative models of color constancy relax one assumption at the expense of others. For example, the illuminant $E(\lambda)$ can be any arbitrary light, not just a weighted sum of three known spectral power distributions, if there are three reference standards rather than one (Brill, 1978; Brill and West, 1986). Each object in the scene is assumed to have a spectral reflectance that is a weighted sum of the three known reflectances of the reference standards: $b_1r_{Std1}(\lambda) + b_2r_{Std2}(\lambda) + b_3r_{Std3}(\lambda)$. In this case the quantal catch of the L cones due to light reflected from an object is

$$Q_L = \Sigma_\lambda\{q_L(\lambda)\ E(\lambda)\ [b_1r_{Std1}(\lambda) + b_2r_{Std2}(\lambda) + b_3r_{Std3}(\lambda)]\}$$
$$= b_1[\Sigma_\lambda\{q_L(\lambda)E(\lambda)r_{Std1}(\lambda)\ \}] + b_2[\Sigma_\lambda\{q_L(\lambda)E(\lambda)r_{Std2}(\lambda)\ \}] + b_3[\Sigma_\lambda\{q_L(\lambda)E(\lambda)r_{Std3}(\lambda)\}].$$

Each term within square brackets of the last equation is the quantal catch of the L cones for one of the three reference standards, and thus has a known value. With two similar equations for Q_S and Q_M, the three equations can be solved for the three unknowns b_1, b_2, and b_3, which specify the reflectance of the object.

An awkward feature of these models of constancy, at least for human vision, is that no reference standard may be available in natural viewing. As mentioned above, the reference standard can be eliminated if one knows (or assumes to know) the average spectral reflectance of the complete scene, but this replaces the problematic reference standard with a questionable assumption. An alternative solution is to assume the surface reflectance of each object in a scene is a weighted sum of two, rather than three, known components of reflectance: $b_1r_1(\lambda) + b_2r_2(\lambda)$. Under this assumption, color constancy can be achieved with trichromatic vision without a reflectance standard by aggregating information from several objects in a scene (Maloney and Wandell, 1986).

The advantage of considering many objects simultaneously is the greater amount of information available from photoreceptors. With N objects there are 3N receptoral quantal absorptions: $Q_{S,x}$, $Q_{M,x}$, and $Q_{L,x}$, for $x = 1, \ldots, N$. Each quantal catch, $\Sigma_\lambda[q_i(\lambda)E(\lambda)R_x(\lambda)]$, will have the form

$$Q_{L,x} = \Sigma_\lambda\{q_L(\lambda)\ [a_1e_1(\lambda) + a_2e_2(\lambda) + a_3e_3(\lambda)]\ [b_{1,x}r_1(\lambda) + b_{2,x}r_2(\lambda)]\}$$

with similar equations for $Q_{M,x}$ and $Q_{S,x}$. The two reflectance weights, $b_{1,x}$ and $b_{2,x}$, are different for each object but the three weights for the illuminant, a_1, a_2, and a_3, do not change from one object to the next because all N objects are illuminated by the same light. The 3N quantal absorptions for the complete scene, therefore, depend on 2N+3 unknown values. With three or more objects, the 3N equations can be solved for the 2N reflectance weights and the 3 illuminant weights (a generalization allows the illuminant to be more complex when there are four or more objects).

The models of color constancy described above are representative of the computational approach to constancy. Other models include alternative assumptions but nearly all seek the spectral reflectance of an object, $R(\lambda)$, from the information available from photoreceptors. The assumptions are an essential element of these models because quantal absorptions alone are insufficient to solve the matrix equation in section 4.4.3. If the assumptions were precisely correct, the human visual system could achieve perfect color constancy. While many of the assumptions are reasonably accurate, none is exactly right. For example, the true spectral reflectance of an object, $R(\lambda)$, and the true power distribution of an illuminant, $E(\lambda)$, usually deviate to some degree from a weighted sum of two or three components.

A computational theory cannot be rejected as a model of the human visual system simply because the assumptions imperfectly describe the spectra of objects and illuminants in natural settings. Moderate inaccuracies in the assumptions usually imply measurable deviations from perfect constancy. These predicted deviations can be a useful test of a theory as a model of human vision because the visual system does not achieve perfect color constancy. A full model of color constancy must account for the variation as well as the stability of the color appearance of objects.

4.4.7 RETINEX MODEL

Land's retinex model (Land and McCann, 1971; Land, 1983; Land, 1986) is another computational theory that considers simultaneously all of the objects in a scene. The quantal absorption of each cone is converted to what is called a 'lightness value,'[4] which depends on only the quanta absorbed by other photoreceptors of the same type (S, M or L). Retinex theory hypothesizes three separate representations of the scene: lightness values for S cones, lightness values for M cones, and lightness values for L cones. The color appearance of an object is determined by the three lightness values at the retinal location corresponding to the object.

The lightness value for a given photoreceptor is constructed from paths through the scene. A path begins at an initial point and then travels through contiguous photoreceptors of the same type (the actual photoreceptor mosaic (Chapter 2) is not considered – each location on the retina is assumed to have an S, M, and L cone). Whenever a path passes through a given receptor, a quantity is calculated. In a widely known version of retinex, the quantity is the logarithm of the ratio

$$\frac{\text{Quantal absorption of given receptor}}{\text{Quantal absorption of receptor at initial point}},$$

unless the ratio is very close to 1 in which case it is taken as exactly 1. The adjustment to exactly 1 is intended to remove the effect of small irregularities in illumination. More than one path can pass through a particular receptor, and a single path can pass through the same receptor more than once. A receptor's final lightness value is the average of the quantity calculated each time a path passes through it.

The retinex model includes elements of randomness and two adjustable parameters. The initial point of the path and the direction of the path from each receptor it crosses are determined randomly. The two parameters are the length of each path and the total number of paths. When the length of the path is short, the lightness values depend on only nearby receptors, while when the path is longer the lightness values are influenced by more remote cones. In the limiting case of arbitrarily many and arbitrarily long paths, the lightness value for a given receptor is determined by the receptor's response relative to the geometric mean of the responses from all other cones of the same type (Brainard and Wandell, 1986).

Retinex theory was the first computational model of color constancy to attract widespread attention. It predicts color appearance fairly accurately in some domains (McCann *et al.*, 1976) but accounts less well for more recent measurements of brightness and color in Mondrian-like displays (Arend and Reeves,

1986; Brainard and Wandell, 1986; Reid and Shapley, 1988; Valberg and Lange-Malecki, 1990). In general, the classical retinex model can be too sensitive to light reflected from distant objects in the scene. For example, a Munsell paper that appears pink in a standard condition is predicted to vary in appearance from beige to purple when other remotely located papers are changed from blue to yellow (Brainard and Wandell, 1986). No such shift in color appearance is observed. A related theoretical point is that many, long paths produce lightness values that are the original receptoral quantal catches adjusted by only a scaling factor, which does not predict perfect constancy (section 4.4.5). Alternative retinex algorithms have been proposed that control the spatial extent over which one object affects the appearance of others, and that operate on multiple levels of spatial resolution (McCann, 1999). The multiresolution retinex model successfully accounts for some fairly large and unintuitive shifts in appearance caused by complex backgrounds.

4.4.8 HUMAN COLOR PERCEPTION WITH CHANGES OF ILLUMINATION

Color perception does not depend strongly on the spectral distribution of illuminating light (section 4.4.1). At the same time, color constancy is not perfect; the appearance of surfaces is affected to some degree by spectral illumination. Studies of color appearance under changes of illumination reveal the precision of human color constancy, and also examine aspects of the visual stimulus that may mediate it.

How good is human color constancy? There is no single answer that applies to all illuminants, surfaces and viewing contexts, but in general the human visual system proficiently gives reasonably stable color percepts of objects. For surfaces presented in a moderately complex scene, constancy is excellent for achromatic appearance (that is, a colorless percept without a hint of redness, greenness, yellowness, or blueness; Brainard, 1998). A color constancy index that ranges from 0 (no constancy) to 1 (perfect constancy) typically was greater than 0.8 in experiments that varied illumination of real surfaces viewed in an experimental room. While constancy indexes must be interpreted and compared cautiously, because they can depend on specific models applied to laboratory measurements and on the color space in which the measurements are represented, a value of 0.8 indicates that the chromaticity of a perceptually achromatic surface closely follows the chromaticity of the illuminant, as expected for color constancy. Simulations of surfaces under illumination presented on a computer video display generally give less good constancy (e.g., Arend *et al.*, 1991). The cause of the difference between real and simulated scenes remains unclear because studies using different types of stimulus displays also differ in other aspects of the experiments. Compared to objects under illumination in real scenes, computer simulations typically present lower light levels, a restricted color gamut, a more limited viewing angle and chromaticities of objects determined from a simplified physical model relating illumination and reflectance to the light reaching the eye.

Measurements of color perception with changes of illumination reveal also whether constancy is mediated by a specific property of a complex scene. Using specially selected sets of illuminants and reflecting surfaces, illumination can be varied while holding constant (i) the local surround of a surface judged in color, (ii) the spatial average across a scene, or (iii) the strongest stimulation of each receptor type by any element within a scene. Conceptually, these three features might be linked to constancy as the possible stimulus property that controls visual adaptation. If any of these features of the stimulus mediates constancy, then changing illumination without altering that feature should eliminate constancy. In experiments using surfaces and illuminants in a real three-dimensional room, removing each of the features in turn was found to reduce but not eliminate color constancy (Brainard, 1998; Kraft and Brainard, 1999). This demonstrates that color constancy cannot be completely explained by a theory that relates the state of visual adaptation to one of these features of a scene. This finding is in accord with studies of color appearance using simpler stimulus configurations, which implicate more complex neural mechanisms (section 4.3.5).

Another approach to evaluating the limits of human color constancy is to assess properties of the visual stimulus that result in a perceived change of illumination. Consider a color Mondrian (section 4.4.1) first presented under one illuminant and then under a different one. The retinal stimulus is affected by the illuminant, of course, but do observers perceive an unvarying color Mondrian under two different illuminants, as required by perfect color constancy? The alternative is that a change in illumination is perceived as a change in the colors of the Mondrian surfaces themselves. When human observers judge whether two Mondrian-like stimuli are (i) a single Mondrian presented under two different illuminants or (ii) two different sets of surfaces, they report the former when the relative cone stimulation *within* each receptor class is the same for both stimuli (for example, identical relative stimulation of L cones in each Mondrian-like stimulus). While within-receptor-type relative stimulation is not strongly altered by illumination changes, it is not precisely preserved. Deviations from identical relative stimulation that result from changing illumination are far larger than discrimination threshold. Yet, two artificially constructed Mondrian-like stimuli that precisely preserve within-receptor-type relative stimulation are more likely to be perceived as the same Mondrian under different illumination than are two stimuli that truly are a single Mondrian under two different illuminants (Nascimento and Foster, 1997). This demonstrates that a change in the retinal stimulus due to a difference in illumination can be readily misperceived as a difference in the objects in view. Further work that isolates to a single cone type the deviations from identical within-receptor-type relative stimulation reveals greater sensitivity to L or M cone deviations than to S cone deviations.

In sum, a change in illumination can result in a perceived difference in the color of objects, though the shift is much less than predicted from the change in the light reflected from each object to the eye. A challenge for the field of color perception is to account for the modest but significant shifts in the color appearance of objects with changes of illumination.

NOTES

1 One approach to estimating this number, which depends strongly on the viewing condition and the state of adaptation, is based on Judd and Kelly (1939) who say 'there are about 10,000,000 surface-colors distinguishable in daylight by the trained human eye . . . (p. 359).' These 10,000,000 colors include variation in hue, saturation, and lightness. A conservatively large estimate of the number of discriminable lightness steps can be made by assuming lightness is discriminated over a 1,000:1 range, with a Weber fraction of 0.5%. This gives a conservatively small number of colors discriminable by only hue and saturation: 10,000,000/1385 = 7220.

2 Exceptions are mixtures within the triangle defined by vertices at (0.33,0.33) and the points for 380 nm and for 700 nm.

3 The spectral reflectance of paper N 6.75 was calculated by interpolation from reflectance spectra for papers N 6 and N 7. The relative spectral reflectances of N 6 and N 7 are very similar. These spectra were weighted according to their total reflectance (30.0% for N 6, 39.5% for N 6.75, 43.1% for N 7).

4 The term 'lightness value' as used in Retinex theory should not be confused with perceptual lightness discussed in section 4.3.1.

REFERENCES

Abney, W.W. (1910) On the change in hue of spectrum colors by dilution with white light. *Proceedings of the Royal Society of London*, 83A, 120–7.

Abramov, I., Gordon, J., and Chan, H. (1991) Color appearance in the peripheral retina: effects of stimulus size. *Journal of the Optical Society of America A*, 8, 404–14.

Adelson, E.H. (1993) Perceptual organization and the judgment of brightness. *Science*, 262, 2042–4.

Ahn, S.J. and MacLeod, D.I.A. (1993) Link-specific adaptation in the luminance and chromatic channels. *Vision Research*, 33, 2271–86.

Arend, L.E. and Reeves, A. (1986) Simultaneous color constancy. *Journal of the Optical Society of America A*, 3, 1743–51.

Arend, L.E., Reeves, A., Schirillo, J., and Goldstein, R. (1991) Simultaneous color constancy: papers with diverse Munsell values. *Journal of the Optical Society of America A*, 8, 661–72.

Bartleson, C.J. (1979) Predicting corresponding colors with changes in adaptation. *Color Research and Application*, 4, 143–55.

Bauml, K.H. (1995) Illuminant changes under different surface collections: examining some principles of color appearance. *Journal of the Optical Society of America A*, 12, 261–71.

Berlin, B. and Kay, P. (1969) *Basic Color Terms: Their*

Universality and Evolution. Berkeley, CA: University of California Press.

Boynton, R.M. and Gordon, J. (1965) Bezold–Brücke hue-shift measured by color-naming technique. *Journal of the Optical Society of America*, 55, 78–96.

Boynton, R.M. and Olson, C.X. (1990) Salience of chromatic basic color terms confirmed by three measures. *Vision Research*, 30, 1311–17.

Brainard, D.H. (1998) Color constancy in the nearly natural image 2. Achromatic loci. *Journal of the Optical Society of America A*, 15, 307–25.

Brainard, D.H. and Wandell, B.A. (1986) Analysis of the retinex theory of color vision. *Journal of the Optical Society of America A*, 3, 1651–61.

Brainard, D.H. and Wandell, B.A. (1992) Asymmetric color matching: how color appearance depends on the illuminant. *Journal of the Optical Society of America A*, 9, 1433–48.

Brill, M.H. (1978) A device performing illuminant-invariant assessment of chromatic relations. *Journal of Theoretical Biology*, 71, 473–8.

Brill, M. H. and West, G. (1986) Chromatic adaptation and color constancy: a possible dichotomy. *Color Research and Applications*, 11, 196–204.

Buchsbaum, G. (1980) A spatial processor model for object colour perception. *Journal of the Franklin Institute*, 310, 1–26.

Burnham, R.W., Evans, R.M., and Newhall, S.M. (1957) Prediction of color appearance with different adaptation illuminations. *Journal of the Optical Society of America*, 47, 35–42.

Burns, S.A., Elsner, A.E., Pokorny, J., and Smith, V.C. (1984) The Abney effect: chromaticity coordinates of unique and other constant hues. *Vision Research*, 24, 479–89.

Chevreul, M.E. (1839) *The Principles of Harmony and Contrast of Colors and Their Applications to the Arts*. (Original English translation, 1854, republished, 1967.) New York: Reinhold.

Chubb, C., Sperling, G., and Solomon, J.A. (1989) Texture interactions determine perceived contrast. *Proceedings of the National Academy of Sciences*, 86, 9631–5.

Cicerone, C.M., Krantz, D.H., and Larimer, J. (1975) Opponent-process additivity-III. Effect of moderate chromatic adaptation. *Vision Research*, 15, 1125–35.

Cohen, J. (1964) Dependency of the spectral reflectance curves of the Munsell color chips. *Psychonomic Science*, 1, 369–70.

Cornelissen, F.W. and Brenner, E. (1995) Simultaneous colour constancy revisited: an analysis of viewing strategies. *Vision Research*, 35, 2431–48.

D'Zmura, M. D. and Lennie, P. (1986) Mechanisms of color constancy. *Journal of the Optical Society of America A*, 3, 1662–72.

De Valois, R.L. and De Valois, K.K. (1993) A multi-stage color model. *Vision Research*, 33, 1053–65.

Ekman, G. (1954) Dimensions of color vision. *Journal of Psychology*, 38, 467–74.

Evans, R.M. (1974) *The Perception of Color*. New York: Wiley.

Fach, C. and Sharpe, L.T. (1986) Assimilative hue shifts in color gratings depend on bar width. *Perception and Psychophysics*, 40, 412–18.

Gordon, J. and Abramov, I. (1988) Scaling procedures for specifying color appearance. *Color Research and Application*, 13, 146–52.

Graham, C. H. and Hsia, Y. (1969) Saturation and the foveal achromatic interval. *Journal of the Optical Society of America*, 59, 993–7.

Guth, S.L. (1991) Model for color vision and light adaptation. *Journal of the Optical Society of America A*, 8, 976–93.

Guth, S.L., Donley, N.J., and Marrocco, R.T. (1969) On luminance additivity and related topics. *Vision Research*, 9, 537–75.

Heinemann, E.G. (1955) Simultaneous brightness induction as a function of inducing- and test-field luminances. *Journal of Experimental Psychology*, 50, 89–96.

Helmholtz, H. von (1866) *Treatise on Physiological Optics* (trans. J.P.C Southall), 2nd edn, 1962. New York: Dover.

Helson, H. (1938) Fundamental problems in color vision. I. The principle governing changes in hue, saturation, and lightness of non-selective samples in chromatic illumination. *Journal of Experimental Psychology*, 23, 439–76.

Helson, H. (1963) Studies of anomalous contrast and assimilation. *Journal of the Optical Society of America*, 53, 179–84.

Hering, E. (1920) *Outline of a Theory of the Light Sense* (trans. L. Hurvich and D. Jameson, 1964). Cambridge, MA: Harvard University Press.

Hurvich, L.M., and Jameson, D. (1957) An opponent-process theory of color vision. *Psychological Review*, 6, 384–404.

Hurvich, L.M. and Jameson, D. (1958) Further development of a quantified opponent-color theory. In *Visual Problems of Colour II*. London: HMSO, pp. 691–723.

Jacobs, G.H. (1967) Saturation estimates and chromatic adaptation. *Perception and Psychophysics*, 2, 271–4.

Jameson, D. and Hurvich, L.M. (1955) Some quantitative aspects of an opponent-colors theory I. Chromatic responses and spectral saturation. *Journal of the Optical Society of America*, 45, 546–52.

Jameson, D. and Hurvich, L. (1959) Perceived color and its dependence on focal, surrounding, and preceding stimulus variables. *Journal of the Optical Society of America*, 49, 890–8.

Jameson, D. and Hurvich, L.M. (1972) Color adaptation: sensitivity control, contrast, after-images. In D. Jameson and L. M. Hurvich (eds), *Handbook of Sensory Physiology*, vol. VII/4. Berlin: Springer-Verlag, pp. 568–81.

Jenness, J.W. and Shevell, S.K. (1995) Color appearance with sparse chromatic context. *Vision Research*, 35, 797–805.

Jordan, G. and Mollon, J.D. (1995) Rayleigh matches and unique green. *Vision Research*, 35, 613–20.

Judd, D.B. (1940) Hue saturation and lightness of surface colors with chromatic illumination. *Journal of the Optical Society of America*, 30, 2–32.

Judd, D.B. and Kelly, K.L. (1939) Method of designating colors (Research Paper RP1239). *Journal of Research of the National Bureau of Standards*, 23, 355–66.

Judd, D.B., MacAdam, D.L., and Wyszecki, G. (1964) Spectral distribution of typical daylight as a function of correlated color temperature. *Journal of the Optical Society of America*, 54, 1031–40.

Kelly, K.L. and Judd, D.B. (1955) The color names dictionary. *Color – Universal Language and Dictionary of Names*. (Vol. Special Publication 440, 1976). National Bureau of Standards.

Kraft, J.M. and Brainard, D.H. (1999) Mechanisms of color constancy under nearly natural viewing. *Proceedings of the National Academy of Sciences, USA*, 96, 307–12.

Krantz, D.H. (1975) Color measurement and color theory: II. Opponent-colors theory. *Journal of Mathematical Psychology*, 12, 304–27.

Land, E.H. (1983) Recent advances in retinex theory and some implications for cortical computation: color vision and the natural image. *Proceedings of the National Academy of Sciences USA*, 80, 5163–9.

Land, E.H. (1986) Recent advances in retinex theory. *Vision Research*, 26, 7–21.

Land, E.H. and McCann, J.J. (1971) Lightness and retinex theory. *Journal of the Optical Society of America*, 61, 1–11.

Larimer, J., Krantz, D.H., and Cicerone, C.M. (1974) Opponent-process additivity: I. Red/green equilibria. *Vision Research*, 14, 1127–40.

Larimer, J., Krantz, D.H., and Cicerone, C.M. (1975) Opponent process additivity: II. Yellow/blue equilibria and non-linear models. *Vision Research*, 15, 723–31.

Maloney, L.T. (1985) Computational Approaches to Color Constancy. Doctoral dissertation, Stanford University.

Maloney, L.T. and Wandell, B.A. (1986) Color constancy: a method for recovering surface spectral reflectances. *Journal of the Optical Society of America A*, 3, 29–33.

Marimont, D.H. and Wandell, B.A. (1994) Matching color images: the effects of axial chromatic aberration. *Journal of the Optical Society of America A*, 11, 3113–22.

McCann, J.J. (1999) Lessons learned from Mondrians applied to real images and color gamuts. *IS&T Reporter*, 14, 1–7.

McCann, J.J., McKee, S.P., and Taylor, T.H. (1976) Quantitative studies in retinex theory: a comparison between theoretical predictions and observer responses to the 'Color Mondrian' experiments. *Vision Research*, 16, 445–58.

Mollon, J. (1985) Studies in scarlet. *The Listener*, 113, 6–7.

Moreland, J.D. and Cruz, A. (1959) Colour perception with the peripheral retina. *Optica Acta*, 6, 117–51.

Munsell Color Company (1929) *Munsell Book of Color*. Baltimore, MD: Munsell Color Co.

Nascimento, S.M.C. and Foster, D.H. (1997) Detecting natural changes of cone-excitation ratios in simple and complex coloured images. *Proceedings of the Royal Society London B*, 264, 1395–402.

Newhall, S.M., Nickerson, D., and Judd, D.B. (1943) Final report of the O.S.A. Subcommittee on the spacing of Munsell Colors. *Journal of the Optical Society of America*, 33, 385–412.

Poirson, A.B. and Wandell, B.A. (1993) Appearance of colored patterns: pattern-color separability. *Journal of the Optical Society of America A*, 10, 2458–70.

Pokorny, J., Shevell, S.K., and Smith, V.C. (1991) Colour appearance and colour constancy. In P. Gouras (ed.), *Vision and Visual Dysfunction, Vol. 6: The Perception of Colour*. London: Macmillan, pp. 43–61.

Purdy, D.M. (1931a) On the saturations and chromatic thresholds of the spectral colours. *British Journal of Psychology*, 21, 283–313.

Purdy, D.M. (1931b) Spectral hue as a function of intensity. *American Journal of Psychology*, 43, 541–59.

Ratliff, F. (1976) On the psychophysiological bases of universal color terms. *Proceedings of the American Philosophical Society*, 120, 311–30.

Reid, R.C. and Shapley, R. (1988) Brightness induction by local contrast and the spatial dependence of assimilation. *Vision Research*, 28, 115–32.

Rubin, M. (1961) Spectral hue loci of normal and anomalous trichromates. *American Journal of Ophthalmology*, 52, 166–72.

Sallstrom, P. (1973) *Color and Physics: Some Remarks Concerning the Physical Aspects of Human Color Vision* (73–09). University of Stockholm: Institute of Physics.

Schiffman, S.S., Reynolds, M. L., and Young, F.W. (1981) *Introduction to Multidimensional Scaling*. New York: Academic Press.

Schirillo, J.A. and Shevell, S.K. (1996) Brightness contrast from inhomogeneous surrounds. *Vision Research*, 36, 1783–96.

Sekiguchi, N., Williams, D.R., and Brainard, D.H. (1993) Efficiency in detection of isoluminant and isochromatic interference fringes. *Journal of the Optical Society of America A*, 10, 2118–33.

Shepard, R.N. (1962) The analysis of proximities: multidimensional scaling with an unknown distance function. II. *Psychometrika*, 27, 219–46.

Shevell, S.K. (1978) The dual role of chromatic backgrounds in color perception. *Vision Research*, 18, 1649–61.

Shevell, S.K. (1982) Color perception under chromatic adaptation: equilibrium yellow and long-wavelength adaptation. *Vision Research*, 22, 279–92.

Shevell, S.K. (1987) Processes mediating color contrast. *Die Farbe*, 34, 261–8.

Shevell, S.K. and Humanski, R.A. (1984) Color perception under contralateral and binocularly fused chromatic adaption. *Vision Research*, 24, 1011–19.

Shevell, S.K. and Humanski, R.A. (1988) Color perception under chromatic adaptation: red/green equilibria with adapted short-wavelength-sensitive cones. *Vision Research*, 28, 1345–56.

Shevell, S.K. and Wei, J. (1998) Chromatic induction: border contrast or adaptation to surrounding light? *Vision Research*, 38, 1561–6.

Shevell, S.K. and Wesner, M.F. (1989) Color appearance under conditions of chromatic adaptation and contrast. *Color Research and Application*, 14, 309–17.

Singer, B. and D'Zmura, M. (1994) Color contrast induction. *Vision Research*, 34, 3111–26.

Stabell, U. and Stabell, B. (1982) Color vision in the peripheral retina under photopic conditions. *Vision Research*, 22, 839–44.

Stevens, J.C. and Stevens, S.S. (1963) Brightness function: effects of adaptation. *Journal of the Optical Society of America*, 53, 375–85.

Stiles, W.S. (1961) Adaptation, chromatic adaptation, colour transformation. *Annales d.t. Real. Soc. Espanola d. Fis. Y. Quinn.*, 57, 149–75.

Valberg, P. and Lange-Malecki, B. (1990) 'Color Constancy' in Mondrian patterns: a partial cancellation of physical chromaticity shifts by simultaneous contrast. *Vision Research*, 30, 371–80.

Vimal, R.L.P., Pokorny, J., and Smith, V.C. (1987) Appearance of steadily viewed lights. *Vision Research*, 27, 1309–18.

von Bezold, W. (1876) *The Theory of Color In Its Relation to Art and Art-Industry* (trans. S.R. Koehler, American edn.). Boston: Prang.

von Kries, J. (1905) Influence of adaptation on the effects produced by luminous stimuli. In D.L. MacAdam (ed.), *Sources of Color Science* (1970). Cambridge, MA: MIT Press, pp. 120–6.

Walraven, J. (1976) Discounting the background – the missing link in the explanation of chromatic induction. *Vision Research*, 16, 289–95.

Wandell, B.A. (1993) Color appearance: the effects of illumination and spatial pattern. *Proceedings of the National Academy of Science USA*, 90, 9778–84.

Ware, C. and Cowan, W.B. (1982) Changes in perceived color due to chromatic interactions. *Vision Research*, 22, 1353–62.

Webster, M.A. and Mollon, J.D. (1995) Colour constancy influenced by contrast adaptation. *Nature*, 373, 694–8.

Wei, J. and Shevell, S.K. (1995) Color appearance under chromatic adaptation varied along theoretically significant axes in color space. *Journal of the Optical Society of America A*, 12, 36–46.

Wesner, M.F. and Shevell, S.K. (1992) Color perception within a chromatic context: changes in red/green equilibria caused by noncontiguous light. *Vision Research*, 32, 1623–34.

Williams, D., Sekiguchi, N., and Brainard, D. (1993) Color, contrast sensitivity, and the cone mosaic. *Proceedings of the National Academy of Sciences, USA*, 90, 9770–7.

Worthey, J.A. and Brill, M.H. (1986) Heuristic analysis of von Kries color constancy. *Journal of the Optical Society of America A*, 3, 1708–12.

Wyszecki, G. (1986) Color Appearance. In K.R. Boff, L. Kaufman, and J.P. Thomas (eds), *Handbook of Perception and Human Performance. Vol. I: Sensory Processes and Perception*. New York: John Wiley and Sons.

Wyszecki, G. and Stiles, W.S. (1982) *Color Science – Concepts and Methods, Quantitative Data and Formulae*, 2nd edn. New York: John Wiley and Sons.

5 Color Appearance and Color Difference Specification

David H. Brainard

Department of Psychology
University of California, Santa Barbara, CA 93106, USA

Present address: Department of Psychology
University of Pennsylvania, 3815 Walnut Street, Philadelphia, PA 19104-6196, USA

CHAPTER CONTENTS

The Science of Color
ISBN 0–444–512–519

5.1 INTRODUCTION

The physical properties of color stimuli may be specified using spectral measurements or tristimulus coordinates. Such specification, however, provides little intuition about how the stimuli will appear. For applications such as color selection we would like to specify color using appearance terms and have an automatic method for computing the corresponding tristimulus coordinates. To do so we need to understand the relation between the physical description of a color stimulus (e.g. its tristimulus coordinates) and a quantitative description of its color appearance.

A second topic of practical importance is to specify the magnitude of differences between colored stimuli. Here we need to understand the relation between changes in the physical description of a color stimulus and corresponding changes in appearance. In specifying color reproduction tolerances, we are likely to be concerned with small color differences: how different must the tristimulus coordinates of two stimuli be before the color difference between them is just barely noticeable? For color coding, on the other hand, we are more likely to be concerned with whether two colors are sufficiently different to be easily discriminable. For example, if we are designing traffic signals we would like to be sure that the red and green lights are easy to tell apart.

There are a number of systematized methods available both for specifying color appearance and for specifying color difference. Unfortunately, no perfect system exists for either purpose. To use the systems successfully, it is necessary to have a firm grasp of the principles underlying their design. The purpose of this chapter is to provide an introduction to color specification systems and some guidance as to their use. A detailed survey of such systems is not attempted here, but a number of excellent reviews are available (Judd and Wyszecki, 1975; Robertson, 1984; Billmeyer, 1987; Hunt, 1987b; Derefeldt, 1991; Fairchild, 1998). This chapter builds on the material introduced in Chapters 3 and 4. Chapter 3 introduces the color matching experiment and describes how tristimulus coordinates may be used to represent the spectral properties of light. Chapter 4 discusses the phenomenology of color appearance and describes the psychological attributes of hue, saturation/chroma, and brightness/lightness.

The chapter begins with a discussion of color order systems. A color order system is a type of color appearance system – that is, a type of system for specifying color appearance. In a color order system, the color appearance of a carefully selected set of color samples is specified. The samples are arranged to make it easy to find a desired color and to allow visual interpolation between samples. To help fix ideas, a detailed review of the popular Munsell color order system is provided, followed by a brief description of a few other systems. Next comes an overview of color difference systems. The overview begins with a concrete example, the CIELAB uniform color space, which is useful for specifying small color differences. Following the example, a few other systems are briefly described. The chapter closes with discussion of a number of issues and topics.

5.2 COLOR ORDER SYSTEMS

5.2.1 EXAMPLE: MUNSELL COLOR ORDER SYSTEM

5.2.1.1 Problem – specifying the appearance of surfaces

The Munsell color order system was originally conceived by A.H. Munsell in 1905 (Munsell, 1992). His goal was to provide a system for specifying colors and for teaching students about the perceptual attributes of color. He devised a symbolic notation for color appearance; this is referred to as Munsell notation. Munsell's system was operationalized as a collection of color samples, so that it was possible to understand visually the relation between Munsell color names and the corresponding color percepts. The Munsell system has been modified several times to improve the correspondence between the actual samples and the underlying perceptual organization (Nickerson, 1940; Berns and Billmeyer, 1985).

Current collections of samples (see http://munsell.com/) implementing the Munsell system are based on the results of an extensive study by an Optical Society of America committee in the 1930s and 40s (Newhall, 1940; Newhall *et al.*, 1943). This committee conducted scaling experiments on samples from an early edition of the Munsell Book of Color. It also made physical measurements of the samples. Based on these data, it generated extensive tables relating Munsell notations to the tristimulus coordinates (under standard conditions of illumination) that a sample of that notation should have. This tabulation now defines the Munsell system, and is sometimes referred to as Munsell renotation.

5.2.1.2 Perceptual ideas

The basic idea underlying the Munsell system is that color appearance may be described in terms of three attributes: hue, chroma, and lightness (see Chapter 4). The system therefore consists of scales for each of these attributes.

Munsell **hue** is a circular scale based on 10 major hues, Red (R), Yellow–Red (YR), Yellow (Y), Green–Yellow (GY), Green (G), Blue–Green (BG), Blue (B), Purple–Blue (PB), Purple (P), and Red–Purple (RP). In addition, the 10 major hues are subdivided further into a scale that ranges from 1 to 10, with 5 denoting the major hue itself. A digit–letter notation is typically used to specify Munsell hue, so that 2.5R would refer to step 2.5 in the major hue category red. Equal steps on the Munsell hue scale are designed to represent equal changes in perceived hue. Thus the 10 subdivisions of the 10 major hues form a 100 point scale for hue.

Munsell **chroma** is specified on a numerical scale starting at 0 and extending out to the maximum possible chroma for each hue. A chroma of zero indicates a black, gray, or white. Increasing chroma numbers indicate progressively more pure color percepts. Samples that differ in Munsell hue but that have the same chroma should be judged to differ equally from an achromatic sample of the same lightness. Equal steps on the chroma scale are meant to represent equal changes in perceived chroma.

The Munsell scale for **lightness** is called value. Munsell value is specified on a numerical scale that ranges from 0 for colors judged to have the same lightness as black to 10 for colors judged to have the same lightness as white. Samples that differ in Munsell hue or chroma but that have the same value should be judged to have the same lightness. Equal steps on the value scale are designed to represent equal changes in perceived lightness.

The notational form used to express Munsell colors begins with the hue, followed by the value and chroma numbers. These latter two are separated by a slash. Thus the notation 2.5R 8/4 refers to a sample with hue 2.5R, value 8, and chroma 4. The letter N is used to denote neutral samples and the chroma value is omitted. Thus N 8/ is used to indicate a neutral sample of value 8 and 0 chroma. In the Munsell scheme, any stimulus (provided it is seen in surface mode) has a color appearance that may be described by the appropriate Munsell notation. See Chapter 4 for a discussion of modes of appearance.

5.2.1.3 Geometric representation

If we hold the attribute of hue constant, it is natural to represent Munsell value and chroma using rectilinear coordinates. A rectilinear representation makes sense for these two attributes because each has a well-defined origin (black for value, neutral for chroma) and because numerical differences on each scale are related monotonically to perceived color difference.

The situation is not so simple for Munsell hue. First, there is no natural origin for hue. Second, there is no linear scale for hue such that numerical differences on the hue scale are monotonically related to perceived differences. It is possible, however, to represent hue geometrically using a polar coordinate system. It turns out that when hue is arranged in a circular fashion, distances between points provide a reasonable approximation to their perceptual differences (see Chapter 4).

The rectilinear representation for chroma and value may be combined with the circular representation for hue to provide a cylindrical coordinate system for the Munsell system. In cylindrical coordinates, the angular coordinate represents hue, the linear coordinate represents value, and the radial coordinate represents chroma. Any stimulus seen in surface mode can thus be thought of as a point in a three-dimensional Munsell space. The geometry of the Munsell system is illustrated in Figure 5.1.

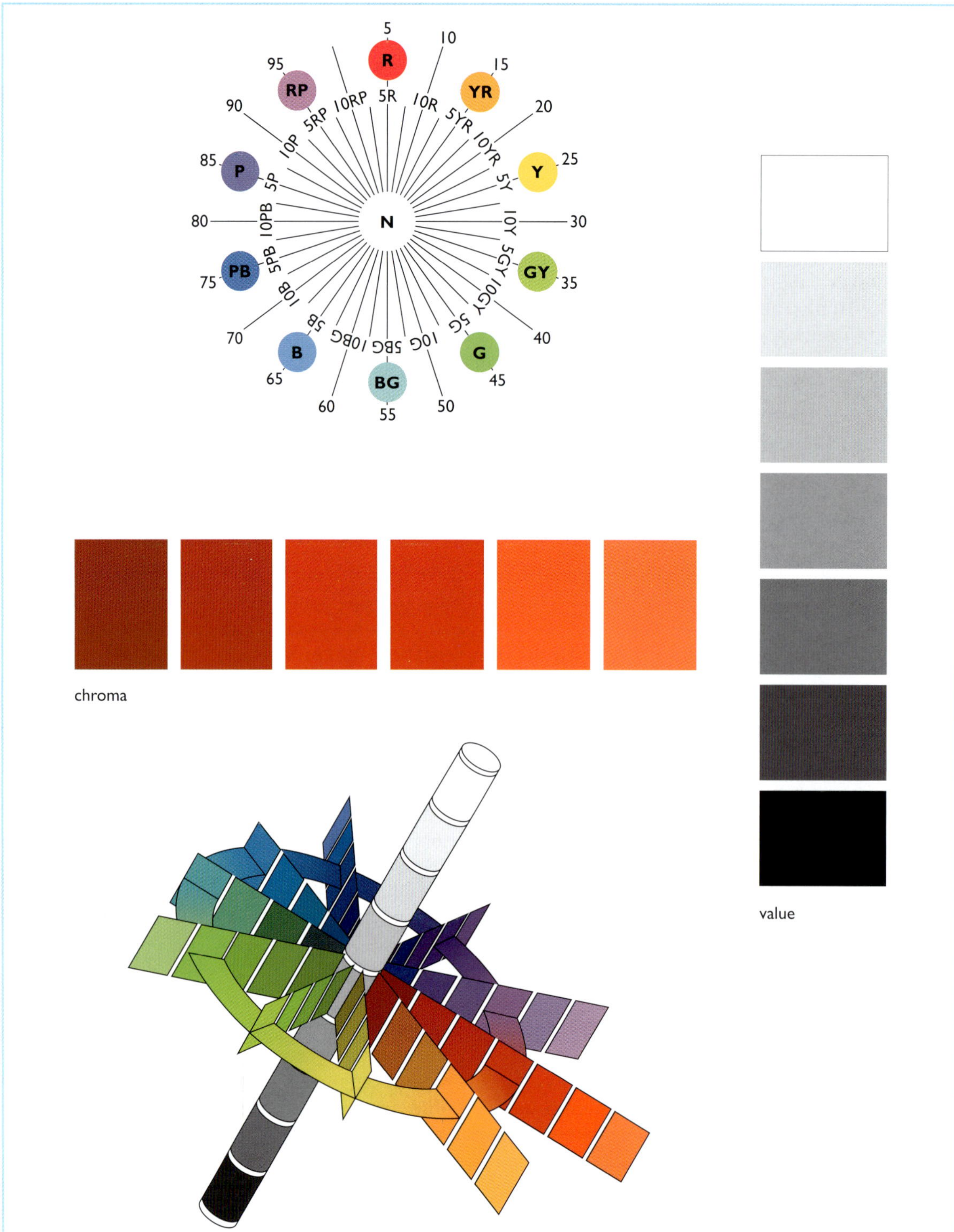

Figure 5.1 **The Munsell color order system. The Munsell hue circle (upper left) is a series of neutral colors that vary in value only (vertical series on right), and a series that varies in chroma at constant hue and value (middle left). As shown at the lower left, the Munsell system may be organized cylindrically, with an angular coordinate representing hue, a linear coordinate representing value, and a radial coordinate representing chroma. (Courtesy of Munsell Color Services, a division of GretagMacbeth.)**

5.2.1.4 Relating Munsell notations to stimuli

Note that the conceptual system described above describes perceptual variables and is independent of any specification of which stimuli elicit particular perceptions (e.g. Figure 5.1). Another way to say this is that, in principle, one can imagine the appearance of any Munsell specification without ever having seen a set of Munsell samples. Thus we can regard the Munsell system as a theory that describes the phenomenology of color perception. No direct experiments justified this theory; it was derived primarily from Munsell's own introspection.

The Munsell system would not have much practical value if it were only an abstract theory of perception. The usefulness of the system arises because there exist a set of samples that exemplify the system. The original implementation of the Munsell scheme was created by A.H. Munsell in conjunction with an artist who carefully painted samples to match Munsell's conception. This led to the production of the Munsell Color Atlas in 1915 (Munsell, 1915). Subsequent work (Munsell *et al.*, 1933; Godlove, 1933) focused on refining the value scale for neutral colors. Thresholds for detecting just-noticeable-differences (JNDs) were measured over a range of stimuli that appeared from black to white, and a scale of equal JND steps was generated from the data. This scale was validated using a variety of other scaling procedures. The value scale thus created formed the backbone of the 1929 *Munsell Book of Color* (Berns and Billmeyer, 1985).

The exact judgments used to determine the samples corresponding to other Munsell notations are not well documented. Basically, however, the following scheme was used (Berns and Billmeyer, 1985). First, judgments were made to equate the lightness of non-neutral colors to those of neutral colors. The result was an assignment of values to a large number of samples. Given a collection of samples of equal value, observers then scaled these according to their hues and chromas. There were two goals of the scalings. The first was to equate the numbers assigned for one attribute across variations in the other, so that within a set of samples with equal value, lines of constant hue and constant chroma were defined. Second, the differences between lines of constant hue and chroma were scaled and the numerical scales adjusted so that equal steps on each scale corresponded to equal perceptual differences. Finally, judgments across colors of differing value were made, so as to equate the hue and chroma scales across variations in value.

The current specification of the relation between Munsell notations and physical samples is based on experiments performed on the 1929 samples by a committee of the Optical Society of America (Newhall, 1940; Newhall *et al.*, 1943). Observers performed two types of tasks in these experiments. In one, they judged whether the 1929 samples in fact satisfied the requirements of the Munsell perceptual scheme. In one experiment, for example, observers viewed a series of samples that had the same nominal hue and value but that varied in chroma. They then indicated whether the samples in fact appeared to have the same hue and scaled the direction and magnitude of any deviations. This type of judgment was used to identify adjustments required to achieve better lines of constant hue, chroma, and value. In a second type of task, observers judged differences between samples from the 1929 book. For example, observers were shown two pairs of samples differing in hue but with the same value and chroma. They were then asked to judge the ratio of the differences between the two pairs. This type of judgment was used to adjust the spacing of the samples in the 1929 judgment to more closely approximate the even perceptual spacing that is the goal of the Munsell scheme.

In addition to scaling experiments on the 1929 samples, the committee also made physical measurements of the samples. By analyzing the relation between perceptual judgments and physical tristimulus coordinates, the committee generated extensive tables relating Munsell notations to the tristimulus coordinates that a sample of that notation should have (under standard conditions of illumination). The actual analysis was performed graphically by plotting the measurements on large pieces of graph paper and fitting smooth curves by hand, so that no analytic expression for the relation between Munsell notation and tristimulus coordinates exists. The tabulation now defines the primary implementation of the Munsell system, and is sometimes referred to as Munsell renotation.

Current implementations of the Munsell system conform closely to the renotation aim points.

5.2.1.5 Discussion

The Munsell color order system may be thought of as consisting of two parts. The first is an abstract perceptual scheme for specifying colors. The second is a large lookup table that defines an instantiation of the Munsell scheme (see Figure 5.2). One side of the table contains tristimulus coordinates of samples. The other side of the table contains the symbolic description corresponding to each sample when it is viewed under standard conditions. Typically these conditions are isolated viewing against a uniform nonselective (gray) background under a specified illuminant. The exact details of the standard viewing conditions vary across color order systems and even for different implementations of the same color order system. The mapping between tristimulus coordinates and symbolic descriptions is defined only for the standard conditions.

As emphasized by McCamy (McCamy, 1985), it is useful to maintain the distinction between a color order system's perceptual scheme and implementations of this scheme. In evaluating a color order system, we can ask two types of questions. First, does the perceptual system on which the system is built provide a useful characterization of color appearance? Second, does a particular instantiation of the system conform to the underlying perceptual ideas? Note, for example, that the mapping between names and tristimulus values is valid only for one set of viewing conditions. These are the conditions under which the scaling experiments that defined the table were performed. For the Munsell system, these were viewing under CIE Standard Illuminant C (an approximation to daylight), with the samples placed against a nonselective background with a reflectance of approximately 18% (Munsell sample N 5/). The mapping is not necessarily valid for other viewing conditions, but that does not mean that the Munsell perceptual scheme could not be applied generally. Rather, it would take another set of scaling experiments or a model of the effect of context on color appearance to provide the appropriate implementation.

The lookup table view of the implementation of color order systems is simplistic, as it neglects the geometric structure that may be imposed on the arrangement of the symbolic names. It does capture the fact that the mapping between tristimulus coordinates and symbolic names is complex. Indeed, an analytic description of this mapping for implementations of the Munsell system has been elusive. Practical translation between tristimulus coordinates and Munsell names is accomplished by lookup table search and interpolation, sometimes with the aid of neural networks (Simon and Frost, 1987; Smith, 1990a; Burns *et al.*, 1990; Usai *et al.*, 1992; Tominaga, 1993). The difficulty with these methods is that they require large databases specifying either the table entries or summaries thereof. Wyszecki and Stiles (1982) provide tabulations of tristimulus coordinates and corresponding symbolic descriptions for the Munsell and other color order systems. A program for performing the conversion is available free of charge from the GretagMacbeth Corporation (http://munsell.com/).

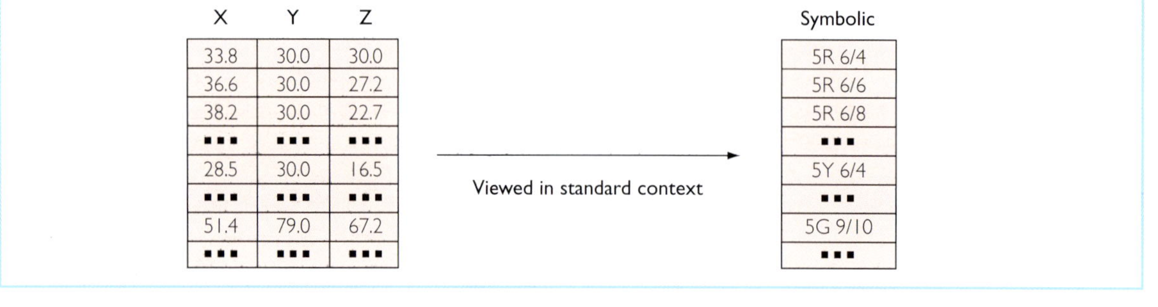

Figure 5.2 Lookup table view of a color order system implementation. One side of the table contains tristimulus coordinates of samples. The other side of the table contains the symbolic description corresponding to each sample when it is viewed under standard conditions. Typically these conditions are isolated viewing against a uniform non-selective (gray) background under a specified illuminant.

The Munsell system is useful for several purposes. First, it allows us to specify colors in appearance terms. With a little training, observers can apparently become proficient at describing colors using Munsell terms (Helson, 1938; Whitfield *et al.*, 1988) so that the Munsell system provides a language for talking about color appearance. In this capacity, the system has been used successfully in scaling experiments that studied the effect of context on color appearance (Helson, 1938; Helson and Jeffers, 1940).

More important, perhaps, is the fact that there exist implementations of the Munsell notational system. Even if a user is unable to name the exact Munsell term for a desired color, he or she can look through the Munsell book of color until a close approximation to the desired color is found. Because the samples are arranged in an orderly way and are evenly spaced, it is possible to interpolate visually between the sample points to specify color more precisely than the sample spacing (Billmeyer, 1988). Once the desired Munsell notation is known, the tables defining the Munsell system in terms of tristimulus coordinates may be used to find a physical specification for the desired color.

Inverse mapping is also possible. A test sample can be compared to the collection of Munsell samples under the standard viewing conditions. It is then possible to interpolate between the near matches and assign a Munsell name to the test sample.

Because of the manner in which it was developed, the Munsell system also provides a metric for the apparent differences between colors. For example, the perceptual difference corresponding to one step of Munsell value should be the same, independent of the hue or chroma of the sample. Note that steps on the three Munsell appearance scales are of different magnitudes. A step of 1 on the value scale is designed to be perceptually equivalent to a step of 2 on the chroma scale and a step of 3 on the hue scale (at chroma 5). Because hue is specified in polar coordinates, the perceptual magnitude of a single hue step varies with chroma.

There are things that the Munsell system does not provide. First, it does not provide any means to take viewing context into account. The same Munsell paper seen in non-standard viewing contexts may appear quite different from what one would expect from its name. If we consider the original Munsell system, based on physical samples, the color constancy of the human visual system will make the specification somewhat robust in the face of changing illumination. Color constancy is not perfect, however, so Munsell notation must be treated carefully in applications where the illuminant is not standard. If we consider Munsell renotation, an additional difficulty arises. Renotation relates tristimulus coordinates of the samples to the Munsell notation. To take changes in illumination into account, it is necessary to calculate how the tristimulus coordinates of an actual sample would change with the illuminant. Some approximations to this calculation are possible (Brainard, 1995). This issue is discussed further in the section on metamerism below.

Second, the Munsell system does not provide a metric for small color differences. Although the Munsell renotation is designed so that equal steps correspond to color differences judged equal, it is important to remember that the color differences judged were well above threshold. For small color differences, one is concerned with visual thresholds, and there is no obvious relation between threshold data and the suprathreshold judgments on which the Munsell system is based (MacAdam, 1974; Robertson, 1977). In addition, it is useful to bear in mind that the Munsell system was based on scaling differences in one of the three color attributes while the others were held fixed. Thus any effects that intrude when all three attributes are covaried are unlikely to be accurately described by the Munsell system.

5.2.1.6 Relation to tristimulus coordinates

The Munsell system may be used to illustrate some of the perceptual effects discussed in Chapter 4. Figure 5.3 shows lines of constant Munsell hue plotted in the CIE 1931 chromaticity diagram. The left panel of the figure shows the plot for Munsell value 2, while the right panel shows the plot for Munsell value 8. Note that in each panel the constant hue lines curve, illustrating the Abney hue shift. Also note that the locations of the lines for particular hues shift considerably between the two panels. The fact that the lines for different value do not superimpose illustrates the Bezold–Brüke

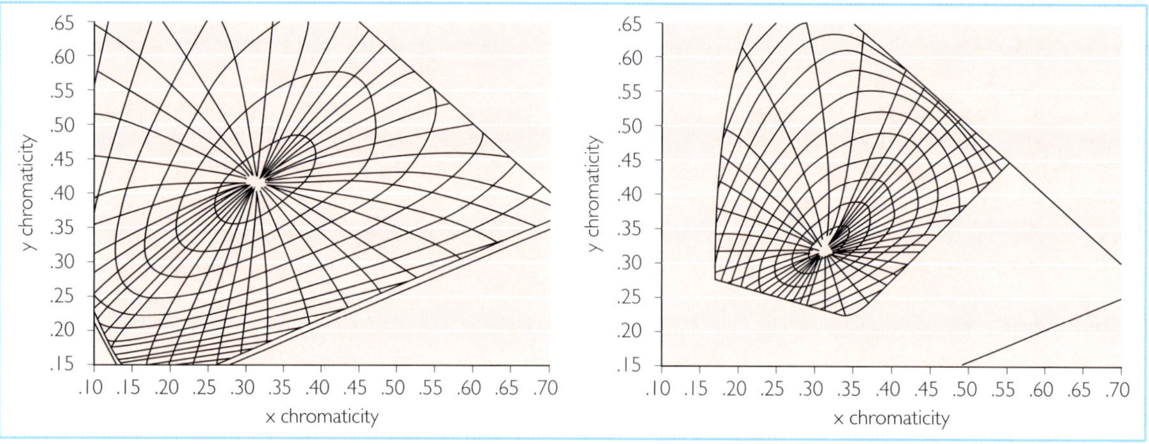

Figure 5.3 (Left) Lines of constant Munsell hue for Munsell value 2, plotted in the CIE 1931 chromaticity diagram. (Right) Lines of constant Munsell hue for Munsell value 8, plotted in the CIE 1931 chromaticity diagram. (From Wyszecki and Stiles, 1982. Copyright © 1982 John Wiley & Sons, Inc., reproduced by permission.)

hue shift. Chapter 4 discusses the Abney and Bezold–Brüke shifts in more detail.

The fact that the constant hue lines curve and are not invariant with changes in value illustrates the basic difficulty in specifying color appearance. Simple models of visual processing do not easily predict the shape of the constant hue lines. The search for models that do is currently an area of active research (see section on color appearance models below).

5.2.2 OTHER COLOR ORDER SYSTEMS

The Munsell color order system is not the only color order system. Other color order systems include the Swedish Natural Color System (NCS), the Optical Society of America Uniform Color Scale (OSA/UCS), the Deutches Institut fur Normung (DIN) system, and the Coloroid system. From the discussion above, one can see that there are two primary ways a system could differ from the Munsell system. First, the perceptual principles on which a system is based could differ. Second, the implementation of the system could differ. For example, a system based on the same perceptual principles as the Munsell system but with samples defined for different viewing conditions might be considered a different system. In practice, it is sometimes difficult to decide whether the perceptual principles of two systems differ because the only way to judge what the words mean is to compare the implementations.

Given this general point, it would be possible to compare the details of a large number of systems. Such detailed comparisons are available elsewhere (Billmeyer and Bencuya, 1987; Derefeldt, 1991). It is of interest, however, to discuss some particular color order systems briefly, both to familiarize the reader with them and to illustrate how a system might be built on principles other than those that underlie the Munsell system. Three systems will be discussed: the Swedish NCS, the OSA/UCS, and the DIN color system. None of these systems denies the role of perceptual dimensions related to hue, saturation, and lightness in our perception of color. The first two differ from the Munsell system primarily in that the judgments used to define the system are not direct scalings of such qualities.

5.2.2.1 Swedish Natural Colour System (NCS)

The fundamental scalings underlying the Munsell color order system are judgments of hue, chroma, and value. These are not the only judgments upon which a color order system can be based. Indeed, the NCS is based on a different set of scalings. In the NCS, the appearance of a color is specified by its resemblance to six elementary colors: red, green, blue, yellow, black, and white. This system was developed from opponent process notions (see Chapter 4), in that it is based on the tenet that in judging the color appearance of stimuli, we have access to the outputs of three independent mechanisms: a red–green mechanism, a blue–yellow mechanism, and a white–black mechanism. (The white–black mechanism is sometimes referred to as the luminance mechanism.) If one accepts this tenet, then judging color in terms related to these mechanisms (by asking subjects about resemblances) is a natural choice. Abramov and Gordon (1994) review basic research on this type of judgment. Samples that implement the NCS system exist as the NCS Colour Atlas, and tristimulus specifications for the NCS notations are available (Swedish Standards Institution, 1982; 1983; 1989; http://www.ncscolour.com/). The detailed description that follows is based primarily on Derefeldt's (1991) review.

Although the subject is asked to judge six resemblances in the scalings for the NCS system, there are some constraints on the judgments they are allowed to make. The first restriction is that no color may be judged as resembling both red and green, and no color may be judged as resembling both blue and yellow. Thus a stimulus may be judged to resemble at most two of red, green, blue, and yellow. The NCS hue is defined in terms of the relative resemblances of the stimulus to these four unique hues. (See Chapter 4 for more on unique hues.) The notation used to specify NCS hue is first a letter specifying one unique hue, then a percentage, and then a second letter specifying a second unique hue. Thus R20B indicates a hue where the ratio of the resemblances to red and green are 80 to 20. The sum of the judged resemblances to the four basic chromatic colors (red, green, blue, and yellow) is referred to in the NCS system as chromaticness. The second restriction is that the sum of chromaticness and the resemblance judgments to black and white must be 100. Because of these restrictions, the six NCS resemblances may be specified using only three numbers. These are the two non-zero hue resemblances and the blackness. Because the hue notation is normalized, however, the overall NCS notation for colors is a number for blackness, a number for chromaticness, and an NCS hue specification. For example, 3060 R20B would represent a color whose individual resemblances were 10 for whiteness, 30 for blackness, 48 for redness, 12 for blueness, and zero each for greenness and yellowness.

Although the basic scaling judgments underlying the NCS are six resemblances, the final specification thus ends up in terms of blackness, chromaticness, and hue. These are conceptual relatives of Munsell lightness (inverted), chroma, and hue. Like the Munsell system, the NCS system may be displayed geometrically. The standard NCS geometry within a particular hue is diagrammed triangularly, as shown on the left of Figure 5.4. Vertical lines represent constant chromaticness. Diagonal lines represent loci of constant blackness. The arrangement of the NCS hue circle is also shown in Figure 5.4. Because of the fundamental role played by red, blue, green, and yellow, these four hues are placed equally around the circle. Other stimuli are then placed proportionately according to their relative resemblances to these four cardinal colors.

Although both the Munsell and NCS systems describe color appearance in terms of similar attributes, it is not clear that the two systems represent the same underlying perceptual dimensions. Indeed, direct comparisons suggest that Munsell and NCS hue are quite different from one another (Billmeyer and Bencuya, 1987; Smith *et al.*, 1990b; see Derefeldt, 1991 for an extended bibliography on this topic). Because the systems differ, one can also ask whether one is more easily learned than the other. It has been claimed that the NCS system is superior in this regard (Derefeldt, 1991), but this remains controversial (Whitfield *et al.*, 1988).

5.2.2.2 OSA Uniform Color Scale (OSA/UCS)

The OSA Uniform Color Scale was designed to provide a specification of stimuli whose appearance is equally spaced perceptually. Its design shares much in common with other color order systems and we describe it here rather than with other uniform color spaces. The goal of the OSA committee that designed the system was to produce a set of samples such that the perceptual spacing between neighboring samples was equal, whether the samples differed in hue, saturation, lightness, or any combination of the three. Thus the fundamental scaling judgments underlying the OSA/UCS are perceptual difference judgments. MacAdam (1974) provides the final report of the OSA committee and describes the history of the creation of the OSA/UCS system.

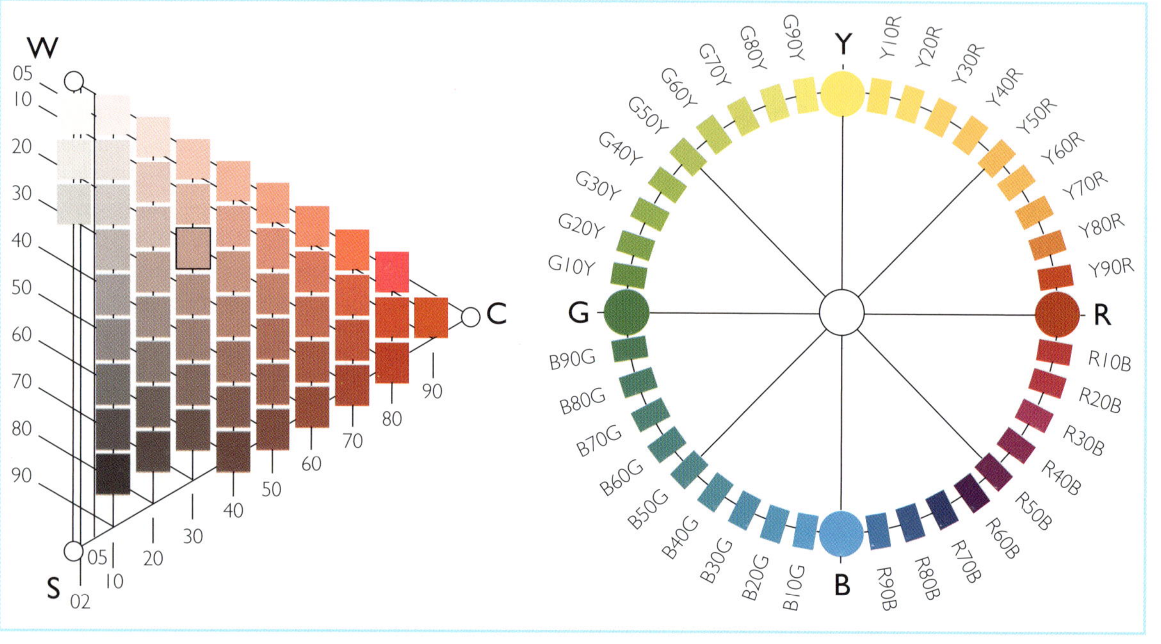

Figure 5.4 (Left) Geometry of constant NCS hue Y90R. The sample outlined in black is 2030 Y90R. (Right) NCS hue circle. (Published with permission from the Scandinavian Colour Institute AB, Stockholm, Sweden. NCS – NATURAL COLOUR SYSTEM, Copyright © and trademark ®, property of Scandinavian Colour Institute AB, Stockholm, Sweden, 2001.)

In the OSA/UCS system, every sample is defined by its values on three coordinates, L, j, and g. Roughly speaking, variation along the L coordinate corresponds to variation in lightness, variation on the j coordinate to variation in blueness/yellowness, and variation on the g coordinate to variation in redness/greenness. For the standard viewing conditions under which the scalings were performed (viewing under CIE illuminant D65 against a nonselective background of 30% reflectance), the Ljg coordinates of a sample may be computed from its CIE 1964 (10°) XYZ tristimulus coordinates. The XYZ coordinates of the sample are specified with respect to CIE illuminant D65 scaled so that a perfect diffuser has a Y coordinate of 100. The formulae for computing L are:[1]

$$L = \frac{(\mathscr{L} - 14.4)}{\sqrt{2}} \qquad (5.1)$$

$$\mathscr{L} = \begin{cases} 5.9[Y_0^{1/3} - 2/3 + 0.042|Y_0 - 30|^{1/3}], & Y_0 > 30 \\ 5.9[Y_0^{1/3} - 2/3 - 0.042|Y_0 - 30|^{1/3}], & Y_0 \leq 30 \end{cases}$$

$$Y_0 = Y(4.4934x^2 + 4.3034y^2 - 4.276xy - 1.3744x - 2.5643y + 1.8103)$$

where x and y are CIE chromaticity coordinates computed from the XYZ tristimulus coordinates. The formulae for computing j and g are:

$$\begin{aligned} j &= C(1.7R^{1/3} + 8G^{1/3} + 9.7B^{1/3}) \\ g &= C(-13.7R^{1/3} + 17.7G^{1/3} - 4B^{1/3}) \end{aligned} \qquad (5.2)$$

with

$$C = \frac{\mathscr{L}}{5.9[Y_0^{1/3} - 2/3]} \qquad (5.3)$$

$$\begin{aligned} R &= 0.7990X + 0.4194Y - 0.1648Z \\ G &= -0.4493X + 1.3265Y + 0.0927Z \\ B &= -0.1149X + 0.3394Y + 0.7170Z \end{aligned}$$

The Ljg coordinate dimensions form a rectilinear coordinate system. An interesting feature of the OSA/UCS system, however, is that the coordinates are intended to be sampled using a regular-rhombohedral scheme. This sounds complex, but may be accomplished by applying the simple rule that the L, j, and g coordinates for any sample are either all even integers or all odd integers, with zero being considered even (MacAdam, 1974). In the OSA/UCS system, chips that are equidistant nearest neighbors on the sampled lattice are designed to be equally salient from one another. One of the features of using this lattice structure is that it may be subsampled by a large number of different planes. Each plane provides a palette that may be useful for color selection (Cowan, personal communication). Figure 5.5 shows such planar sampling from the OSA/UCS space.

The size of color steps in the OSA/UCS lattice is about 20 just-noticeable-differences under the viewing conditions used by the committee. The committee concluded, however, that judgments of color discriminations are fundamentally non-Euclidean, so that they did not recommend their system for specification of color differences generally. That is, the committee recommended against using Euclidean distance in the Ljg coordinate space as a general color metric. Indeed, they concluded that no such metric could exist (MacAdam, 1974; see also Indow, 1980). This emphasis may have led to a lack of interest in the system, but one should bear in mind that the committee's conclusion applies not just to their own space but to any color difference space.

Note that the OSA/UCS system makes no explicit use of the concepts of color appearance. The scaling judgments used to define the space are entirely those of color difference. Although this may be a weakness for applications where intuitive descriptions of color are required, the space may still be used for appearance specification. Because the arrangement of colors in the space is regular, users may visually locate a desired sample in the space and find its OSA/UCS coordinates by interpolation.

5.2.2.3 DIN color system

The DIN system was developed as a German standard for color specification; a readable

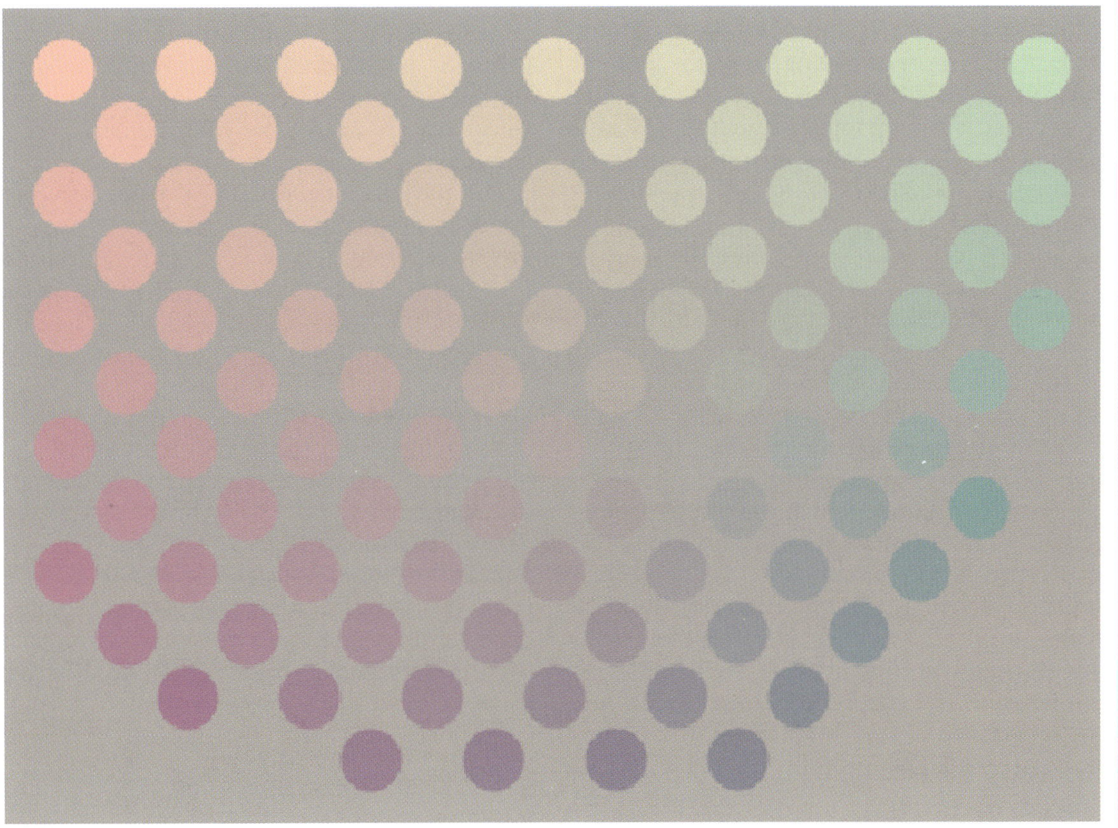

Figure 5.5 **A plane of regularly spaced colors in the OSA/UCS space. The plane is constrained by the requirement that L = j. All coordinate values are integral. L values run from –5 to 6 (bottom to top) while g values run from –10 to 6 (left to right).**

description may be found in a historical review by Richter and Witt (1986). The principles underlying the DIN system are very similar to those of the Munsell system, with the interesting variation that a number of colorimetric constraints were imposed to make the system more convenient to use (Richter and Witt, 1986; Billmeyer, 1987; Derefeldt, 1991). As with the Munsell, NCS, and OSA/UCS systems, the DIN system is implemented in a color atlas (DIN, 1980).

The three perceptual variables of the DIN system are hue, saturation, and darkness. The DIN hue scale for a single saturation and darkness was constructed from scaling data, much in the same way as Munsell hue. Rather than extending the scale to other saturations and lightnesses through further scaling experiments, however, DIN hue was defined to be constant for lines of constant dominant and complementary wavelength (with respect to CIE Illuminant C: Richter and Witt, 1986; Billmeyer, 1987). This simplification makes the transformation between tristimulus coordinates and DIN hue straightforward, at the cost of making DIN hue only an approximate measure of perceived hue. A similar compromise was used to construct the DIN saturation scale. Lines of constant saturation were measured for a single darkness level, and the scale was then extended under the assumption that lines of constant saturation are the same for all darkness degrees (Robertson, 1984; Richter and Witt, 1986; Billmeyer, 1987). Thus the DIN hue and saturation of a sample may be calculated directly from its chromaticity coordinates. DIN darkness degree is an inverse scale for lightness. DIN darkness was determined by scaling for neutral colors. For non-neutral colors, the darkness for a sample is determined as a direct function of the sample's relative luminance factor relative to CIE Illuminant C. The relative luminance factor is the luminance of a sample divided by the luminance of an optimal color with the same chromaticity of the sample. An optimal color is a theoretical construct. Its surface reflectance is such that it has the highest luminance of any physically realizable surface of the same chromaticity (Schrodinger, 1920; Rosch, 1928; MacAdam, 1935; Wyszecki and Stiles, 1982; Richter and Witt, 1986). Again, this is a convenient approximation which simplifies the calculation of DIN darkness degree.

5.3 COLOR DIFFERENCE SYSTEMS

5.3.1 EXAMPLE: CIELAB COLOR SPACE

5.3.1.1 Problem – specifying color tolerances

In writing contracts for color reproduction, it is important to be able to specify how accurately a color must be reproduced. To do this, it is necessary to have an objective metric for measuring color differences. There are several levels at which one might want to specify color tolerances. For precise applications, one might want to know how large a measured color difference has to be before observers can reliably detect it. This size of difference is often referred to as a just-noticeable-difference. On the other hand, if one is worried about reproducing the characteristic color associated with, say, a particular brand, one might want to know how large a measured color difference has to be before it is classified differently by customers. Detectable color differences do not necessarily cause any change in the color name given to a stimulus.

The purpose of the CIELAB color space is to quantify small color differences. By small is meant differences typical of color reproduction tolerances – larger than a JND under optimal viewing conditions, but smaller than the differences typically scaled in color appearance systems. As discussed in Chapter 3, when stimuli are expressed in tristimulus coordinates, the distance between the coordinates of two colored stimuli does not correlate well with their discriminability. The CIELAB color space was derived from the CIE 1931 XYZ coordinate system in an attempt to provide coordinates for colored stimuli so that the distance between the coordinates of any two stimuli is predictive of the perceived color difference between them.

5.3.1.2 Definition of CIELAB

The CIELAB coordinates of a light are referred to as the CIE 1976 $L^*a^*b^*$ coordinates. These may be obtained from the light's CIE 1931 XYZ coordinates according to the equations

$$L^* = \begin{cases} 116\left(\frac{Y}{Y_n}\right) - 16, & \frac{Y}{Y_n} > 0.008856 \\ 903.3\left(\frac{Y}{Y_n}\right), & \frac{Y}{Y_n} \leq 0.008856 \end{cases}$$

$$a^* = 500\left[f\left(\frac{X}{X_n}\right) - f\left(\frac{Y}{Y_n}\right)\right] \quad (5.4)$$

$$b^* = 500\left[f\left(\frac{Y}{Y_n}\right) - f\left(\frac{Z}{Z_n}\right)\right]$$

where the function f(s) is defined as

$$f(s) = \begin{cases} s^{1/3}, & s > 0.008856 \\ 7.787(s) + \frac{16}{116}, & s \leq 0.008856 \end{cases} \quad (5.5)$$

In this equation, the quantities X_n, Y_n, and Z_n are the tristimulus coordinates of a white point. Little guidance is available as to how to choose an appropriate white point. In the case where the stimuli being judged are illuminated samples, the tristimulus coordinates of the illuminant may be used. In the case where the lights being judged are displayed on a color monitor, the sum of the tristimulus coordinates of the three monitor phosphors stimulated at their maximum intensity may be used.

The Euclidean distance between the CIELAB coordinates of two lights provides a rough guide to their discriminability. The symbol ΔE^*_{ab} is used to denote distance in the uniform color space and is defined as

$$\Delta E^*_{ab} = \sqrt{(\Delta L^*)^2 + (\Delta a^*)^2 + (\Delta b^*)^2} \quad (5.6)$$

where the various Δ quantities on the right represent the differences between the corresponding coordinates of the two stimuli.

5.3.1.3 Underlying experimental data

It is difficult if not impossible to go back through the literature and discover the fundamental data used to derive the CIELAB system. The formula is a simplification of the Adams–Nickerson color difference formula that was used in industrial practice prior to 1976 (McLaren, 1970, 1971). Robertson (1977) compares the CIELAB formula with two fundamental data sets. The first of these is the spacing of the Munsell colors. Figure 5.6 plots the CIELAB a*b* coordinates of contours of equal Munsell chroma and lines of constant Munsell hue. If the two spaces were consistent with each other, the contours of constant chroma would be circles and the radial spacing between lines of constant hue would be constant at each chroma. As the figure illustrates, the agreement between the two spaces is only approximate. Another comparison data set is the MacAdam ellipses, which measure the just-noticeable color differences (MacAdam, 1942; see Chapter 3). If CIELAB accurately represents uniform color differences, these should plot as circles in the CIELAB space. Figure 5.6 also shows the MacAdam ellipses plotted in the CIELAB space. Clearly these are not circular. As Robertson (1977) points out, the lack of agreement between CIELAB and the Munsell/MacAdam data could arise because CIELAB is designed to handle color differences of a magnitude intermediate between the spacing of Munsell samples and just-noticeable-differences.

To provide a feel for the scale of ΔE^*_{ab}, we can compute the average ΔE^*_{ab} value corresponding to measured just-noticeable color differences. Wyszecki and Stiles (1982) provide the parameters for color difference ellipses measured around 25 different chromaticities by MacAdam (1942). The ellipses represent variability in observers' color matches. From the ellipse parameters it is possible to compute the value of ΔE^*_{ab} that corresponds to traversing 1.96 standard deviations along the major and minor axis of each ellipse. The average resulting value is 3.6, with a range of 0.9 to 9.9. Consistent with this, Stokes, Fairchild, and Berns (1992) report that when the average (taken over image locations) ΔE^*_{ab} difference between two images is below about 2.2, the images are not discriminably different from each other. To give a visual sense for the scale of ΔE^*_{ab}, Figure 5.7 shows several series of colors separated by constant CIELAB differences.

5.3.1.4 Discussion of the CIELAB system

There is general agreement that using the CIELAB system is an improvement over using the Euclidean distance between XYZ tristimulus coordinates as a color difference metric. To emphasize the difference between CIELAB and

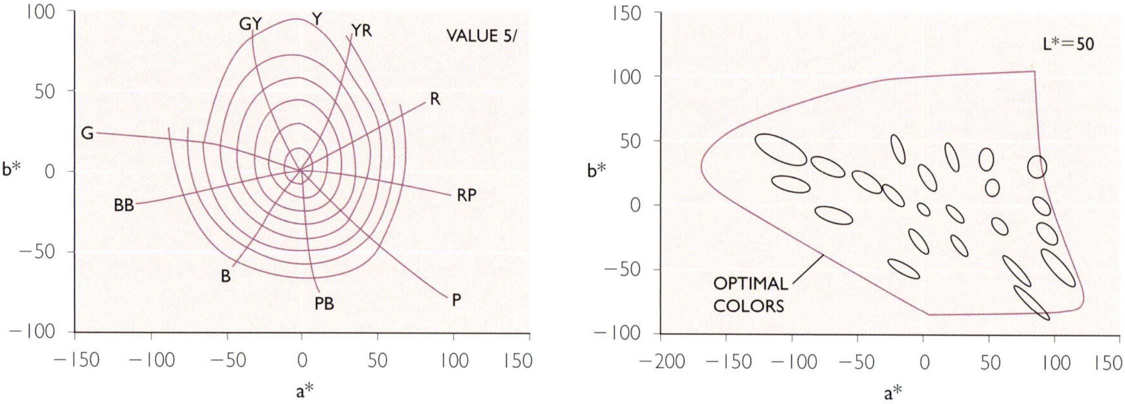

Figure 5.6 **(Left) Contours showing equal Munsell chroma and iso-hue lines plotted in CIELAB coordinates. (Right) A plot of the CIELAB coordinates of isodiscrimination contours measured by MacAdam. The scale of each ellipse has been expanded to improve the visibility of its shape. (From Robertson, 1977. Copyright © 1984 John Wiley & Sons, Inc., reproduced by permission.)**

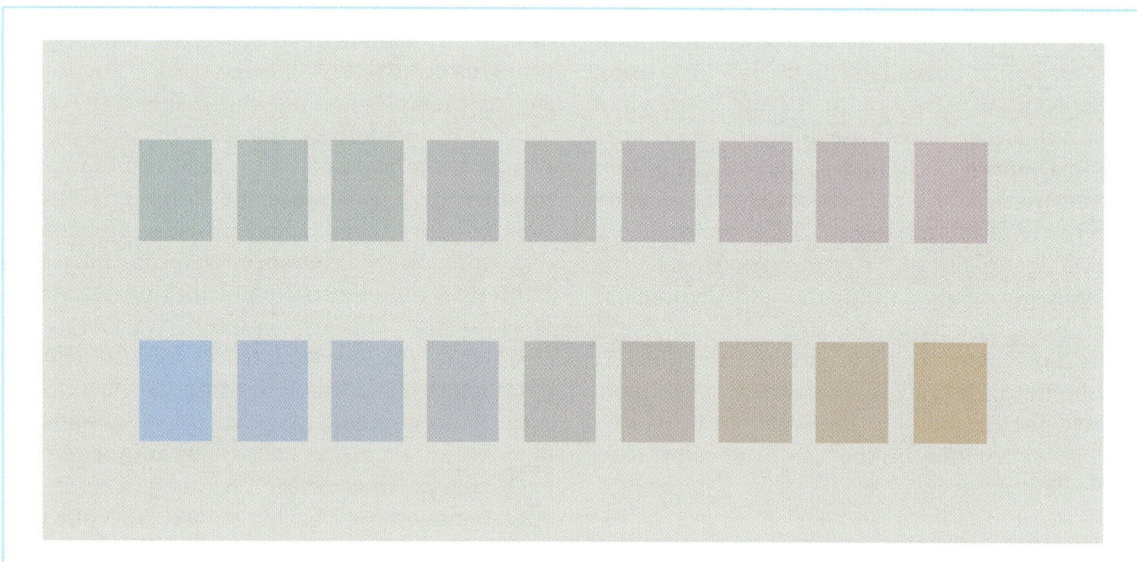

Figure 5.7 **Each row shows a series of colors separated by constant CIELAB differences. First row shows CIELAB $\Delta E^*_{ab} = 4$ along the a* dimension, second row shows CIELAB $\Delta E^*_{ab} = 12$ along the b* dimension. CIELAB coordinates were computed with respect to a white point defined by the background of the figure.**

tristimulus coordinates, Figure 5.8 shows isodiscrimination contours calculated using equal ΔE^*_{ab} values. The contours are plotted in the equiluminant XZ plane of the CIE XYZ color space. If the two distances in XYZ and CIELAB both represented perceptual color differences, the contours would plot as circles. Clearly, they do not.

Since its initial standardization, predictions of the CIELAB system have been compared to new measurements. These have led to a revision of the original system. The CIE has recommended one of these revisions, CIE94 (CIE, 1995; Hung and Berns, 1995). A second revision in widespread use is the CMC formula (Clark *et al.*, 1984). In the CIE94 system, a distance measure ΔE^*_{94} is substituted for ΔE^*_{ab}. To understand the computation of ΔE^*_{94}, first note that we can rewrite Eqn. 6 as

$$\Delta E^*_{ab} = \sqrt{(\Delta L^*)^2 + (\Delta C^*_{ab})^2 + (\Delta H^*_{ab})^2} \quad (5.7)$$

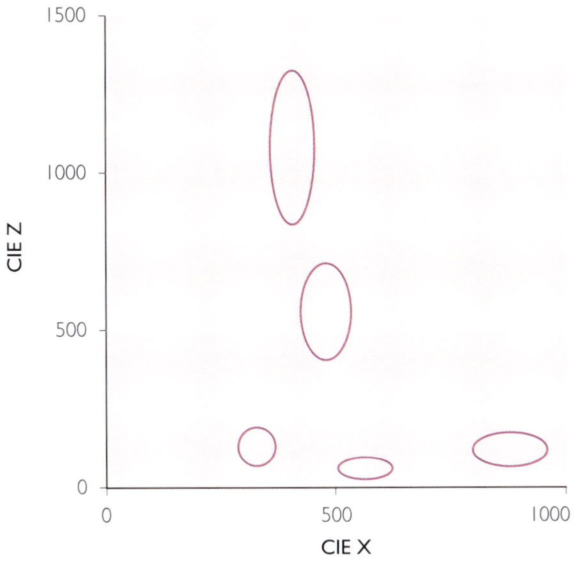

Figure 5.8 Isodiscrimination contours calculated using equal ΔE^*_{ab} values plotted in the XZ plane of the CIE XYZ color space. The points on each of the five contours were calculated to have a constant ΔE^*_{ab} difference of 15 from a base stimulus. The conversion from XYZ coordinates to CIELAB coordinates was done with respect to a white point with the same chromaticity as CIE D65 daylight and a luminance of 1000 cd/m². The luminance of the base stimuli was always taken to be 500 cd/m². The contours were computed in the equiluminant XZ plane. If CIELAB and CIE XYZ agreed about color differences, the contours would plot as circles.

where the chroma coordinate C^*_{ab} is defined by $C^*_{ab} = \sqrt{(a^*)^2 + (b^*)^2}$, where ΔC^*_{ab} denotes the difference in the C_{ab} coordinate of the two stimuli, and where the hue difference ΔH^*_{ab} is defined by $\Delta H^*_{ab} = \sqrt{\Delta E^*_{ab} - \Delta L^* - \Delta C^*_{ab}}$. The CIE94 difference measure ΔE^*_{94} is computed as a modification of Eqn. 7:

$$\Delta E^*_{94} = \sqrt{\left(\frac{\Delta L^*}{k_L S_L}\right)^2 + \left(\frac{\Delta C^*_{ab}}{k_C S_C}\right)^2 + \left(\frac{\Delta H^*_{ab}}{k_H S_H}\right)^2}. \quad (5.8)$$

In equation 5.8 the S weighting factors are defined as, $S_L = 1$, $S_C = 1 + 0.045C^*_{ab\_s}$ and $S_H = 1 + 0.015C^*_{ab\_s}$ where $C^*_{ab\_s}$ is the chroma coordinate of the standard sample from which differences are being computed.[2] The k weighting factors are all set to 1 for the reference viewing conditions[3] but may be modified at the user's discretion for other viewing conditions. Further refinement of CIELAB-based systems can be expected and future versions may provide more precise guidance about the choice of the k weighting factors.

Although the CIELAB system was designed for specification of color tolerances, it has been used to assess color differences in other contexts (Carter and Carter, 1981; Silverstein and Merrifield, 1981). In the absence of better formulae, this is a reasonable thing to do. However, it should be stressed that the formulae are not grounded in empirical data that support these other uses. Figure 5.6 gives useful comparisons to keep in mind.

As noted above, one of the chief difficulties in developing a color difference specification system is to take the viewing conditions into account. Color discrimination thresholds depend heavily on factors other than the differences in tristimulus coordinates. These factors include the adapted state of the observer (Stiles, 1959), the spatial and temporal structure of the stimulus (deLange, 1958a, 1958b; Mullen, 1985; Sekiguchi *et al.*, 1993) and the perceptual task being performed by the observer (Carter and Carter, 1981; Silverstein and Merrifield, 1985; Poirson and Wandell, 1990; Nagy and Sanchez, 1990). The basic CIELAB formulae include normalization to a white point which is designed to take the first of these factors into account. At present, however, our understanding of observer adaptation is not sufficiently well developed to make us believe that the CIELAB formulation is satisfactory (see Brainard and Wandell, 1991; Fairchild, 1998).

Zhang and Wandell (1997) have developed an extension of CIELAB, called S-CIELAB, which takes the spatial structure of the stimulus into account. S-CIELAB is based on psychophysical measurements showing that visual sensitivity to spatial gratings falls off more rapidly with grating spatial frequency when the gratings are modulated in some color directions (e.g. red–green and blue–yellow gratings) than when they are modulated in others (e.g. black/white gratings: Mullen, 1985; Sekiguchi *et al.*, 1993). The S-CIELAB metric is computed in two separable stages, based on the data and model of Poirson and Wandell (Poirson and Wandell, 1996). The first stage computes the effect of spatial structure on the discriminability of different chromatic components of an image. The second stage applies the standard CIELAB metric to the output of the first stage. The S-CIELAB metric does a better job of predicting observers' judgments of the perceptual differences between color images than the unmodified CIELAB metric, but it is clear that further development is required (Zhang and Wandell, 1998).

The CIELAB system was not designed to be a color appearance system. Although it does define scales for hue, chroma, and lightness, these scales are only approximate and are not as well grounded in appearance data as most color order systems or color appearance models.

5.3.2 OTHER COLOR DIFFERENCE SYSTEMS

5.3.2.1 CIELUV

At the time the CIELAB standard was introduced, the CIE also introduced a second system for specifying small color differences. This is called the CIELUV system, and coordinates in this system are referred to as the CIE 1976 L*u*v* coordinates. Like the CIELAB system, the CIELUV system was derived from systems used widely in practice prior to the standardization. CIELUV coordinates are derived from tristimulus coordinates as well. The formulae for computing CIELUV coordinates may be found in numerous publications (Wyszecki and Stiles, 1982; CIE, 1986). At the time of standardization, the CIE recognized that it was difficult to choose between the two systems, as each worked better on different validation data sets and each had its proponents. Indeed, the general feeling in the color community was that no color difference system explained more that about 80% of the variance in color discrimination data, and that each system explained a different 80% (Cowan, personal communication). More recently, opinion has tended to favor the CIELAB system and its successor CIE94, and the CIELUV system is no longer widely recommended (Fairchild, 1998).

5.3.2.2 Color order systems

The OSA/UCS color order system may be thought of as a color difference system. This system was designed to apply larger color differences than either CIELAB or CIELUV. It is discussed under color order systems above. As with CIELAB and CIELUV, this system is designed to handle cases where samples vary in both chromaticity and luminance. Other color order systems (e.g. Munsell, DIN) are based at least in part on scalings of color differences, as when observers are asked to pick a chip whose saturation is halfway between that of two reference samples. These systems are more difficult to interpret as full color difference systems, however, because they are not based on data where multiple stimulus attributes are covaried. Nonetheless, they are sometimes used in this fashion (Richter and Witt, 1986).

5.4 CURRENT DIRECTIONS IN COLOR SPECIFICATION

5.4.1 CONTEXT EFFECTS

As illustrated in Figure 5.2, implementations of color order systems may be thought of as lookup tables that specify the relation between color appearance and physical samples. As such, these implementations embody knowledge about the psychology of color appearance. The implementations, however, depend on scaling experiments conducted using a well-specified viewing context. This is emphasized in Figure 5.2 by the fact that the viewing conditions are specified along the arrow linking the two sides of the table. Clearly, it would be useful to be able to specify color appearance for conditions other than the standard. Of particular interest is the prediction of the appearance of images, where the stimulus at each location is viewed in the complex surround defined by the rest of the image. Because the effects of context can be quite large (Figure 5.9), neglecting them can lead to large prediction errors.

In general, both the appearance and discriminability of colored stimuli depend on the context in which the stimuli are viewed (see Chapters 3 and 4). Because our understanding of context effects is incomplete, it is not yet possible to incorporate precisely the effects of context into color specification systems. It is possible to lay out a general framework that allows us to incorporate what is known about the effect of

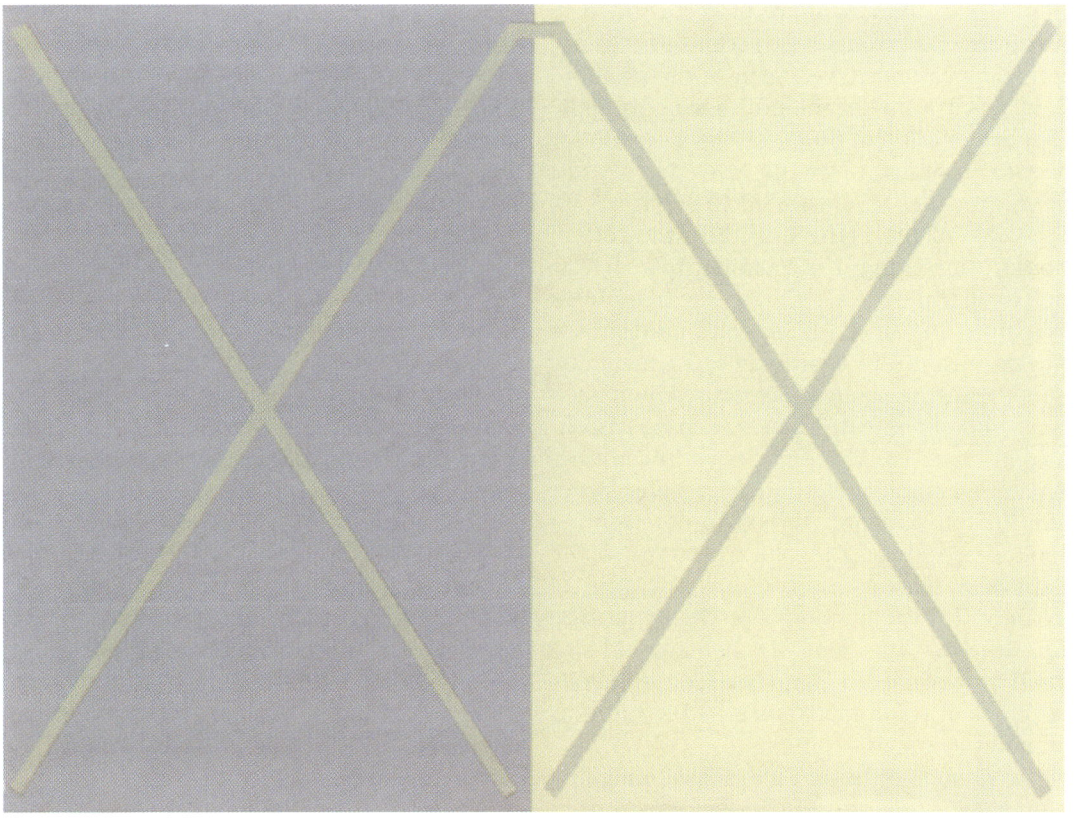

Figure 5.9 **Illustration of context effects. The x-shaped intersections on the two sides of the figure appear quite different. The light reaching the eye from these two regions is the same, however. This can be seen by tracing from one x-shaped region to the other. (From Albers, 1975. Copyright © 1975 Yale University Press, reproduced with permission.)**

context into current color order and discrimination systems. This framework provides the foundation for current work towards developing color appearance models. The key to this framework is asymmetric color matching.

Asymmetric color matching is an experimental procedure that may be used to establish pairs of stimuli that match across changes in viewing context (von Kries, 1902; Burnham *et al.*, 1957; Stiles, 1967; Krantz, 1968; Brainard and Wandell, 1992; Poirson and Wandell, 1993; Webster and Mollon, 1995). In an asymmetric matching experiment, the observer adjusts the color of one stimulus, seen in some arbitrary context, to match the appearance of a standard stimulus seen in a standard context. By setting such matches, the observer establishes pairs of stimuli that, across contexts, have the same appearance. The two contexts may be separated spatially or in time, but in either case the observer need only judge identity of color appearance; the complex structure of appearance scaling judgments does not intrude into the experiment.

Let us use the term standard context to refer to a set of viewing conditions for which we have implemented a color order system. Typically, the standard context consists of viewing a single sample at a time against a uniform gray background, under a well-specified illuminant. Let us use the term test context to refer to some other set of viewing conditions for which we would like to specify color appearance. Suppose that we are able to develop a descriptive model that predicts observers' asymmetric matches between any two contexts. In particular, this model should allow us to relate the tristimulus coordinates of any stimulus seen in the test context to the tristimulus coordinates of a stimulus that has the same appearance when seen in the standard context. Such a model then allows us to apply the implementation of the color order system for the standard context to stimuli viewed in the test context. This idea is illustrated in Figure 5.10. The left side of the figure illustrates the role of asymmetric matching. The asymmetric matching model would allow us to map the tristimulus coordinates of a test stimulus seen in a test context to the tristimulus coordinates of a matching stimulus with the same appearance when seen in the standard context. These matching tristimulus coordinates could then be used in conjunction with an implementation of a color order system for the standard context to determine a symbolic description of the color appearance of the test stimulus in the test context. The role of the color order system is shown on the right of the figure. Note that this general scheme could also be used in reverse to map between symbolic descriptions of color appearance and tristimulus coordinates in the test context.

The advantage of using asymmetric matching to extend color order system implementations to general viewing contexts is that it separates the problem of understanding context from the problem of implementing a color order system. On the one hand, the asymmetric matching experiments may be conducted without reference to color names and hence results from them may be used to generalize any color order system. On the other hand, color order systems may be developed carefully for single context with the knowledge that they may be generalized once an acceptable theory of asymmetric matching is developed.

The approach outlined above relies on the assumption that the effect of context measured by asymmetric matching correctly predicts the effect of context on color appearance for other measures (e.g. color scaling and naming). Recent empirical work by Speigle and Brainard (Speigle and Brainard, 1996; Speigle, 1997; Speigle and Brainard, 1999) lends support to this assumption.

At present, no general theory of asymmetric matching exists. Most current theories attempt to explain asymmetric matching by developing a model of how color signals originating in the cone photoreceptors are processed by subsequent visual mechanisms and of how this processing varies with viewing context (von Kries, 1902; Burnham *et al.*, 1957; Hurvich and Jameson, 1957; Stiles, 1967; Krantz, 1968; Brainard and Wandell, 1992; Fairchild and Berns, 1993; Poirson and Wandell, 1993; Webster and Mollon, 1995; Delahunt and Brainard, 2000). The simplest model goes back to von Kries, who suggested that the effect of context was simply to scale the cone signals independently for each

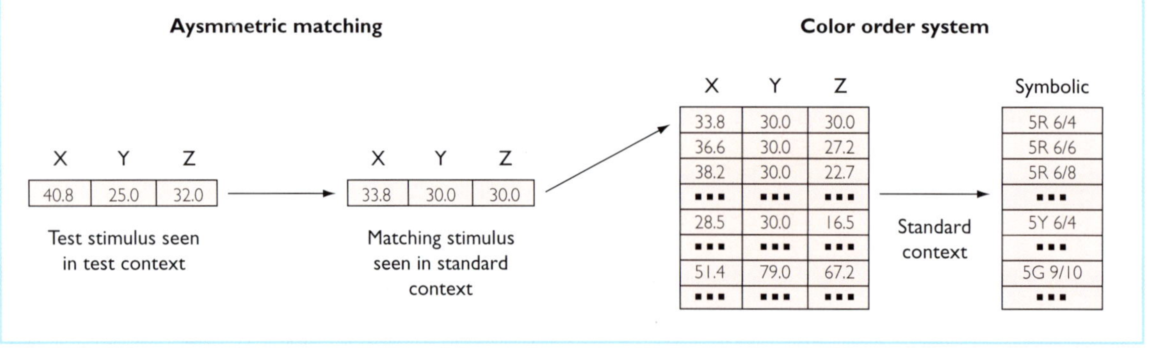

Figure 5.10 **Schematic of how asymmetric matching can be used to extend a color order system to other contexts. The left side of the figure illustrates the role of asymmetric matching. A general characterization of asymmetric matching would allow us to map the tristimulus coordinates of a test stimulus seen in a test context to the tristimulus coordinates of a matching stimulus with the same appearance when seen in the standard context. These matching tristimulus coordinates could then be used in conjunction with an implementation of a color order system for the standard context to determine a symbolic description of the color appearance of the test stimulus in the test context. The role of the color order system is shown on the right of the figure.**

cone type (von Kries, 1905). This class of model accounts well for a subset of color context effects (Brainard and Wandell, 1992; Chichilnisky and Wandell, 1997) and Land's well-known retinex theory of context vision is a special case of the general von Kries scheme (Land and McCann, 1971; Land, 1986; Brainard and Wandell, 1986). A von Kries type of transform cannot account for all color context effects, however (Krauskopf *et al.*, 1982; Poirson and Wandell, 1993; Webster and Mollon, 1995). Chapter 4 discusses basic research on this topic in more detail.

5.4.1.1 Color appearance models

The goal of color appearance models is to provide an analytic relation between a specification of a stimulus and the context in which it is viewed and its color appearance (in terms of numerical correlates of appearance attributes). As such, color appearance models must contain components for both sides of Figure 5.10. One component of the model must account for the effect of context on appearance, while a second must provide an analytic description of the mapping between tristimulus coordinates and symbolic names for a standard context.

An early attempt at developing a color appearance model was made by Judd (Judd, 1940). Second generation models were developed by Hunt (Hunt, 1982; Hunt and Pointer, 1985; Hunt, 1987a, 1987b, 1991) and by Nayatani and his coworkers (Nayatani, Takahama, and Sobagaki, 1981; Nayatani, Sobagaki, and Takahama, 1986; Nayatani *et al.*, 1987; Nayatani *et al.*, 1990). More recently, several other color appearance models have been developed, and the CIE has recently standardized an interim color appearance model, CIECAM97s, recommended for use at the current time (CIE, 1998; Fairchild, 1998). For illustrative purposes, we provide an overview of the CIECAM97s model. Although this model is likely to be further refined, its design synthesizes a great deal of our current knowledge about color appearance. Fairchild (1998) provides a thorough review of recent color appearance models.

5.4.1.2 CIECAM97s

The CIECAM97s model is illustrated in Figure 5.11. The initial stage of the model (shown on the top of the figure) starts with the encoding of a test stimulus (called the source in the CIE documents) by the visual system. This is accomplished in the model by computing the CIE XYZ tristimulus coordinates of the test. These coordinates are indicated in the figure by the grouped rectangles. The next step is to take the viewing context into account. This is done by transforming the tristimulus coordinates to coordinates that represent the adapted cone responses of a stimulus that would match the source, when it was seen under standardized reference viewing conditions. The transformation takes context into account and results in a representation of

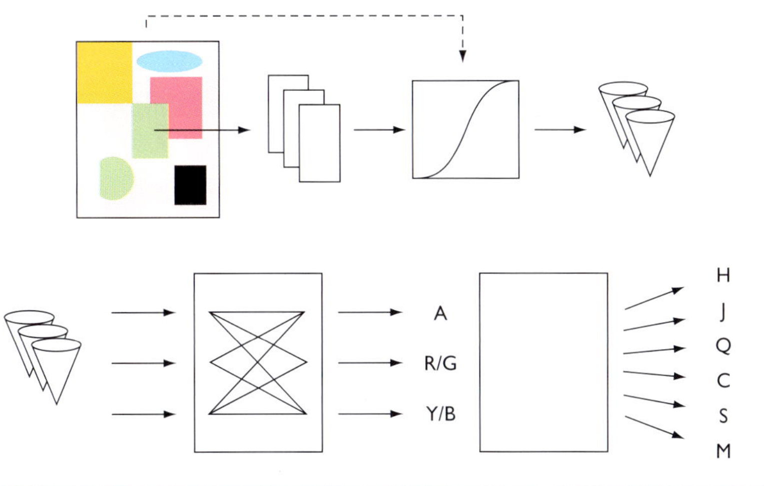

Figure 5.11 Schematic illustration of the CIECAM97s color appearance model. See description in the text.

the test in terms of the L, M, and S cone photoreceptor responses. The actual calculation of the adapted cone responses is somewhat involved and depends on the context in which the test is seen. It is illustrated in the figure by the sigmoidal nonlinearity. The arrow from the context to the nonlinearity indicates that the transformation depends on the context. To apply the model in practice involves a certain degree of art, as the user must set a number of parameters that specify the completeness of adaptation to the viewing context. The adapted cone responses are the output of the first stage of the model and are shown schematically in the figure by the grouped cones.

The first stage of the CIECAM97s model is analogous to the first stage in the asymmetric matching framework described above. The only difference is that rather than mapping the tristimulus coordinates of the test to those of a matching stimulus, it maps the tristimulus coordinates of the test to adapted cone responses. The adapted cone responses can, however, be associated with the tristimulus coordinates of a matching stimulus in the reference context by applying the inverse of the first stage with the parameters set for the reference context.

The purpose of the second stage of CIECAM97s is to provide an analytic description of how the adapted cone coordinates relate to color appearance attributes. It is based on an opponent process model of how subsequent visual mechanisms process the adapted cone signals. The key idea is that signals originating in the three classes of cones are recombined to form a non-opponent achromatic signal and opponent chromatic signals. The opponent process model was articulated in the modern literature by Hurvich and Jameson (Hurvich and Jameson, 1957; Jameson and Hurvich, 1955, 1964), who used it to explain a large number of color appearance phenomena. It is lent credence by the fact that observers can make judgments that may be interpreted as tapping solely the chromatic mechanisms (Jameson and Hurvich, 1955, 1964; Larimer *et al.*, 1974, 1975; Krantz, 1975; Walraven, 1976; Shevell, 1978; Werner and Walraven, 1982; Shevell and Wesner, 1989). In the model, each of the opponent signals is formed as a weighted combination of the adapted cone signals. The achromatic signal (indicated by A in the figure) is formed as the weighted sum of the three adapted cone signals. The red/green signal (R/G) is obtained by opposing signals from adapted L and S cones with signals from adapted M cones. The yellow/blue signal (Y/B) is obtained by opposing signals from adapted L and M cones with signals from adapted S cones.

To produce color appearance descriptions, the model provides a set of transformations between A, R/G, and Y/B and scales for appearance attributes. Included are scales for hue (H), lightness (J), brightness (Q), chroma (C), saturation (S), and colorfulness (M).

The second stage of the CIECAM97s model is analogous to the second stage of the asymmetric matching framework described above. Note, however, that the lookup table description has been replaced by an analytic characterization between the adapted cone responses and the appearance scales. A second difference, neglected above, is that in CIECAM97s the relation between adapted cone responses and the appearance scales does contain a dependence on viewing context. For example, the scale for lightness depends on a comparison of the achromatic signal of the test and the achromatic signal for an image region designated by the user as white. This dependence means that in CIECAM97s, there is not complete separation between the effect of context and the transformation between adapted cone signals and appearance scales. This separation could be restored if the model of asymmetric matching accurately predicts the match to a white sample, since then the adapted cone signals for a white seen in the reference context could be substituted for the adapted cone signals of an image region designated by the user as white.

5.4.1.3 Discussion

CIECAM97s is interesting in that it attempts to bridge basic research on the nature of visual processing with applied research on color order systems. The greatest difficulty for testing and developing this (or any other) color appearance model is the huge array of possible viewing contexts that must be studied. Contextual factors that influence color appearance include both the size and shape of the stimulus itself, its local and global surround, and the adapted state of the observer. Our current understanding is based primarily on experiments where isolated test stimuli are viewed against uniform backgrounds of varying chromaticities and luminances. The difficulty is that it is not clear how to generalize from these experiments to more complicated viewing situations. Overcoming this difficulty is a prerequisite for a complete color appearance model and research on methods for doing so is ongoing (see Chapter 4). Note that if a color appearance model contains a successful model of context effects, this model could be used together with the asymmetric matching framework described above to extend color order systems to multiple contexts.

A particularly important area of application for color appearance models is to describe the appearance of stimuli presented on CRT displays. A great deal of image previewing and manipulation is now done using such displays, with the ultimate goal of printing a hard copy of the image. Ideally, it would be possible to make a reproduction of the CRT image that had exactly the same appearance as the original. This goal will probably not become easily achievable, however, until it is possible to describe both original and reproduced images in color appearance terms. As color appearance models are refined, they are likely to play increasing roles in automated color reproduction. (See Chapter 8 for a discussion of color reproduction.)

5.4.2 METAMERISM

5.4.2.1 The problem of metamerism

An important issue that arises in using color specification systems is the following. Current color specification systems are based on tristimulus coordinates. This presents no difficulties if one's goal is to use the system to produce a sample that will be viewed only under a single illuminant. One designs the sample to produce the desired tristimulus coordinates under the desired illuminant and the actual reflectance function of the sample is irrelevant (see Chapters 3 and 4). But what if the sample is to be viewed under more than one illuminant? For example, what if the specification is for the color of a car, which will be seen under a variety of daylights (and perhaps under artificial lighting at night)? The stability of the color appearance will depend on which reflectance function is chosen initially. How should the designer make this choice? This is the problem of metamerism.

5.4.2.2 Colorant order systems?

A brute force approach is provided by colorant order systems (Judd and Wyszecki, 1975). These are systems that are in many ways like color order systems. The difference is that these systems are not implemented in terms of tristimulus coordinates. Rather, their implementation is provided directly in terms of amounts of particular pigments, dyes, or inks. The advantage of a colorant order system is that a designer may choose a sample from it and be guaranteed that the final production will behave under different illuminants exactly as the sample. Thus the designer is restricted a priori to choosing among a set of producible samples, rather than choosing from a set of specifications that have multiple possible implementations. By investigating how various samples appear under different illuminants, the designer may use samples from colorant order systems to produce acceptable results.

The disadvantage of colorant order systems is that their use is confined to the output medium for which they were implemented. This limits the amount of effort that can go into their implementations and tends to make each such system idiosyncratic.

5.4.2.3 Metamerism indices

The goal of a metamerism index is to help designers reproduce a target sample so that the behavior of the reproduction under changes of illumination closely matches that of the target (Wyszecki and Stiles, 1982). A metamerism index is always based on a metric that defines how different two stimuli appear (e.g. CIELAB). To compute the metamerism index between two samples that have identical tristimulus coordinates under a reference illuminant, one chooses a test illuminant. Often the reference illuminant is CIE D65 and the test illuminant is CIE Illuminant A. One then computes or measures the tristimulus coordinates of the two samples under the test illuminant and computes the color difference between these using the chosen color metric. The smaller the difference, the more similarly the two samples appear under the change of illumination. Wyszecki and Stiles (1982) provide discussion and an example calculation.

5.4.2.4 Linear models

Another approach to the problem of metamerism is to specify colors in terms of their physical properties rather than in terms of their tristimulus coordinates. This seems at first like a radical proposal, as it suggests neglecting the economy of specification offered by the color matching experiment. However, as the problem of metamerism itself makes clear, there is sometimes a need to preserve more information about samples than their tristimulus coordinates under a particular illuminant.

A promising theoretical development that might allow such specification is the notion that small-dimensional linear models may be used to describe many surface reflectance functions to a high degree of accuracy. Linear models approximate spectral data as weighted sums of a small number of fixed basis functions (see Chapter 4; Brainard, 1995).

The number of basis functions used in a linear model is called the dimension of the model. This nomenclature emphasizes the fact that basis functions may be interpreted as describing the dimensions along which spectra may vary. The insert in Figure 5.12 shows the basis functions for a three-dimensional linear model for surfaces. The first basis function reflects fairly evenly across the visible spectrum. By varying the weight assigned to this basis function, we can capture variation in overall reflectance from one surface to another. The second basis function reflects positively at the long wavelength end of the spectrum and negatively at the short wavelength end. By assigning a positive weight to this basis function, we capture the fact that some surfaces (e.g. ones that tend to appear red) reflect best at longer wavelengths. By assigning a negative weight to this basis function, on the other hand, we capture the fact that some surfaces (e.g. ones that tend to appear green) reflect best at the middle and short wavelengths. The third basis function, which reflects positively in the middle region of the spectrum and negatively at either end, shows another dimension along which surface reflectances within the model can vary.

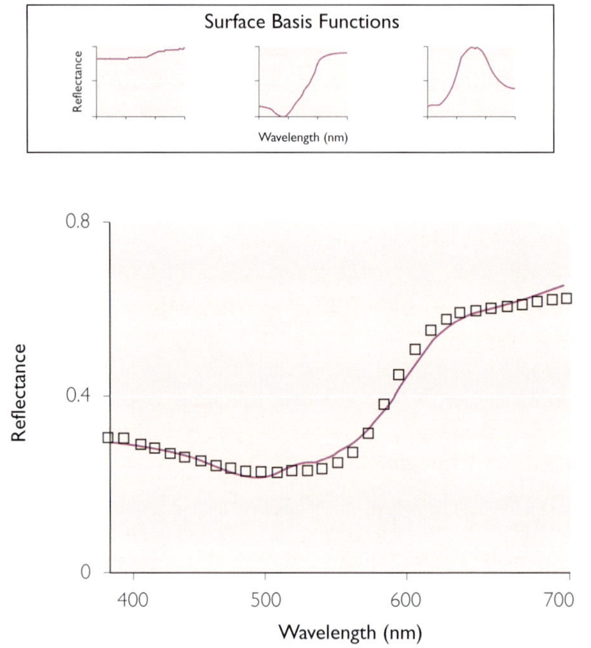

Figure 5.12 The open squares in the figure show a measured surface reflectance function. The solid line shows an approximation to this function obtained using a three-dimensional linear model. The insert shows the reflectance spectra of the linear model's basis functions. (From Brainard *et al.*, 1993. Copyright © 1993 American Psychological Society, reproduced by permission of Blackwell Publishers.)

The basis functions shown in Figure 5.12 were obtained by performing a principal components analysis of the reflectance functions of a large set of colored papers (Cohen, 1964). Similar analyses have been performed for other collections of surfaces and for measured daylight spectral power distributions (Judd *et al.*, 1964; Maloney, 1986; Jaaskelainen, Parkkinen, and Toyooka, 1990; Marimont and Wandell, 1992). The results indicate that linear models with a small number of basis functions provide an excellent description of naturally occurring spectra. The main portion of Figure 5.12 shows a typical surface reflectance function and its linear model approximation.

Linear models provide an efficient description for surface reflectance functions, since specifying the weights on each basis function provides enough information to reconstruct a close approximation to the full reflectance function. Brainard and Wandell (Wandell and Brainard,

1989; Brainard and Wandell, 1990) have outlined schemes to incorporate linear model specifications into color reproduction systems. The basic idea as it applies to color order systems is very simple, however. Rather than defining a color order system in terms of the relation between sample tristimulus coordinates and symbolic descriptors, the system could be defined in terms of the relation between linear model weights and the same descriptors. Since it is always possible to compute sample tristimulus coordinates from reflectance spectra (under the standard viewing conditions for which the color order system is defined), the linear model formulation loses no information. The formulation provides extra information, however, since the full spectrum of each sample is available. As methods for accurately controlling sample spectra become available, color order systems using spectral sample specification could provide reproduction whose appearance changes with illumination were well defined. Moreover, with such a scheme, the system's sample spectra might even be designed to have roughly constant appearance across common changes in illumination (Berns *et al.*, 1985).

ACKNOWLEDGMENTS

I thank P. Alessi, R. Berns, W. Cowan, M. Fairchild, D. Post, S. Shevell, L. Silverstein, W. Swanson, and B. Wandell for useful discussions or comments on the manuscript.

NOTES

1 Formulae for the conversion are provided by MacAdam (MacAdam, 1974). The published formulae, however, contain an error. MacAdam's Equation 1 for the computation of $\mathscr{L}$ works only for stimuli with values of Y_0 >30. The formulae published here correct for this problem and work for all values of Y_0. They were inferred by examining Semmelroth (1970) whose Equation 3 provides the basis for MacAdam's Equation 1. The formulae published here were checked by implementing them as MATLAB functions and verifying that they correctly reproduce tabulated values (MacAdam, 1978). The implementation is available as part of the freely distributed Psychophysics Toolbox (http://psychtoolbox.org/, release 2.45 and later). Note also that in addition to propagating the error introduced by MacAdam (1974), the formulae provided in the widely used reference by Wyszecki and Stiles (1982) contain additional errors: they do not incorporate the transformation between $\mathscr{L}$ and L, and the definitions of j and g are reversed.

2 In many applications there is no a priori reason to designate either of the two stimuli being compared as the standard. The effect of arbitrarily choosing one or the other as standard is small as long as small color differences are being evaluated. An alternative is to use the geometric mean of the chroma coordinate: $C^*_{ab\_s} = \sqrt{C^*_{ab\_1} C^*_{ab\_2}}$. This issue is discussed in more detail in the CIE technical report (CIE, 1995).

3 The reference viewing conditions specify, among other things, viewing samples under CIE illuminant D65 against a nonselective background with L* = 50. A complete description of the reference conditions is available in several sources (CIE, 1995; Hung and Berns, 1995; Fairchild, 1998).

REFERENCES

Abramov, I. and Gordon, J. (1994) Color appearance: on seeing red – or yellow, or green, or blue. *Annual Review of Psychology*, 45, 451–85.

Albers, J. (1975) *Interaction of Color*. New Haven, CT: Yale University Press.

Berns, R.S. and Billmeyer, F.W., Jr (1985) Development of the 1929 Munsell Book of Color: a historical review. *Color Research and Application*, 10, 246–50.

Berns, R.S., Billmeyer, F.W., Jr, and Sacher, R.S. (1985) Methods for generating spectral reflectance functions leading to color-constant properties. *Color Research and Application*, 10, 73–83.

Billmeyer, F.W., Jr (1987) Survey of color order systems. *Color Research and Application*, 12, 173–86.

Billmeyer, F.W., Jr (1988) Quantifying color appearance visually and instrumentally. *Color Research and Application*, 13, 140–5.

Billmeyer, F.W., Jr and Bencuya, A.K. (1987) Interrelation of the Natural Color System and the Munsell color order system. *Color Research and Application*, 12, 243–55.

Brainard, D.H. (1995) Colorimetry. In M. Bass (ed.), *Handbook of Optics: Volume 1. Fundamentals, Techniques, and Design*. New York: McGraw-Hill, pp. 26.1–26.54.

Brainard, D.H. and Wandell, B.A. (1986) Analysis of the retinex theory of color vision. *Journal of the Optical Society of America A*, 3, 1651–61.

Brainard, D.H. and Wandell, B.A. (1990) Calibrated processing of image color. *Color Research and Application*, 15, 266–71.

Brainard, D.H. and Wandell, B.A. (1991) Evaluation of CIE Luv and CIE Lab as perceptual image representations. *Society for Information Display International Symposium Technical Digest*, 22, 799–801.

Brainard, D.H. and Wandell, B.A. (1992) Asymmetric color-matching: how color appearance depends on the illuminant. *Journal of the Optical Society of America A*, 9, 1433–48.

Burnham, R.W., Evans, R.M., and Newhall, S.M. (1957) Prediction of color appearance with different adaptation illuminations. *Journal of the Optical Society of America*, 47, 35–42.

Burns, S.A., Cohen, J.B., and Kuznetsov, E.N. (1990) The Munsell color system in fundamental color space. *Color Research and Application*, 15, 29–51.

Carter, E.C. and Carter, R.C. (1981) Color and conspicuousness. *Journal of the Optical Society of America*, 71, 723–9.

Chichilnisky, E.J. and Wandell, B.A. (1997) Increment-decrement asymmetry in adaptation. *Vision Research*, 37, 616.

CIE (1986) *Colorimetry*, 2nd edn. Bureau Central de la CIE. Publication 15.2.

CIE (1995) *Industrial Color Difference Evaluation*. Bureau Central de la CIE. Publication 116–95.

CIE (1998) *The CIE 1997 Interim Colour Appearance Model (Simple Version), CIECAM97s*. Bureau Central de la CIE. Publication 131–98.

Clark, F.J.J., McDonald, R., and Rigg, B. (1984) Modification to the JPC79 colour-difference formula. *Journal of the Society of Dyers and Colourists*, 100, 128–32.

Cohen, J. (1964) Dependency of the spectral reflectance curves of the Munsell color chips. *Psychonomic Science*, 1, 369–70.

Delahunt, P.B. and Brainard, D.H. (2000) Control of chromatic adaptation: signals from separate cone classes interact. *Vision Research*, 40, 2885–903.

deLange, H. (1958a) Research into the dynamic nature of the human fovea–cortex systems with intermittent and modulated light. I. Attenuation characteristics with white and coloured light. *Journal of the Optical Society of America*, 48, 777–84.

deLange, H. (1958b) Research into the dynamic nature of the human fovea–cortex systems with intermittent and modulated light. II. Phase shift in brightness and delay in color perception. *Journal of the Optical Society of America*, 48, 784–9.

Derefeldt, G. (1991) Colour appearance systems. In P. Gouras (ed.), *The Perception of Colour*. Boca Raton, FL: CRC Press, Inc., pp. 218–61.

DIN (1980) *DIN 6164 Part 1: DIN color chart. System based on the 2-degree standard colorimetric observer*. Berlin: Beuth-Verlag.

Fairchild, M.D. (1998) *Color Appearance Models*. Reading, MA: Addison-Wesley.

Fairchild, M.D. and Berns, R.S. (1993) Image color-appearance specification through extension of Cielab. *Color Research and Application*, 18, 178–90.

Godlove, I.H. (1933) Neutral value scales. II. A comparison of results and equations describing value scales. *Journal of the Optical Society of America*, 23, 419–25.

Helson, H. (1938) Fundamental problems in color vision. I. The principle governing changes in hue, saturation and lightness of non-selective samples in chromatic illumination. *Journal of Experimental Psychology*, 23, 439–76.

Helson, H. and Jeffers, V.B. (1940) Fundamental problems in color vision. II. Hue, lightness, and saturation of selective samples in chromatic illumination. *Journal of Experimental Psychology*, 26, 1–27.

Hung, P.C. and Berns, R.S. (1995) Determination of constant hue loci for a CRT gamut and their predictions using color appearances. *Color Research and Application*, 20, 285–95.

Hunt, R.W.G. (1982) A model of colour vision for predicting colour appearance. *Color Research and Application*, 7, 95–112.

Hunt, R.W G. (1987a) A model of colour vision for predicting color appearance in various viewing conditions. *Color Research and Application*, 12, 297–314.

Hunt, R.W.G. (1987b) *The Reproduction of Colour*, 4th edn. Tolworth, England: Fountain Press.

Hunt, R.W.G. (1991) Revised colour-appearance model for related and unrelated colours. *Color Research and Application*, 16, 146–65.

Hunt, R.W.G. and Pointer, M.R. (1985) A colour-appearance transform for the CIE 1931 standard colorimetric observer. *Color Research and Application*, 10, 12–19.

Hurvich, L.M. and Jameson, D. (1957) An opponent-process theory of color vision. *Psychological Review*, 64, 384–404.

Indow, T. (1980) Global color metrics and color appearance systems. *Color Research and Application*, 5, 5–12.

Jaaskelainen, T., Parkkinen, J., and Toyooka, S. (1990) A vector-subspace model for color representation. *Journal of the Optical Society of America A*, 7, 725–30.

Jameson, D. and Hurvich, L.M. (1955) Some quantitative aspects of an opponent-colors theory. I. Chromatic responses and spectral saturation. *Journal of the Optical Society of America*, 45, 546–52.

Jameson, D. and Hurvich, L.M. (1964) Theory of brightness and color contrast in human vision. *Vision Research*, 4, 135–54.

Judd, D.B. (1940) Hue saturation and lightness of surface colors with chromatic illumination. *Journal of the Optical Society of America*, 30, 2–32.

Judd, D.B., MacAdam, D.L., and Wyszecki, G.W. (1964) Spectral distribution of typical daylight as a function of correlated color temperature. *Journal of the Optical Society of America*, 54, 1031–40.

Judd, D.B. and Wyszecki, G. (1975) *Color in Business, Science, and Industry*. New York: John Wiley and Sons.

Krantz, D. (1968) A theory of context effects based on cross-context matching. *Journal of Mathematical Psychology*, 5, 1–48.

Krantz, D.H. (1975) Color measurement and color theory: II. Opponent-colors theory. *Journal of Mathematical Psychology*, 12, 304–27.

Krauskopf, J., Williams, D.R., and Heeley, D.W. (1982) Cardinal directions of color space. *Vision Research*, 22, 1123–31.

Land, E.H. (1986) Recent advances in retinex theory. *Vision Research*, 26, 7–21.

Land, E.H. and McCann, J.J. (1971) Lightness and retinex theory. *Journal of the Optical Society of America*, 61, 1–11.

Larimer, J., Krantz, D.H., and Cicerone, C.M. (1974) Opponent-process additivity – I. Red/green equilibria. *Vision Research*, 14, 1127–40.
Larimer, J., Krantz, D.H., and Cicerone, C.M. (1975) Opponent process additivity – II. Yellow/blue equilibria and non-linear models. *Vision Research*, 15, 723–31.
MacAdam, D.L. (1935) The theory of the maximum visual efficiency of colored materials. *Journal of the Optical Society of America*, 25, 249–52.
MacAdam, D.L. (1942) Visual sensitivities to color differences in daylight. *Journal of the Optical Society of America*, 32, 247–74.
MacAdam, D.L. (1974) Uniform color scales. *Journal of the Optical Society of America*, 64, 1691–702.
MacAdam, D.L. (1978) Colorimetric data for samples of OSA uniform color scales. *Journal of the Optical Society of America*, 68, 121–30.
Maloney, L.T. (1986) Evaluation of linear models of surface spectral reflectance with small numbers of parameters. *Journal of the Optical Society of America A*, 3 (10), 1673–83.
Marimont, D.H. and Wandell, B.A. (1992) Linear models of surface and illuminant spectra. *Journal of the Optical Society of America A*, 9, 1905–13.
McCamy, C.S. (1985) Physical exemplification of color order systems. *Color Research and Application*, 10, 20–5.
McLaren, K. (1970) The Adams–Nickerson colour-difference formula. *Journal of the Society of Dyers of Colourists*, 86, 354–66.
McLaren, K. (1971) Adams–Nickerson colour-difference formula: correction and addenda. *J. Soc. Dyers Colourists*, 87, 159.
Mullen, K.T. (1985) The contrast sensitivity of human colour vision to red–green and blue–yellow chromatic gratings. *Journal of Physiology (London)*, 359, 381–400.
Munsell, A.E.O., Sloan, L.L., and Godlove, I.H. (1933) Neutral value scales. I. Munsell neutral value scale. *Journal of the Optical Society of America*, 23, 394–411.
Munsell, A.H. (1915) *Atlas of the Munsell Color System*. Malden, MA: Wadsworth–Howland & Company.
Munsell, A.H. (1992) *A Color Notation*, 17th edn. Newburgh, NY: Macbeth.
Nagy, A.L. and Sanchez, R.R. (1990) Critical color differences determined with a visual search task. *Journal of the Optical Society A*, 7, 1209–17.
Nayatani, Y., Hashimoto, K., Takahama, K., and Sobagaki, H. (1987) A non-linear color-appearance model using Estevez–Hunt–Pointer primaries. *Color Research and Application*, 12, 231–42.
Nayatani, Y., Sobagaki, H., and Takahama, K. (1986) Prediction of color appearance under various adapting conditions. *Color Research and Application*, 11, 62–71.
Nayatani, Y., Takahama, K., and Sobagaki, H. (1981) Formulation of a nonlinear model of chromatic adaptation. *Color Research and Application*, 6, 161–71.
Nayatani, Y., Takahama, K., Sobagaki, H., and Hashimoto, K. (1990) Color–appearance model and chromatic adaptation transform. *Color Research and Application*, 15, 210–21.
Newhall, S.M. (1940) Preliminary report of the O.S.A. subcommittee on the spacing of the Munsell colors. *Journal of the Optical Society of America*, 30, 617–45.
Newhall, S.M., Nickerson, D., and Judd, D.B. (1943) Final report of the O.S.A. subcommittee on the spacing of Munsell Colors. *Journal of the Optical Society of America*, 33, 385–412.
Nickerson, D. (1940) History of the Munsell color system and its scientific application. *Journal of the Optical Society of America*, 30, 575–86.
Poirson, A.B. and Wandell, B.A. (1990) Task-dependent color discrimination. *Journal of the Optical Society of America A*, 7, 776–82.
Poirson, A.B. and Wandell, B.A. (1993) Appearance of colored patterns – pattern color separability. *Journal of the Optical Society of America A*, 10, 2458–70.
Poirson, A.B. and Wandell, B.A. (1996) Pattern–color separable pathways predict sensitivity to simple colored patterns. *Vision Research*, 36, 515–26.
Richter, M. and Witt, K. (1986) The story of the DIN color system. *Color Research and Application*, 11, 138–45.
Robertson, A.R. (1977) The CIE 1976 color-difference formulae. *Color Research and Application*, 2, 7–11.
Robertson, A.R. (1984) Colour order systems: an introductory review. *Color Research and Application*, 9, 234–40.
Rosch, S. (1928) Die Kennzeichnung der Farben. *Physikalische Zeitschrift*, 29, 83–91.
Schrödinger, E. (1920) Theorie der pigmente von grosster leuchtkraft. *Annalen der Physik (Leipzig)*, 62, 603–22.
Sekiguchi, N., Williams, D.R., and Brainard, D.H. (1993) Efficiency for detecting isoluminant and isochromatic interference fringes. *Journal of the Optical Society of America A*, 10, 2118–33.
Semmelroth, C.J. (1970) Prediction of lightness and brightness on different backgrounds. *Journal of the Optical Society of America*, 60, 1685–9.
Shevell, S.K. (1978) The dual role of chromatic backgrounds in color perception. *Vision Research*, 18, 1649–61.
Shevell, S.K. and Wesner, M.F. (1989) Color appearance under conditions of chromatic adaptation and contrast. *Color Research and Application*, 14, 309–17.
Silverstein, L.D. and Merrifield, R.M. (1981) Color selection and verification testing for airborne color CRT displays. *Fifth Advanced Aircrew Display Symposium, Naval Air Test Center, Patuxent River, MD.*
Silverstein, L.D. and Merrifield, R.M. (1985) The development and evaluation of color systems for airborne applications. *DOT/FAA/PM-85-19, US Department of Transportation, Federal Aviation Administration.*
Simon, F.T. and Frost, J.A. (1987) A new method for the conversion of CIE colorimetric data to Munsell notations. *Color Research and Application*, 12, 256–61.
Smith, N. S., Whitfield, T.W.A., and Wiltshire, T.J. (1990a) A colour notation conversion program. *Color Research and Application*, 15, 338–43.

Smith, N.S., Whitfield, T.W.A., and Wiltshire, T.J. (1990b) Comparison of the Munsell, NCS, DIN, and Coloroid colour order systems using the OSA–UCS model. *Color Research and Application*, 15, 327–37.

Speigle, J.M. (1997) Testing whether a common repersentation explains the effects of viewing context on color appearance. Unpublished PhD Thesis, University of California, Santa Barbara.

Speigle, J.M. and Brainard, D.H. (1996) Is color constancy task independent? *IS&T/SID Color Imaging Conference: Color Science, Systems, and Applications, Scottsdale, AZ*, pp. 167–72.

Speigle, J.M. and Brainard, D.H. (1999) Predicting color from gray: the relationship between achromatic adjustment and asymmetric matching. *Journal of the Optical Society of America A*, 16, 2370–6.

Stiles, W.S. (1959) Color vision: The approach through increment threshold sensitivity. *Proceedings National Academy of Sciences (USA)*, 45, 100–14.

Stiles, W.S. (1967) Mechanism concepts in colour theory. *Journal of the Colour Group*, 11, 106–23.

Stokes, M., Fairchild, M.D., and Berns, R.S. (1992) Precision requirements for digital color reproduction. *ACM Transactions on Graphics*, 11, 406–22.

Swedish Standards Institution (1982) *Swedish Standard SS 01 91 03 CIE tristimulus values and chromaticity coordinates for colour samples in SS 01 91 02*. Stockholm.

Swedish Standards Institution (1983) *Swedish Standard SS 01 91 01 CIE tristimulus values and chromaticity coordinates for some 16000 colour notations according to SS 01 91 00*. Stockholm: SSI.

Swedish Standards Institution (1989) *Swedish Standard SS 0191 02 colour atlas*, 2nd edn. Stockholm: SSI.

Tominaga, S. (1993) Color notation conversion by neural networks. *Color Research and Application*, 18, 253–9.

Usai, S., Nakaguchi, S., and Nakano, M. (1992) Reconstruction of Munsell color space by a five-layer neural network. *Journal of the Optical Society of America A*, 9, 516–20.

von Kries, J. (1902) Chromatic adaptation. Originally published in *Festschrift der Albrech-Ludwigs-Universitat*, pp. 145–8. Translated in D.L. MacAdam (ed.), *Sources of Color Vision*. Cambridge, MA: MIT Press.

von Kries, J. (1905) Influence of adaptation on the effects produced by luminous stimuli. In *Handbuch der Physiologie des Menschen*, Vol. 3, pp. 109–282. Translated in D.L. MacAdam (ed.), *Sources of Color Vision*. Cambridge, MA: MIT Press.

Walraven, J. (1976) Discounting the background: The missing link in the explanation of chromatic induction. *Vision Research*, 16, 289–95.

Wandell, B.A. and Brainard, D.H. (1989) Towards cross-media color reproduction. Proceedings: OSA applied vision topical meeting, San Francisco, CA.

Webster, M.A. and Mollon, J.D. (1995) Colour constancy influenced by contrast adaptation. *Nature*, 373, 694–8.

Werner, J.S. and Walraven, J. (1982) Effect of chromatic adaptation on the achromatic locus: the role of contrast, luminance and background color. *Vision Research*, 22, 929–44.

Whitfield, T.W.A., Powell, A.S., O'Connor, M., and Wiltshire, T.J. (1988) The conceptual NCS: an empirical investigation. *Color Research and Application*, 13, 119–23.

Wyszecki, G. and Stiles, W.S. (1982) *Color Science – Concepts and Methods, Quantitative Data and Formulae*, 2nd edn. New York: John Wiley & Sons.

Zhang, X. and Wandell, B.A. (1997) A spatial extension of CIELAB for digital color-image reproduction. *Journal of the Society for Information Display*, 5, 61–3.

Zhang, X. and Wandell, B.A. (1998) Color image fidelity metrics evaluated using image distortion maps. *Signal Processing*, 70, 201–14.

6 The Physiology of Color Vision

Peter Lennie

Center for Neural Science, New York University, New York, NY 10003, USA

CHAPTER CONTENTS

The Science of Color
ISBN 0–444–512–519

6.1 INTRODUCTION

Most of what we know about color vision has been learned from psychophysical investigations, most of what we know about the underlying physiology has been discovered with the explicit guidance of theories grounded in psychophysical observation, and mostly the physiological findings have confirmed expectations. One might therefore be forgiven for supposing that to discuss the physiology of color vision is merely to provide an account of the mechanics of systems whose operating principles we understand well. To some extent that is true, particularly for the earliest stages of color vision, but modern physiological investigations have also revealed an organization that could not be suspected from psychophysical observations.

This chapter first reviews briefly the gross anatomy of the visual pathway, from the retina to the occipital cortex. Then it examines the physiology of the different stages, beginning with a look at the techniques used to explore it. Relatively little of this work has been undertaken on the human visual system, but a great deal has been done on the visual system of the macaque monkey, which, because its structure is similar to that of the human, is widely thought to be a good model.

6.1.1 BASIC ANATOMY OF THE VISUAL SYSTEM

6.1.1.1 The retina

The image is formed on the retina, shown in vertical cross-section in Figure 6.1. This highlights very clearly the layers that comprise a structure less than 0.5 mm thick.

The general organization of the retina is broadly the same in all vertebrates: there are

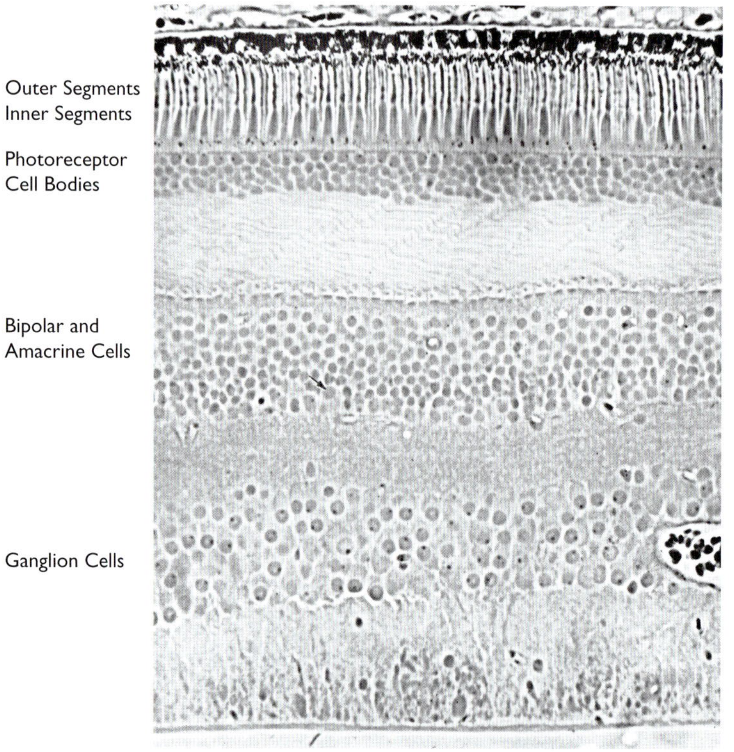

Figure 6.1 Vertical section through the primate retina, showing its layered structure. Light enters the retina from the bottom of the picture, passing through all layers before being absorbed in the outer segments of photoreceptors. The three principal layers of cells are identified. The rods and the cones lie nearest the top of the figure, with their different parts identified. Bipolar cells and amacrine cells lie in the inner nuclear layer. Ganglion cells lie in the ganglion cell layer. (From Boycott and Dowling, 1969, reproduced with permission.)

three vertical stages, with interconnecting horizontal pathways at the junctions between stages. Figure 6.2 shows this diagramatically. The photoreceptors, rods and cones, which form the most peripheral stage, lie farthest from the pupil, and light must pass through the thickness of the retina before being absorbed. Since the neural retina is transparent, this is visually inconsequential. The inverted organization seems to be an adaptation to the demands of the photoreceptors – metabolically the most active cells in the body – which derive their nutrients from the nearby choroid. Structurally, rods and cones are grossly similar, consisting of two clearly defined parts, the inner and outer segments. The outer segment, nearest the choroid, contains the photopigment, and within it originate the light-evoked signals. The inner segment contains the biological support mechanisms.

Until relatively recently most anatomical work on the retina used vertical sections of the kind shown in Figure 6.1. These make clear the vertical strata and also some structural features such as the fovea (Figure 6.3), which contains no rods and where all neurons beyond the cones are displaced, forming a pit over the very densely packed cones.

Although neuroanatomists working with vertical sections have been able to identify some sub-classes of the major neuron groups identified in Figure 6.2 (principally through scrutiny of the levels at which their dendrites and axons branch), the clearest indications of different sub-classes have often emerged through examination

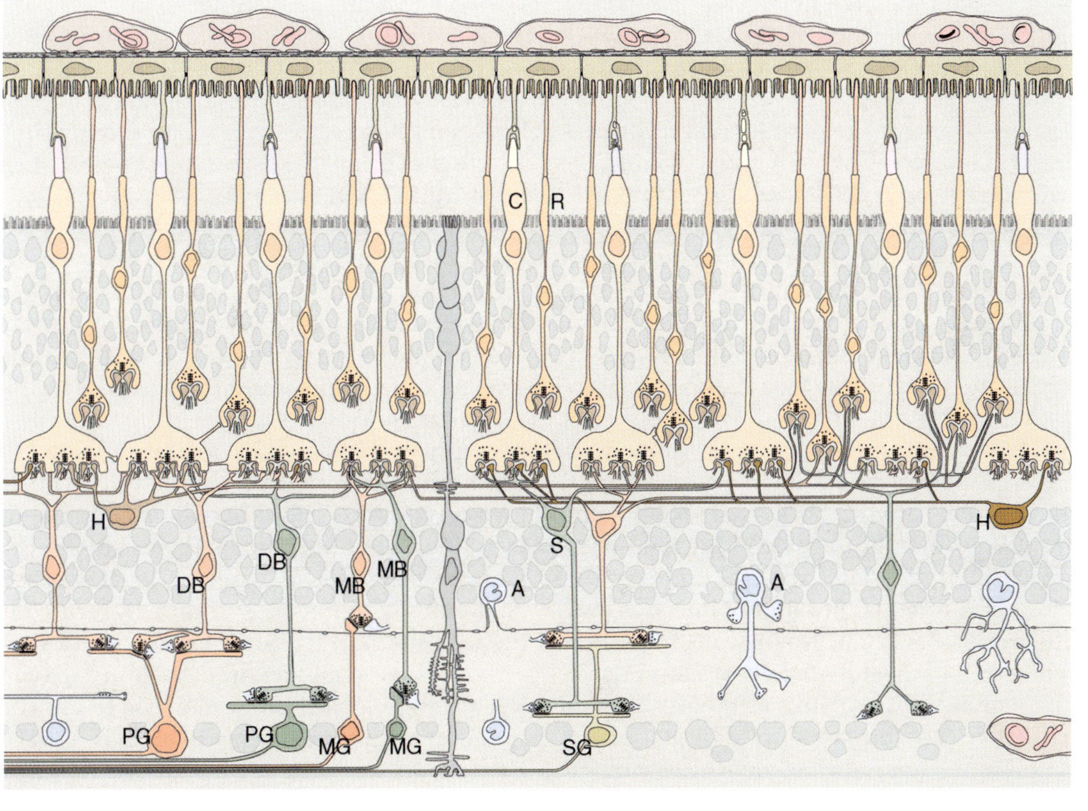

Figure 6.2 Diagram of the neurons and their principal connections in the primate retina. C, cone; R, rod; MB, midget bipolar cell; DB, diffuse bipolar cell; S, S cone bipolar cell; H, horizontal cell; A, amacrine cell; MG, midget ganglion cell; PG, parasol ganglion cell; SG, S cone ganglion cell. Bipolar cells and ganglion cells colored red are off-center types; those colored green are on-center types. (Adapted from Rodieck, 1998, with corrections by R.W. Rodieck.)

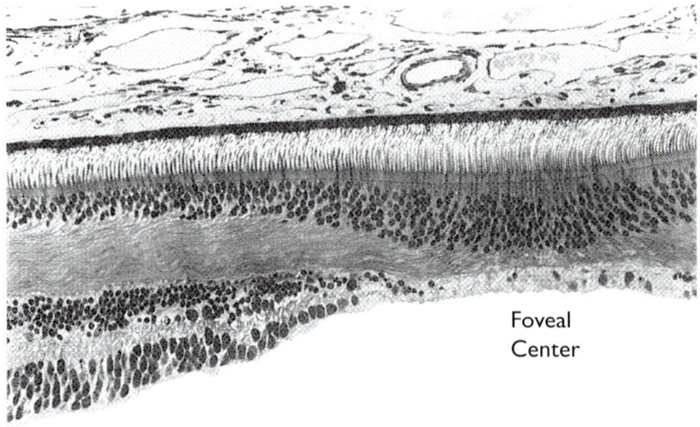

Figure 6.3 Vertical section through the human fovea, showing the elongation of the cones, and the absence of the other neurons, which lie outside the center of the fovea and to which the cones are connected through long fibers. (Photograph courtesy of Anita Hendrickson.)

of horizontal sections of retina – sometimes whole-mounted retinas – in which one can view the retina in the plane of the image, and which reveal the pattern and spread of a neuron's dendritic field.

It is now clear that the primate retina contains several kinds of bipolar cells, several kinds of horizontal cells, several kinds of ganglion cells, and perhaps many kinds of amacrine cells. We will consider some of these in detail later, but for the moment the important idea is that the existence of several types among each major class of cell suggests the retina forms multiple representations of the image. This idea draws clear support from an examination of ganglion cells, whose axons form the optic nerve. Anatomical classes of ganglion cells are characterized principally by the pattern, horizontal extent, and depth of branching of their dendritic fields. The characteristic dimensions vary, of course, with position on the retina, but at any one spot cells of different classes can be robustly distinguished. Ganglion cells of the different classes form quasi-regular mosaics of sampling elements, each of which conveys a (presumably) different representation of the image to the brain. These different arrays project differently into the brain. Their relevance to color vision stems from the fact that different classes of ganglion cells are connected in different ways to the cone photoreceptors.

In the primate retina there are two major and several minor classes of ganglion cells. The two major classes, now widely known as *P cells* and *M cells*,[1] together constitute about 90% of the 1.25 million ganglion cells in each eye. P cells alone probably constitute 80% of all ganglion cells. The most distinctive anatomical difference between them is size: at any one eccentricity the P cells have much smaller cell bodies, smaller dendritic fields, and smaller axons. P and M cells are connected to cones through different kinds of bipolar cells (they both also make indirect connections with rods, but these are not relevant here). In and near the fovea each P cell contacts a single *midget bipolar cell*, which in turn contacts a single cone (Wässle and Boycott, 1991). In the fovea, there are two midget ganglion cells and two midget bipolar cells for every cone. Each cone drives two midget bipolar cells, which in turn drive two P cells. These dual contacts made by a single cone seem to be the origin of distinct pathways, for the two midget bipolar cells are anatomically different, and they in turn contact their counterpart P cells in different planes in the retina. As we shall see, these pathways have different physiological properties. There are corresponding pathways feeding two kinds of M cells. Each M cell contacts a single *diffuse bipolar cell*, which in turn contacts several cones. Other, rarer, kinds of ganglion cells are clearly distinguished anatomically (Rodieck *et al.*, 1993), but except for a bistratified cell that is associated with signals from S cones (Dacey and Lee, 1994), little is known about their function, and their central projections, discussed below, suggest that most have no substantial role in color vision.

The horizontal pathways in the retina, represented by horizontal cells and (to some extent) amacrine cells, seem to be organized to permit the infusion of remote signals into the direct vertical pathways. Horizontal cells, of which there are at least two types, make connections directly with cones at their junctions with bipolar cells, and near the fovea each horizontal cell makes contact with most of the cones that lie in its dendritic field (Wässle *et al.*, 1989; Ahnelt and Kolb, 1994). Amacrine cells exist in many more discernible forms than do other retinal neurons. Some have an identified special role in the transmission of rod signals from bipolar cells to ganglion cells, but beyond some involvement in shaping the responses of ganglion cells, the roles of most are unclear.

6.1.1.2 Central projections

Ganglion cells project to several centers in the brain, notably the superior colliculus (SC) in the midbrain and the lateral geniculate nucleus (LGN) in the thalamus (Figure 6.4). Each optic nerve branches at the optic chiasm, and approximately half of the nerve fibers (representing ganglion cells in the nasal retina) cross to the other hemisphere. The representation of the retinal image is split vertically through the fovea, each half being represented in one hemisphere. The peculiarity of the projection results in the left visual field being represented in the right hemisphere, and *vice-versa*. This brings the representation of visual space broadly into register with the representations provided by other senses, which are all crossed.

The SC is phylogenetically older, and is the more important center in lower mammals; in primates it receives inputs from only a small fraction of the retinal ganglion cells. These cells are of the rarer types found in the retina (i.e., neither P nor M cells). The SC has clear roles in directing eye movements and in intersensory localization (Sparks and Nelson, 1987), but all that we know about it, including the physiology of neurons in it, suggests that it has no consequential role in color vision.

The LGN in primates is a highly developed, laminated, structure to which the retinal P cells and M cells project. The prototypical LGN in the primate has six layers, organized in two distinct groups (Figure 6.5).

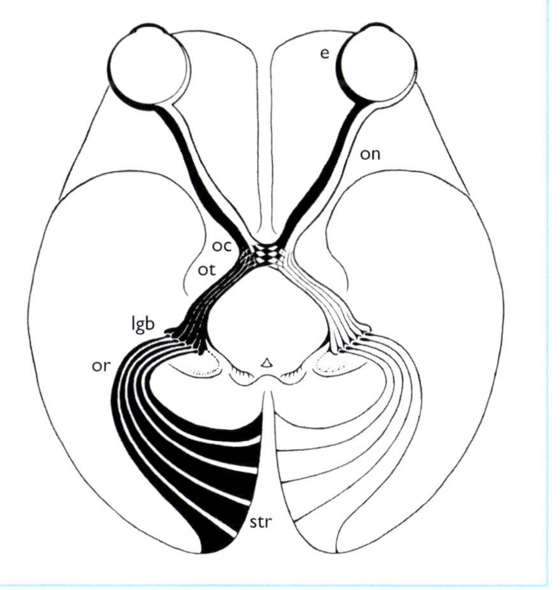

Figure 6.4 **Major visual centers in the brain. The optic nerve (ON) from each eye (E) divides at the optic chiasm (OC), sending half its fibers into the optic tract (OT) of each hemisphere, which projects to the lateral geniculate nucleus (LGB). The lateral geniculate nucleus in turn projects via the optic radiation (OR) to the striate cortex (STR). The projection into each hemisphere originates in the half-retina on that side of the head. (Reproduced with permission from Polyak, 1957. Copyright © 1957, University of Chicago Press.)**

The four dorsal, *parvocellular*, layers receive inputs from the retinal P cells, with those from the left and right eyes being interleaved. The two ventral, *magnocellular*, layers receive inputs from the M cells, separately from each eye. There are no discernible connections among layers, and physiological evidence suggests no function connections. The topography of the retinal image is preserved on the LGN, each layer of which contains an orderly though distorted map. The distortions in the map are broadly consistent with each projecting ganglion cell occupying a fixed territory in the LGN, so that the representation of the central visual field is large – a convenience for physiologists.

6.1.1.3 Visual cortex

Neurons in the LGN project to *striate cortex* (also known as *primary visual cortex* or *V1*), an anatomically distinctive cortical region in the occipital

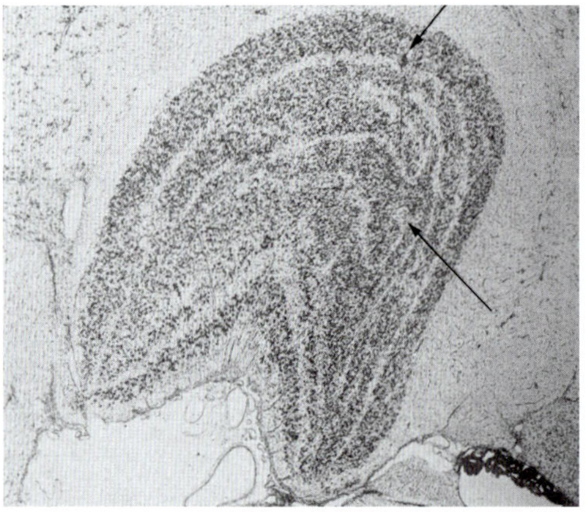

Figure 6.5 Section through the lateral geniculate nucleus (LGN), showing its laminated structure. The prototypical LGN has six layers – four dorsal (parvocellular) layers and two ventral (magnocellular) layers – though this arrangement is not always present. The magnocellular layers are thinner and contain larger cells. The LGN contains a topographical map of the half of the retina that projects to it. The arrows in this figure mark the path of a microelectrode that recorded the discharges of individual neurons. (From Wiesel and Hubel, 1966, reproduced with permission.)

lobe, at the back of the brain. The cortex as a whole is a large, thin (~2 mm) sheet containing several clearly defined layers of neurons, and in the human brain (and to a lesser extent the monkey brain) is deeply folded to fit into the cranial cavity. Cortex is functionally specialized, but, with a few exceptions, its structure provides little evidence of this and almost everywhere is similar anatomically. Figure 6.6 shows the major laminar subdivisions of striate cortex. It differs from cortex elsewhere in the brain by having a much thicker layer 4, to which the incoming fibers from the LGN project.

The general organization of cortex is as follows: inputs from lower levels of the visual pathway arrive in layer 4, ascending outputs to higher levels of the pathway arise in the upper layers (above layer 4), and descending (feedback) outputs to lower levels arise in the lower layers (below layer 4).

The anatomical distinctiveness of striate cortex (the thick layer 4 produces a texture visible to the naked eye) makes it relatively easy to discover that in each hemisphere it contains a single map of the left or right half of the visual field. As would be expected from the topography of the earlier map in the LGN, this contains a large representation of the central visual field and a progressively reduced representation of the peripheral field. Beyond this cortex lies a great deal more that is intimately coupled to vision. Because it is not structurally distinctive, its organization has been less easy to discern, but modern work, using both anatomical and physiological methods, shows unequivocally that it contains multiple maps of the visual field. These maps (at least twenty-two have now been identified) cover the whole of the occipital lobe of the brain, and substantial parts of the temporal and parietal lobes. The fraction of the brain they occupy, and their general arrangement, are most easily seen in representations that unfold the cortex and lay it flat. Figure 6.7 (Felleman and Van Essen, 1991) shows this done for the macaque monkey, and makes clear how large a fraction (around 50%) of cortex is devoted to visual analysis. In the human brain the fraction is considerably smaller, perhaps around 15%.

By tracing the connections among visual areas, and knowing from which layers in cortex these connections originate and to which layers they project, it becomes possible to discover a hierarchical structure that can accommodate, somewhat loosely, all the areas (Figure 6.8). This hierarchy has its origin in striate cortex, ascends through the second visual area, V2, and then on through perhaps seven further levels. Beyond V2 each level contains more than one area, so the general picture that emerges is one of multiple parallel streams organized hierarchically.

The parallel organization of cortical streams reflects to some degree, but by no means fully, the parallel organization of signals conveyed by the M and P pathways through the LGN. The M and P cells project to different subdivisions of layer 4, and these in turn project to other layers within striate cortex. The separate identities of the pathways are generally not well-preserved beyond this level, although a small but distinctive projection that appears to be dominated by signals from the M pathway has been traced from striate cortex to an extrastriate region known as the middle temporal area (MT).

Within the collection of extrastriate cortical areas concerned with vision, there appears to be

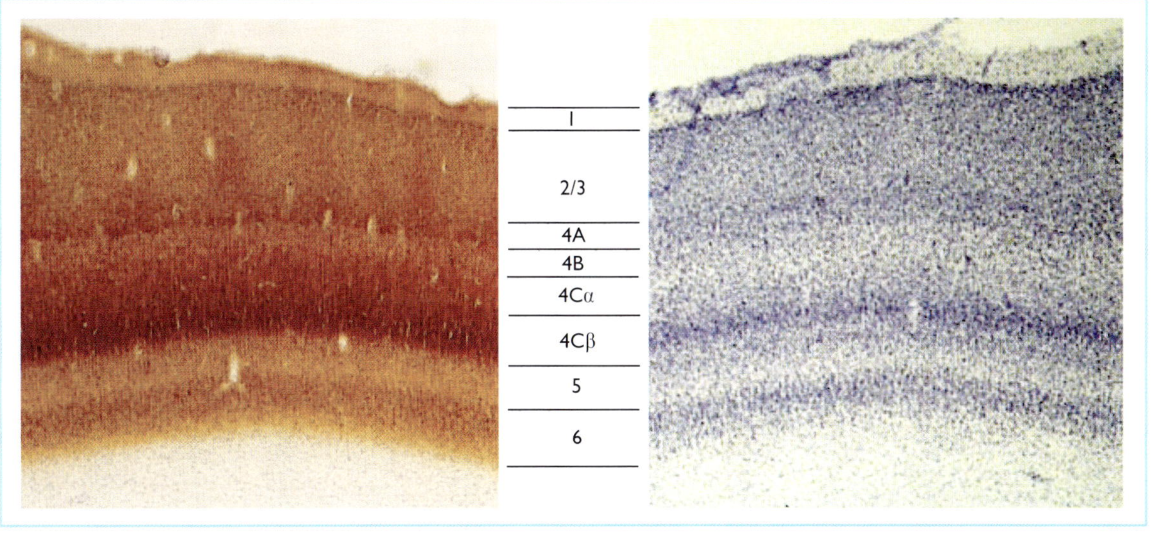

Figure 6.6 **The arrangement of layers in striate cortex, revealed by two stains that highlight different aspects of the organization. (Right) A stain that reveals the locations of the cell bodies of neurons. (Left) A stain for the enzyme cytochrome oxidase, which labels densely the input layers in the middle of cortex, and also shows the 'blobs' in layer 2/3 that are a distinctive feature of the upper layers.**

a broad division into two groups. One contains a set of heirarchically connected areas that form a conduit from striate cortex, through area V2, into the parietal lobe of the brain. The other contains a set of areas that carry information from striate to the temporal lobe. Experimental and clinical studies of parietal cortex show it to have important roles in spatial orientation and visual localization, and perhaps also with the analysis of self-movement, but there are no indications that it is important for color vision. Temporal cortex is for object vision, and damage to it, or to the visual areas that lead to it, can bring about profound disruption of various aspects of object vision, including color vision.

6.1.2 EXPLORING FUNCTION

Some useful inferences about function can be drawn from our knowledge of the structure of the visual pathway (for example, one can infer that P cells are probably important for visual acuity), but a great deal more can be learned by examining activity in the nervous system. Physiologists have available to them a powerful armament of methods. For the purposes of understanding mechanisms of color vision, and particularly how these give rise to perceptual phenomena, most of the activity we need to pursue occurs on a time scale of tens of msec, and on a spatial scale that involves groups of neurons. The following paragraphs review briefly some of the more important methods that are relevant to exploration on these scales, and outline their strengths and weaknesses.

6.1.2.1 Recording signals from individual neurons

Within an individual neuron signals are propagated electrically, and between neurons, chemically, via *neurotransmitters*. In their resting states most neurons maintain a steady potential difference of ~60 mv across the cell membrane. A reduction in this potential difference (depolarization) constitutes the neural signal. The membrane potential is controlled by neurochemical events at the synapses (junctions) between the cell and those from which it receives signals. A neuron receives most of its synaptic connections on its dendrites and soma (Figure 6.9).

Each neuron receives thousands of synaptic connections from other neurons, and each synapse, when active, gives rise to a brief event, a *postsynaptic potential*, that tends either to excite (depolarize) or inhibit (hyperpolarize) the neuron. The aggregate weight of the postsynaptic

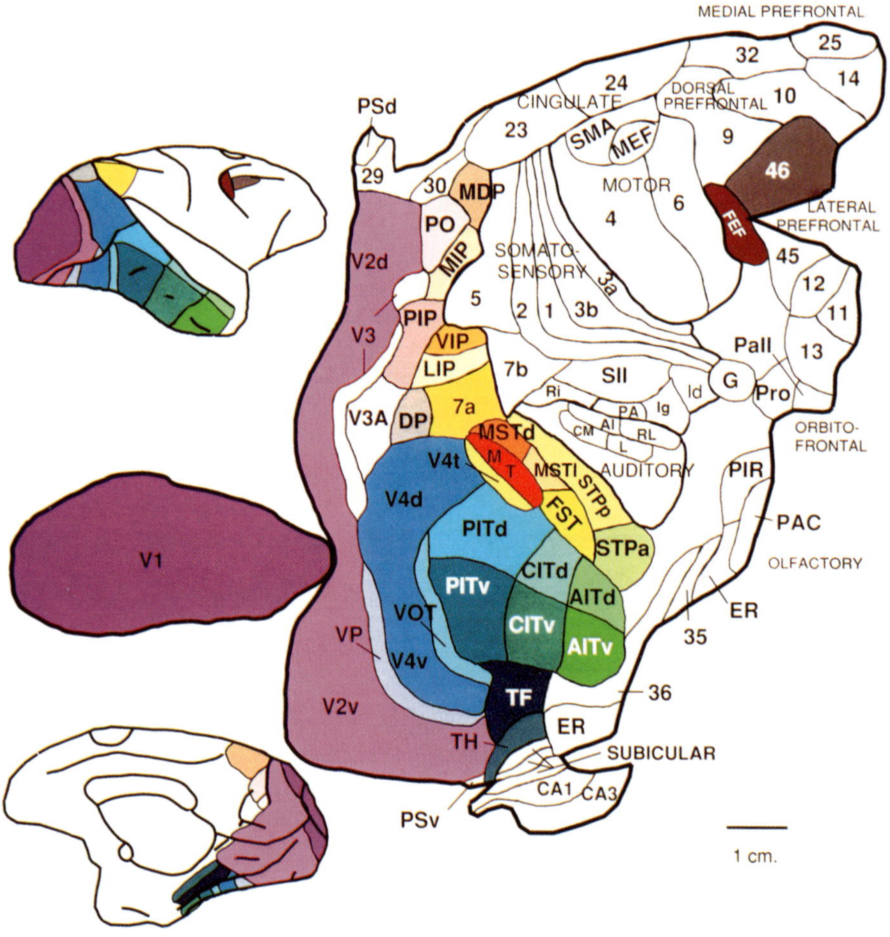

Figure 6.7 **Diagram of the cortex unfolded from one hemisphere of the monkey, showing identified visual areas. The areas that are colored are recognized as being visual sensory areas, or areas closely associated with them. V1 is the primary visual (striate) cortex, which receives input from the lateral geniculate nucleus. V1 projects principally to area V2. Many of these visual areas contain topographically organized maps of the half of the retina that sends a projection to the hemisphere. Visual areas constitute about half of the monkey's cortex. Corresponding areas in the human cortex undoubtedly account for a smaller fraction of the total. (From Felleman and Van Essen, 1991. Reproduced by permission of Oxford University Press.)**

potentials within a certain integration time (and over a certain integration distance) determines the resulting change in the membrane potential of the cell. In most neurons, if the cell becomes sufficiently depolarized (taking the membrane potential from perhaps 60 mv to 50 mv) a large impulsive depolarization *(action potential)* is triggered and propagated rapidly along the membrane. When this action potential reaches the axon terminals, it causes the release of neurotransmitter at synapses making contact with other neurons. Activity at the synaptic connections between cells thus controls the propagation and transformation of signals in the nervous system.

The impulsive nature of most neural communication permits signals to be transmitted rapidly and reliably (within broad limits the existence of an action potential is the important event, rather than its size), and almost all neurons propagate signals via action potentials. A drawback, however, is that the dynamic range of a neuron is limited (the rates at which action potentials are discharged vary from a few per second to, at most,

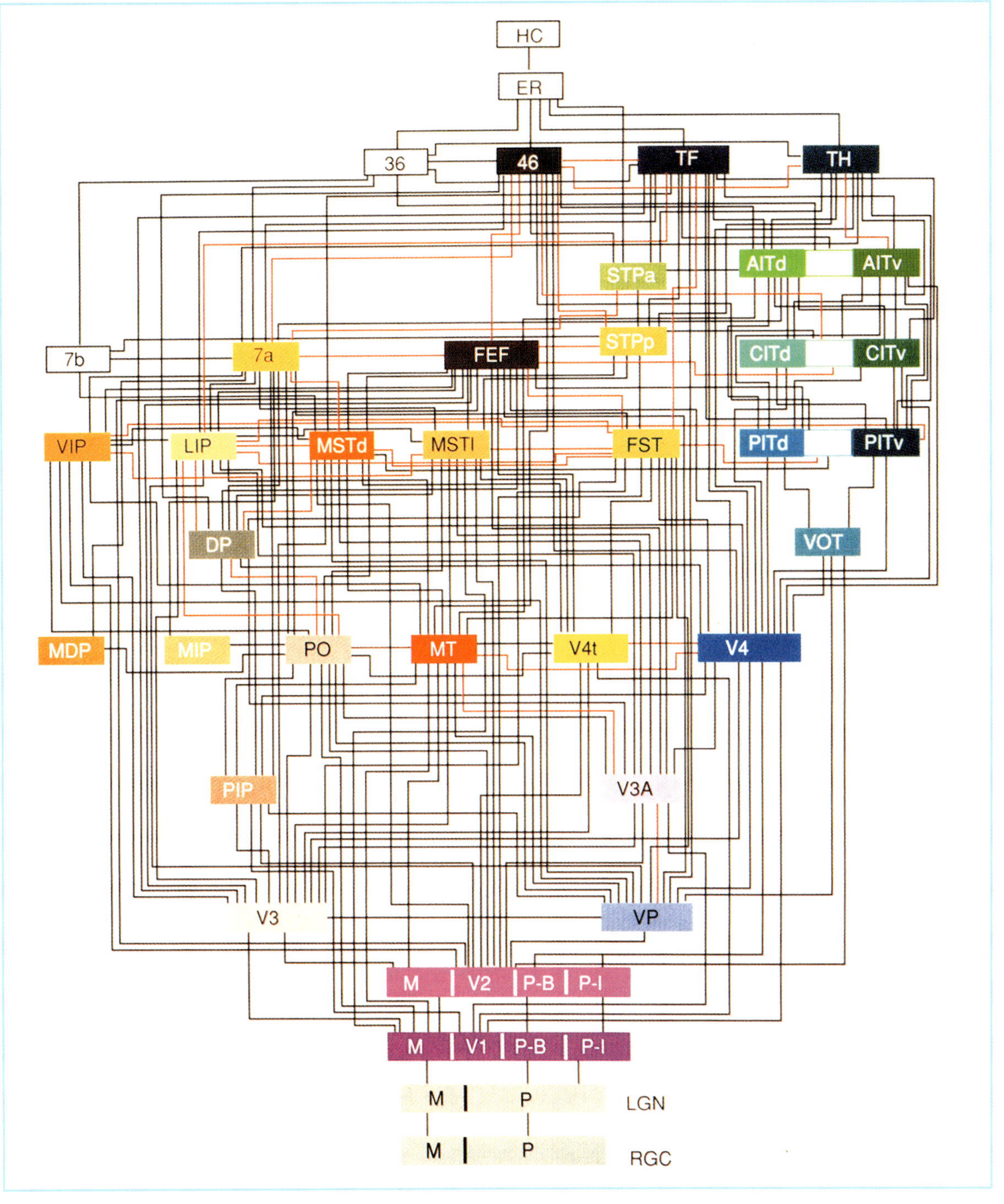

Figure 6.8 Diagram showing the hierarchical organization of visual cortical areas and the known connections among them. The areas at the highest level are at the top. The hierarchy is inferred from the polarities of the connections between areas. Each element in the diagram corresponds to an area identified in Figure 6.7. (From Felleman and Van Essen, 1991. Reproduced by permission of Oxford University Press.)

a few hundred per second). In rarer kinds of neurons, found particularly in sensory systems, the changes in membrane potential induced by synaptic events are propagated passively along the membrane, as relatively slowly changing potentials. This mechanism of transmission is

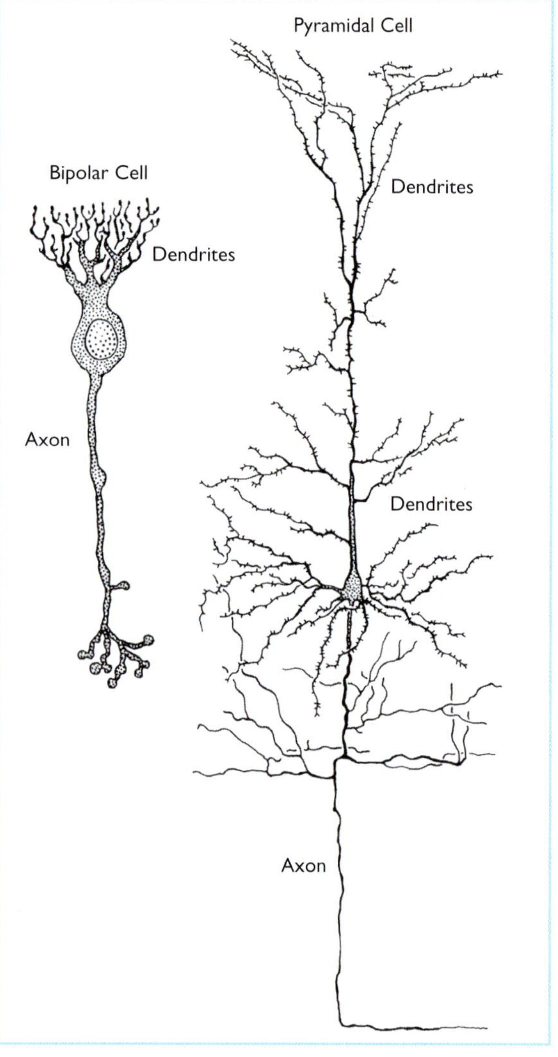

Figure 6.9 **Diagram of the general structure of neurons, and their specializations. (Left) Bipolar cell in the retina. (Right) Pyramidal cell in cortex. The neuron accumulates signals from other cells mostly through synaptic connections on its dendrites. The action potential usually originates at the junction of the cell body and axon, and is propagated down the axon to the axon terminal system where it causes the release of neurotransmitter at synapses. (Adapted from Kuffler and Nichols, 1976.)**

used by all retinal neurons except ganglion cells. It provides neurons with a larger dynamic range than would be possible were action potentials used, but at the cost of slower and less reliable signal transmission over distances.

In many parts of the nervous system individual neurons are large enough to withstand penetration by a microelectrode that can record the potential difference across the membrane. Even where this is not the case microelectrodes that sit just outside the membrane can record (extracellularly) the local electrical disturbance produced by an action potential, though not any slow potentials. Intracellular methods are usually most practicable *in vitro*, when the neurons are not subject to movement by the pulse and other small body movements, but extracellular methods are much more robust, and can record signals from individual neurons in moving animals. The small size of neurons in the primate retina makes it exceptionally difficult to record their activity with intracellular electrodes. Some special techniques have been developed for studying the signals generated by photoreceptors (see the next section), but apart from photoreceptors only ganglion cells have been studied exhaustively in primates, because they generate action potentials that can be recorded with extracellular electrodes. Much of what we know directly about the function of other retinal neurons has been learned through studying reptiles and fish, in which cells are much larger. Elsewhere in the primate's visual system, extracellular recordings provide valuable information about the characteristics of individual neurons.

6.1.2.2 Recording larger scale electrical activity

Gross electrical activity evoked by light can be recorded from several places in the nervous system. The electroretinogram (ERG) is a composite signal that can be recorded either with electrodes placed on the retina, or with surface electrodes on the intact eye. Elements of the composite light-evoked signal can be attributed to different stages of signal analysis in the nervous system. The ERG has been particularly helpful in the analysis of signals generated by photoreceptors.

Gross electrical signals evoked by visual stimuli can be recorded with electrodes placed on the scalp, or on the surface of the cortex. Although large signals can be evoked by time-varying changes in color, they are often difficult to interpret, because the source of the signals is hard to localize.

6.1.2.3 Direct imaging of activity

Active neurons consume more oxygen than inactive ones, and as a result provoke local increase in the circulation of blood. Several recently developed techniques can record these stimulus-induced local changes in the circulation, and have been exploited in attempts to reveal cortical structures that might be involved in the analysis of color. In cortex that can be viewed directly following removal of the skull, one can record changes in the composition of light reflected from the cortical surface to produce a map that shows local regional specialization (Roe and Ts'o, 1995). Positron emission tomography can be used to measure local changes in circulation in the human brain, and has been used to identify regions that are engaged in the analysis of color. The attraction of this method, and similar methods that exploit magnetic resonance imaging (Engel *et al.*, 1997), is that they reveal activity on a scale of millimeters. The drawback is that they measure changes in circulation occurring on a time scale of seconds.

6.2 PHOTORECEPTORS

6.2.1 RECEPTOR SIGNALS

Many of the important steps in the transduction of light to electrical signals in the nervous system are now understood, and have been clearly described (see, for example, Baylor 1987; Torre *et al.*, 1995). The general functional principles are the same in rods and cones, although there are important differences of detail between them, notably in the speed of responses, and in their time-courses. In the dark the receptor maintains a steady potential of ~ −40 mv across its membrane. When the receptor is illuminated, the potential becomes hyperpolarized to as much as −70 mv. This hyperpolarization by an effective stimulus makes photoreceptors unique among vertebrate neurons, which normally become depolarized when excited. Primate cones are too small to accommodate microelectrodes that can measure change in membrane potential, but Baylor and colleagues (Schnapf *et al.*, 1990) have characterized the electrical responses *in vitro* by drawing the outer segment of a cone into a micropipette and measuring the current flow through the outer segment. In darkness, there is a steady inward current (the *dark current*) of 30–50 pA. This arises from the flow of $Na+$ ions through the permeable membrane of the outer segment, and a flow of $K+$ ions out of the inner segment. The current is maintained by pumps in the inner segment that drive $Na+$ ions out and $K+$ ions in. During illumination, the $Na+$ permeability of the outer-segment membrane is reduced, and the current flow correspondingly reduced, resulting in hyperpolarization of the membrane. These light-induced changes in outer-segment membrane conductance result from a recently discovered cascade of biochemical events inside the outer segment (Pugh and Lamb, 1993; Torre *et al.*, 1995). In darkness, the photoreceptors release neurotransmitter continuously from their terminals, which contact bipolar cells and horizontal cells. The absorption of light and consequent hyperpolarization of the cell reduces the amount of transmitter released.

6.2.2 VISUAL PROPERTIES

Figure 6.10 shows the change in current flowing through the outer segment of a single monkey cone induced by a series of brief flashes of progressively increased intensity, at three wavelengths.

Several important principles can be inferred. First, over a substantial range of progressively increasing flash intensities, the cone's responses have exactly the same shape, and can be superimposed if scaled by the flash intensity. This linear relationship between light intensity and response breaks down at high flash intensities, where the responses saturate. Second, the cones generate sets of responses of identical shape regardless of the wavelength of light that excites them – they are univariant. Third, the responses are biphasic, and last considerably longer than the flash.

6.2.2.1 Spectral sensitivity

Given the univariance of a cone, demonstrated very clearly by Baylor *et al.* (1987), its spectral sensitivity can be readily measured by finding, at each of several wavelengths, the flash intensity required to evoke a response of a specified size. Figure 6.11 shows the result of essentially this kind of measurement made on a sample of cones from the macaque retina (Baylor *et al.*, 1987).

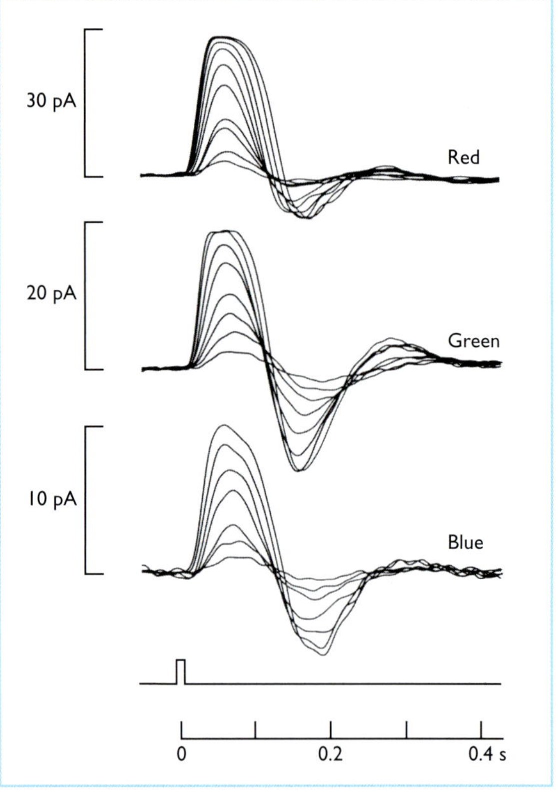

Figure 6.10 Current flow induced in the outer-segment of the three kinds of primate cones. Each set of traces shows the responses to brief flashes (identified by the pulse at bottom) at a series of intensities stepped by factors of 2. The responses of low and middle amplitudes would be superimposed if scaled by the flash intensity. (From Schnapf *et al.*, 1990, reproduced with permission.)

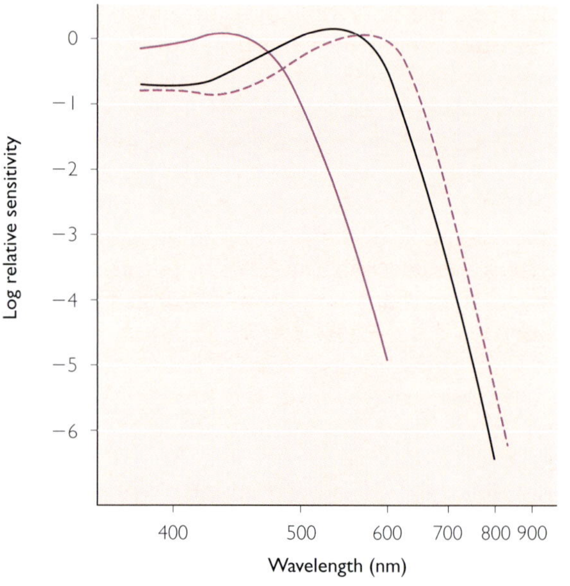

Figure 6.11 Spectral sensitivities of cones in the retina of the macaque monkey. From left to right the curves show the averaged spectral sensitivities of small samples of S, M, and L cones. (From Baylor *et al.*, 1987, reproduced with permission.)

These measurements, remarkable for the range of wavelengths over which they can be made, show higher sensitivity at short wavelengths than is found in curves of cone fundamentals measured psychophysically. Differences of this kind would be expected from the different circumstances under which measurements are made – the psychophysically derived fundamentals include the effects of selective absorption of light by passive filters in the eye, and of self-screening by photopigment. After correcting for the effects of these other absorbing filters, a linear transformation of the cone spectral sensitivities describes well the shapes of the color-matching functions measured by Stiles and Burch (1959).

The measurements in Figure 6.11 are averages from populations of cones that fall very tightly into three distinct groups. No electrophysiological measurements have revealed cones with *anomalous* spectral sensitivities, neither have spectrophotometric methods that measure directly the absorption spectrum of the photopigment in the outer segment, and which have been applied to larger numbers of cones from retinas of old-world primates. Anomalous pigments have been found in the cones of new-world primates (Mollon *et al.*, 1984).

6.2.2.2 Light adaptation

The small dynamic range of impulse-discharging neurons requires that the retina map an enormous range of light levels on to a small range of signal amplitudes in optic nerve fibers. We know something of the general principles that govern this relationship between output and input: the retina as a whole preserves little information about the absolute level of illumination, and at any moment the range of outputs is mapped on to a small part of the input range around the ambient level of illumination; the input range represented in the output is larger at higher levels of illumination. The upshot is that the signal entering the optic nerve conveys information about the local *contrast* in the image. To achieve this requires two kinds of regulating mechanisms: a subtractive one to discard the signal about the ambient level of illumination, and a multiplicative one to reduce the gain of signal transmission (Walraven *et al.*, 1989). Cones contribute something to the normalization of these signals.

Because each cone – at least in and near the fovea – appears to have an essentially private pathway through the retina, and does not pool its signals with those from other cones, there would appear to be some advantage in regulating sensitivity at the receptors. Psychophysical measurements demonstrate light-adaptation in mechanisms that have spectral sensitivities close to those of individual cones (Stiles, 1939); physiological measurements, made by recording extracellular current flow across outer segments (Valeton and van Norren, 1983), *in vivo*, measurements of current flow in single cones *in vitro* (Schnapf *et al.*, 1990), and measurements of the *a*-wave of the electroretinogram (Hood and Birch, 1993) show that steady illumination reduces the sensitivity of cones through a multiplicative gain reduction, and possibly also some response compression. At high levels of illumination (above 10^4 td), photopigment bleaching contributes substantially to the reduction in sensitivity. It is not clear from physiological measurements that the regulation of sensitivity within cones is sufficient to explain gain changes measured psychophysically; the latter are evident at low levels of illumination that do not desensitize cones, and implicate mechanisms beyond cones, perhaps at the synaptic connections between cones and bipolar cells.

There appears also to be some subtractive mechanism within the cones, for over much of their operating range the *steady-state* responses to standing background illumination vary little with level of illumination. Figure 6.12, which shows how flash responses vary with the strength of background and flash, illustrates the effects of both desensitizing gain changes and subtractive changes that stabilize the responses to standing backgrounds.

6.2.2.3 Dynamics

A cone's biphasic response to a flash (Figure 6.10) implies a band-pass frequency characteristic. The Fourier transform of the response to a pulse can be used to reveal a cone's sensitivity to different temporal frequencies. When this is done to a moderately light-adapted cone (Figure 6.13) we see that it has a pass-band that peaks near 5 Hz, with sensitivity falling on either side.

The extent to which cones limit the temporal resolving power of the visual system is unclear. The temporal characteristics of vision depend on the spatial (Robson, 1966), and chromatic

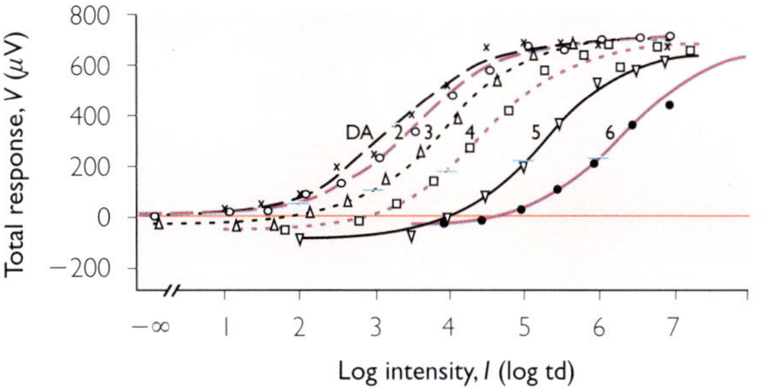

Figure 6.12 **Responses of primate cones to a series of flashes of different intensity, recorded in the presence of backgrounds at a range of intensities. Each curve represents the set of responses obtained on a single background, whose intensity is marked by the short horizontal bar on that curve. Points to the left of the bar represent responses to decremental flash, points to the right, responses to incremental flashes. The operating range of the cones is set by the background. (Reprinted from Valeton and van Norren, 1983. Copyright © 1983, with permission from Elsevier.)**

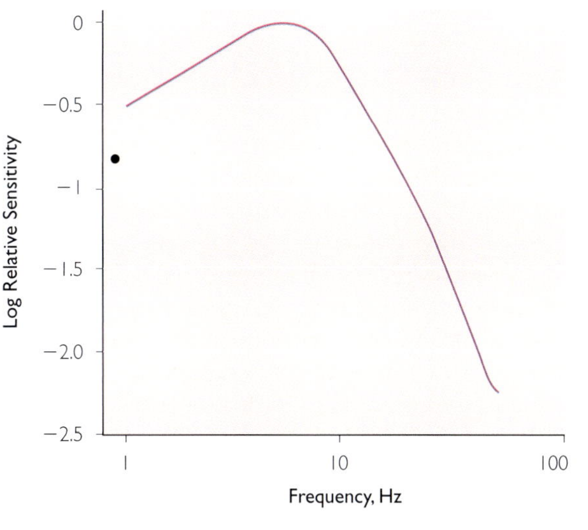

Figure 6.13 **Temporal modulation transfer function of primate cones, obtained by Fourier transform of the impulse response. (Courtesy of W. Makous.)**

(Estévez and Spekreijse, 1974) attributes of stimuli in ways that suggest that cones seldom limit the temporal resolving power of the visual system; measurements of the late receptor potential (a component of the electroretinogram attributed to photoreceptors) point to the same conclusion (Boynton and Baron, 1975).

The kinetics of the cone's photocurrent response to flashes vary little with level of light-adaptation (Schnapf *et al.*, 1990), so the adaptation-dependent changes observed psychophysically (Kelly, 1961) apparently must reflect action at later sites.

6.3 INTERMEDIATE RETINAL NEURONS

6.3.1 HORIZONTAL CELLS AND BIPOLAR CELLS

6.3.1.1 Connections to cones

Horizontal cells and bipolar cells make synaptic contacts with cones through a specialized connection (the 'triad') that seems designed to permit horizontal cells to regulate the transmission of signals from cones to bipolar cells. The triad consists of a central bipolar cell dendrite flanked by two horizontal cell dendrites. Each cone accommodates 20–30 triads in invaginations in its pedicle (foot).

Two morphological classes of horizontal cells (H1, H2) have been identified in the primate retina; a third class (H3) might also be present (Kolb *et al.*, 1994). The H2 cell contacts only cones; the H1 horizontal cell contacts both rods and cones: dendrites contact cones, axon terminals contact rods. The axon is long and thin and apparently provides rather poor communication between the two ends of the cell, which are often considered to operate relatively independently. Each horizontal cell appears to contact every L and M cone within its dendritic field (in the fovea covering perhaps six or seven cones, in the periphery perhaps two to three times as many), but only H2 cells contact all S cones (Wässle *et al*, 1989; Ahnelt and Kolb, 1994). H1 cells make very few contacts with S cones (Ahnelt and Kolb, 1994; Goodchild *et al.*, 1996).

Two morphologically distinctive types of bipolar cells contact cones: *diffuse* bipolar cells and *midget* bipolar cells (other types contact rods). Diffuse bipolars contact 5–7 cones (Boycott and Wässle, 1991); a midget bipolar cell contacts a single cone, everywhere in the retina (Wässle *et al.*, 1994). Each class of bipolar cell appears to exist in two sub-types, named for the characteristic morphology of their cone connections. An *invaginating* bipolar cell inserts a dendritic terminal into the cone pedicle, forming the central element of a triad; a *flat* bipolar cell makes contacts with the surface of the pedicle. In the central retina each cone probably makes contact with four bipolar cells, one of each kind (Wässle and Boycott, 1991).

6.3.1.2 Functional organization

Primate horizontal cells have not been studied *in vivo*, but single-unit recordings in cat, where horizontal cells resemble in form and connections the H1 type in primate, show some mixing of rod and cone signals at levels of illumination where both receptor types are active (Lankheet *et al.*, 1991). *In vitro* recordings from H1 cells in primate (Verweij *et al.*, 1999) show that they too receive rod input.

The dense connections horizontal cells make with the cones underlying their dendritic fields implies mixing of signals from cones of different types. *In vitro* recordings from horizontal cells in the intact retina (Dacey, 1996; Dacey *et al.*, 1996) show that H1 cells receive signals of the same polarity from L cones and M cones, but not S cones; H2 cells receive signals from all cone classes, with that from S cones being conspicuous.

Bipolar cells receive direct signals from cones and perhaps directly from horizontal cells. Each bipolar cell is connected to a region of retina (or, equivalently, it views a region of visual space) within which light will evoke some physiological response. This is known as the *receptive field*. Receptive fields in vertebrates typically consist of two concentrically organized regions, a circular center and enclosing, overlapping, surround (Naka, 1976), and the primate is no exception (Dacey *et al.*, 2000). Center and surround generate signals of opposite polarity, so that when both are illuminated together, the bipolar cell responds poorly. The receptive field surround appears to originate in H1 horizontal cells, which influence the bipolar cell either directly, or by regulating transmission of signals from cones

(Dacey *et al.*, 2000). The midget bipolar cell in the primate will therefore have a receptive field in which the center and surround have different spectral sensitivities: the spectral sensitivity of the center is that of a single cone, while the spectral sensitivity of the surround is that of horizontal cells that accumulate signals from both L and M cones. The spectral sensitivities of the center and surround of a diffuse bipolar cell are probably more alike, because each mechanism draws inputs from several cones.

L and M cones, and their associated pathways, are not distinguishable by modern histological methods, but Kouyama and Marshak (1992) have identified an immunocytochemically distinct class of invaginating midget bipolar cells that are connected only to S cones. In most instances each bipolar cell contacts a single cone, although each S cone contacts more than one bipolar cell (Mariani, 1984; Kouyama and Marshak, 1992).

There are two functional types of bipolar cells: one in which illumination of the center depolarizes the cell and illumination of the surround hyperpolarizes it (often known as ON-bipolar cells), another in which illumination of the center hyperpolarizes the cell, and illumination of the surround depolarizes it (OFF-bipolar cells). These two fundamental types seem to exist in all retinas, and provide the first stages of on- and off-pathways that remain distinct as far as visual cortex.

The on- and off- types of bipolar cell appear to be the physiological expression of an anatomical distinction we noted earlier: on-bipolar cells make invaginating contacts with cones; off-bipolar cells make flat contacts with cones (Stell *et al.*, 1977). In general, each cone therefore provides a signal to two on-pathways (midget and diffuse), and two off-pathways. The organization of connections to S cones might be different: a presumed on-pathway is known to exist, but although a counterpart off-pathway might be inferred from the presence of some flat bipolar cell contacts that appear on S cones (Kouyama and Marshak, 1992), the bipolar cells making these contacts have not been identified.

6.3.1.3 Amacrine cells

Amacrine cells (named by Cajal for their lack of an axon) lie in the inner retina and make connections with bipolar cells and ganglion cells. They exist in a wide variety of morphological types (Masland, 1988; Wässle and Boycott, 1991). With rare exceptions, little is known about their roles. Some amacrine cells might have little to do directly with vision, instead controlling functions such as eye-growth (Schaeffel *et al.*, 1995). One class of amacrine cell (AII) provides an essential link in the chain from rod photoreceptor to ganglion cell: it links the rod bipolar cell through an inhibitory synapse to a diffuse cone off-bipolar cell, and through an excitatory synapse to an on-bipolar cell. These cone bipolar cells in turn contact ganglion cells (Sterling *et al.*, 1988). Amacrine cells that contact midget bipolar cells and midget ganglion cells make indiscriminate contacts with all midget bipolar cells within reach. These include bipolar cells driven by both L and M cones (Calkins and Sterling, 1996). Most types of amacrine cells are not directly interposed between bipolar and ganglion cells, and the general organization of their connections suggests that they modulate the transmission of information from bipolar cells to ganglion cells, or add components to the receptive fields of ganglion cells.

No physiological recordings have been obtained *in vivo* from amacrine cells in primates, but where recordings have been obtained from other species amacrine cells have often exhibited complex behaviors (for example giving depolarizing responses to both light onset and light offset) that suggest an important role in the formation of some distinctive nonlinear behaviors in kinds of ganglion cells that project to the superior colliculus (see below). Where receptive fields have been characterized (Kaneko, 1973) they are circular, but have no center-surround organization.

6.4 GANGLION CELLS AND LGN CELLS

Neurons in LGN are, in their general behavior, almost indistinguishable from the ganglion cells that drive them, so it is convenient to consider both kinds together. Because different classes of LGN neuron are segregated in different layers of the nucleus, and can be selected for study, LGN neurons are more often studied than ganglion cells.

6.4.1 STRUCTURAL ISSUES

In primate retina the principal classes of bipolar cells, midget and diffuse, make specific connections in the *inner plexiform layer* (IPL) with the two kinds of ganglion cells known as parasol and midget cells. A midget bipolar cell in the fovea (Calkins *et al.*, 1994), and to eccentricities of perhaps 6°, makes exclusive contact with a single midget ganglion cell, providing each cone with a private pathway through the retina. A parasol cell in the fovea receives inputs, via diffuse bipolar cells, from perhaps 30–50 cones (Grünert *et al.*, 1993).

The on- and off- types of each of the major classes of bipolar cell contact their counterpart ganglion cells at different depths within the retina, permitting the identification of on- and off-center ganglion cells in anatomical sections (Perry *et al.*, 1984; Watanabe and Rodieck, 1989). The on-bipolars contact on-center ganglion cells in a stratum of the IPL closer to the ganglion cells (Famiglietti and Kolb, 1976).

Recent anatomical evidence points to reliable structural differences among midget pathways that might be associated with the L and M cones. Calkins *et al.* (1994) found that (within each of the major classes, on- and off-) most midget bipolar cells in the monkey retina made one of two different kinds of synaptic connections with midget ganglion cells: either the synapse had around 50 synaptic ribbons, or it had around 30, with no overlap between the distributions. There is a corresponding disparity in the numbers of synaptic ribbons each kind of bipolar cell makes with the cone that drives it. The bipolar cells making the two kinds of connections were randomly distributed on the retina. Among the bipolar-ganglion connections studied, 44% had the larger number of synaptic ribbons. These different synaptic connections might reflect differences between the pathways conveying signals from L and M cones, although it is not known which kind of cone might be associated with each pathway.

It is not known if any midget ganglion cells convey S cone signals, but these signals are known to be carried by another, relatively rare, kind of ganglion cell described by Rodieck (1991) and Dacey (1993). This *small bistratified* cell has dendrites that branch in two planes in the IPL, one in the region where off-bipolars contact midget ganglion cells, and the other in the region where on-bipolars contact midget ganglion cells. The span of the bistratified cell's dendrites matches that of the parasol cell, so in the fovea might cover 30–50 cones, and the cell might receive signals from 3–5 S cones. Small bistratified cells constitute less than 2% of ganglion cells in and near the fovea (Dacey, 1994), and probably provide a mosaic that is too coarse to account for the spatial resolving power of the S cone system measured psychophysically (Williams and Collier, 1983). This and other evidence to be reviewed below suggests that the retina must contain additional S cone pathways.

Parasol and midget cells project respectively to the magnocellular and parvocellular divisions of the LGN (Perry *et al.*, 1984); small bistratified cells project to the parvocellular layers (Rodieck, 1991). The internal organization of the LGN is locally complex with afferent fibers from ganglion cells making contact with relay neurons that convey signals to cortex, and with interneurons. The LGN also receives projections from several other parts of the brain. Nothing that we know of the internal organization helps us understand color vision.

6.4.2 FUNCTION ORGANIZATION

The action potentials discharged by a ganglion cell or LGN cell can be recorded with an electrode that sits outside the neuron, and this makes it possible to record from individual neurons in an intact animal, and to study their visual sensitivities. Where the visual properties of ganglion cells have been compared with those of the LGN neurons to which they project, they have been found to be essentially identical, except perhaps for differences in sensitivity that probably reflect the action of regulatory mechanisms in the LGN (Sherman, 1996). In the following discussion ganglion cells and LGN neurons are therefore distinguished only when their properties are known to differ. The physiological counterparts of the anatomically identified parasol and midget cells are named for their projections to magnocellular and parvocellular layers in the LGN, and are known as M and P cells, respectively. This terminology provides some potential for confusion, for it does not accommodate the small bistratified cells that project to the parvocellular layers.

6.4.2.1 Receptive field organization

Both P (parvocellular) and M (magnocellular) cells have receptive fields organized into two concentric antagonistic regions: a center (on- or off-) and a surrounding region of opposite sense. This arrangement is common in vertebrates. The receptive fields of small bistratified cells appear to lack clear center–surround organization (Dacey and Lee, 1994).

The distributions of sensitivity within center and surround mechanisms are usually represented by Gaussian profiles of different extents and opposite polarity (Figure 6.14A; Rodieck, 1965); the properties of these mechanisms are commonly inferred from a neuron's spatial modulation transfer function (or contrast-sensitivity function (Enroth-Cugell and Robson, 1966)) measured with grating patterns whose luminance is modulated sinusoidally about a constant mean (see Figure 6.14B).

Neurons respond to moving or counterphase-flickering gratings with a modulated discharge that reflects the time-varying changes of luminance locally within the receptive field. Contrast sensitivity is typically measured by finding, as a function of the spatial frequency of a grating, the contrast required to evoke a modulated discharge of specified amplitude (Figure 6.14C). Such measurements show that, to a close approximation, both center and surround accumulate cone signals linearly, and the cell responds to the sum of the signals aggregated from the two mechanisms (Kaplan and Shapley, 1982; Derrington and Lennie, 1984). It is important to note that this linear behavior is observed when neurons are stably adapted to the average luminance of the grating and are driven by modulations about this mean; changing mean luminance leads to the expression of nonlinearities (see below).

As one would expect from the anatomy of their connections, M cells have larger receptive fields than P cells. Although anatomical evidence points to the center of a P cell receptive field originating in a single cone, conventional measurements of contrast sensitivity only rarely hint at this (Derrington and Lennie, 1984; Blakemore and Vital-Durand, 1986). Measurements made with interference fringes formed directly on the

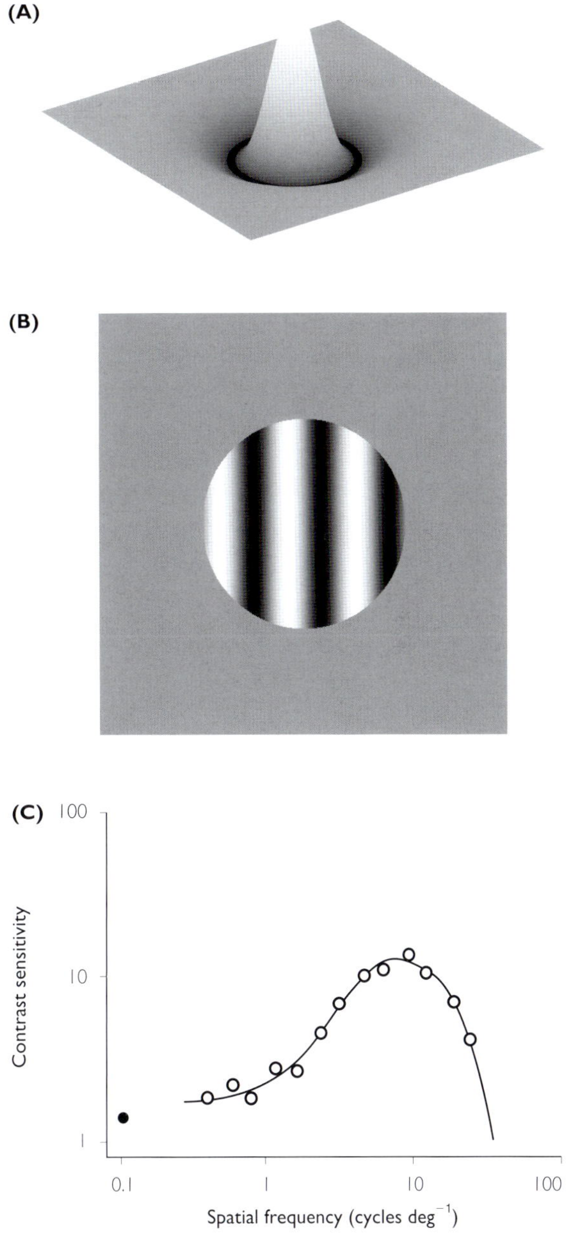

Figure 6.14 **(A) Diagram showing the distribution of sensitivity within the center and surround mechanisms of a ganglion cell's receptive field. The peak sensitivity of the center greatly exceeds that of the surround, but because the center is much smaller than the surround, the center only slightly dominates when both regions of the receptive field are illuminated. (B) Sinusoidal grating patterns of the kind used to explore the spatiotemporal transfer characteristics of visual neurons. (C) Contrast sensitivity function obtained from a parvocellular neuron in LGN. (From Derrington and Lennie, 1984, reproduced with permission)**

retina (by-passing the optics of the eye) are consistent with the center receiving signals from a single cone (McMahon *et al.*, 2000).

6.4.2.2 Contrast sensitivity

M and P cells differ in their sensitivities to contrast, M cells having several times greater contrast sensitivity to achromatic gratings (Kaplan and Shapley, 1982; Derrington and Lennie, 1984). Over a range of low to moderate contrasts, the responses of both M and P cells to stimuli of optimal spatial frequency grow linearly with contrast, but the greater sensitivity of M cells leads to their giving responses of saturating amplitude to high-contrast stimuli (Derrington and Lennie, 1984). Moreover, the temporal frequency at which sensitivity peaks is around 20 Hz in M cells and around 10 Hz in P cells (Derrington and Lennie, 1984). This, coupled with the higher contrast sensitivity of M cells, results in M cells responding to a range of high frequency signals that are apparently never seen by P cells.

Signals from the center and surround of a receptive field travel through different pathways to reach a neuron, and are subject to different delays and attenuation, so it is not surprising that the interaction between center and surround varies with the temporal frequency of visual stimulation. As temporal frequency is raised, center–surround antagonism is apparently reduced, so the spatial contrast sensitivity curve (Figure 6.14C) tends to lose its distinctive band-pass shape, becoming instead low-pass. This behavior is consistent with surround signals lagging center signals by several milliseconds (Derrington and Lennie, 1984).

6.4.3 CHROMATIC PROPERTIES

In the M cell's receptive field, center and surround generally have different spectral sensitivities, although the differences are not often conspicuous. The center has a spectral sensitivity close to that of $V\lambda$ (see Chapter 2), therefore drawing its inputs from L and M cones, while the surround draws on some different mix of cone signals (Derrington *et al.*, 1984; Kaiser *et al.*, 1990), possibly even having some local chromatically opponent structure within it (Schiller and Colby, 1983; Lee *et al.*, 1989).

In the P cell's receptive field, center and surround have overtly different spectral sensitivities (Wiesel and Hubel, 1966; Gouras, 1968; Dreher *et al.*, 1976; Derrington *et al.*, 1984). The different spectral sensitivities of center and surround endow the P cell with curious properties: the spatial contrast sensitivity curve measured with achromatic gratings has a characteristic bandpass shape that reflects that antagonistic interaction between center and surround (Figure 6.14), but the curve measured with chromatic gratings (sinusoidal modulation of chromaticity rather than luminance) has a lowpass shape, so that sensitivity to chromatic modulation is highest when a spatially uniform field of light is modulated in time. For this reason a spatially uniform field is now often used to characterize the chromatic properties of receptive fields. The luminance and/or chromaticity of this field are usually modulated in time about some point near the center of the chromaticity diagram.

P cells fall into two chromatic classes, loosely red–green and yellow–blue (De Valois *et al.*, 1966; Wiesel and Hubel, 1966; Gouras, 1968). The analysis of cone inputs reveals one class that receives opposed inputs from L and M cones only, and a second class that receives inputs from S cones opposed to some unspecified combination of signals from L and M cones (Derrington *et al.*, 1984; Figure 6.15).

The techniques now used to characterize the chromatic properties of P cells show that the neurons receive opposed inputs from different cone classes, but do not reveal the spatial distribution of these inputs. Until recently, it was presumed that the different kinds of cones whose signals were opposed were cleanly segregated in center and surround of the receptive field (bearing in mind possible exceptions for cells driven by S cones), but several lines of evidence have recently prompted a closer look at alternatives. First, if indeed the P cell receives its center input from a single cone, it will have a chromatically opponent receptive field even if its surround draws indiscriminately on all cone classes (Lennie, 1980). Second, the recently discovered similarity of the genes that encode L and M cone pigments, and the very similar structures of the cone pigments themselves (Nathans *et al.*, 1992), raise the possibility that the visual system might not distinguish them during development; third,

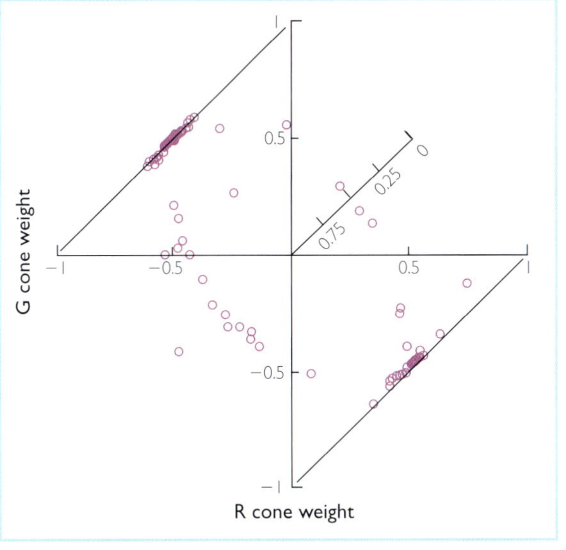

Figure 6.15 Distribution of weights that P cells in LGN attach to inputs from the different classes of cones. The weights attached to signals from L and M cones are represented explicitly; cells that receive inputs from only L and M cones are represented by points that lie on the unit diagonals; cells that receive inputs from S cones are represented by points inside the diagonals. The unsigned S cone weight can be read from the internal scale. (From Derrington *et al.*, 1984, reproduced with permission.)

the connections horizontal cells make with cones (Wässle *et al.*, 1989), and the physiological signals recorded from horizontal cells (Dacey, 1996) suggest that they receive mixed signals from the different classes of cones. Fourth, the amacrine cells that contact midget bipolar cells and midget ganglion cells make indiscriminate contact with the bipolar cells driven by both kinds of cones (Calkins and Sterling, 1996). Lennie *et al.* (1991) showed that the properties of L–M opponent neurons were consistent with either pure cone input to the surround, or mixed cone input from L and M cones, but not S cones. Reid and Shapley (1992) have argued that the P cell's surround receives inputs from a single class of cone. Given the mixing of cone signals present in horizontal cells and amacrine cells, this would require some elaborate organization that segregates cone signals again. *In vitro* recordings from midget ganglion cells in the periphery show mixed cone input to both center and surround (Dacey and Lee, 1999); no recordings have yet been made from central retina.

Dacey and Lee (1994) showed that the small bistratified ganglion cell that projects to parvocellular LGN receives 'on' (depolarizing) signals from S cones and 'off' signals from L and M cones. Neurons that receive strong 'off' (hyperpolarizing) signals from S cones, and 'on' signals from L and M cones, also exist, although they are encountered less frequently (de Monasterio and Gouras, 1975; Derrington *et al.*, 1984; Valberg *et al.*, 1986). Their anatomical substrate has not yet been found. As was noted in an earlier section, there are probably yet other kinds of neurons that carry signals from S cones, for in and near the fovea the sampling density of the small bistratified system is too low to account for the visual acuity of the S cone system.

Just as the different temporal characteristics of center and surround make the spatial properties of receptive fields depend on the temporal frequency of visual stimulation, so too do they affect the chromatic properties. At high temporal frequencies the phase difference between center and surround signals is reduced, so the mechanisms tend to act synergistically rather than antagonistically. In P cells this leads to some loss of chromatic opponency (Gouras and Zrenner, 1979; Derrington *et al*, 1984; Smith *et al.*, 1992). However, up to frequencies of 20 Hz or more the effect is small (Derrington *et al.*, 1984; Lee *et al.*, 1990) – too small to contribute significantly to the rapid decline in sensitivity to chromatic flicker found psychophysically (Wisowaty and Boynton, 1980), which must therefore originate in cortex.

6.4.3.1 Chromatic adaptation

The two-color adaptation methods developed by Stiles (1939) to isolate chromatic mechanisms psychophysically have been used to isolate the chromatic mechanisms in ganglion cells and LGN cells (Wiesel and Hubel, 1966; Gouras, 1968), but have not been employed to explore details of chromatic adaptation. We know that a change in mean illumination causes a ganglion cell's sensitivity to decline approximately in proportion to the level of illumination (Purpura *et al.*, 1990; Lee *et al.*, 1990). The mechanism almost certainly lies before the ganglion cells themselves, for the gain change proceeds independently in rod and cone pathways that converge on the same ganglion cells. Less attention has been paid to the changes in ganglion cell behavior that result from changing the mean chromaticity of illumination. DePriest *et al.* (1991) found that, at constant luminance, a modest step change in the chromaticity of a background brought about a long-lasting change in the maintained discharge of a P cell, a step in the 'on' color direction increasing the discharge, a step in the 'off' color direction decreasing the discharge. A step in luminance that provided a similar change in cone excitation had little effect upon the maintained discharge. Yeh *et al.* (1996) described similar behavior. These long-lasting changes in discharge provide cortex with a persisting signal about the ambient chromaticity.

In addition to changing the maintained discharge, the step change in background color perturbs the cell's sensitivity, although different investigations do not fully agree on the nature of the change. DePriest *et al.* (1991) found a rapid, paradoxical, increase in sensitivity to chromatic probe stimuli following a change in background that would have been expected to reduce sensitivity. Yeh *et al.* (1996), who used larger background steps, found prolonged disturbances of sensitivity, possibly reflecting saturation of an opponent site. These experiments point to possibly complex mechanisms of sensitivity regulation involving sites at which signals from the different classes of cones have converged.

6.4.4 CANDIDATE CHROMATIC AND ACHROMATIC PATHWAYS

The two different types of chromatically opponent P cells, a 'red–green' one and a 'blue–yellow' one, together with M cells, whose spectral sensitivities are close to that of $V\lambda$, provide plausible substrates of the three kinds of post-receptoral mechanisms postulated by psychophysicists.

There seems little doubt that the P cells provide signals to two chromatically opponent visual channels, but the role of M cells in the third channel is less secure. Modern psychophysical work attributes to this mechanism high spatial and temporal resolution, and a spectral sensitivity close to that of $V\lambda$ (for a review, see Lennie *et al.*, 1993). The temporal resolving power of M cells (and also of P cells) considerably exceeds that measured psychophysically, but the spatial resolving power of the mosaic of M cells is demonstrably too low to explain psychophysical performance (Lennie, 1993). Moreover, having a $V\lambda$-like spectral sensitivity does not necessarily implicate M cells as the third post-receptoral mechanism. Lennie *et al.* (1993) argue that although M cells are a plausible substrate of luminous efficiency functions measured with heterochromatic flicker photometry, similar functions can be obtained from linear transformations of the signals carried by P cells, and this provides a more probable account of luminous efficiency functions derived by other means, such as acuity measurements.

The above considerations encourage one to explore the possibility that the P pathway carries signals for all three chromatic dimensions of vision. Several observations, puzzling when considered in isolation, become more intelligible in that context. First, around 90% of P cells (about 80% of all ganglion cells) are of the 'red–green' type that receive opponent signals from L and M cones – many more than are needed to account for visual acuity for colored objects, but the right number to explain visual acuity for achromatic objects. Second, the center–surround organization of their receptive fields ensures that they respond well to chromatic changes at low spatial frequencies and to achromatic stimuli at high spatial frequencies. Simply put, a single P cell is equally capable of conveying information about the chromatic and achromatic content of the image, albeit in different frequency bands. Its response is ambiguous, but this ambiguity can be resolved by comparing, at some higher level, signals from different neurons (Lennie and D'Zmura, 1988). This kind of account leaves M cells little role in color vision, save possibly in heterochromatic flicker matches. Lee (1996) attributes to M cells a larger role in object vision.

6.5 CORTEX

6.5.1 STRUCTURAL ISSUES

In primates, V1 is the only cortical area that receives projections from LGN. Those from magnocellular and parvocellular layers arrive in different anatomical subdivisions of layer 4: M cells project principally to layer 4Cα, and P cells project mainly to layers 4Cβ and 4A (see Figure 6.6). The incoming fibers from the LGN are segregated

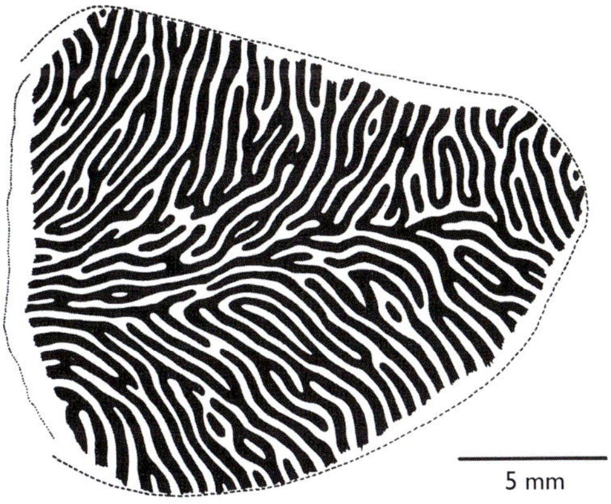

Figure 6.16 **The organization of ocular dominance columns in striate cortex of the macaque monkey. The cortex here has been unfolded as a flat sheet. Radioactive tracer injected into one eye is deposited in striate cortex, in regions to which that eye projects. This results in the distinctive pattern of stripes. (From Hubel and Wiesel, 1977, reproduced with permission.)**

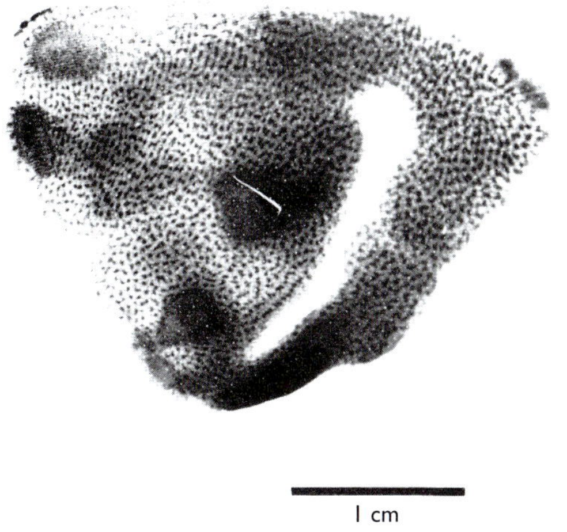

Figure 6.17 **Distribution of cytochrome oxidase 'blobs' in the unfolded striate cortex of the macaque monkey. The blobs are spaced almost uniformly throughout striate cortex, and fall within the separate ocular dominance columns that define the territories dominated by the two eyes. (From Livingstone and Hubel, 1984. Copyright © 1984 by the Society for Neuroscience.)**

by eye of origin into strips about 0.5 mm wide. These strips, known as *ocular dominance columns*, can be readily identified anatomically by examining the uptake in cortex of the radioactive amino acid proline injected into one eye. This is transported to cortex and deposited in layer 4 (Figure 6.16). This anatomical segregation of signals from the two eyes is not well maintained in layers above and below layer 4, and ocular dominance columns are less sharply defined.

V1 contains a topographically organized map of half of the visual field, with a large representation of the fovea and a much smaller representation of the periphery. Most of the distortion in the map can be explained by the variation in the density of retinal ganglion cells from fovea to periphery; each ganglion cell projects, via LGN, to a roughly constant volume of cortex. The arrangement and size of distinctive anatomical features such as ocular dominance columns does not vary from place to place in the map.

Within the overall pattern established by the ocular dominance columns, other repeating structures can be discerned in V1. Cortex stained for the presence of the enzyme cytochrome oxidase displays a regular pattern of patches where the enzyme is concentrated (Figure 6.17). These 'blobs,' which are more prominent above and below layer 4, lie securely within the separate domains of left- and right-eye columns.

The existence of repeating structures in V1 suggests a modular organization, assembled from units of a certain size. It is widely believed that the fundamental organizing unit spans the width of a pair of adjacent strips of input from left and right eyes, and therefore occupies about 1 mm^2 of cortical surface and has a depth of about 2 mm. This unit, known as a *hypercolumn* (Hubel and Wiesel, 1974), contains perhaps 200 000 cells. Within a hypercolumn there are further organizational regularities that can be discerned physiologically but not anatomically.

Signals from different subdivisions of layer 4 are delivered to different places within V1. Layer 4Cα, which receives its input from M cells, makes a distinctive projection to layer 4B, which sends an equally distinctive projection out of striate cortex to extrastriate regions that appear to be particularly concerned with the analysis of image movement (Zeki, 1974; Newsome *et al.*, 1985), and which ultimately send major projections to the parietal lobe. Neurons in layers 4Cβ and 4A, which receive input from P cells, project principally to the upper layers of striate cortex.

Neurons in the upper layers of striate cortex send projections principally to area V2.

6.5.2 FUNCTIONAL ORGANIZATION

6.5.2.1 Striate cortex

The earliest studies showed that receptive fields of V1 neurons often differ profoundly from those of neurons in retina and LGN. The most prominent differences lay in the spatial organization of receptive fields, which instead of being concentrically organized, were often elongated, sometimes having no distinct excitatory and inhibitory regions (Hubel and Wiesel, 1977). The result is that most neurons in V1 are selective for the orientation of visual stimuli that fall within their receptive fields; they are also often sharply selective for the size of the stimulus (Figure 6.18), and for its direction of movement. The uniformity of receptive field properties in retina and LGN thus gives way to great heterogeneity in cortex.

Hubel and Wiesel (1962, 1968) drew a broad distinction, generally upheld by subsequent work, between two major kinds of cortical cell that they called *simple* and *complex*. These have similar orientation, spatial, and directional selectivities, but differ sharply in the form of their responses. A simple cell generates a response that reflects the quasi-linear addition of signals (excitatory or inhibitory) arising in different parts of the receptive field. A map of the excitatory and inhibitory regions in a simple receptive field provides a reasonable guide to the visual selectivity of the cell. A complex cell is inherently nonlinear: the receptive field generally cannot be parsed into distinct excitatory and inhibitory regions, and the cell will respond with an increased discharge to either a localized increase or decrease in illumination. The behavior of the complex cell represents an important change in the way the visual system analyzes the image, for, unlike the simple cell or a neuron at an earlier stage in the pathway, it gives a response from which the image cannot be reconstructed. It is unclear whether or not complex cells derive their inputs from simple cells, or receive the same inputs as simple cells.

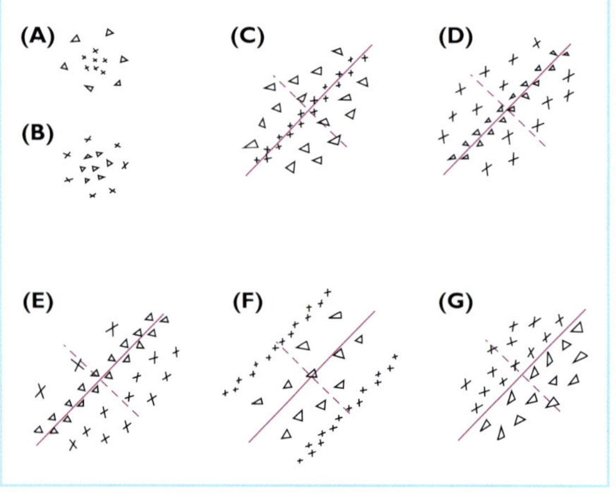

Figure 6.18 **Diagram of the receptive field organization often found in cells in striate cortex. Crosses represent excitatory regions giving 'on' responses; triangles represent inhibitory regions giving 'off' responses. (A) and (B) illustrate the arrangement of regions in concentrically-organized receptive fields typical of ganglion cells and LGN cells, but relatively rare in cortex. (C–G) represent arrangements of excitatory and inhibitory regions in different simple cells. (From Hubel and Wiesel, 1962, reproduced with permission.)**

Cells with different properties tend to be concentrated at different depths within cortex. Complex cells are most often found in layers 2/3 and in layer 5. Simple cells are found in layers 2/3 and in layer 4. Neurons with concentrically organized receptive fields are found in layer 4, where inputs from LGN arrive. Above and below layer 4, neurons can often be excited by stimulation through either eye, although rarely are both eyes equally effective. If a cell can be driven binocularly, it is often sensitive to the relative position of the stimuli presented to the two eyes, responding well when the stimuli fall on corresponding points, much less well otherwise. This makes neurons sensitive to binocular depth (Poggio and Talbot, 1981).

Neurons with different visual preferences are placed in an orderly arrangement in cortex. From any point on the cortical surface, extending perpendicularly through the depth of the cortex, neurons prefer stimuli of the same orientation. On an adjacent, parallel, trajectory neurons prefer a slightly different orientation. A set of 'orientation columns,' covering the range of orientations around the circle, is contained within the width of a pair of ocular dominance columns (a hypercolumn; Hubel and Wiesel, 1977).

Beyond layer 4 of striate cortex the distinct identities of the incoming M and P pathways are not well preserved. Neurons in layer 4B tend to have higher contrast sensitivities than neurons elsewhere (Hawken and Parker, 1984), presumably reflecting their close association with inputs from the sensitive M cells, but neurons in other layers give few explicit indications of the sources of their driving signals.

Neurons in striate cortex respond best to contrast modulations at temporal frequencies distributed around 12 Hz, a lower and more variable frequency than characterizes neurons in LGN (Hawken *et al.*, 1996), but one that better matches psychophysical measurements. As temporal frequency is lowered below the peak, the sensitivity of a cortical neuron often declines sharply.

6.5.2.2 Extrastriate cortex

The visual characteristics of neurons in regions beyond striate cortex have been less thoroughly studied, but some general characteristics are well known. Among the collection of visual areas that lead toward the temporal lobe, and are the most likely to be important for color vision, receptive fields of neurons grow progressively larger as one moves towards the temporal lobe, and nearly all neurons can be driven by inputs through either eye, but the general properties of receptive fields – spatial selectivity, orientation, and direction selectivity – change little from area to area. There is some physiological evidence that different areas are specialized for different kinds of analysis; this issue is taken up in a later section.

6.5.3 CHROMATIC PROPERTIES

In exploring the properties of cortical neurons, investigators have concentrated on aspects of color vision that cannot be easily explained by the known properties of neurons at earlier stages in the pathway.

6.5.3.1 Separation of chromatic and achromatic signals

It was noted earlier that P cells driven by signals from L and M cones must be the substrate of the achromatic pathway that supports visual acuity, and presumably also a red–green opponent pathway, but that in any individual cell the chromatic and achromatic signals are confounded. In cortex one might expect to find mechanisms whose behavior better reflects what is observed psychophysically, namely substantial independence of chromatic and achromatic mechanisms.

There is a profound change in the general chromatic characteristics of cells as one moves from LGN to cortex. The ubiquitous color-opponent P cells in LGN give way to a dearth of overtly color-opponent neurons in V1. Hubel and Wiesel (1968) commented on this in their first investigation of primate visual cortex, and it has been confirmed regularly since (Gouras, 1974).

Neurons with receptive fields in and near the fovea often have sharply defined preferences for stimuli containing relatively high spatial frequencies – high enough that chromatic aberration removes much of the chromatic contrast from the image. This preference for high spatial frequencies undoubtedly accounts for the weak responses of many neurons to stimuli containing spatio-chromatic contrast, and as a result, most investigations of the chromatic properties of neurons concentrate on cells that prefer stimuli containing low spatial frequencies.

Overtly color-opponent neurons are found in all layers of striate cortex, but more often in layer 4 than elsewhere. In layer 4 and layer 6 particularly, the most responsive neurons often, but by no means always, have receptive fields with poorly defined orientation selectivity, and low-pass spatial frequency tuning (Lennie *et al.*, 1990). These receptive fields are reminiscent of receptive fields in LGN, with the following important difference: their chromatic characteristics depend little upon the spatial configuration of the stimulus. Cortical neurons therefore do not confound different dimensions of stimulus variation in the way that LGN neurons do.

In the upper layers of cortex, where simple and complex cells predominate, few neurons are overtly color-opponent. Most of those that can be excited by colored patterns can also be excited by patterns defined by brightness contrast; cells that respond best to isoluminant chromatic contrasts are rare (Gouras and Krüger, 1979; Thorell *et al.*, 1984; Lennie *et al.*, 1990). When a neuron's receptive field properties can be established with stimuli defined by either color or brightness contrast, the spatial and orientational selectivities are generally similar (Thorell *et al.*, 1984; Lennie *et al.*, 1990).

The general picture to emerge from studies of striate cortex is that for the first time there appear in large numbers neurons whose receptive field properties are indifferent to the chromatic composition of the stimulus – they may be conceived as analyzing spatial structure with little regard for the spectral composition of the stimulus. Most of these neurons respond best when stimulus patterns are defined by brightness rather than color contrast. In this sense cortex might be viewed as having formed an achromatic pathway. The standing of independent chromatic pathways is less clear.

Neurons that respond preferentially to stimuli defined by color rather than brightness contrast are also found in areas V2, V3, and V4, and in parts of the temporal lobe.

6.5.3.2 Number of chromatic channels

Psychophysical evidence reviewed in Chapter 3 grants a special status to two chromatic axes in color space (loosely a red–green axis and a yellow–blue one), but at the same time that evidence is not consistent on the locus of these special (cardinal) directions. Moreover, studies that have examined aftereffects of habituating to modulations of chromaticity along different directions in color space (Krauskopf *et al.*, 1986; Webster and Mollon, 1991) reveal more mechanisms than just the two tuned to the cardinal directions – mechanisms tuned to intermediate directions exist too.

P cells in LGN fall neatly into just two chromatic classes. Moreover, their sensitivities are not changed by prolonged exposure to habituating stimuli of the kind used to reveal multiple chromatic mechanisms in psychophysical experiments. These multiple mechanisms must originate in cortex.

Several studies have examined the distribution of chromatic preferences among cells in striate cortex. Although they do not agree on details, these investigations do agree that chromatic preferences are not clustered in two groups. Vautin and Dow (1985), in recordings made from awake monkeys, found that, when chromatic preferences were explored with monochromatic lights, neurons in layer 4 fell into four loosely defined clusters (blue, green, yellow, red), identified by their wavelengths of peak excitability. Thorell *et al.* (1984) and Lennie *et al.* (1990) found a similar modest tendency for cells' chromatic preferences to be aligned along the red–green and yellow–blue axes (properly an axis of exclusively L and M cone modulation and one of exclusively S cone modulation) of color space. In the upper layers of cortex, chromatic preferences are broadly distributed.

To the extent that cells' chromatic preferences are broadly distributed, neurons in striate cortex are a candidate substrate for the multiple chromatic mechanisms inferred from psychophysical experiments. However, it is hard to tell from physiological observations which of the neurons that respond to colored stimuli are important for color vision – that is, which neurons might have a role in perceptual judgments about color. Attempts to identify the relevant neurons have generally sought to demonstrate physiological properties that mirrored those of the psychophysical mechanisms. One such attempt, to explore habituation to chromatically modulated stimuli, showed that although some cortical neurons habituate (and neurons in LGN never do), others become more responsive following prolonged stimulation (Lennie *et al.*, 1994). Another approach has been to examine whether or not color-opponent neurons are concentrated in particular places – pathways specialized for the analysis of color.

6.5.3.3 Spatial contrast effects

Some of the most distinctive phenomena of color vision – for example, the uniform color induced in a neutral patch by enclosing it in a colored region – depend upon spatial interactions between nearby regions of visual field. These remote influences have a longer reach than can plausibly be associated with any mechanisms in retina or LGN, and have generally been thought to originate in cortex. In area V1, long-range contrast effects have been observed in the domains of orientation and direction of movement (Blakemore and Tobin, 1972; Knierim and Van Essen, 1992; Lamme, 1995), but not consistently in the domain of color. In their first discussion of neurons in striate cortex, Hubel and Wiesel (1968) described a rare 'double-opponent' receptive field, in which a core region with co-extensive color-opponent mechanisms (for example, red-on, green-off) was enclosed by an outer region containing color-opponent mechanisms of the opposite sense. Neurons with such properties could perhaps account for induced color phenomena (Daw, 1984), but they are rare, and their receptive fields are small. Livingstone and Hubel (1984) and Ts'o and Gilbert (1988) later studied neurons, perhaps differing from those explored by Hubel and Wiesel, in which the region enclosing the core of the receptive field was not itself color-opponent, but always suppressed the response to a stimulus applied to the core region. It is unclear what such cells might do for color vision.

In seeking physiological accounts of color induction, physiologists have looked most carefully at area V4 (the fourth visual cortical area). Zeki (1973, 1977) discovered that this contains an unusually large proportion of cells with sharp chromatic selectivities. Moreover, Zeki (1983) later found that the response of a V4 cell to a colored stimulus in the middle of its receptive field depended on the color of light falling in surrounding regions, in a manner that was correlated with the colored appearance the stimulus to a human observer. Schein and Desimone (1990) later described a mechanism that might be responsible for this behavior: the receptive field of a V4 cell is enclosed by a region that has the same spectral characteristics as the receptive field proper, but when illuminated always suppresses the response to a stimulus falling within the receptive field.

6.5.3.4 Private pathways for color

Two kinds of evidence bear on the question of whether there exist cortical pathways specialized for color. The first comes from physiological studies that have looked for special concentrations of color-opponent cells in different parts of cortex. The second comes from studies that have attempted to localize color centers in human cortex.

All investigators seem to agree that area V4 contains neurons with interesting chromatic properties, but there is much less agreement on whether V4 is an area specialized for analysis of the chromatic attributes of objects. V4 is the principal conduit of information from lower visual cortical regions to the temporal lobe, a region crucially involved in all aspects of object vision, not just the analysis of color (Heywood and Cowey, 1987; Heywood *et al.*, 1992). It therefore seems unlikely that V4 could be devoted exclusively to the analysis of color. Nevertheless, subdivisions of V4 might have differently specialized functions, undertaking analyses of different attributes of the image; one of these might be the analysis of color.

This issue has been explored in studies that have traced pathways projecting from earlier stages of visual cortex to V4. Most of the work that has attempted to trace a specialized color pathway has concentrated on the projections that originate in the cytochrome oxidase 'blobs' in V1. Livingstone and Hubel (1984) first drew attention to properties of cells in blobs, finding that they tended to have concentrically organized receptive fields, more than half being color-opponent – a much higher proportion than is typically found elsewhere in V1. Neurons in the blobs project to the second visual area, V2. When stained for cytochrome oxidase, V2 shows a pattern not of blobs, but of three alternating stripes, often called thick, thin, and pale (Tootell *et al.*, 1983). The projections from blobs in V1 end preferentially in the thin stripes (Livingstone and Hubel, 1983). Neurons in the thin stripes and the pale stripes project to V4 (Shipp and Zeki, 1985; DeYoe and Van Essen, 1985), where their terminations seem to be segregated (DeYoe *et al.*, 1994).

Physiological explorations of the pathway that originates in blobs are equivocal on the question of it being specialized for color. Ts'o and Gilbert (1988) corroborated Livingstone and Hubel's (1984) finding of a concentration of color-opponent cells in blobs, but Lennie *et al.* (1990) and Leventhal *et al.* (1995) found no concentrations of this kind. In area V2, Hubel and Livingstone (1987) described a concentration of color-opponent cells in the thin stripes to which blobs project. Later studies in which cells were characterized quantitatively (Levitt *et al.*, 1994; Gegenfurtner *et al.*, 1996) have found only a slight tendency for cells with different properties to be clustered in different stripes.

Although work on monkeys provides no firm pointers to the existence of a specialized color pathway, studies of people with cortical lesions (usually resulting from stroke) that cause selective impairment of color vision, without (or with little) concomitant impairment of other dimensions of vision, suggest the existence of a cortical region specialized for the analysis of color (Zeki, 1990). However, it is often unclear from these studies whether the impairment affects the capacity to identify colors, or the capacity to distinguish surfaces of different color. Where this question has been examined (Mollon *et al.*, 1980; Victor *et al.*, 1989; Barbur *et al.*, 1994), achromatopsic subjects often are able to use chromaticity to segment surfaces, and sometimes have near normal hue discrimination, but are much impaired in naming colors and grouping of items of similar color.

Recently developed methods can identify in cortex the local changes in blood flow and blood volume associated with increased neural activity. Two of these kinds of measurement, positron emission tomography (PET) and functional magnetic resonance imaging (fMRI), have been used to investigate whether or not mechanisms of color vision are localized in particular cortical regions (Zeki *et al.*, 1991; Corbetta *et al.*, 1991). The results show that a region in the fusiform gyrus, which lies between the occipital and temporal lobes, seems to be unusually active during the perception of colored patterns, though the degree to which it is specialized for the analysis of color has not been fully explored.

ACKNOWLEDGMENTS

This work was supported by NIH grants EY04440 and EY01319.

NOTES

1 Other terms are sometimes used. The cell types were originally distinguished by Polyak (1941), who called them 'midget' and 'parasol' cells. Perry *et al.* (1984) have called them Pβ and Pα cells.

REFERENCES

Ahnelt, P. and Kolb, H. (1994) Horizontal cells and cone photoreceptors in primate retina: a Golgi-light microscope study of spectral connectivity. *Journal of Comparative Neurology*, 343, 387–405.

Barbur, J.L., Harlow, A.J., and Plant, G.T. (1994) Insights into the different exploits of colour in the visual cortex. *Proceedings of the Royal Society of London B*, 258, 327–34.

Baylor, D.A. (1987) Photoreceptor signals and vision. *Investigative Ophthalmology and Visual Science*, 28, 34–49.

Baylor, D.A., Nunn, B.J., and Schnapf, J.L. (1987) Spectral sensitivity of cones of the monkey *Macaca fascicularis*. *Journal of Physiology (London)*, 390, 145–60.

Blakemore, C. and Tobin, E.A. (1972) Lateral inhibition between orientation detectors in the cat's visual cortex. *Experimental Brain Research*, 15, 439–40.

Blakemore, C. and Vital-Durand, F. (1986) Effects of visual deprivation on the development of the monkey's lateral geniculate nucleus. *Journal of Physiology (London)*, 380, 493–512.

Boycott, B.B. and Dowling, J.E. (1969) Organization of the primate retina: light microscopy. *Philosophical Transactions of the Royal Society of London B*, 255, 109–94.

Boycott, B.B. and Wässle, H. (1991) Morphological classification of bipolar cells of the primate retina. *European Journal of Neuroscience*, 3, 1069–88.

Boynton, R.M. and Baron, W.S. (1975) Sinusoidal flicker characteristics of primate cones in response to heterochromatic stimuli. *Journal of the Optical Society of America*, 65, 1091–100.

Calkins, D.J., Schein, S.J., Tsukamoto, Y., and Sterling, P. (1994) M and L cones in macaque fovea connect to midget ganglion cells by different numbers of excitatory synapses. *Nature*, 371, 70–2.

Calkins, D.J. and Sterling, P. (1996) Absence of spectrally specific lateral inputs to midget ganglion cells in primate. *Nature*, 381, 613–15.

Corbetta, M., Miezin, F.M., Dobmeyer, S., Schulman, G.L., and Petersen, S.E. (1991) Selective and divided attention during visual discriminations of shape, color and speed: functional anatomy by positron emission tomography. *Journal of Neuroscience*, 11, 2383–402.

Dacey, D.M. (1993) Morphology of a small-field bistratified ganglion cell type in the macaque and humn retina. *Visual Neuroscience*, 10, 1081–98.

Dacey, D.M. (1994) Physiology, morphology and spatial densities of identified ganglion cell types in primate retina. In *Higher-order Processing in the Visual System*. Chichester: Wiley, pp. 12–28.

Dacey, D.M. (1996) Circuitry for color coding in the primate retina. *Proceedings of the National Academy of Sciences (USA)*, 93, 582–8.

Dacey, D.M. and Lee, B.B. (1994) The blue-on opponent pathway in the primate retina originates from a distinct bistratified ganglion cell. *Nature*, 367, 731–5.

Dacey, D.M. and Lee, B.B. (1999) Functional architecture of cone signal pathways in the primate retina. In K.R. Gegenfurtner and L.T. Sharpe (eds), *Color Vision: From Genes to Perception*. Cambridge: Cambridge University Press, pp. 181–202.

Dacey, D.M., Lee, B.B., Stafford, D.K., Pokorny, J., and Smith, V.C. (1996) Horizontal cells of the primate retina: cone specificity without spectral opponency. *Science*, 271, 656–9.

Dacey, D., Packer, O.S., Diller, L., Brainard, D., Peterson, B., and Lee, B. (2000) Center surround receptive field structure of cone bipolar cells in primate retina. *Vision Research*, 40, 1801–11.

Daw, N.W. (1984) The psychology and physiology of colour vision. *Trends in Neuroscience*, 7, 330–35.

de Monasterio, F.M. and Gouras, P. (1975) Functional properties of ganglion cells of the rhesus monkey retina. *Journal of Physiology (London)*, 251, 167–95.

De Valois, R.L., Abramov, I., and Jacobs, G.H. (1966) Analysis of response patterns of LGN cells. *Journal of the Optical Society of America*, 56, 966–77.

DePriest, D.D., Lennie, P., and Krauskopf, J. (1991) Slow mechanisms of chromatic adaptation in macaque. *Investigative Ophthalmology and Visual Science*, 32 (Suppl.), 1252.

Derrington, A.M., Krauskopf, J., and Lennie, P. (1984) Chromatic mechanisms in lateral geniculate nucleus of macaque. *Journal of Physiology (London)*, 357, 241–65.

Derrington, A.M. and Lennie, P. (1984) Spatial and temporal contrast senstivities of neurones in lateral geniculate nucleus of macaque. *Journal of Physiology (London)*, 357, 219–40.

DeYoe, E.A., Felleman, D.J., Van Essen, D.C., and McClendon, E. (1994) Multiple processing streams in occipitotemporal visual cortex. *Nature*, 371, 151–4.

DeYoe, E.A. and Van Essen, D.C. (1985) Segregation of efferent connections and receptive field properties in visual area V2 of the macaque. *Nature*, 317, 58–61.

Dowling, J.E. and Boycott, B.B. (1966) Organization of the primate retina: electron microscopy. *Proceedings of the Royal Society of London B*, 166, 80–111.

Dreher, B., Fukuda, Y., and Rodieck, R.W. (1976) Identification, classification and anatomical segregation of cells with X–like and Y–like properties in the lateral geniculate nucleus of old-world primates. *Journal of Physiology (London)*, 258, 433–52.

Engel, S., Zhang, X., and Wandell, B. (1997) Color tuning in human visual cortex measured with functional magnetic resonance imaging. *Nature*, 388, 68–71.

Enroth-Cugell, C. and Robson, J.G. (1966) The contrast sensitivity of retinal ganglion cells of the cat. *Journal of Physiology (London)*, 187, 517–52.

Estévez, O. and Spekreijse, H. (1974) A spectral compensation method for determining the flicker characteristics of the human colour mechanisms. *Vision Research*, 14, 823–30.

Famiglietti, E.V., Jr and Kolb, H. (1976) Structural basis for on- and off-center responses in retinal ganglion cells. *Science*, 194, 193–5.

Felleman, D.J. and Van Essen, D.C. (1991) Distributed hierarchical processing in the primate cerebral cortex. *Cerebral Cortex*, 1, 1–47.

Gegenfurtner, K.R., Kiper, D.C. and Fenstemaker, S.B. (1996) Processing of color, form, and motion in macaque area V2. *Visual Neuroscience*, 13, 161–72.

Goodchild, A.K., Chan, T.L. and Grünert, U. (1996) Horizontal cell connections with short wavelength sensitive cones in macaque monkey retina. *Visual Neuroscience*, 13, 833–45.

Gouras, P. (1968) Identification of cone mechanisms in monkey ganglion cells. *Journal of Physiology (London)*, 199, 533–47.

Gouras, P. (1974) Opponent-colour cells in different layers of foveal striate cortex. *Journal of Physiology (London)*, 238, 583–602.

Gouras, P. and Krüger, J. (1979) Response of cells in foveal visual cortex of the monkey to pure color contrast. *Journal of Neurophysiology*, 42, 850–60.

Gouras, P. and Zrenner, E. (1979) Enhancement of luminance flicker by color-opponent mechanisms. *Science*, 205, 587–9.

Grünert, U., Greferath, U., Boycott, B.B., and Wässle, H. (1993) Parasol (Pα) ganglion-cells of the primate fovea: immunocytochemical staining with antibodies against GABAA-receptors. *Vision Research*, 33, 1–14.

Hawken, M.J. and Parker, A.J. (1984) Contrast sensitivity and orientation selectivity in lamina IV of the striate cortex of old world monkeys. *Experimental Brain Research*, 54, 367–72.

Hawken, M.J., Shapley, R.M., and Grosof, D.H. (1996) Temporal-frequency selectivity in monkey visual cortex. *Visual Neuroscience*, 13, 477–92.

Heywood, C.A. and Cowey, A. (1987) On the role of cortical visual area V4 in the discrimination of hue and pattern in macaque monkeys. *Journal of Neuroscience*, 7, 2601–16.

Heywood, C.A., Gadotti, A., and Cowey, A. (1992) Cortical area V4 and its role in the perception of color. *Journal of Neuroscience*, 12, 4056–65.

Hood, D.C. and Birch, D.G. (1993) Human cone receptor activity: the leading edge of the *a*-wave and models of receptor activity. *Visual Neuroscience*, 10, 857–71.

Hubel, D.H. and Livingstone, M.S. (1987) Segregation of form color and stereopsis in primate area 18. *Journal of Neuroscience*, 7, 3378–415.

Hubel, D.H. and Wiesel, T.N. (1962) Receptive fields, binocular interactions, and functional architecture in the cat's visual cortex. *Journal of Physiology (London)*, 160, 106–54.

Hubel, D.H. and Wiesel, T.N. (1968) Receptive fields and functional architecture of monkey striate cortex. *Journal of Physiology (London)*, 195, 215–43.

Hubel, D.H. and Wiesel, T.N. (1974) Sequence regularity and geometry of orientation columns in the monkey striate cortex. *Journal of Comparative Neurology*, 158, 267–94.

Hubel, D.H. and Wiesel, T.N. (1977) The Ferrier lecture. Functional architecture of macaque monkey visual cortex. *Proceedings of the Royal Society of London B*, 198, 1–59.

Kaiser, P.K., Lee, B.B., Martin, P.R., and Valberg, A. (1990) The physiological basis of the minimally distinct border demonstrated in the ganglion cells of the macaque retina. *Journal of Physiology (London)*, 422, 153–83.

Kaneko, A. (1973) Receptive field organization of bipolar and amacrine cells in the goldfish retina. *Journal of Physiology (London)*, 235, 133–53.

Kaplan, E. and Shapley, R.M. (1982) X and Y cells in the lateral geniculate nucleus of the macaque monkey. *Journal of Physiology (London)*, 330, 125–44.

Kelly, D.H. (1961) Visual responses to time-dependent stimuli. II. Single-channel model of the photopic visual system. *Journal of the Optical Society of America*, 51, 747–54.

Knierim, J.J. and Van Essen, D.C. (1992) Neuronal responses to static texture patterns in area V1 of the alert macaque monkey. *Journal of Neurophysiology*, 67, 961–80.

Kolb, H., Fernandez, E., Schouten, J., Ahnelt, P., Linberg, K.A., and Fisher, S. K. (1994) Are there three types of horizontal cell in the human retina? *Journal of Comparative Neurology*, 343, 370–86.

Kouyama, N. and Marshak, D.W. (1992) Bipolar cells specific for blue cones in the macaque retina. *Journal of Neuroscience*, 12, 1233–52.

Krauskopf, J., Williams, D.R., Mandler, M.B., and Brown, A.M. (1986) Higher order color mechanisms. *Vision Research*, 26, 23–32.

Kuffler, S.W. and Nicholls, J.G. (1976) *From Neuron to Brain*. Sunderland: Sinauer.

Lamme, V.A.F. (1995) The neurophysiology of figure–ground segregation in primary visual cortex. *Journal of Neuroscience*, 15, 1605–15.

Lankheet, M.J.M., van Wezel, R.J.A., and van de Grind, W.A. (1991) Effects of background illumination on cat horizontal cell responses. *Vision Research*, 31, 919–32.

Lee, B.B. (1996) Receptive field structure in the primate retina. *Vision Research*, 36, 631–44.

Lee, B.B., Martin, P.R., and Valberg, A. (1989) Nonlinear summation of M– and L–cone inputs to phasic ganglion cells of the macaque. *Journal of Neuroscience*, 9, 1433–42.

Lee, B.B., Pokorny, J., Smith, V.C., Martin, P.R., and Valberg, A. (1990) Luminance and chromatic modulation sensitivity of macaque ganglion cells and human observers. *Journal of the Optical Society of America A*, 7, 2223–6.

Lennie, P. (1980) Parallel visual pathways: a review. *Vision Research*, 20, 561–94.

Lennie, P. (1993) Roles of M and P pathways. In R.M. Shapley and D.M.K. Lam (eds), *Constrast Sensitivity*.Cambridge, MA: MIT Press, pp. 201–13.

Lennie, P. and D'Zmura, M. (1988) Mechanisms of color vision. *CRC Critical Reviews in Neurobiology*, 3, 333–400.

Lennie, P., Haake, P.W., and Williams, D.R. (1991) The design of chromatically opponent receptive fields. In M.S. Landy and J.A. Movshon (eds), *Computational Models of Visual Processing*. Cambridge, MA: MIT Press, pp. 71–82.

Lennie, P., Krauskopf, J., and Sclar, G. (1990) Chromatic mechanisms in striate cortex of macaque. *Journal of Neuroscience*, 10, 649–69.

Lennie, P., Lankheet, M.J.M., and Krauskopf, J. (1994) Chromatically selective habituation in monkey striate cortex. *Investigative Ophthalmology and Visual Science (Supplement)*, 35, 1662.

Lennie, P., Pokorny, J., and Smith, V. C. (1993) Luminance. *Journal of the Optical Society of America A*, 10, 1283–93.

Leventhal, A.G., Thompson, K.G., Liu, D., Zhou, Y., and Ault, S. J. (1995) Concomitant sensitivity to orientation, direction, and color of cells in layers 2, 3, and 4 of monkey striate cortex. *Journal of Neuroscience*, 15, 1808–18.

Levitt, J.B., Kiper, D.C., and Movshon, J.A. (1994) Receptive fields and functional architecture of macaque V2. *Journal of Neurophysiology*, 71, 2517–42.

Livingstone, M.S. and Hubel, D.H. (1983) Specificity of cortico-cortical connections in monkey visual system. *Nature*, 304, 531–4.

Livingstone, M.S. and Hubel, D.H. (1984) Anatomy and physiology of a color system in the primate visual cortex. *Journal of Neuroscience*, 4, 309–56.

Mariani, A.P. (1984) Bipolar cells in monkey retina selective for the cones likely to be blue-sensitive. *Nature*, 308, 184–6.

Masland, R.H. (1988) Amacrine cells. *Trends in Neuroscience*, 11, 405–10.

McMahon, M.J., Lankheet, M.J.M., Lennie, P., and Williams, D. (2000) Fine structure of parvocellular receptive fields in the primate fovea revealed by laser interferometry. *Journal of Neuroscience*, 20, 2043–53.

Mollon, J.D., Bowmaker, J.K., and Jacobs, G.H. (1984) Variations of colour vision in a New World primate can be explained by a polymorphism of retinal photopigments. *Proceedings of the Royal Society of London B*, 222, 373–99.

Mollon, J.D., Newcombe, F., Polden, P.G. and Ratcliff, G. (1980) On the presence of three cone mechanisms in a case of total achromatopsia. In G. Verriest (ed.), *Colour Vision Deficiencies*. Bristol: Hilger, pp. 130–5.

Naka, K.I. (1976) Functional organization of the catfish retina. *Journal of Neurophysiology*, 40, 26–43.

Nathans, J., Merbs, S.L., Sung, C.H., Weitz, C.J., and Wang, Y. (1992) Molecular genetics of human visual pigments. *Annual Review of Genetics*, 26, 403–24.

Newsome, W.T., Wurtz, R.H., Dürsteler, M.R., and Mikami, A. (1985) Deficits in visual motion processing following ibotenic acid lesions of the middle temporal visual area. *Journal of Neuroscience*, 5, 825–40.

Perry, V.H., Öhler, R., and Cowey, A. (1984) Retinal ganglion cells that project to the dorsal lateral geniculate nucleus in the macaque monkey. *Neuroscience*, 12, 1101–23.

Poggio, G.F. and Talbot, W.H. (1981) Mechanisms of static and dynamic stereopsis in foveal cortex of the rhesus monkey. *Journal of Physiology (London)*, 315, 469–92.

Polyak, S.L. (1941) *The Retina*. Chicago: University of Chicago Press.

Polyak, S.L. (1957) *The Vertebrate Visual System*. Chicago: University of Chicago Press, p. 289.

Pugh, E.N., Jr and Lamb, T.D. (1993) Amplification and kinetics of the activation steps in phototransduction. *Biochim Biophys Acta*, 1141, 111–49.

Purpura, K., Tranchina, D., Kaplan, E., and Shapley, R.M. (1990) Light adaptation in the primate retina: analysis of changes in gain and dynamics of monkey retinal ganglion cells. *Visual Neuroscience*, 4, 75–93.

Reid, R.C. and Shapley, R.M. (1992) Spatial structure of cone inputs to receptive fields in primate lateral geniculate nucleus. *Nature*, 356, 716–18.

Robson, J.G. (1966) Spatial and temporal contrast sensitivity functions of the visual system. *Journal of the Optical Society of America*, 56, 1141–2.

Rodieck, R.W. (1965) Quantitative analysis of cat retinal ganglion cell response to visual stimuli. *Vision Research*, 5, 583–601.

Rodieck, R.W. (1991) Which cells code for color? In A. Valberg and B.B. Lee (eds), *From Pigments to Perception*. New York: Plenum Press, pp. 83–94.

Rodieck, R.W. (1998) *The First Steps in Seeing*. Sunderland: Sinauer Associates.

Rodieck, R.W., Brening, R.K., and Watanabe, M. (1993) The origin of parallel visual pathways. In R. Shapley and D. M.-K. Lam (eds), *Contrast Sensitivity*. Cambridge, MA: MIT Press, pp. 117–47.

Roe, A.W. and Ts'o, D.Y. (1995) Visual topography in primate V2: multiple representation across functional stripes. *Journal of Neuroscience*, 15, 3689–715.

Schaeffel, F., Bartmann, M., Hagel, G., and Zrenner, E. (1995) Studies on the role of the retinal dopamine/melatonin system in experimental refractive error in chickens. *Vision Research*, 35, 1247–64.

Schein, S.J. and Desimone, R. (1990) Spectral properties of V4 neurons in the macaque. *Journal of Neuroscience*, 10, 3369–89.

Schiller, P.H. and Colby, C.L. (1983) The responses of single cells in the lateral geniculate nucleus of the rhesus monkey to color and luminance contrast. *Vision Research*, 23, 1631–41.

Schnapf, J.L., Nunn, B.J., Meister, M., and Baylor, D.A. (1990) Visual transduction in cones of the monkey *Macaca fascicularis*. *Journal of Physiology (London)*, 427, 681–713.

Sherman, S.M. (1996) Dual response modes in lateral geniculate neurons: mechanisms and functions. *Visual Neuroscience*, 13, 205–13.

Shipp, S. and Zeki, S.M. (1985) Segregation of pathways leading from area V2 to areas V4 and V5 of macaque monkey visual cortex. *Nature*, 315, 322–5.

Smith, V.C., Lee, B.B., Pokorny, J., Martin, P.R., and Valberg, A. (1992) Responses of macaque ganglion cells to the relative phase of heterochromatically modulated lights. *Journal of Physiology (London)*, 458, 191–221.

Sparks, D.L. and Nelson, J.S. (1987) Sensory and motor maps in the mammalian superior colliculus. *Trends in Neuroscience*, 10, 312–17.

Stell, W.K., Ishida, A.T., and Lightfoot, D.O. (1977) Structural basis for on- and off-center responses in retinal bipolar cells. *Science*, 198, 1269–71.

Sterling, P., Freed, M.A., and Smith, R.G. (1988) Architecture of rod and cone circuits to the ON-beta ganglion cell. *Journal of Neuroscience*, 8, 623–42.

Stiles, W.S. (1939) The directional sensitivity of the retina and the spectral sensitivities of the rods and cones. *Proceedings of the Royal Society of London B*, 127, 64–105.

Stiles, W.S. and Burch, J.M. (1959) NPL colour-matching investigation: final report. *Optica Acta*, 6, 1–26.

Thorell, L.G., De Valois, R.L. and Albrecht, D.G. (1984) Spatial mapping of monkey V1 cells with pure color and luminance stimuli. *Vision Research*, 24, 751–69.

Tootell, R.B.H., Silverman, M.S., De Valois, R.L., and Jacobs, G.H. (1983) Functional organization of the second cortical visual area (V2) in the primate. *Science*, 220, 737–9.

Torre, V., Ashmore, J.F., Lamb, T.D., and Menini, A. (1995) Transduction and adaptation in sensory receptor cells. *Journal of Neuroscience*, 15, 7757–68.

Ts'o, D.Y. and Gilbert, C.D. (1988) The organization of chromatic and spatial interactions in the primate striate cortex. *Journal of Neuroscience*, 8, 1712–27.

Valberg, A., Lee, B.B., and Tigwell, D.A. (1986) Neurones with strong inhibitory S-cone inputs in the macaque lateral geniculate nucleus. *Vision Research*, 26, 1061–4.

Valeton, M.J. and van Norren, D. (1983) Light adaptation of primate cones: an analysis based on extracellular data. *Vision Research*, 23, 1539–47.

Vautin, R.G. and Dow, B.M. (1985) Color cell groups in foveal striate cortex of the behaving macaque. *Journal of Neurophysiology*, 54, 273–92.

Verweij, J., Dacey, D.M., Peterson, B.B., and Buck, S.L. (1999) Sensitivity and dynamics of rod signals in H1 horizontal cells of the macaque monkey retina. *Vision Research*, 39, 3662–72.

Victor, J.D., Maiese, K., Shapley, R., Sidtis, J., and Gazzaniga, M.S. (1989) Acquired central dyschromatopsia: analysis of a case with preservation of color discrimination. *Clinical Vision Sciences*, 4, 183–96.

Walraven, J., Enroth-Cugell, C., Hood, D.C., MacLeod, D.I.A., and Schnapf, J. (1989) The control of visual sensitivity: receptoral and postreceptoral processes. In L. Spillmann and J. Werner (eds), *Visual Perception: The Neurophysiological Foundations*. New York: Academic Press, pp. 53–101.

Wässle, H. and Boycott, B.B. (1991) Functional architecture of the mammalian retina. *Physiological Reviews*, 71, 447–80.

Wässle, H., Boycott, B.B., and Röhrenbeck, J. (1989) Horizontal cells in the monkey retina: cone connections and dendritic network. *European Journal of Neuroscience*, 1, 421–35.

Wässle, H., Grünert, U., Martin, P.R., and Boycott, B.B. (1994) Immunocytochemical characterization and spatial distribution of midget bipolar cells in the macaque monkey retina. *Vision Research*, 34, 561–79.

Watanabe, M. and Rodieck, R.W. (1989) Parasol and midget ganglion cells of the primate retina. *Journal of Comparative Neurology*, 289, 434–54.

Webster, M.A. and Mollon, J.D. (1991) Changes in colour appearance following post-receptoral adaptation. *Nature*, 349, 235–8.

Wiesel, T.N. and Hubel, D.H. (1966) Spatial and chromatic interactions in the lateral geniculate body of the rhesus monkey. *Journal of Neurophysiology*, 29, 1115–56.

Williams, D.R. and Collier, R.J. (1983) Consequences of spatial sampling by a human photoreceptor mosaic. *Science*, 221, 385–7.

Wisowaty, J.J. and Boynton, R.M. (1980) Temporal modulation sensitivity of the blue mechanism: measurements made without chromatic adaptation. *Vision Research*, 20, 895–909.

Yeh, T., Lee, B.B., and Kremers, J. (1996) The time course of adaptation in macaque retinal ganglion cells. *Vision Research*, 36, 913–31.

Zeki, S.M. (1973) Colour coding in rhesus monkey prestriate cortex. *Brain Research*, 53, 422–7.

Zeki, S.M. (1974) Functional organization of a visual area in the posterior bank of the superior temporal sulcus of the rhesus monkey. *Journal of Physiology (London)*, 236, 549–73.

Zeki, S.M. (1977) Colour coding in the superior temporal sulcus of rhesus monkey visual cortex. *Proceedings of the Royal Society of London B*, 197, 195–223.

Zeki, S.M. (1983) Colour coding in the cerebral cortex: the responses of wavelength-selective and colour-coded cells in monkey visual cortex to changes in wavelength composition. *Neuroscience*, 9, 767–81.

Zeki, S.M. (1990) A century of cerebral achromatopsia. *Brain*, 113, 1721–77.

Zeki, S.M., Watson, J.D.G., Lueck, C.J., Friston, K.J., Kennard, C., and Frackowiak, R.S.J. (1991) A direct demonstration of functional specialization in human visual cortex. *Journal of Neuroscience*, 11, 641–9.

7 The Physics and Chemistry of Color: the 15 Mechanisms

Kurt Nassau

16 Guinea Hollow Road, Lebanon, NJ 08833, USA

Every gaudy color
Is a bit of truth.

Nathalia Crane

CHAPTER CONTENTS

The Science of Color
ISBN 0–444–512–519

7.1 OVERVIEW: 15 CAUSES OF COLOR

Fifteen causes of color originating in a variety of physical and chemical mechanisms can be sorted into five groups. (I) *Vibrations and simple excitations* produce the colors of incandescence (e.g. flames), gas excitations (neon tube, aurora), and vibrations and rotations (blue ice and water). (II) *Ligand field effects* produce color in transition metal compounds (turquoise, chrome green) and as impurities in otherwise colorless substances (ruby, emerald). (III) *Molecular orbital effects* produce the colors of organic compounds (indigo, chlorophyll), and of charge transfer compounds (blue sapphire, lapis lazuli). (IV) *Energy band effects* give the colors seen in metals and alloys (gold, brass), in semiconductors (cadmium yellow, vermillion), in doped semiconductors (blue and yellow diamond), and in color centers (amethyst, topaz). (V) *Geometrical and physical optic* effects produce colors from dispersive refraction (rainbow, prism spectroscope), scattering (blue sky, blue eyes, red sunset), interference (soap bubble, iridescent beetles), and diffraction (the corona aureole, opal). In essentially all of these 15 mechanisms it is the interaction of light with the electrons in matter that produces color.

7.2 INTRODUCTION TO THE PHYSICS AND CHEMISTRY OF COLOR

Color is perceived when the wavelengths constituting white light are absorbed, reflected, refracted, scattered, or diffracted by matter on their way to our eyes; alternatively, a non-white distribution of light may be emitted by some system. Fifteen specific physical or chemical mechanisms are outlined in Table 7.1, based on the book *The Physics and Chemistry of Color* (Nassau, 2001). More detailed descriptions and applications can be found there, together with many detailed references for further reading. Some selected references are also given at the end of this chapter.

As in any attempt at classification, there is an element of choice in the construction of Table 7.1, with some overlaps and some almost arbitrary assignments. The classification uses five groups based on the fundamental mechanisms involved: three of these – vibrations and simple excitations, energy bands, and geometrical and physical optics – are normally part of the physics curriculum; molecular orbitals are normally part of chemistry; and ligand fields are covered in both disciplines. It is unusual, however, for even an extended academic treatment of most of these topics to concern itself with the colors produced as such.

In the limited space available, it is not possible to cover any of these topics with full scientific rigor. Analogously, it is not possible to explain all technical terms for nontechnical readers. Full understanding is not usually required for significant insight: the context will usually supply an approximate meaning and the general reader will at least come away with a feel for the technical language used in each field. Recommendations for further reading are given at the end of this chapter.

There are some widely repeated color attributions such as that blue and green are caused by copper, dark blue by cobalt, and so on, but such assumptions are only rarely correct. Even in a highly restricted field such as the dark blue gemstones of Figure 7.1, cobalt can indeed be the cause, yet six other mechanisms not involving cobalt can also produce such colors. (Regrettably,

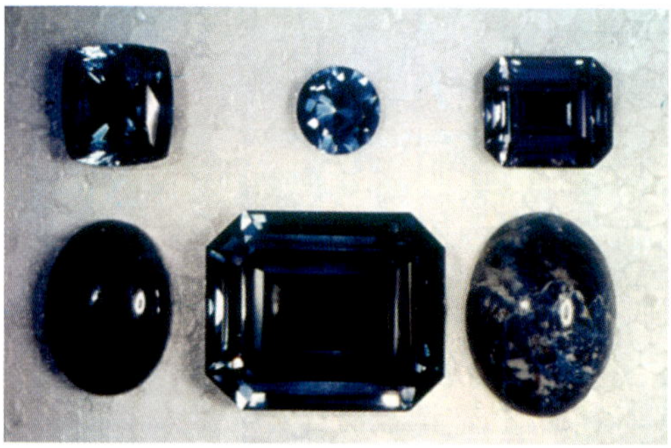

Figure 7.1 **Six blue gemstones with different causes of color. (Left to right, above) Maxixe-type beryl (radiation-induced color center), blue spinel (ligand field color from a cobalt impurity), spinel 'doublet' (colorless spinel containing a layer of organic dye); (below) shattuckite (ligand field in an idiochromatic copper compound), blue sapphire (Fe-Ti intervalence charge transfer), lapis lazuli (S_3 anion-anion charge transfer); the largest stone is 2 cm across.**

Table 7.1 Examples of the 15 causes of color

Vibrations and simple excitations	
1	Incandescence
	Hot objects, the sun, flames, filament lamps, carbon arcs, limelight, pyrotechnics*
2	Gas excitations
	Vapor lamps, neon signs, corona discharge, auroras, lightning*, lasers*
3	Vibrations and rotations
	Blue water and ice, iodine, bromine, chlorine gas, blue gas flame
Transitions involving ligand field effects	
4	Transition metal compounds
	Turquoise, malachite, chrome green, rhodochrosite, smalt, copper patina, fluorescence*, phosphorescence*, lasers*, phosphors*
5	Transition metal impurities
	Ruby, emerald, alexandrite, aquamarine, citrine, red iron ore, jade*, glasses*, dyes*, fluorescence*, phosphorescence*, lasers*
Transition between molecular orbitals	
6	Organic compounds
	Dyes*, biological colorations*, fluorescence*, phosphorescence*, lasers*
7	Charge transfer
	Blue sapphire, magnetite, lapis lazuli, ultramarine, chromates, Painted Desert, Prussian blue
Transitions involving energy bands	
8	Metals
	Copper, silver, gold, iron, brass, 'ruby' glass
9	Pure semiconductors
	Silicon, galena, cinnabar, vermillion, cadmium orange and yellow, diamond
10	Doped semiconductors
	Blue and yellow diamonds, light-emitting diodes, lasers*, phosphors*
11	Color centers
	Amethyst, smoky quartz, desert 'amethyst' glass, fluorescence*, phosphorescence*, lasers*
Geometrical and physical optics	
12	Dispersive refraction, polarization, etc.
	Rainbows, halos, sun dogs, photoelastic stress analysis, 'fire' in gemstones, prism spectrum
13	Scattering
	Blue sky, red sunset, blue moon, moonstone, Raman scattering, blue eyes, skin, butterflies, bird feathers*, other biological colors*
14	Interference without diffraction
	Oil slick on water, soap bubbles, coatings on camera lenses, biological colors*
15	Diffraction
	Aureole, glory, diffraction grating spectrum, opal, liquid crystals biological colors*

*Only in part

the dark blue Hope diamond was not available for inclusion in this figure!) Detailed study may be needed to establish the specific cause of the color of an unknown material.

The scientific understanding of color began in 1666, when Newton first used the word 'spectrum' for the array of colors produced by a glass prism. He recognized that the colors comprising white light are 'refracted' (bent) by different amounts and also understood that there is no 'colored' light – the color being in the brain of the beholder. There is merely present in the light a range of energies (or the proportional frequencies, or the inversely proportional wavelengths, and so on). The specific system of units employed depends on whether the user is a chemist, physicist, spectroscopist, etc. For convenience, energy in electron volts (eV) and wavelength in nanometers (nm) are used as the variables in this chapter:

$$(\text{wavelength in nm}) \times (\text{energy in eV}) = 1239.9.$$

It should be noted that when a band of wavelengths is removed from white light, e.g. by absorption, then the color complementary to that removed will be perceived. Thus if the red-appearing end of the visible spectrum (long wavelengths, low energies) is removed, then a blue color is seen. If the blue-appearing end (short wavelengths, high energies) is removed, then a yellow is seen. Removing the central green-appearing wavelengths produces a reddish purple.

It seems remarkable that so many distinct causes of color should apply to the small band of electromagnetic radiation to which the eye is sensitive: less than one 'octave' in an electromagnetic spectrum of more than 80 octaves, ranging from alternating current, radio waves, and the infra-red through the visible to the ultra-violet, x-rays, gamma rays, and cosmic rays. So much happens in this narrow visible band because this is the energy range where the interaction of radiation with electrons first becomes important. Radiation at just lower energies than the visible range (i.e. infra-red) induces motions in atoms and molecules which we sense as heat, if at all. Radiation at just higher energies than the visible range (i.e. ultra-violet) can ionize atoms, that is completely remove one or more electrons, and can permanently alter molecules, as in suntans and sunburns. Only in the narrow optical region, just that region to which the human eye is sensitive, is the energy of light well attuned to nondestructive interactions with the electronic structure of matter with a wide diversity of colorful results.

Electrons are involved in the interactions of our 15 mechanisms and we could claim that we 'see' electrons whenever we perceive color.

The increase of the refractive index with increasing energy (decreasing wavelength) which leads to Newton's spectrum is only the small central region of the full so-called dispersion curve, shown for a colorless glass in Figure 7.2. At low energies in the infra-red (left) there are features derived from the absorption of infrared energy which produce excited lattice vibrations, originating in the molecular framework derived from the bonding between atoms. At high energies (right) there are features derived from the unpairing and excitation of previously paired electrons on individual atoms which lead to absorptions in the ultra-violet. It is the interaction of the distant effects from both of these sets of absorptions that produces the gently sloping central region of Figure 7.2, as discussed below under Mechanism 12.

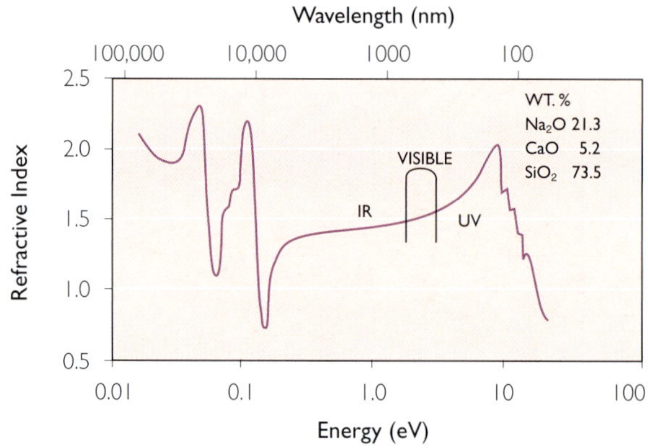

Figure 7.2 The extended refractive index curve of a colorless crown glass.

The infra-red absorptions of Figure 7.2 can be shifted into the visible region with light, strongly bonded atoms, as in the vibrations and rotations of Mechanism 3 of Table 7.1. Similarly, the ultraviolet absorptions of Figure 7.2 can be shifted into the visible region in a wide variety of situations leading to color from Mechanisms 1, 2, and 4 through 11 of Table 7.1.

Quantum theory applies when the energy of a photon (also quantum, the smallest unit of light that can exist) is absorbed or emitted by an electron, atom, or group of atoms. Such a system can only absorb or emit certain quantities of energy and we can represent such a system by an energy diagram as in Figure 7.3. It takes energy to raise the ball up the steps, one or more steps at a time. Energy is again released when the ball falls back downwards. There may be 'selection rules' which 'allow' or 'forbid' certain of these single or multiple steps, so that absorption A and emission C in this diagram may be allowed and will occur strongly, while emission B may be forbidden and will not occur or only weakly.

7.3 MECHANISM 1: COLOR FROM INCANDESCENCE

Colloquially we speak of 'red hot' 'white hot,' and so on. These colors are parts of the sequence black, red, orange, yellow white, and bluish white seen as an object is heated to successively higher temperatures. The light produced consists of photons given off by electrons, atoms, and molecules when part of their thermal vibration

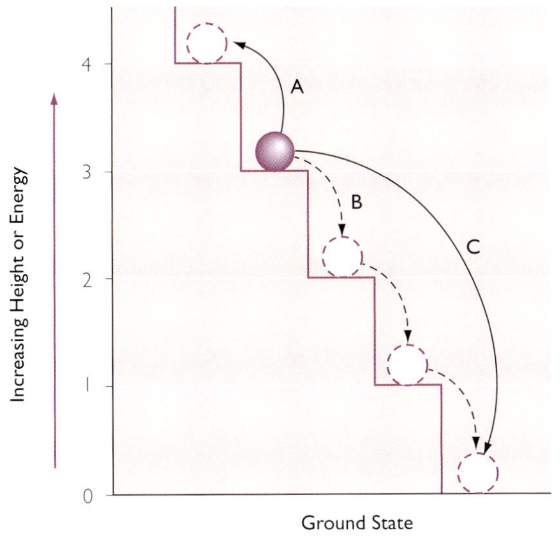

Figure 7.3 **Schematic representation of a quantum system that can only exist at discreet energy levels; only some transitions are allowed.**

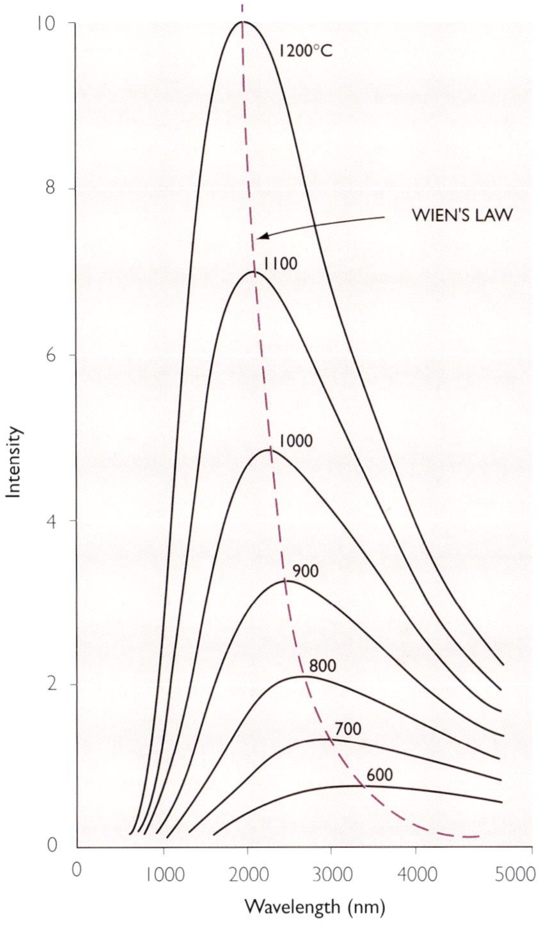

Figure 7.4 **Planck's black body curves for different temperatures, also showing Wien's law.**

energy is emitted as radiation. Max Planck found in 1900 that the quantization of energy was necessary to explain the idealized 'black body' radiation, thus producing the quantum theory. Planck's equation for the energy E (in W/cm^2) radiated into a hemisphere at wavelength λ (in nm) and in interval $d\lambda$, at temperature T (in K) is given by:

$$E\,d\lambda = 37{,}415 d\lambda \,/\, \lambda^5\,[\exp(14{,}338/\lambda T) - 1].$$

The total radiated energy E_T (in W) is given by:

$$E_T = 5.670 \times 10^{-12}\,T^4.$$

At any given temperature there is a peak in the intensity of the emitted radiation. This peak shifts toward shorter wavelengths (higher energies) with increasing temperature, as can be seen in the curves of Figure 7.4. Wien's law gives the peak wavelength A_m as: 2,897,000/T.

Our definition of 'white' is derived from emission from the 5700 °C temperature of the surface of the sun. Its peak near 550 nm (2.25 eV) is paralleled in the maximum sensitivity of our eyes in the same region usually attributed to our evolution in the vicinity of our sun. The sequence of incandescence colors is shown on a color triangle in Figure 7.5. No matter how high the temperature, a blue–white is the 'hottest' color there can be.

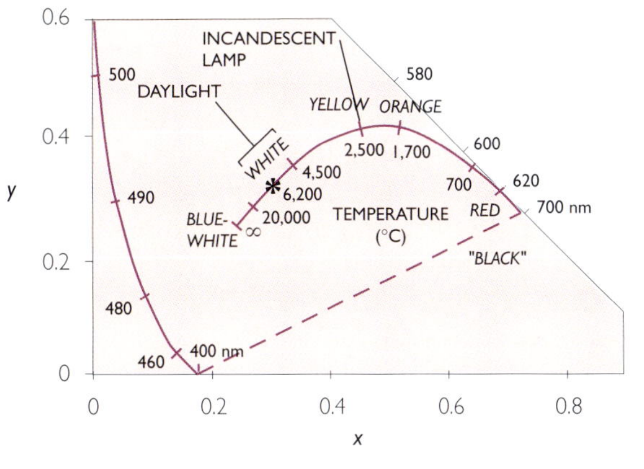

Figure 7.5 **Black body colors shown on a chromaticity diagram.**

The color of incandescence is used in radiation pyrometers to measure temperature. Lighting sources from the primitive candle through limelight, arc lamps, incandescent filament lamps, and flash bulbs all are based on incandescence, the usual aim being to avoid color. Part of the light from pyrotechnic devices is also derived from incandescence, originating from high temperatures produced by chemical reactions.

7.4 MECHANISM 2: COLOR FROM GAS EXCITATION

The incandescence of Mechanism 1 applies to the color of any substance when heated. Specific chemical elements, present as a vapor or a gas have their electrons excited into higher energy levels in gas excitations. Light is emitted when the excess energy is released as photons. Examples of various forms of excitations include electrical excitations as in arcs, sparks, lightning, neon tubes, and sodium and mercury vapor lamps; chemical excitations as in the chemist's flame test for sodium, potassium, copper, and a few other elements; and high energy particles as in the northern aurora borealis and southern aurora australis displays.

Unusual is triboluminescence, seen when we crunch a wintergreen 'Lifesaver' candy in front of a mirror in the dark. The high voltage field produced during the formation of electrically charged sugar crystal surfaces accelerates electrons which then excite nitrogen gas molecules in the air to produce the ion N_2^+ which emits light as a blue luminescence. Some ultra-violet is also produced and causes the oil of wintergreen (methyl salicilate) vapor to fluoresce with a particularly intense blue color.

Some of the energy levels for a sodium atom in the gaseous state are shown in Figure 7.6. In a sodium vapor lamp a high voltage produces ionization from the initial 'ground state' into the sodium ion Na^+ plus one electron at or above the top line of this figure. As the electron recombines with the ion, the sodium atom passes along allowed transitions, only some of which are shown as arrows in Figure 7.6, with the emission of heat and/or photons. The position of the various levels shown, as well as the specific allowed transitions are given by quantum theory. All paths terminate in the lowest two arrows which correspond to the emission of the well-known yellow 'sodium doublet' at 589.7 nm and 589.0 nm.

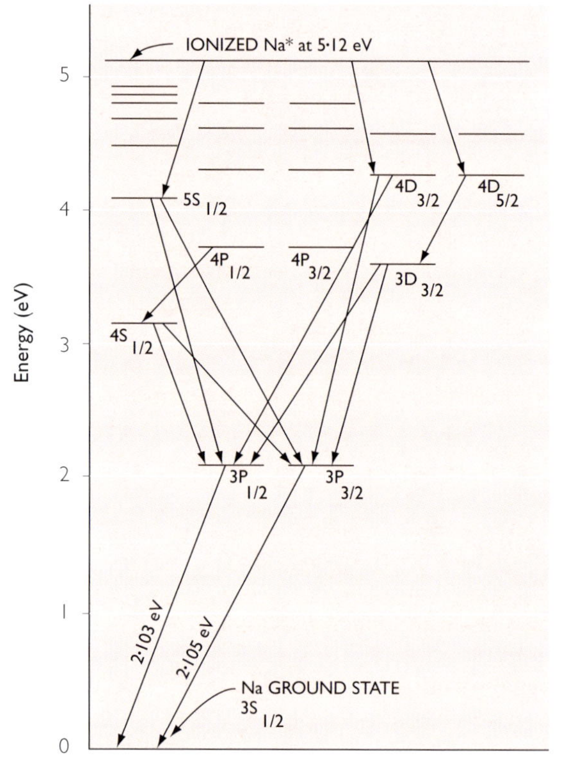

Figure 7.6 **Energy level scheme of an isolated atom of sodium, showing some allowed transitions.**

Sodium and mercury vapor lamps very efficiently emit middle and short wavelengths, that are perceived as yellow and blue, respectively. These are often used in parking lots, where their unaccustomed color disguises the color of our automobiles. Mercury vapor lamps also produce much ultra-violet which is converted by a phosphor coating inside fluorescent tube lamps into lower energy wavelengths in the yellow-, orange-, and red-appearing parts of the visible spectrum to yield a better color balance for indoor lighting. In gas lasers, such as the helium–neon laser, electrical gas excitation produces coherent light with optical feedback from mirrors at each end of the tube; all the photons have almost exactly the same frequency and are in step both in space and in time.

7.5 MECHANISM 3: COLOR FROM VIBRATIONS AND ROTATIONS

As discussed above in connection with Figure 7.1, most vibrations between atoms absorb only at very low energies in the infra-red. The pitch of a vibrating string in a musical instrument is raised both if the mass of the string is reduced and if the tension applied to the string is increased. Analogously, the highest vibrational frequencies occur with the lightest atoms, as with hydrogen, when most strongly bonded, as in the H-bond-strengthened bonding among water molecules.

The isolated water molecule is bent and has three fundamental vibrations, as in Figure 7.7. When individual water molecules are trapped in the gemstone emerald (beryl containing both water and chromium $Be_3Al_2Si_6O_{18}.xCr_2O_3.yH_2O$), the absorption spectrum of Figure 7.8 clearly shows at the left absorptions which can be identified with these v_1, v_2, and v_3 vibrations of Figure 7.7. In addition, there are overtones, combinations of two or more vibrations at somewhat higher frequencies (higher energies, shorter wavelengths). All of these vibrations result in absorptions in the ultra-violet region as shown. Note that the spectrum of pure beryl, also given in Figure 7.8 does not show these absorptions.

In liquid water or solid ice, the hydrogen bonding between adjacent molecules raises the energies of these vibrations and leads to very weak combination absorptions at the long-wavelength end of the visible spectrum. As a result, pure water and ice have a complementary very pale blue color. This is best seen in tropical white-sand beaches and in ice caves in glaciers. A green color in water or ice generally derives from the presence of algae. The usually cited reflections from a blue sky do occur, but are not a significant cause of blue, as already shown in 1922 by C.V. Raman, who used a polarizer to eliminate reflections. Also note the blue color

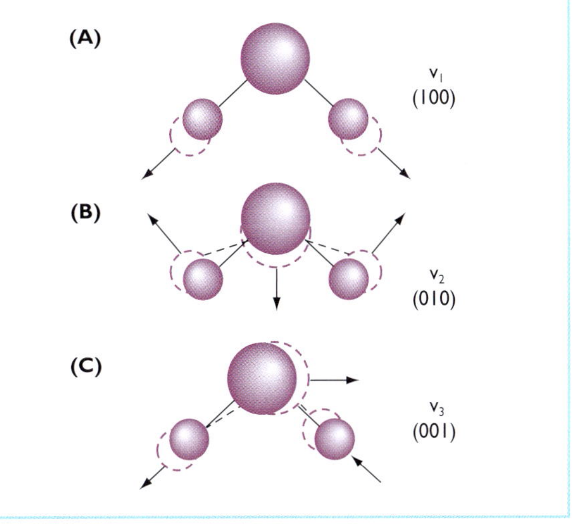

Figure 7.7 **The three fundamental vibrations of the bent water molecule: the symmetrical stretch (A), the symmetrical bend (B), and the antisymmetrical bend (C).**

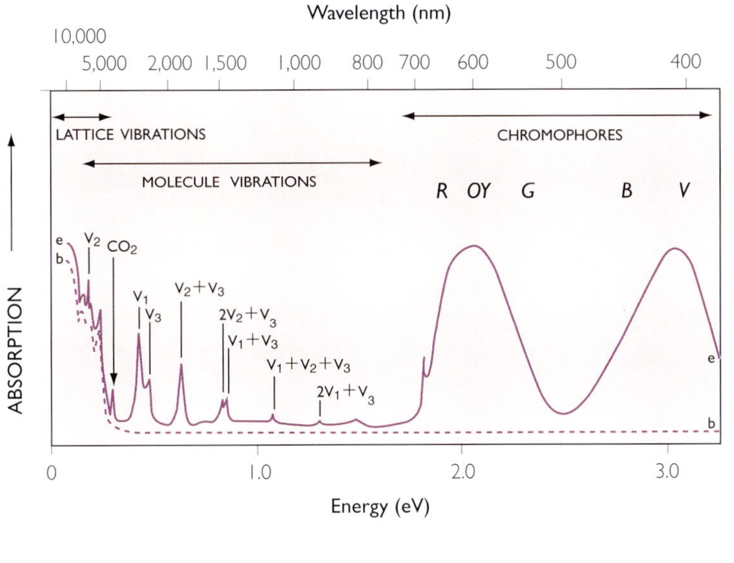

Figure 7.8 **The absorption spectrum of colorless beryl (b) and emerald (e), the latter showing vibrational absorptions derived from water molecules and carbon dioxide CO_2 in the infra-red and from Cr^{3+} in the visible. (After D.L. Wood and K. Nassau (1968) *American Mineralogist*, 53, 777.)**

seen in indoor pools, as well as the difference in color between the pale blue of a shallow lagoon and the deep blue of the adjacent deep ocean. The gray seen in bad weather does not derive from reflection but from light scattered from foam and air bubbles close to the surface, which prevent the deeper penetration required to show a blue. An extended discussion is given by Nassau (2001).

Excited vibrational states of a molecule, as well as the related excited rotational states of the molecule, can be superimposed on the electronic excitations of the previous section. These are involved in the violet color of iodine vapor as in Figure 7.9, the reddish-brown of bromine liquid and vapor, and the green of chlorine gas. The blue–green emitted by an oxygen-rich gas flame seen on a kitchen range or a bunsen burner also involves such superimposed vibrational, rotational, and electronic excitations in unstable molecules such as CH and C_2.

7.6 MECHANISMS 4 AND 5: COLOR FROM LIGAND FIELD EFFECTS

A large energy is required to excite one of a pair of electrons in most inorganic substances, hence electronic absorptions generally occur in the ultra-violet as in Figure 7.1. Unpaired electrons are present in transition metal compounds, usually in d or f orbitals, as in salts of the d transition elements such as chromium (see Figure 7.10), iron, cobalt, nickel, and copper; of the 4f lanthanides such as cerium and neodymium; and of the 5f actinides such as uranium. Light absorption can then occur at lower energies in the visible region of the spectrum. This leads to the ligand field colors of Mechanism 4 and provides the colors of many minerals and paint pigments.

This same explanation applies to Mechanism 5, where the transition metal is only an impurity, typically present at about the one percent level in an otherwise colorless substance. This provides some of the colors in minerals, gemstones, ceramics, glass, glazes, and enamels.

Consider a crystal of the aluminum oxide corundum Al_2O_3, also known as colorless sapphire when in gem quality form. Each aluminum is surrounded by six oxygens in the form of a slightly distorted octahedron as shown in Figure 7.11. All electrons are paired and there is no absorption in the visible region. Now replace one out of every hundred aluminums by a trivalent chromium ion, which has 18 paired and three unpaired electrons. These unpaired electrons are situated in 3d orbitals which have the capacity to hold ten electrons, two in each of the

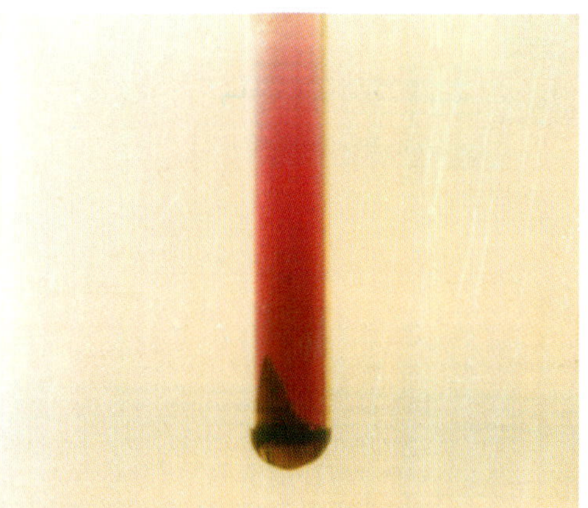

Figure 7.9 Iodine vapor produced by heating iodine crystals (combined electronic-vibration-rotation color).

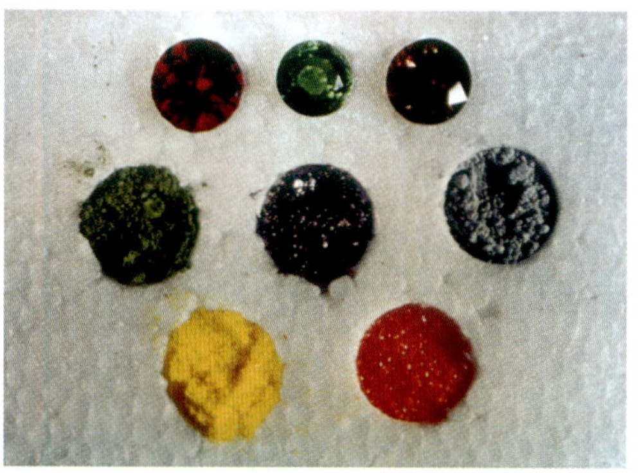

Figure 7.10 Some colors produced by chromium. (Left to right, above) alexandrite, emerald, and ruby (all three Cr^{3+} allochromatic ligand field colors); (center) chromium carbonate, chromium chloride, and chromium oxide (all three Cr^{3+} idiochromatic ligand field colors); (below) ammonium dichromate and potassium chromate (both Cr^{6+} charge transfer colors).

five orbitals customarily designated d_{xy}, d_{yz}, d_{xz}, $d_{x^2-y^2}$, and d_{z^2}. In a free chromium ion all the 3d electrons would occupy levels having the same energy as in the central part of Figure 7.12, so that again light-absorbing transitions could not occur.

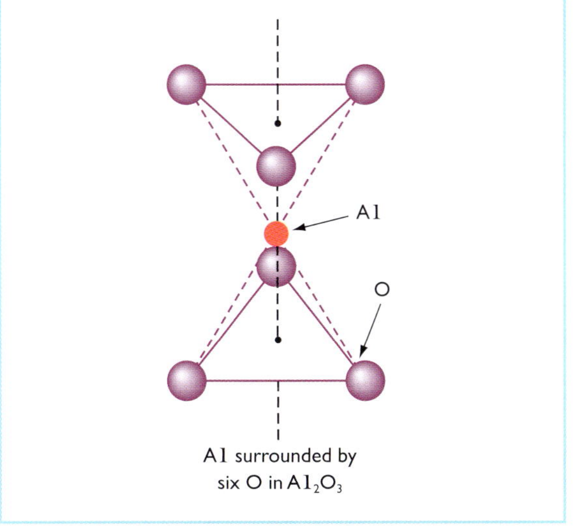

Figure 7.11 The distorted octahedral oxygen ligand environment around an Al ion in sapphire Al_2O_3.

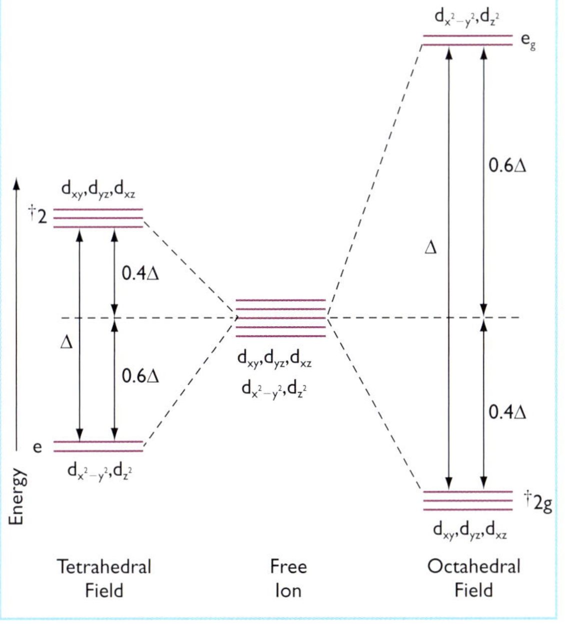

Figure 7.12 The splitting of the five 3d orbitals in a tetrahedral and an octahedral ligand field.

In corundum, however, such energy levels are perturbed by the existence of the six neighboring oxygens – the 'ligands' – in Figure 7.11. The spacing of the levels as at the left and right in Figure 7.12 is affected by two factors: the geometrical distribution of the ligands (here distorted octahedral) and the strength of the bonding, the ligand field (or the crystal field, the equivalent size of the electric field produced by the oxygen ions), here very large. This is covered by ligand field theory (an earlier, less sophisticated version was crystal field theory). Ligand field theory can also be viewed as a special case of the molecular orbital theory discussed next.

Consider now ruby, which is Al_2O_3 containing 1% or so chromium in the form Cr^{3+} replacing Al^{3+}. The symmetry of the ligand field and its strength give the energy level scheme at (A) and transition scheme at (B) in Figure 7.13. Here the short-wavelength violet and medium-wavelength yellow–green regions of the spectrum passing through ruby are absorbed in the two upward arrows in (B). This produces the absorption spectrum shown at (C), giving ruby its predominantly long-wavelength transmission and therefore its deep red color seen in Figures 7.10 and 7.14. The Cr^{3+} must pass through the energy level labeled ^2E in losing its energy again, with the emission of some heat. When it returns from ^2E back down to the ground state, a photon of long-wavelength light is emitted, giving ruby a red fluorescence, best seen under ultra-violet illumination as in Figure 7.14. This fluorescence is harnessed in the ruby laser.

Consider now a Cr^{3+} present in the emerald of Figure 7.8 discussed above. Here too the symmetry is distorted octahedral, but the ligand field is a little weaker, being 2.05 eV instead of the 2.23 eV of ruby at (A) to (C) in Figure 7.13. Although this is a relatively small change, it produces a significant shift in the absorption bands as shown at (D) in Figure 7.13 (and also seen in the upper curve of Figure 7.8). The dominant transmission is in the medium-wavelength region, producing the change from the red color of ruby to the green color of emerald, seen in Figures 7.10 and 7.14! Interestingly enough, the position of the ^2E level does not change significantly with the ligand field, as can be seen at (A) in Figure 7.13 so that the same red fluorescence

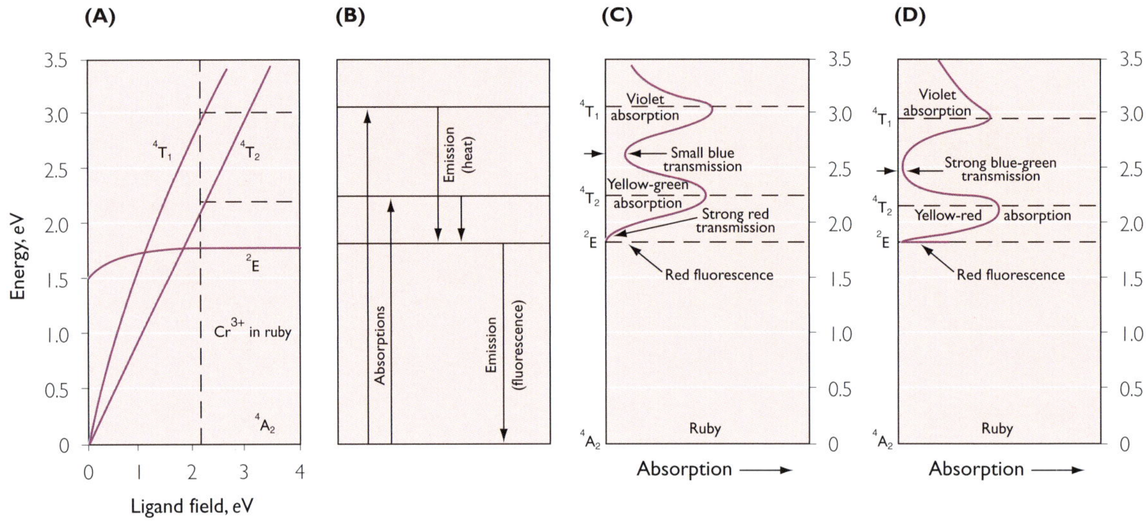

Figure 7.13 The term diagram of Cr^{3+} in a distorted octahedral field (A), the energy levels and transitions in ruby (B), and the resulting absorption spectra and fluorescence of ruby (C) and emerald (D).

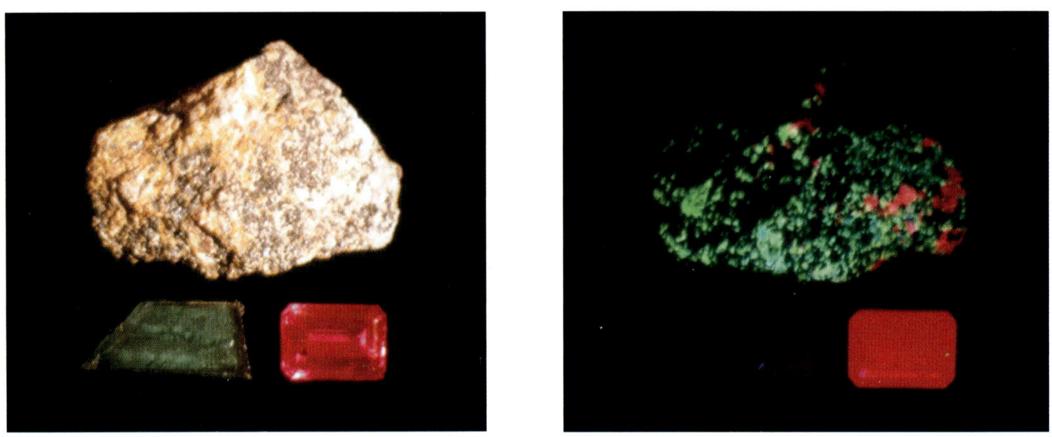

Figure 7.14 White light (left) and ultra-violet light (right) views of a mineral specimen from Franklin, New Jersey, containing calcite $CaCO_3$ (tan color with red fluorescence) and willemite $ZnSiO_4$ (brown with green fluorescence), both containing MnO^{2+}, as well as green emerald $Be_3Al_2Si_60_{18}$:Cr and red ruby Al_2O_3:Cr, both showing the red Cr^{3+} fluorescence; ruby is 2 cm across (all derived from allochromatic ligand field effects).

is present in both red ruby and green emerald, as just barely visible in Figure 7.14.

What then might be the color of a ligand field intermediate between that of green emerald and that of red ruby? Nature has provided for us an answer in the form of the extremely rare and precious gemstone alexandrite, an answer that demonstrates how she can confound our expectations and yet turn out to be perfectly reasonable in retrospect. The medium- and long-wavelength absorption bands are so delicately balanced in alexandrite that in daylight (rich in short wavelengths) or the similar quality light from a fluorescent tube lamp we see a blue–green color, somewhat resembling emerald, while in candle light or the light from an incandescent lamp (rich in long wavelengths) we perceive a red color, somewhat resembling a ruby, as shown in Figure 7.15.

As the chromium concentration of colorless

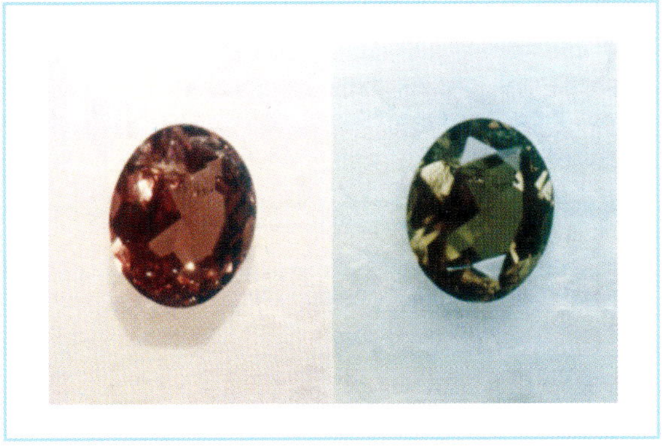

Figure 7.15 A synthetic alexandrite gemstone, 5 mm across, changing from a reddish color in the light from an incandescent lamp to a greenish color in the light from a fluorescent tube lamp (allochromatic ligand field effects).

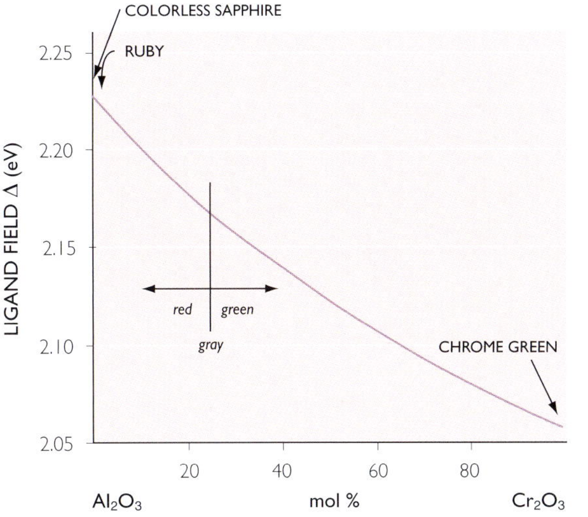

Figure 7.16 The variation of the ligand field and the color in the solid solution system between colorless sapphire Al_2O_3 and chrome green Cr_2O_3. (After D. Reinen (1969) *Structure and Bonding*, 6, 39.)

to pink sapphire is increased to form ruby and beyond, the ligand field becomes weaker. The result is a change from colorless through red and gray to the dark green of pure chromium oxide Cr_20_3, the pigment chrome green, as shown in Figure 7.16. A specimen on the red side of gray (including ruby itself) can be turned green by heating it, which causes the atoms to move apart from thermal expansion, producing a reduction of the ligand field as in 'thermochromism.' In the reverse process, a specimen on the green side of gray can be turned red by the application of pressure in 'piezochromism.'

Mechanism 4 colors comprise most transition metal compounds (sometimes called 'idiochromatic,' i.e. self-colored) including pigments such as the chrome green mentioned above, green viridian $Cr_2O(OH)_4$; blue smalt glass $K_2CoSi_30_8$, and Thenard's blue Al_2CoO_4; gemstones such as pink rhodochrosite $MnCO_3$ and green malachite $Cu_2(CO_3)$ $(OH)_2$; and minerals and ores such as brown manganite $MnO(OH)$, red iron ore Fe_2O_3, yellow goethite $FeO(OH)$, and green bunsenite NiO. The idiochromatically colored copper mineral shattuckite $Cu_5(SiO_3)_4(OH)_2$ is shown in Figure 7.1.

Small amounts of these same transition metals give color in otherwise colorless substances in Mechanism 5 (sometimes called 'allochromatic,' i.e. other-colored). Examples include many minerals and gemstones including the chromium-based ruby, emerald, and alexandrite seen in Figures 7.10, 7.14, 7.15 and discussed above; the manganese-colored pink morganite form of beryl; the iron-colored blue to green aquamarines and tourmalines, yellow citrine, green jade (in part); and so on. The red fluorescence of chromium in ruby and emerald as well as the red and green fluorescence of divalent manganese in calcite and willemite, respectively, can be seen in Figure 7.14. Some colors in ceramics, glass, glazes, and enamels are also based on transition metal impurities. The allochromatic mineral spinel can be colored a deep blue by cobalt, as shown in Figure 7.1.

7.7 MECHANISM 6: COLOR FROM MOLECULAR ORBITALS

Here color derives from organic compounds involving electrons belonging to several atoms within a molecule. The related charge transfer colors are discussed separately in the next section.

A 'conjugated' organic compound is one that contains alternating single and double bonds in chains and/or rings of (mostly) carbon atoms. Such an arrangement contains 'pi-bonded' electrons located in molecular orbitals which belong to the whole chain and/or ring system. If such systems are large enough, the excited states of these electrons occur at energies similar to those of the unpaired electrons in transition metal compounds and can therefore absorb and emit photons. The absorptions of the conjugated cyclic benzene C_6H_6 or the linear 2,4 hexadiene C_6H_{10}, $CH_3—CH{=}CH—CH{=}CH—CH_3$ are still in the ultra-violet, but with the conjugated linear ten carbon chain 2,4,6,8 decatetraene $C_{10}H_{14}$, the absorption has moved into the short-wavelength end of the spectrum and produces a complementary pale yellow color.

In addition to extending the length of the conjugated chain, there are a variety of other means of obtaining the desired 'bathochromic' shift of the absorptions to longer wavelengths (lower energies). Such shifts are produced by the presence of electron donor groups which push electrons into the conjugated system, such as the $-NH_2$ group in the dye crystal violet $C(C_6H_4NH_2)_3$ shown in Figure 7.17, or electron acceptor groups which pull electrons out of the conjugated system, such as the NO_2 group. An example of a molecule containing both is one of the nitrophenylenediamine dyes also shown in Figure 7.17. This dye absorbs in the short-wavelength part of the spectrum and gives a complementary yellow to brown color. It is used in hair dyes where it can penetrate into the hair because of its small size. Molecules that have many resonance structures tend to provide large bathochromic shifts. Two of the resonance forms of crystal violet are shown in Figure 7.17. A large multi-ring molecule is the red–violet dye violanthrone which is attractive to look at even in the formula, shown in Figure 7.18.

A 'spinel doublet,' an imitation of blue sapphire, consists of two pieces of colorless spinel held together with a layer of cement containing an organic blue dye, shown in Figure 7.1.

A useful conjugated 'chromophore' (color-bearing) group is that of the blue dye indigo, also shown in Figure 7.18. This has been used since antiquity, from the woad of the 'Picts' (painted people) whom Julius Caesar fought in Britain in 58 BC, up to today's all-pervading blue jeans. With two bromine atoms added, the result is Tyrian purple, laboriously extracted from certain sea shells and used exclusively by Roman emperors as a status symbol.

Molecular orbital dye colors occur widely in

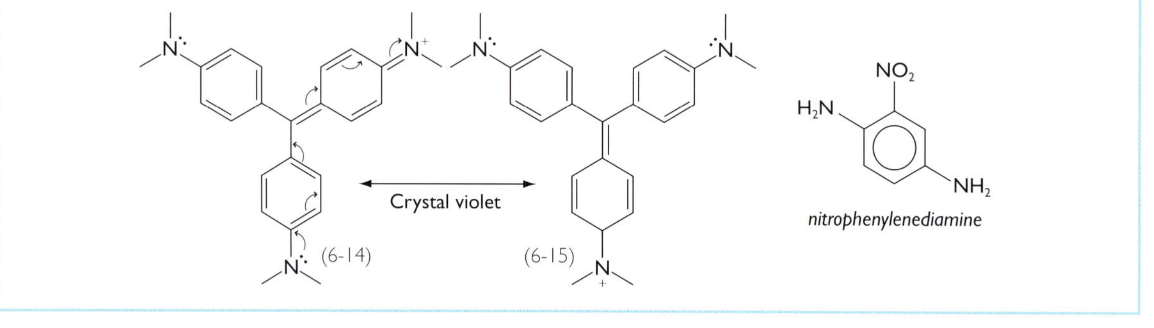

Figure 7.17 **Two resonance structures of crystal violet (left) and the structure of a nitrophenylenediamine hair dye (right).**

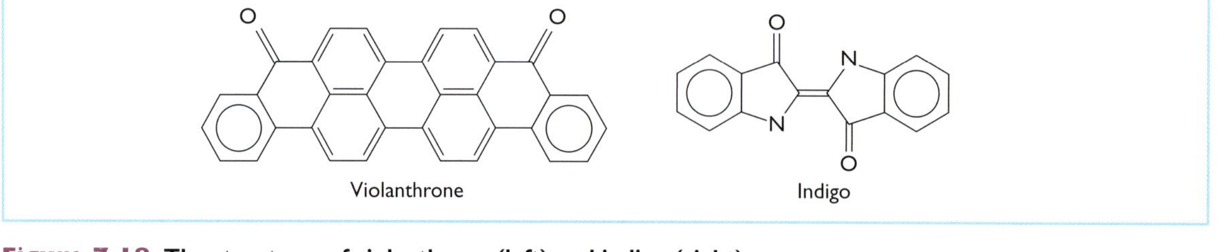

Figure 7.18 **The structures of violanthrone (left) and indigo (right).**

the plant and animal kingdoms as well as in the products of the modern synthetic dye and pigment industry. Just as with ligand field energy levels, some of the absorbed energy may be re-emitted in the form of fluorescence. This is used in dye lasers, where tuning of the wavelength of the laser light is possible because of the broad nature of the fluorescence peaks as shown in Figure 7.19. Chemical energy can also excite such a system and lead to fluorescence (or to a much slower phosphorescence) as in the bioluminescence of fireflies and angler fishes and in the chemoluminescent 'lightsticks' of Figure 7.20. Here a slow chemical reaction emits the fluorescence from organic molecules over a period of several hours.

If the conjugated aspect of the framework of an organic colorant molecule is destroyed, then the color will be lost. This can happen in bleaching, where a double bond may be converted to a single bond by the chlorine or peroxide in chemical bleaches or by oxidizing pollutants in the atmosphere. In photochemical bleaching or fading, ultra-violet present in sunlight and other illuminations provides the energy to permit even the oxygen in the air to produce the same conversion. This is why museums take care to avoid ultra-violet in their illumination.

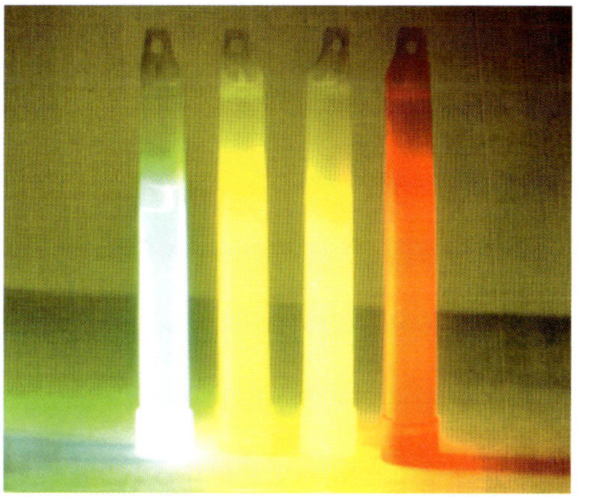

Figure 7.20 **Four chemoluminescent 'Cyalume' light sticks, 15 cm long, made by the American Cyanamid Company (molecular orbital effects).**

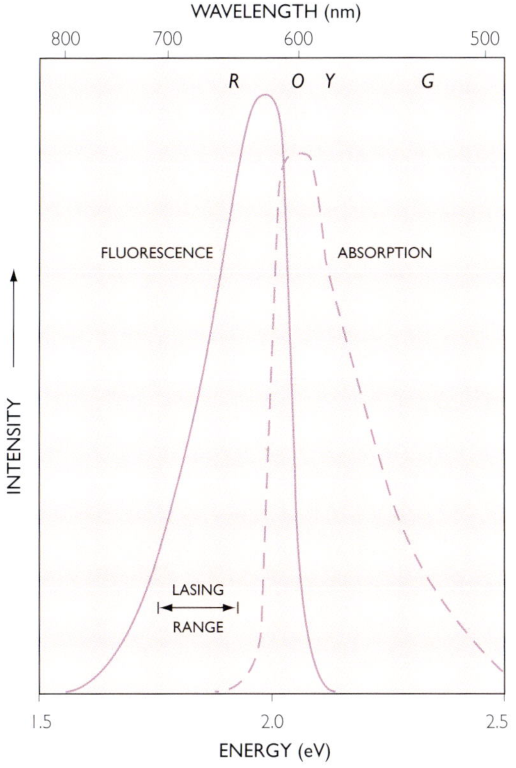

Figure 7.19 **Absorption and fluorescence spectra of cresyl violet, also known as the laser dye oxazine 9, dissolved in ethanol. (After K.H. Drexhage (1973) in F.P. Schafer (ed.), *Dye Lasers*. New York: Springer-Verlag.)**

7.8 MECHANISM 7: COLOR FROM CHARGE TRANSFER

A crystal of sapphire Al_2O_3 containing a few hundredths of one percent of titanium is colorless. If, instead, it contains a similar amount of iron, a pale yellow color is seen. However, when both impurities are present together they produce a magnificent deep blue color, that of blue sapphire, as seen in Figure 7.1. The mechanism at work is intervalence charge transfer, the motion of an electron from one transition metal ion to another produced by the absorption of the energy of a photon, resulting in a temporary change in the valence state of both ions. This also causes the black or dark colors of many variable valence transition metal oxides such as the iron oxide magnetite Fe_3O_4. This mechanism is sometimes also called electron hopping or cooperative charge transfer.

Consider two adjacent Al sites in corundum

occupied by Fe^{2+} and Ti^{4+} as in Figure 7.21. The transfer of an electron from the Fe to the Ti changes the valence state of both ions:

$$Fe^{2+} + Ti^{4+} \rightarrow Fe^{3+} + Ti^{3+}.$$

This process requires energy, as shown in Figure 7.22. Since the energy of 2.1 eV corresponds to the absorption of a medium-wavelength photon in the yellow region of the spectrum, the complementary color blue results.

Blue sapphire is an example of 'heteronuclear' intervalence charge transfer with two different transition metal ions involved. In black magnetite Fe_3O_4 or $Fe^{2+}O{\cdot}(Fe^{3+})_2O_3$, there is 'homonuclear' intervalence charge transfer with two valence states of the same metal in two different sites A and B:

$$(Fe^{2+})A + (Fe^{3+})B \rightarrow (Fe^{3+})A + (Fe^{2+})B.$$

The right-hand side of this equation has a higher energy than the left-hand side. The result is a broadband light absorption and the black color.

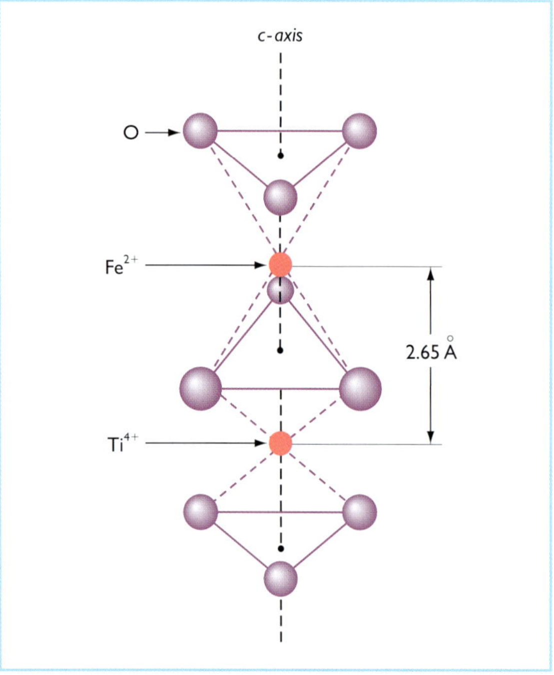

Figure 7.21 Two adjacent distorted octahedral sites containing Fe^{2+} and Ti^{4+} in blue sapphirel (compare with Figure 7.11).

In sapphire this mechanism is also present, but there it absorbs only in the infra-red.

This same mechanism gives the 'carbon–amber' brown beer-bottle color in glass made with iron sulfide and charcoal, and the brilliant blue color to the pigment Prussian blue $(Fe^{3+})_4[Fe^{2+}(CN)_6]_3$. The yellow/brown/red colors of many rocks, e.g. in the Painted Desert, derive from charge transfer involving small traces of iron.

Charge transfer can also involve ligand atoms. One example is the oxygen-to-chromium charge transfer in the yellow chromate K_2CrO_4. and the orange dichromate $(NH_4)_2(Cr^{6+})_2O_7$, both shown in Figure 7.10. Note that here the formal valence of 6+ on the Cr leaves no unpaired electrons and therefore prevents ligand field colors as occur in the trivalent Cr^{3+} of Figures 7.10, 7.14, and 7.15. In blue sapphire the charge transfer mechanism is also present, but absorbs only in the ultra-violet.

A final example of charge transfer is the deep blue gemstone lapis lazuli of Figure 7.1, which is the single crystal form of the pigment ultramarine, approximately $CaNa_7Al_6Si_6O_{24}S_3SO_4$. This color derives from charge transfer within groups of sulfur triplets $(S_3)^-$.

Charge transfer transitions are strong because they are 'allowed' by the selection rules, hence intense colors are produced by as little as 1/100 percent Fe and Ti in blue sapphire. By contrast the 'forbidden' transitions in the ligand field colored ruby are so weak that one percent or more Cr is required to produce an intense red color.

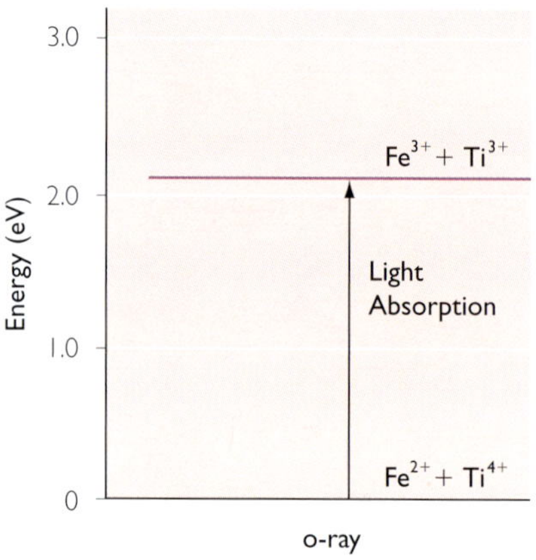

Figure 7.22 Transition from the ground state to the excited state in the blue sapphire of Figure 7.21.

7.9 MECHANISM 8: METALLIC COLORS FROM BAND THEORY

Consider two hydrogen atoms coming together to form a bond as shown Figure 7.23. Two equal energy atomic orbitals, one from each hydrogen atom, interact to form two molecular orbitals. One of these, the bonding molecular orbital, has a lower energy, while the other, the antibonding orbital, has a higher energy. The molecular orbitals can accommodate exactly the same number of electrons as the atomic orbitals from which they were formed, namely two per orbital. For the normal bonding distance d between the two atoms, Figure 7.23 leads from atomic orbitals at (A) in Figure 7.24 to the two molecular orbitals at (B).

If we now consider four atoms, we expect to see four separate energy molecular orbitals as at (C) in Figure 7.24. Extrapolating this approach to a piece of metal containing some 10^{23} strongly interacting atoms per cubic centimeter, we can reasonably expect the bonding to involve 10^{23} molecular orbitals in an 'energy band' as at (D) in Figure 7.24. Here there are so many levels that the band may be viewed as being occupied in an essentially continuous manner. If the band has an energy range of 1 eV then the spacing between adjacent levels would be 10^{-23} eV, an immeasurably small quantity for all practical purposes.

Band theory gives a full explanation of the properties of the metals of the periodic table and of the alloys formed by mixtures of them. The exact shape of the energy band depends on the atomic orbitals involved (3d and 4s for the first row transition elements, as in Figure 7.25), on the relative amounts of the atoms present, on the geometrical packing arrangement of the atoms, and on the spacing between the atoms. The total number of electrons involved is the sum of the valence electrons for all the atoms present, that is those electrons outside the full shells and therefore available for bonding. These electrons now occupy the band from the bottom upward, just as if one were pouring a liquid into an oddly shaped container, as in the shading for iron Fe in Figure 7.25. This 'density of states' diagram shows that the capacity to hold electrons varies at different energies within the band. The highest energy filled level is called the Fermi surface, usually designated E_f, and is illustrated for iron and copper Cu in Figure 7.25. The bonding electrons no longer belong to individual atoms, but to the piece of metal as a whole. They are 'delocalized.' In copper, which has three more conduction electrons per atom than iron, the band is filled to a higher level.

The good electrical and thermal properties of metals immediately follow from this arrangement. An electric field raises the energy of an electron from below the Fermi surface to a high energy level in the empty part of the band, as indicated for iron by the vertical arrows in Figure 7.25. This creates a negatively charged electron above E_f and a positively charged 'hole', which is

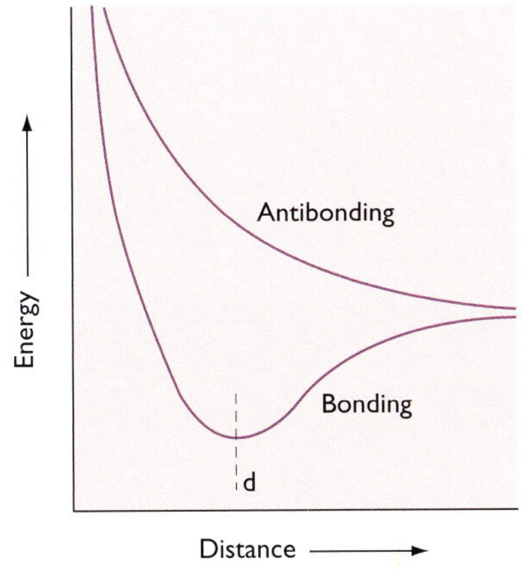

Figure 7.23 The energy of bonding and antibonding molecular orbitals of the hydrogen molecule He.

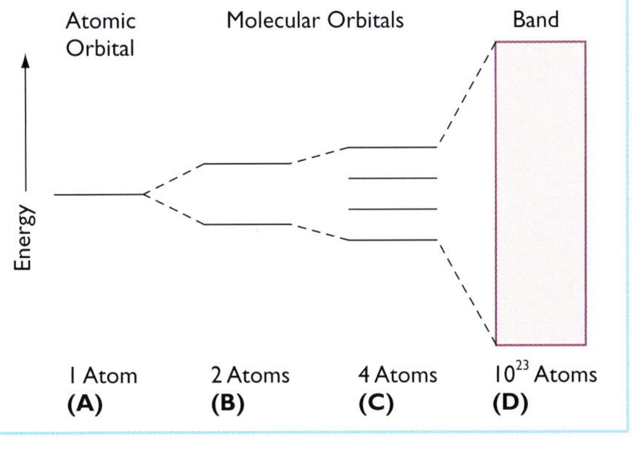

Figure 7.24 The conversion of atomic orbitals (A) into molecular orbitals (B and C) and into a band (D).

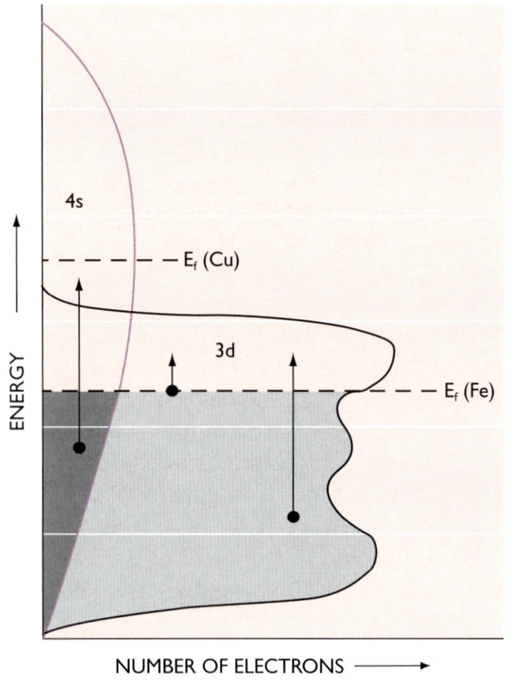

Figure 7.25 Schematic density of states diagram for the metals iron Fe and copper Cu. (After J. Slater (1951) *Quantum Theory of Matter.* New York: McGraw-Hill.)

a missing electron in the otherwise continuous electron sea below E_f. In the applied electric field these two species move in opposite directions, the result being an electric current; the two species generally move at different speeds. A similar excitation by heat also produces electrons and holes, both of which diffuse away from the hot region toward the cold region, thus producing a flow of energy. This results in the thermal conductivity, where there is no net charge movement.

When light falls onto a metal, the electrons below the Fermi surface can also become excited into higher energy levels in the empty part of the band by absorbing the energy from the light, producing electron-hole pairs, again as indicated by the arrows in Figure 7.25. The light is so intensely absorbed that it can penetrate to a depth of only a few hundred atoms, typically less than a single wavelength. Since the metal is a conductor of electricity, this absorbed light which is, after all, an electromagnetic wave, will induce alternating electrical currents in the metal surface. Electromagnetic theory shows that these currents immediately re-emit the light back out of the metal, thus providing the strong reflection of a smooth (polished) metal surface.

The efficiency of this process depends on the selection rules which apply to the atomic orbitals from which the energy band had formed. If the efficiency of the absorption and re-emission processes is approximately equal at all optical energies, then the different wavelengths present in white light will be reflected equally well, thus leading to the silvery colors of the smooth surfaces of metals such as iron, chromium, and silver. However, if the efficiency decreases with increasing energy, as is the case for gold and copper, the slightly reduced reflectivity at the higher energy end of the spectrum results in the observed yellow and reddish colors, respectively. The colors of alloys follow the same general pattern but are difficult to predict. For example, the addition of 25% copper to pure gold produces an alloy with a reddish color, while a similar amount of silver produces a greenish one.

The direct light absorption of a metal in the absence of reflection can be observed only rarely. Gold is extremely malleable and can be beaten into gold leaf less than 100 nm thick. This is less than the thickness necessary to support fully the electric currents which produce the metallic reflection. Under these circumstances a bluish green color is additionally seen in transmitted light. When gold is in a colloidal form, however as in the 10 nm diameter particles which give the color to 'ruby glass,' the complex scattering theory originated by Mie explains the unexpected red color. A yellow color in glass also derives from Mie scattering, but here from metallic colloidal silver particles. Both of these colors can be seen in Figure 7.26.

7.10 MECHANISM 9: COLOR IN SEMICONDUCTORS

In some band theory materials it is possible for a gap, the 'band gap,' to occur within the band, with important consequences for color. This happens when there are exactly four valence electrons per atom on average available for entry into the band in a chemical element or compound. The result is that the lower energy band, now called the valence band, is exactly filled with electrons to its capacity and the upper band, called the conduction band, is exactly empty, as shown at the left in Figure 7.27. The size of the energy spacing between the edges of the two bands is the band-gap energy (or energy gap), usually designated E_g.

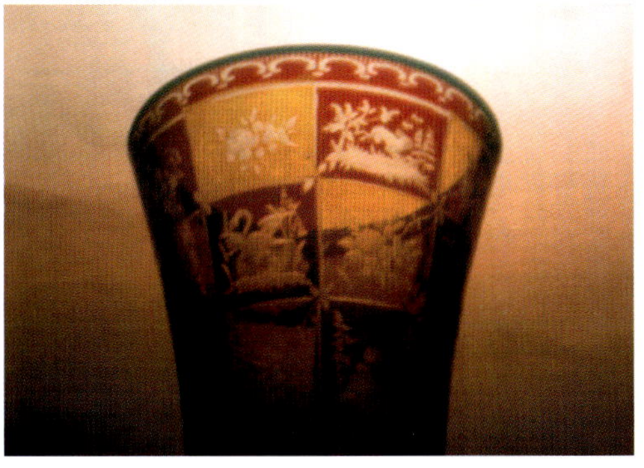

Figure 7.26 Antique engraved Czechoslovakian glass colored yellow with silver and red with gold (both Mie scattering from colloidal metal particles).

Consider the absorption of light as represented by the vertical arrows A, B, and C in Figure 7.27. Since there are no electron energy levels within the band gap, the lowest energy light that can be absorbed corresponds to arrow A, involving the excitation of an electron from the top of the valence band to the bottom of the conduction band. The energy of this light of course corresponds to the band-gap energy E_g. Light of any higher energy can also be absorbed as indicated by arrows B and C.

If the substance represented by this figure has a large band gap, that is large on the scale of optical energies, such as the 5.4 eV of diamond or the similar value of pure sapphire, then none of the energies of the visible spectrum can be absorbed. These substances are indeed colorless when pure, as in Figure 7.28. Such

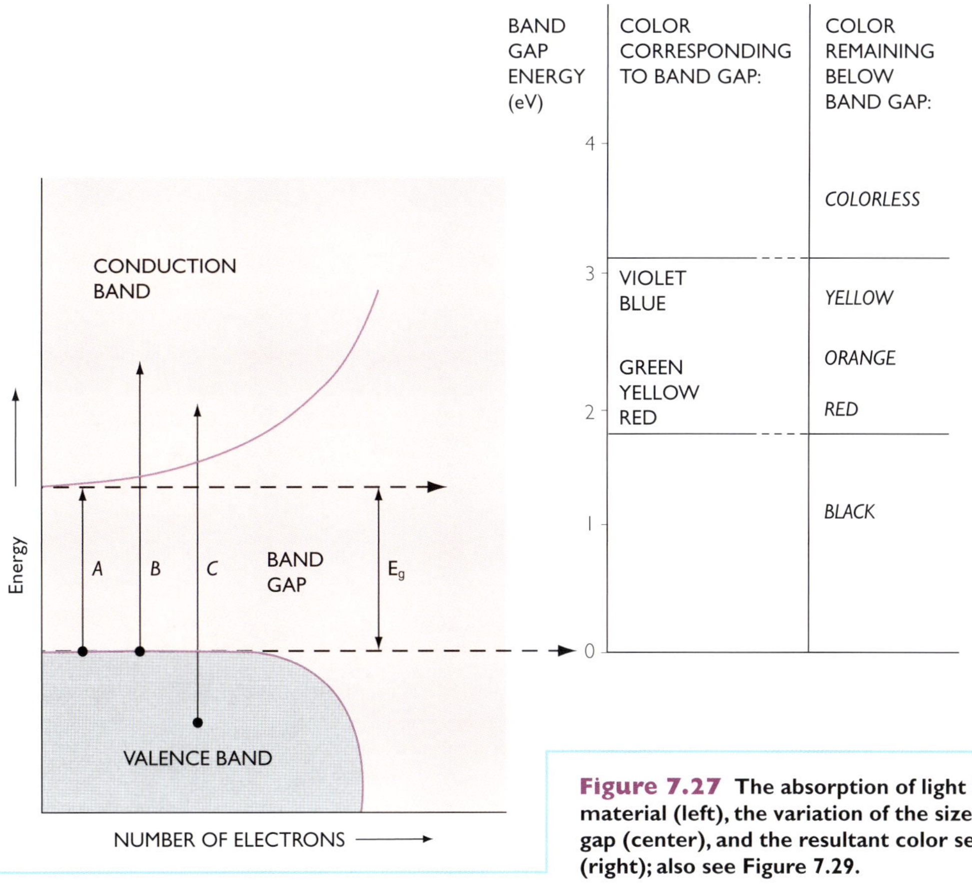

Figure 7.27 The absorption of light in a band-gap material (left), the variation of the size of the band gap (center), and the resultant color sequence (right); also see Figure 7.29.

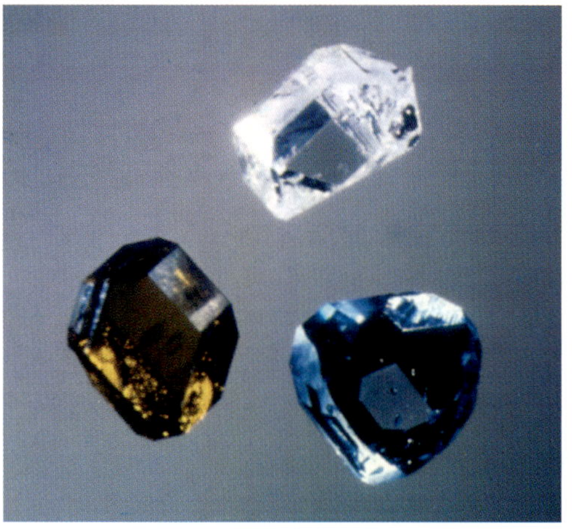

Figure 7.28 **Synthetic diamond crystals: colorless (pure, large band-gap semiconductor), yellow (doped semiconductor containing nitrogen donor), and blue (doped semiconductor containing boron acceptor) grown at the General Electric Co.; the largest is 3 mm across.**

'large band-gap semiconductors' are excellent electrical insulators because a very large voltage would be required to excite an electron across the energy gap. They can also be viewed as covalently to ionically bonded materials, as is usually done in chemistry.

Consider now a 'medium band-gap semiconductor,' a material with a somewhat smaller band gap with energy E_g within the visible spectrum. An example is the compound cadmium sulfide CdS, which is also known as the pigment cadmium yellow and the mineral greenockite. The 2.6 eV band-gap energy listed in Table 7.2 permits absorption of the highest energy (shortest wavelengths) part of the visible spectrum, but of none of the other wavelengths. This leads to the complementary yellow color as can be deduced from the color scales at the right of Figure 7.27.

A somewhat smaller band gap of 2.3 eV permits absorption of the medium to large energy wavelengths of the visible spectrum and produces the complementary orange color as shown in Figure 7.27. A yet smaller band gap as in the pigment vermillion, also known as the mineral cinnabar HgS, with a band gap of 2.0 eV, results in all energies except the lowest being absorbed and thus leads to a red color. All visible energies are absorbed when the band-gap energy is less than the 1.77 eV (700 nm) limit of the visible spectrum. These 'narrow band-gap semiconductors' are therefore black, as in the last three materials of Table 7.2.

An illustration of this change in the band-gap size is shown by mixed crystals of yellow cadmium sulfide CdS, E_g = 2.6 eV, and black cadmium selenide CdSe, 1.6 eV; these compounds have the same structure and form a continuous solid solution series. Figure 7.29 illustrates the yellow-orange-red-black sequence of these mixed crystals as the band-gap energy decreases following the sequence at the right in Figure 7.27. Mixed crystals such as Cd_4SSe_3 form the painter's pigment cadmium orange and are also used to provide a range of orange colors in opaque glass and plastic. Mercuric sulfide HgS exists in two different crystalline forms. Cinnabar (the pigment vermillion) with E_g = 2.0 eV is a deep red but can transform on exposure to light in an improperly formulated paint to the black metacinnabar with E_g = 1.6 eV. This has happened in a number of old paintings in as little as five years.

Table 7.2 Colors of some band-gap semiconductors

Substance	Mineral name	Pigment name	Band gap energy (eV)	Color
C	Diamond		5.4	Colorless
ZnO	Zincite	Zinc White	3.0	Colorless
CdS	Greenockite	Cadmium Yellow	2.6	Yellow
$CdS_{1-x}Se_x$		Cadmium Orange	2.3	Orange
HgS	Cinnabar	Vermillion	2.0	Red
HgS	Metacinnabar		1.6	Black
Si			1.1	Black
PbS	Galena		0.4	Black

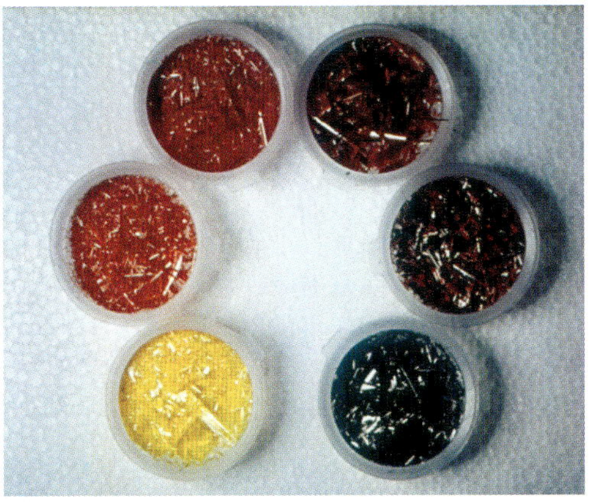

Figure 7.29 **Mixed solid solution crystals of yellow cadmium sulfide CdS and black cadmium selenide CdSe showing the intermediate band-gap colors as in Figure 7.27.**

7.11 MECHANISM 10: COLOR FROM IMPURITIES IN SEMICONDUCTORS

If an added substance or 'dopant' forms an 'impurity level' within the band gap, then light can be absorbed by (or emitted from) a wide band-gap semiconductor at energies less than the band gap. A pure diamond crystal is composed of carbon atoms, each of which contributes four valence electrons to the valence band. It is colorless, as in Figure 7.28. Now consider a diamond in which just a few carbon atoms out of a million have been replaced by nitrogen atoms, each containing five valence electrons. The structure of the diamond is not significantly disturbed. The extra electrons enter a donor level, so-called because these electrons can be donated from it to the empty conduction band during the absorption of energy, as shown at the left in Figure 7.30. Note that the valence band remains completely filled and the impurity levels are fully localized, so that there are no movable electrons or holes that could provide electrical conductivity.

The donor level is broadened by thermal vibrations and other factors, as at the right of Figure 7.30. The resulting absorption at the high energy, short-wavelength end of the visible spectrum leads to the complementary yellow color seen in both natural and synthetic (man-made) nitrogen-containing diamonds, as in Figure 7.28.

Boron has one less electron than carbon, and the presence of just a few boron atoms per million carbon atoms in diamond produces holes in the band gap as shown in Figure 7.31. The resulting energy level is called an 'acceptor' level since it can accept electrons from the full valence band. The energy required for this change in boron-doped diamond is very small and, because of broadening, absorbs only at the low energy, long-wavelength end of the visible spectrum, leading to the complementary blue color as in Figure 7.28. Since the acceptor level energy is so small, even the thermal energy at room temperature can produce this excitation. The resulting holes in the valence band can now move in the presence of an electric field. Accordingly blue boron-doped diamonds, including the famous Hope diamond, conduct electricity at room temperature.

Some double-doped materials contain both donors and acceptors, as in Figure 7.32. Under suitable circumstances these can absorb ultra-violet or electrical energy to produce the transition a from the valence band up to the conduction band. If the return path proceeds via steps f, g, and d, then light may be emitted corresponding to the energy release from one of these downward steps, such as g. This is then fluorescence or electroluminescence, respectively, depending on the nature of the excitation. The former occurs in 'phosphor' powders, for example in zinc sulfide ZnS containing Cu and other additives, used as an internal coating in the fluorescent tube lamps discussed above. These phosphors convert the ultra-violet produced by the mercury into visible light, particularly into low energy, longer wavelength light so as to produce a more reddish 'warmer' light approximating daylight. Phosphors are also used inside the screen of a television tube, activated by a stream of electrons (cathode rays) in cathodoluminescence.

Electroluminescence can use a similar powder deposited onto a thin sheet of metal and covered with a transparent conducting electrode to produce lighting panels, often used as nightlights.

Some phosphors contain impurities which form 'trapping' levels, as at the right in Figure

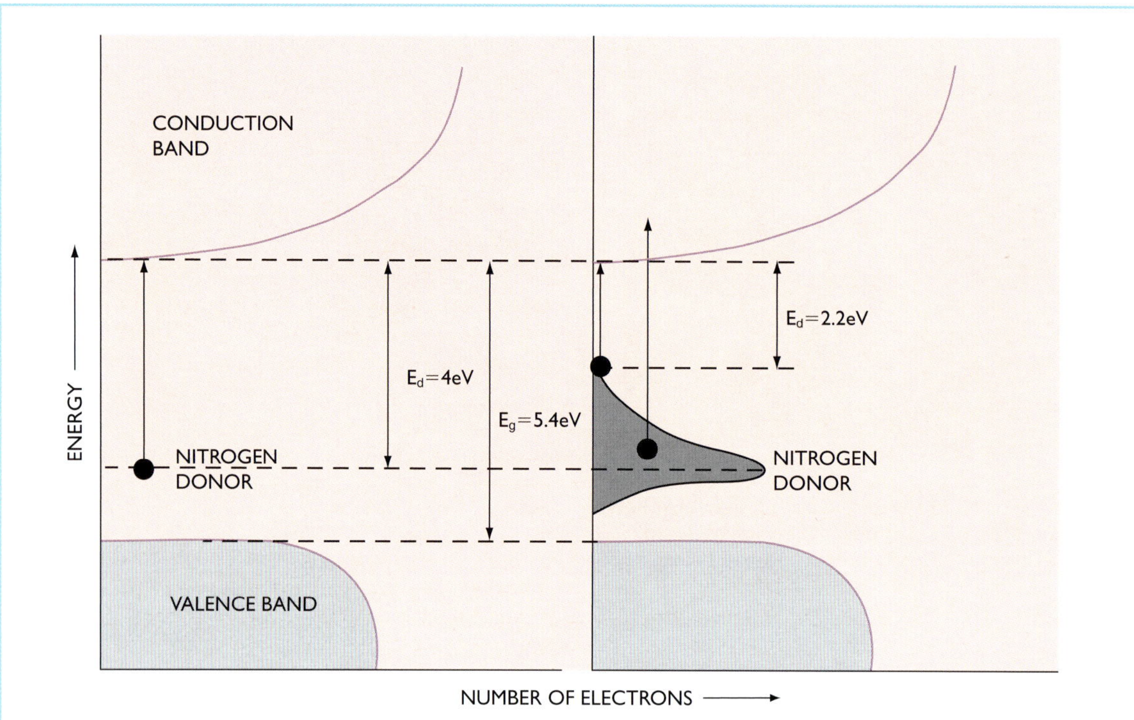

Figure 7.30 The nitrogen donor energy level in the band gap of diamond (left) forms a broadened band and results in the absorption of light (right) to give a yellow color.

7.32. An excited electron may land in a trap, as by steps a and j in this figure, and can then only be released when additional energy is added to permit step k and subsequent light emission via f, g, and d as above. If the trap level is close to the conduction band, then even the thermal energy of room temperature may be able to supply the energy required for release from the trap by step k slowly, thus resulting in phosphorescence, lasting seconds to many minutes. If the energy required for release is a little larger, then infra-red light may permit the escape, so that higher energy visible light is then produced as in a pre-excited infra-red detecting screen.

Finally, there is injection luminescence, which can occur in a crystal containing a junction between differently doped semiconductor regions. An electric current can then produce recombination between electrons and holes in the junction region, giving light from tiny light-emitting diodes (LEDs). These are widely used in alphanumeric display devices (usually red) in electronic equipment, in fiber-optic communication systems, in compact disc players, and so on. With a suitable geometry, the emitted light can be coherent in the similarly functioning semiconductor lasers.

7.12 MECHANISM 11: COLOR FROM COLOR CENTERS

If a century old glass bottle is exposed in the desert to the ultra-violet radiation present in the strong (because of unpolluted desert air) sunlight for ten years or so, the glass will have acquired an attractive purple color. If such a bottle is instead exposed to an intense source of energetic radiation, such as in a cobalt-60 gamma-ray cell, then an even deeper purple color appears within a few minutes, as shown at upper left in Figure 7.33. Either color disappears on heating the bottle in a medium-hot baking oven.

The color in this 'desert amethyst glass' derives from a color center associated with a manganese impurity that was used at one time to decolorize greenish iron-containing glass. Similar color centers explain the colors of the gemstones

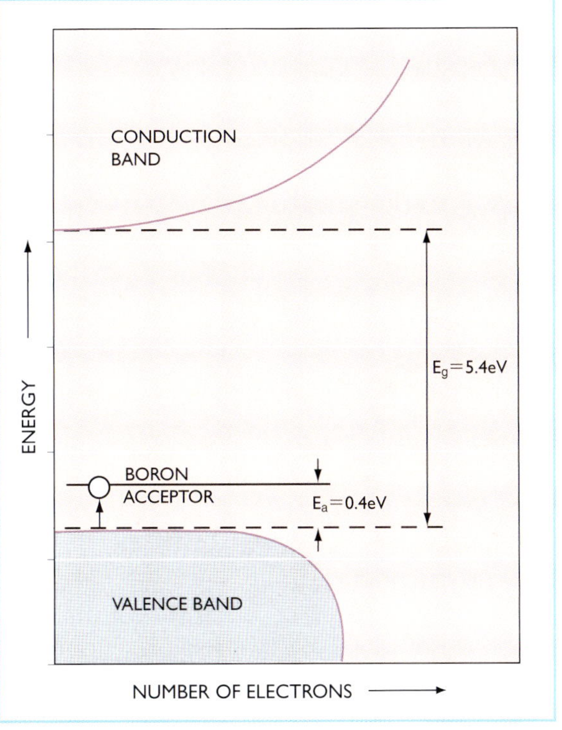

Figure 7.31 **The boron acceptor energy level in the band gap of diamond, resulting in a blue color and in electrical conductivity as in the Hope diamond.**

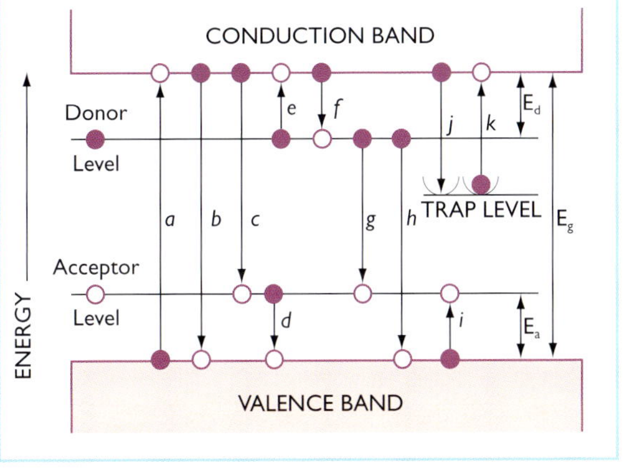

Figure 7.32 **Possible absorption and emission transitions in the band gap of a phosphor containing acceptor, donor, and trapping levels.**

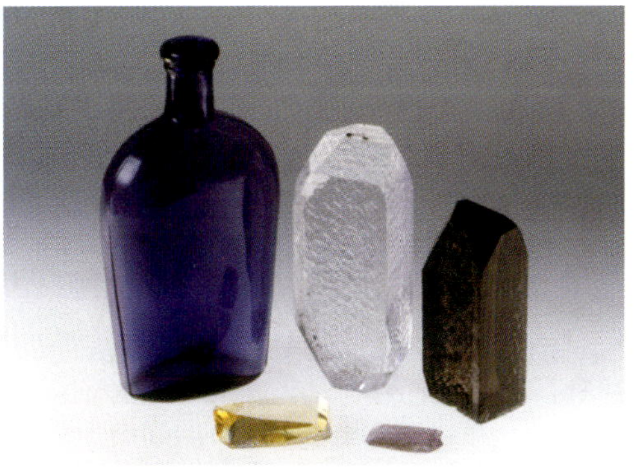

Figure 7.33 **(Left to right, above) century-old glass bottle, irradiated to form 'desert amethyst glass' (color center); colorless synthetic quartz crystal as grown, and one that has been irradiated to form smoky quartz (color center); below: a synthetic citrine quartz colored yellow by Fe (transition metal impurity) and one that has been additionally irradiated to form amethyst (color center).**

amethyst, smoky quartz, and yellow to orange to brown and blue topaz. Many other materials, both natural and man-made, can be irradiated to produce color centers, including irradiated diamonds of various colors. All the specific color centers mentioned so far are perfectly stable, losing their color only when heated. Other color centers exist that are unstable and fade when exposed to light, while yet others fade even during storage in the dark.

The term color center is sometimes used so loosely that even transition metal and band-gap colorations are incorporated. This rare usage ignores the unique characteristics of color centers; the conventional academic usage is followed here.

Consider an ionic crystal such as ordinary table salt, the alkali halide sodium chloride NaCl. This consists of a three-dimensional array of Na^+ and Cl^- ions. A single Cl^- can be missing in two different ways: if a compensating Na^+ is also missing, then the crystal remains electrically neutral and color is not produced. If, however, a Na^+ is not missing, then another way of maintaining electrical neutrality is for a free electron, designated e^-, to occupy the site vacated by the Cl^-. This entity is called an F-center, after the German 'Farbe' (color). One can view the lone electron as if it were part of an imaginary negatively charged transition metal ion located in the ligand field of the surrounding K^+ ions, or one can view this electron as consisting of a trapping energy level within the band gap of this transparent wide band-gap semiconductor material, exactly as at the right in Figure 7.32.

Some form of exciting energy, such as irradiation by ultra-violet or by high-energy electrons, x-rays, or gamma rays, can now excite an electron from the valence band into the conduction band and from there into the trap by steps a and j in Figure 7.32. There are, usually, excited energy levels within the trap itself, such as the level at 2.7 eV for NaCl, which can absorb a photon, leading to a yellow/brown color in irradiated NaCl; this defect is then called a color center. Note that the electron is still within the trap even when in the excited energy level. The photon energy can be lost as fluorescence or as heat, with the electron still remaining in the trap. Another photon can then again be absorbed.

Only by supplying energy corresponding to step k, more than 3 eV for sodium chloride, can the electron leave the trap and return via the conduction band directly to the valence band. This can happen if the crystal is heated and then results in destruction of the color center and bleaching of the color. If the energies for absorption and for destruction are about the same size, then bleaching can occur merely while the material is being illuminated, leading to optical bleaching or fading.

If the energy of step k is sufficiently small, the color may even fade at room temperature. This occurs in self-darkening sun glasses, where the ultra-violet present in sunlight produces the darkening and room temperature leads to fading as soon as there is no ultra-violet to maintain the coloration. Other color centers, designated F′ (involving two electrons trapped at a Cl^- vacancy), M (two adjacent F vacancies), V_K, etc. are possible in alkali halides, which may absorb in the visible, the ultra-violet, or the infra-red regions. Some of these color centers show fluorescence and some are used as laser materials. As an alternative to irradiation, growth in the presence of excess metal or solid state electrolysis have also been used to generate some color centers.

The general description of a material capable of supporting a color center is given in Figure 7.34, where the colorless state is shown above and the colored state below. Two kinds of precursors are present in the colorless state: a hole precursor A which can lose an electron, e.g. when absorbing energetic radiation as shown, to form a hole center A^+, and an electron precursor B which can absorb the electron ejected from A to form the electron center B^-. Either the A^+ or the B^- in the lower part of Figure 7.34 can be the color center that absorbs light to give color; even both may do so in some materials. On heating, the electron is released from B^- and returns to A^+, with the system returning to the colorless state of A plus B.

Several gemstone materials derive their attractive colors from color centers. Colorless 'rock-crystal' quartz, shown center above in Figure 7.33, is composed of silicon oxide SiO_2, shown schematically at A in Figure 7.35. All natural and synthetic quartz contains some aluminum as an impurity, an Al^{3+} typically replacing one out of every 10 000 Si^{4+}. For electrical neutrality a hydrogen ion H^+ or a Na^+ is also present nearby. Such quartz is colorless, but irradiations either natural in the ground over thousands of years or man-provided in a few minutes, e.g. in a Cobalt-60 gamma-ray cell, produces smoky quartz, shown at upper right in Figure 7.33. As illustrated at B in Figure 7.35, irradiation ejects an

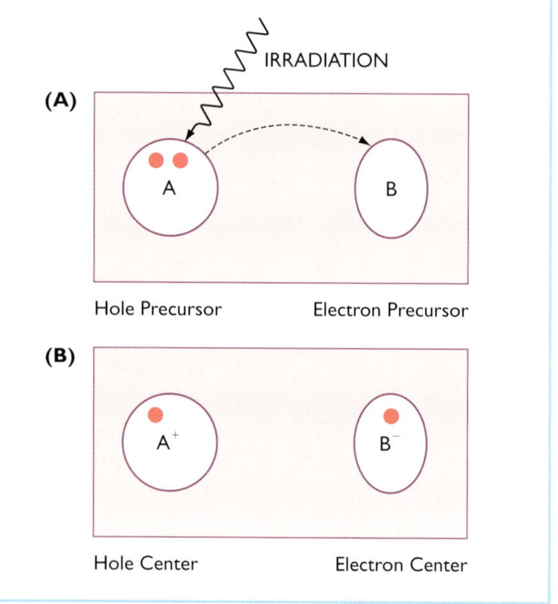

Figure 7.34 The irradiation of hole and electron precursors (A) to form hole and electron centers (B), either or both of which could be color centers.

electron from an oxygen adjacent to the Al^{3+}. The whole $[AlO_4]^{5-}$ entity acts as the hole precursor and converts to the hole center $[AlO_4]^{4-}$. The electron is trapped by the H^+ electron precursor, producing the neutral H atom electron center. Here it is the hole center that is the light-absorbing color center and provides the gray to brown to black color of smoky quartz seen in Figure 7.33. Also shown in this figure at lower left is the yellow citrine form of quartz (often incorrectly called smoky topaz) which contains Fe^{3+} instead of Al^{3+} as an impurity. The yellow color derives from the ligand field impurity, Mechanism 5. Irradiation of this material can now produce the color of the purple amethyst form of quartz, shown at lower right in Figure 7.33, containing the hole color center $[FeO_4]^{4-}$, exactly analogously to that in smoky quartz.

The color centers in both amethyst and smoky quartz are stable to light but the color is lost on being heated to 300–500 °C. If not overheated, the color centers and the colors can then be restored by another irradiation.

Natural yellow to orange to brown so-called 'precious' topaz contains a color center that again is stable to light. Any colorless topaz can be irradiated to produce a similarly colored but different color center which, however, is unstable and fades in a few days in light. Blue topaz also contains a stable color center. The precise chemical nature of most such color centers is unknown. Interestingly, the irradiation of colorless diamonds can produce color centers giving yellow, blue, brown, green, and rarely red colors. Although the first two of these are similar in appearance to the N-caused yellow and the B-caused blue band-gap-impurity colors discussed above, they represent much less valued materials which can be distinguished by absorption spectroscopic and other features.

The color center in deep blue Maxixe beryl, shown in Figure 7.1, is unstable and fades very slowly when exposed to light at room temperature.

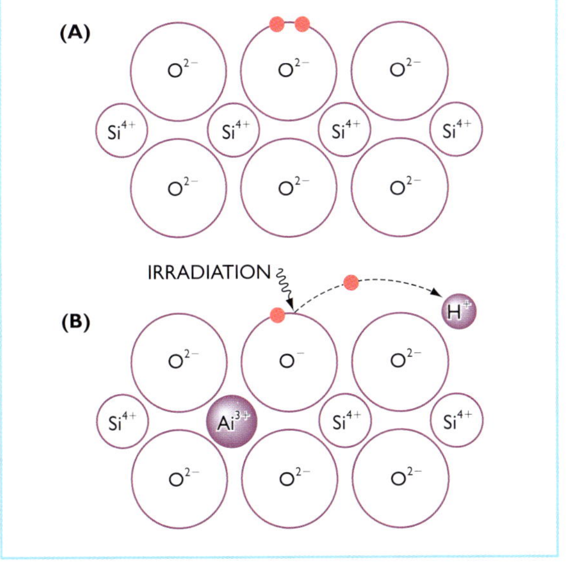

Figure 7.35 Schematic representation of the structure of pure quartz (A) and the formation by irradiation of the smoky quartz color center in Al-containing quartz (B).

7.13 MECHANISM 12: COLOR FROM DISPERSION

The discovery by Newton of this phenomenon and its dependence on the ultra-violet electronic and infra-red vibrational features was discussed at the beginning of this chapter. Dispersion is also known as dispersive refraction. In the visible region of a colorless transparent substance, the refractive index n at wavelength λ is given by the Sellmeier dispersion formula

$$n^2 - 1 = a\lambda^2(\lambda^2 - A^2)^{-1} + b\lambda^2(\lambda^2 - B^2)^{-1}$$

where A, B,. . . are the wavelength of the individual infra-red and ultra-violet absorptions seen in Figure 7.21, and a, b,. . . are constants representing the strengths of these absorptions. Only two or three terms, corresponding to the absorptions closest to the visible region, are required for an excellent fit in this region.

Anomalous dispersion results when there is a light absorption in the visible region of an otherwise transparent medium. Instead of n in the Sellmeier dispersion formula it is now necessary to use the complex refractive index $n = N + ik$, where i is the imaginary $\sqrt{-1}$ and k is the absorption coefficient. The variation of n and k in a glass having a violet color derived from an absorption at 550 nm (in the central part of the visible spectrum) is shown in Figure 7.36. In the absorption region, the natural resonating frequency of the absorbers interacts with the vibration of the light in a complicated manner

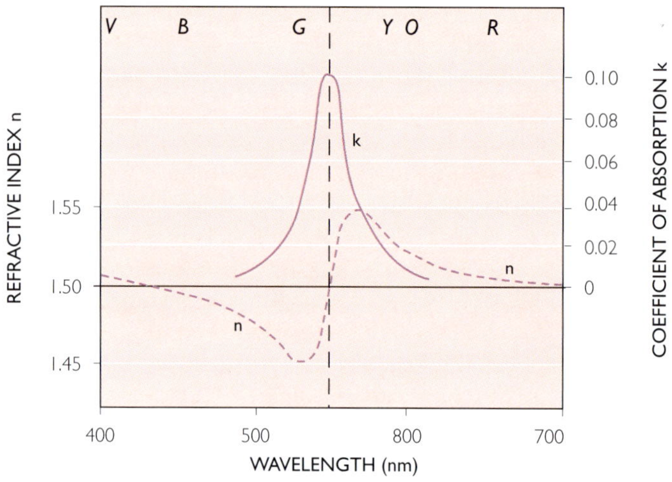

Figure 7.36 Refractive index and absorption coefficient in a violet crown glass having an absorption band at 550 nm.

involving the phase velocity and the phase angle, producing a speeding up of the light, thus giving a lower n, on the short-wavelength side of the absorption, and a slowing down, with a higher n, on the other side. In the central region of the absorption, the refractive index increases with the wavelength, instead of decreasing as usual. This region may, of course, be difficult to observe since it occurs exactly where the light is most strongly absorbed.

If a beam of light is passed through a prism cut out of the colorless glass of Figure 7.2, then the sequence of colors seen is the normal spectral sequence shown at the top of Figure 7.37. The glass of Figure 7.36, absorbing at 550 nm in the green-appearing part of the spectrum, therefore has the complementary color violet; here the sequence in the lower half of Figure 7.37 applies. The red to yellow–green sequence at (a) follows normal behavior as above in Figure 7.37 and at the right in Figure 7.36, as does the blue–green to violet sequence at (c), again corresponding to the color sequence above in Figure 7.36 and at the left in Figure 7.37. The yellow–green to blue–green sequence at (b) in Figure 7.37 is reversed. The 550 nm 'green' itself at refractive index n = 1.50 does not appear here since it is totally absorbed. The overall color sequence that is observed from this prism is shown at (d) in Figure 7.37. Compared to the normal spectrum this is truly 'anomalous,' both in the sequence of colors as well as in the width of the spectrum.

If either the refractive index variation or the coefficient of absorption variation is known for all wavelengths for a substance, then the other one can be calculated by use of the Kramers–Krönig dispersion relationships. Usually we think of the absorption as the 'cause' and the dispersion as the 'effect,' but the two are inextricably interdependent: one cannot exist without the other.

In addition to the spectrum produced by a prism, there are a variety of dispersion-produced color phenomena. A ray of light passing into the top of a faceted gemstone follows a path controlled by total internal reflections and is seen coming back out of the top of the stone as the 'brilliance.' Since the geometry of the path corresponds to that in a prism, these transmitted rays are also dispersed into a spectrum, leading to flashes of color, the 'fire.' The amount of brilliance depends on the magnitude of the refractive index and the amount of fire depends on the magnitude of the dispersion. Diamond is paramount in both among naturally occurring gemstones.

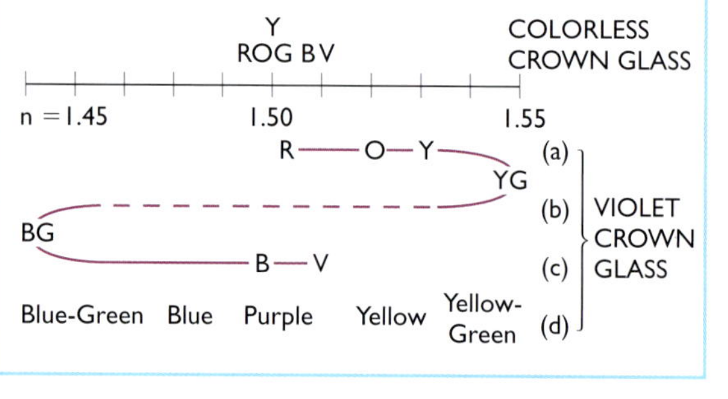

Figure 7.37 Color sequences produced by dispersion in the colorless crown glass of Figure 7.2 (above) and the violet crown glass of Figure 7.36 (below).

The refracted paths through a raindrop produce the primary and secondary rainbows as in Figure 7.38. Higher order rainbows can be seen in the laboratory but cannot be observed in nature. The refracted paths through hexagonal ice crystals produce the 22° and the 45° halos around the sun and moon, the parhelia such as sundogs or moondogs, as well as a variety of other white and colored arcs.

Finally there is the green flash, seen rarely at the setting of the sun. Here the density gradient of the atmosphere acts as a prism, separating the colors as shown in Figure 7.39. Since the shortest wavelengths, which appear violet and blue, are scattered from the beam as described below, a green image is seen just at the final setting under favorable circumstances for just a brief moment.

A more complicated case than dispersive refraction is 'double refraction,' which provides color when certain anisotropic crystals are viewed between crossed polarizers. Here the light on entering the crystal is resolved into ordinary ray (or o-ray or ω-ray) and the extraordinary ray (or e-ray or ε-ray) as shown for a calcite crystal in Figure 7.40. These rays move at different velocities through the crystal and can be recombined in the second polarizer to produce color by interference (see below). An example is a thinned ice cube viewed between crossed polarizers in Figure 7.41.

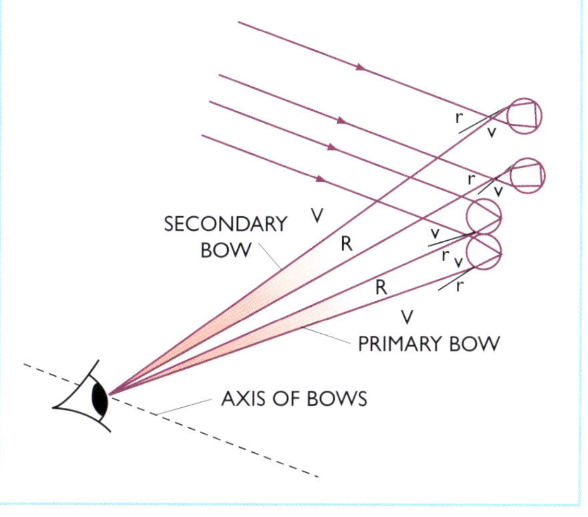

Figure 7.38 Formation of the primary and secondary rainbows by single and double reflections inside raindrops, respectively.

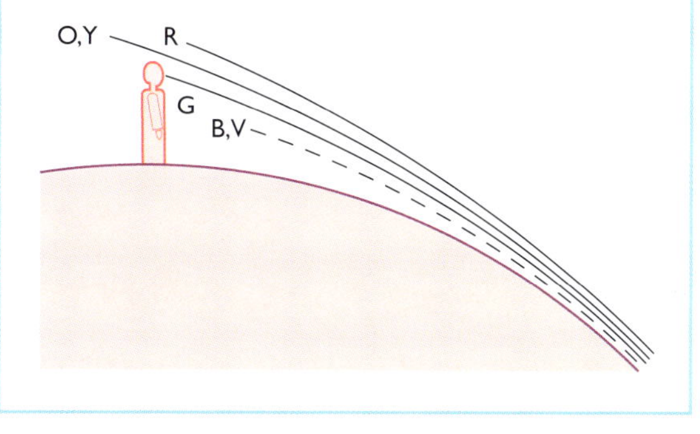

Figure 7.39 The formation of the green flash at sunrise or sunset from a combination of dispersion and scattering.

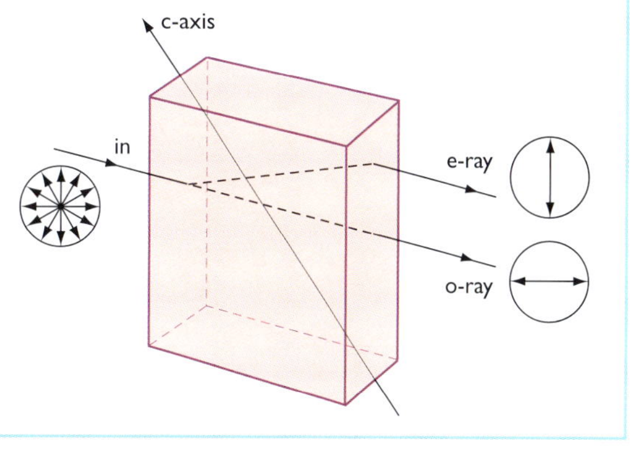

Figure 7.40 The separation of a beam of light in a calcite crystal into polarized ordinary and extraordinary rays.

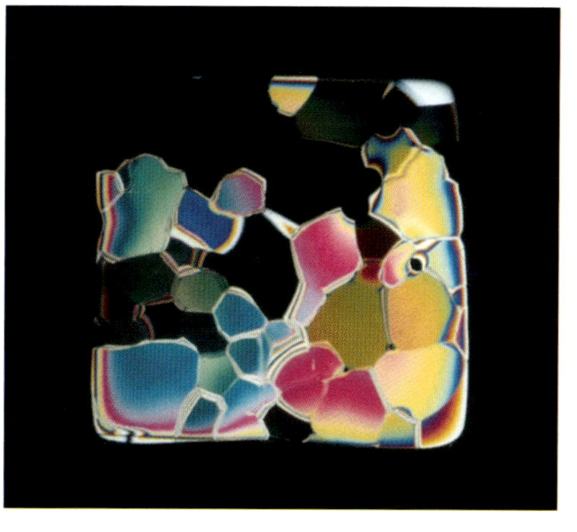

Figure 7.41 A thinned ice cube, 3 cm across, viewed between crossed polarizers (interference colors). (Photograph courtesy of R.L. Barns.)

7.14 MECHANISM 13: COLOR FROM SCATTERING

Perfectly clean air does not normally seem to scatter light. Sunbeams may reveal themselves in the presence of dust, most spectacularly in cathedrals. Yet even the purest substances, including gases, liquids, crystals, and glasses, are found to scatter light when carefully examined.

Leonardo da Vinci had observed that a fine water mist produced light scattering, but for many centuries there was only confusion and misleading ideas abounded. The English experimentalist John Tyndall (1820–93) first showed that the extent of scattering from particles small compared to the wavelength of light depends on the wavelength, with the short-wavelength blue-appearing end of the spectrum being much more strongly scattered than the long-wavelength red-appearing end.

Lord Rayleigh was the first to understand that scattering particles were not necessary since even the purest of substances have fluctuations in their refractive index which can scatter light. He showed that the intensity of the scattered light I_s is related to that of the incident light I_o by the inverse fourth power of the wavelength I_s/I_o = const. λ^{-4}. If we take the intensity of scattered light at the 400 nm end of the spectrum to be 100, then light at the 700 nm end is scattered only at an intensity of 10.7, as shown in Figure 7.42. The terms 'Rayleigh scattering' and 'Tyndall blues' are often applied to the scattered blue colors. A dark background, such as the dark of outer space, is required for an intense blue scattered color to be perceived, as in Figure 7.43, where the orange to red color of the rising and setting sun also results from the removal of the shorter wavelengths by scattering. Sunrise and sunset colors are particularly spectacular when volcanic eruptions inject dust into the upper atmosphere.

The atoms and molecules in a gas, liquid, crystal, or glass, are evenly distributed on a macroscopic scale, yet at the atomic level there is considerable nonrandom distribution. As one example, in a gas or a liquid individual molecules as well as small clusters of a few molecules continuously come together in collision for a brief instant before dispersing again. This produces fluctuations in density which act as light-scattering entities much as do particles of dust. In a glass there will be similar density and refractive index variations, both from imperfect mixing of the various ingredients of the glass as well as from the frozen-in liquid density fluctuations. Even in what might be thought of as a perfectly ordered single crystal, there usually will be a variety of point defects (impurity atoms, vacancies, and clusters of these) and line and plane defects (dislocations, disclinations, low angle grain boundaries, stacking faults, and the like). There are also local density fluctuations from the thermal vibrations of the atoms or molecules. All of these entities scatter light.

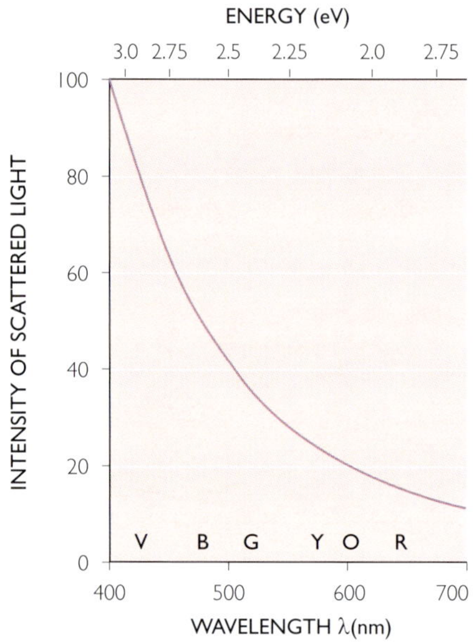

Figure 7.42 The intensity of Rayleigh scattered light varies with λ^{-4}.

The Rayleigh scattering process itself involves light-scattering entities that are very small compared to the wavelength of light; they absorb photons and re-emit them. Since light is a transverse oscillation, the scattered light is polarized, as indicated in Figure 7.44. Exactly perpendicular to the beam the scattered light is completely polarized in a direction perpendicular to the incident beam, while in other directions, such as at the angle θ shown in Figure 7.44, there is an additional component of the polarization parallel to the incident beam direction of $\cos^2\theta$. The combination $(1 + \cos^2\theta)$ gives the total light-scattering intensity distribution. The blue of the overhead sky at sunset, corresponding to

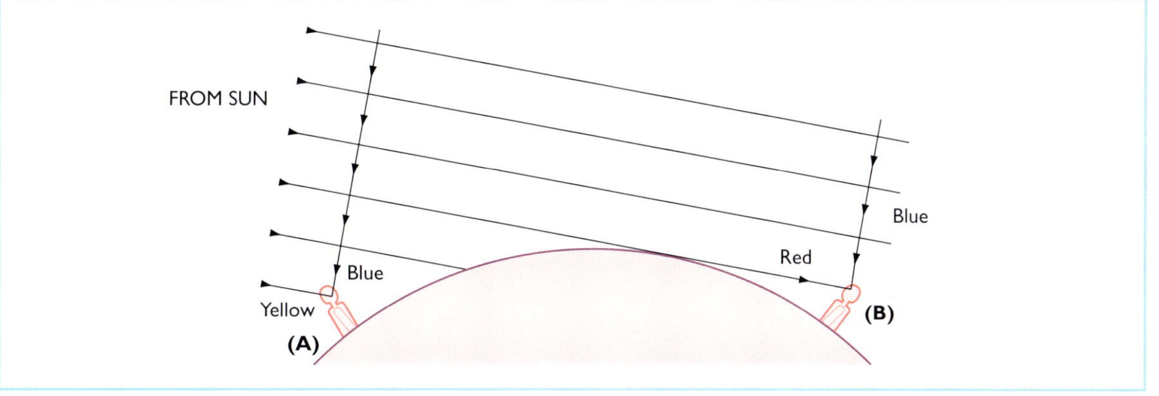

Figure 7.43 **The formation of the blue sky (A) and red sunset colors (B) from scattering in the atmosphere.**

$\theta = 90°$, is however not completely polarized as might be expected. In its long path toward us, some of the initially scattered light is scattered again with a resulting partial randomizing of the polarization. As much as one-fifth of the light from a clear sky has undergone multiple scattering.

Some of our most spectacular atmospheric phenomena derive from various types of scattering: the blue of the sky, the red of the sunset, the white of clouds and, that epitome of rare occurrences, the blue moon, involving oil droplet clouds from forest fires (calendric explanations for this rarity have been shown to be incorrect; see Nassau, 2001).

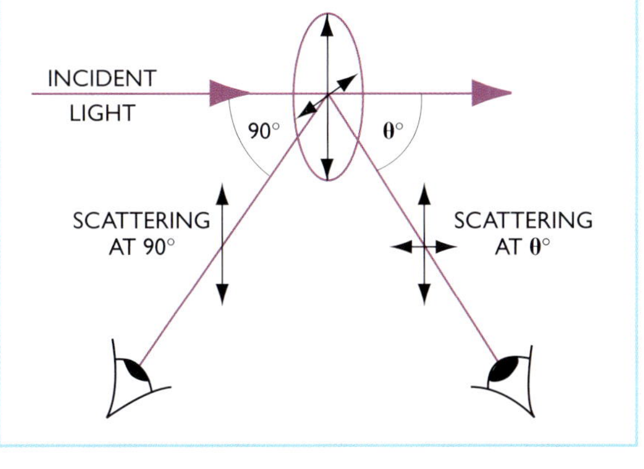

Figure 7.44 **Rayleigh scattered light at 90° is fully polarized; at other angles it is only partly polarized.**

Most blue and green bird feather colors involve scattering, as do many animal and some vegetable blues. The same scattering phenomenon is seen in the blue color of eyes, particularly in the intense blue of most infants, where the yellow to dark brown to black pigments such as melanin have formed only partially and Rayleigh scattering in the iris is seen against the dark interior of the eye. Combined with some yellow coloration from melanin, a green color of the iris results. If melanin dominates, brown to black colors appear. Melanin is absent in albinos, in whose eyes the Rayleigh scattering adds to the color of the underlying red blood vessels to produce pink. The pink skin color of light-skinned individuals originates similarly from scattering in the skin combined with the red blood vessels just below the surface.

If the size of the scattering particles approaches the wavelength of light or exceeds it, then the complicated Mie scattering theory applies and colors other than blue can occur. Mie theory also applies to scattering particles which are electrically conducting as previously mentioned under Mechanism 8. All wavelengths are scattered equally by the largest size particles, giving white as in fogs and clouds. Rayleigh and Mie scattering are called elastic scattering, because there is no change of the wavelength. Inelastic scattering with a shift in the wavelength of the scattered light includes Raman scattering and Brillouin scattering, both of which can be used for laser operation, as well as several other forms of scattering.

7.15 MECHANISM 14: COLOR FROM INTERFERENCE WITHOUT DIFFRACTION

Two light waves of the same wavelength can interact under appropriate circumstances in two different ways: they can add so as to reinforce if they are in phase, as shown at (A) in Figure 7.45. Alternatively, they can subtract if they are out of phase, cancelling as at (B). In this section are covered only those causes of color which involve interference without diffraction. The combination of interference with diffraction is deferred to the following section.

The first observation of interference without the simultaneous occurrence of diffraction was performed about 1815 by the French scientist A. Fresnel. A monochromatic light source was reflected in two mirrors made of black glass so as to reflect light only at the front surface. The mirrors were inclined at a small angle to each other to produce two overlapping beams of light on a screen. The result was a series of 'interference fringes' consisting of alternating bands of light and dark. If either mirror was covered or removed, the fringes disappeared and only the uniform illumination derived from the other mirror remained.

With the availability of monochromatic (single wavelength) light from a laser, the observation and study of interference has been greatly facilitated. This has led to the widespread use of a variety of interference-based devices, including Twyman–Green and multiple-reflection interferometers, such as the Fabry–Perot etalons used for precision measurements, as well as interference filters.

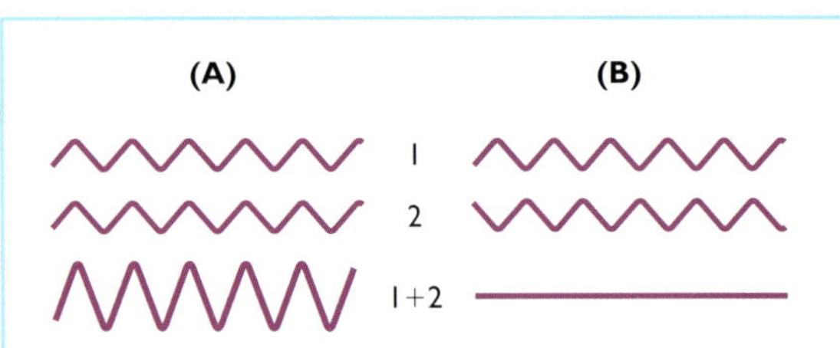

Figure 7.45 Equal intensity equal wavelength light waves 1 and 2 produce constructive reinforcement if they are in phase (A) or destructive cancellation if they are out of phase (B).

When a plane, coherent, monochromatic beam of light A–A in Figure 7.46 is incident at an angle onto a thin film such as a sheet of glass or plastic, then part of the wave will enter the film as shown at B. Part of this beam will be reflected at the back surface at C and a part of this reflected beam will leave the film in direction D. Part of a second wave in beam A–A passing through E will be reflected at the upper surface of the film so that it too leaves in direction D. As drawn in Figure 7.46, there is an extra path length of exactly five wavelengths while beam B traverses the distance 2b within the glass, while beam E travels only one wavelength a in the air. The net path difference is thus four wavelengths, so that the two beams might be expected to be exactly in phase with each other. However, reflection at a medium of higher refractive index as at the top surface produces a phase change equivalent to one-half wavelength. This does not happen at the lower surface, which is reflection at a medium of lower refractive index. The two beams appearing in direction D are therefore out of phase as shown and will undergo total destructive cancellation, as at B in Figure 7.45 if the intensities are equal.

As either the angle, the thickness, or the wavelength changes, alternating bands from cancellations and from reinforcements will result. A tapered film with monochromatic light produces a series of dark and light bands. With white light, however, the sequence of overlapping light and dark bands from all the spectral wavelengths leads to Newton's color sequence. Starting with

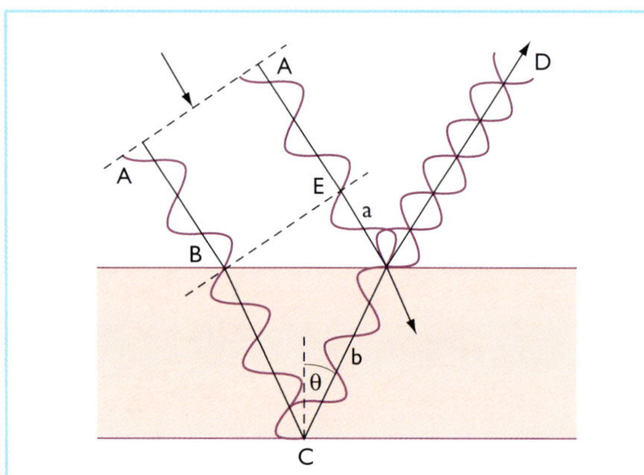

Figure 7.46 Interference of light reflected from the front and back surfaces of a thin parallel film.

the thinnest film, there appear black, gray, white, yellow, orange, red (end of the first 'order'); violet, blue, green, yellow, orange–red, violet (end of the second 'order'); and so on. These colors are seen in the tapered air gap between touching non-flat sheets of glass, in cracks in glass or in crystals, in a soap bubble, in an oil slick on a water surface, and in the petrological microscope. Direct sunshine or a bright light are required for the most spectacular colors.

Antireflection coatings on camera lenses employ this effect. A coating is applied that has a refractive index geometrically intermediate between the refractive indexes of the glass and air, with a coating thickness of one-quarter the wavelength of light. Such a coating reduces the overall reflected light to less than one half. The reflected light can be reduced to less than one-tenth by multiple-layer coatings, which usually appear purple to the eye.

There are many instances of structural colorations in biological systems that owe their color to thin film interference, usually involving multiply layered structures. The layers may be composed of keratin, chitin, calcium carbonate, mucus, and so on. There is frequently a backing layer of very dark melanin that enhances the color by absorbing the nonreflected light.

Biological interference colorations are usually 'iridescent,' which designation implies that multiple colors are seen as in the rainbow (Latin *iris*) and also that the colors change as the viewing angle is changed. Examples include pearl and mother-of-pearl, the transparent wings of house and dragon flies, iridescent scales on beetles and butterflies, and iridescent feathers on hummingbirds and peacocks. An example of the complexity that can be involved is given in Figure 7.47, which shows the color-causing structure on the surface of scales on the wings of the brilliant blue butterfly *Morpho rhetenor*, seen in Figure 7.48, where a drop of acetone also changes the refractive index involved in the interference process and hence the color. The eyes of many nocturnal animals contain multilayer structures that improve night vision and produce green iridescent metallic-like reflections. This color is often seen at night as the roadside reflections of automobile headlights from animal eyes or in flash photos, as in Figure 7.49.

Interference of polarized white light in an optically anisotropic substance, such as crumpled cellophane viewed between crossed polarizers, derives from the double refraction discussed above and also leads to color. Photoelastic stress analysis is the use of this effect to check glass for strains and, in deformed plastic models, to study the stresses in machinery and in medieval cathedrals.

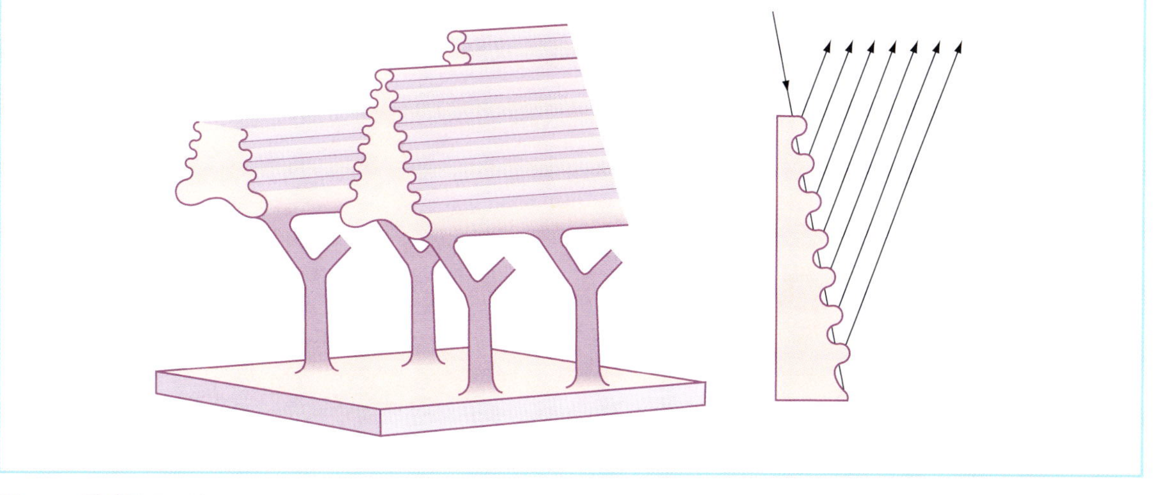

Figure 7.47 **(Left) structure of the vanes on the surface of scales on the wings of *Morpho rhetenor*; (right) multiple interference produced by the ridges on these vanes. (After T.F. Anderson and A.G. Richards (1959) *Journal of Applied Physics*, 13, 748, and F. Mijhout (1981) *Scientific American*, 245, 140.)**

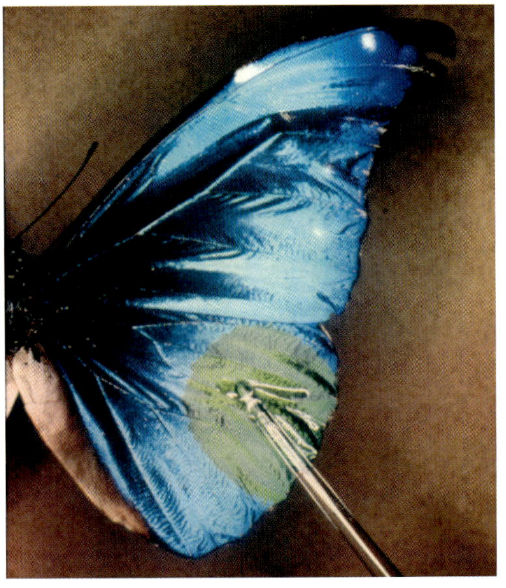

Figure 7.48 Iridescent metallic-like colors on the 8 cm long wing of the butterfly *Morpho rhetenor*, showing the change in color produced by a drop of acetone (multiple thin film interference). Note that the metallic-like characteristic does not show in color printing (Photograph courtesy of F. Mijhout).

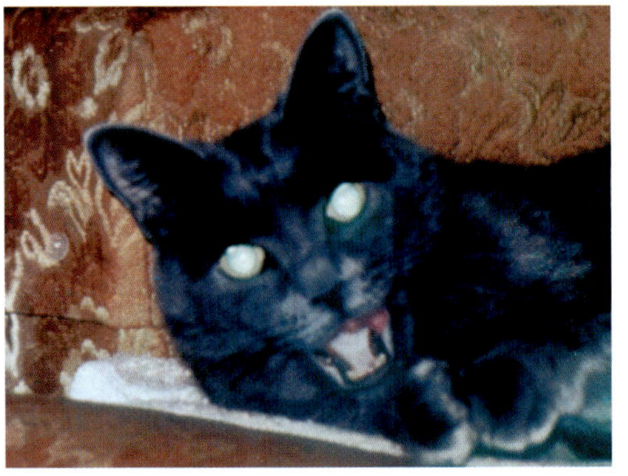

Figure 7.49 Green metallic-like reflection of a photographic flash from the eyes of a cat (multiple thin film interference). Note that the metallic-like characteristic does not show in color printing.

7.16 MECHANISM 15: COLOR FROM DIFFRACTION

Diffraction describes the spreading of light at the edges of an obstacle. It ultimately supplied the incontrovertible proof for the wave aspect of light. Diffraction was first described in detail in the 1665 posthumous book by the Italian mathematician F. Grimaldi. He studied the shadow of small objects using a small opening in a window shutter, just as did Newton to obtain the spectrum a few years later. He observed that the shadows were larger than could be explained by geometrical optics and also showed colored fringes, as in Figure 7.50, not only outside but even inside the shadow under certain conditions. Grimaldi used the word 'diffraction' for the effects that he was unable to explain. It remained for the three contemporaries Thomas Young (1773–1829), Joseph von Fraunhofer (1787–1826), and Augustin Fresnel (1788–1827) to provide adequate descriptions and explanations.

Consider sunlight passing through a large opening in a shutter with the transmitted light falling on a screen. As the opening is made smaller, so the patch of light on the screen becomes smaller and its edges appear to become sharper. Beyond a certain point, however, the edges become indistinct and begin to show colored fringes. The mechanism involves the spreading of a wave into the geometrical shadow region of an object, as shown in Figure 7.51, and interference of the spreading part of the wave with the undisturbed part of the wave. A sequence of light and dark bands is produced by a single edge in monochromatic light, while with white light a sequence of colors appears much as in the Newton color sequence discussed above. Such fringes can easily be observed by viewing one hand, held about a foot from one's eye, against a bright window. Fringes will be seen when the fingers are squeezed together so that only a little light passes between them.

Interference can result from light beams diffracted from opposite sides of small particles, producing a sequence of colored rings called the 'corona' (not to be confused with the 'solar corona' seen only during an eclipse). The corona can frequently be seen surrounding the sun (using very dark sunglasses), derived from cloud particles. In Figure 7.52 the path difference between the two rays diffracted from opposite edges of the particle at A is zero, thus producing

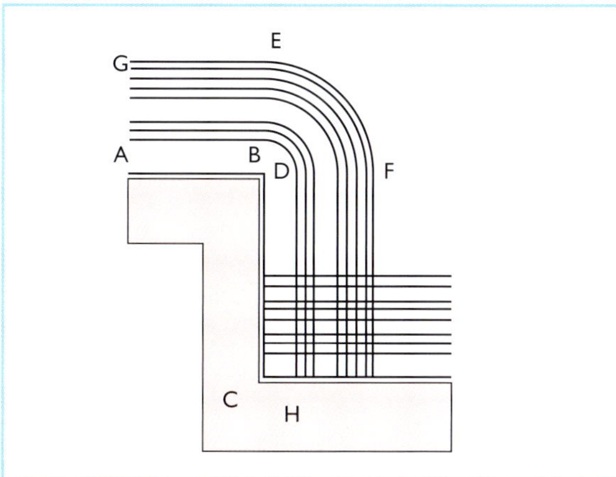

Figure 7.50 **Drawing of diffraction given in Grimaldi's 1665 book; H is the geometrical shadow and the thin lines represent colored fringes.**

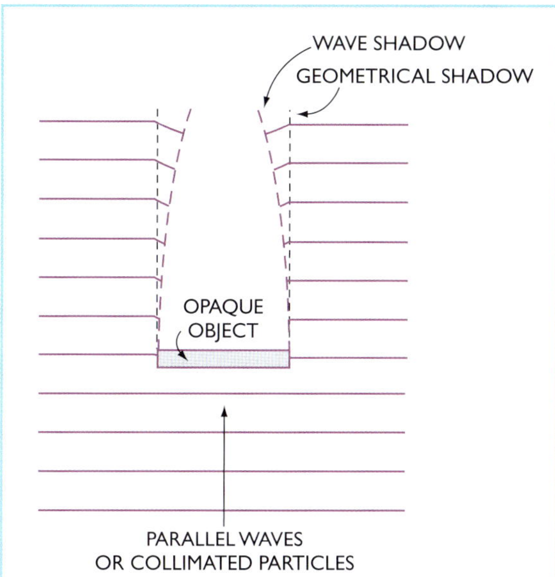

Figure 7.51 **The geometrical and wave shadows of an opaque object produced by particles and waves, respectively.**

reinforcement. At B the path difference is d sinθ. When this is a whole wavelength, that is when

$$n\lambda = \sin\theta$$

where n is an integer, reinforcement occurs, while half-way between there will be cancellation for any wavelength λ. The size of the cloud

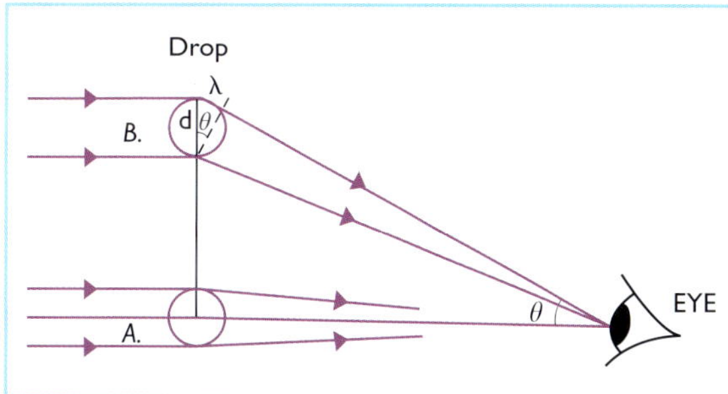

Figure 7.52 **Diffraction by the edges of drops of water leading to the corona.**

particles can be deduced from measuring the angular diameter of the corona. For uniformly sized particles there is the usual interference color sequence. With many sizes of particles present, merely a bluish disk, the 'corona aureole,' is seen surrounding the sun. This same mechanism occurs in Bishop's ring, the glory, and the specter of the Brocken. Translucent clouds having uniform particle sizes may show a range of pastel colors, then called iridescent or luminescent clouds, when viewed near the sun (use very dark sunglasses).

A regular two- or three-dimensional array of scattering objects or openings forms a diffraction grating. This is most familiar when used in a spectroscope, as in Figure 7.53, where the path difference is again $n\lambda = \sin\theta$. Diffraction gratings provide colors in the animal kingdom, as in the beetle *Serica sericae* and the indigo or gopher snake *Drymarchon corais couperii*, which show spectral colors in direct sunlight. This effect can also be seen by viewing at a glancing angle across a phonograph record or compact disc or by looking at a distant streetlamp or flashlight through a black cloth umbrella, as in Figure 7.54, taken at a distance with a telephoto lens.

The epitome of diffraction gratings is the gemstone opal, showing on a white or a black background flashes of varied colors called the 'play of color' as in Figure 7.55 ('opalescence' is merely a milky-white translucent appearance). At one time this was believed to involve thin film interference, but electron microscope photographs taken of an opal revealed its secret, demonstrating a regular three-dimensional array of equal-size spheres, as shown in Figure 7.56. The actual composition of the spheres is amorphous silica,

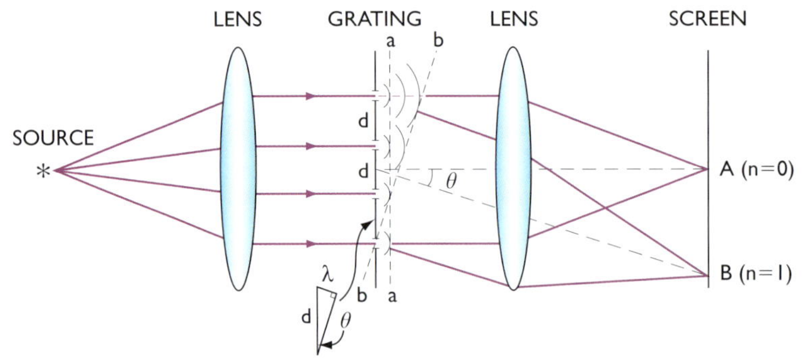

Figure 7.53 Schematic diagram for a diffraction grating spectroscope showing constructive reinforcement for the undeflected beam at n = θ and for the first order spectrum at n = 1.

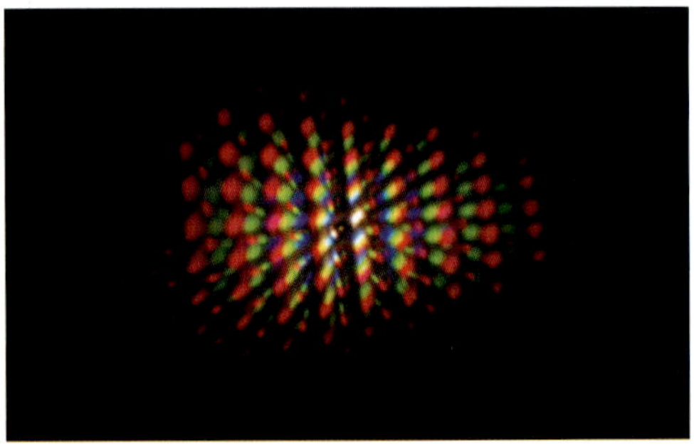

Figure 7.54 A distant flashlight viewed through a black umbrella fabric (diffraction).

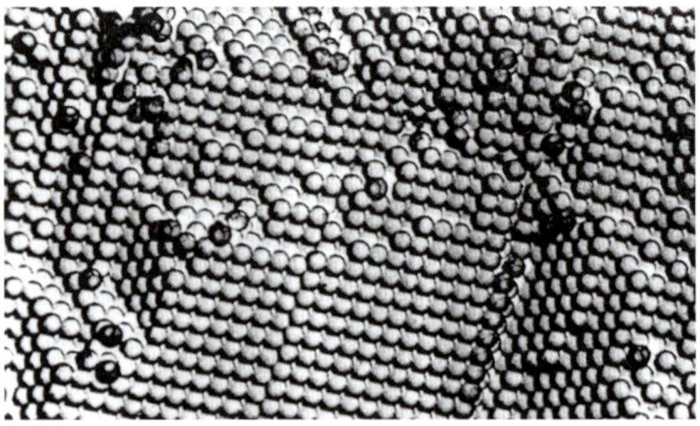

Figure 7.56 Electron microscope view of a synthetic opal; individual spheres are about 250 nm (0.00001 in.) across. (Photograph courtesy Ets. Ceramiques Pierre Gilson.)

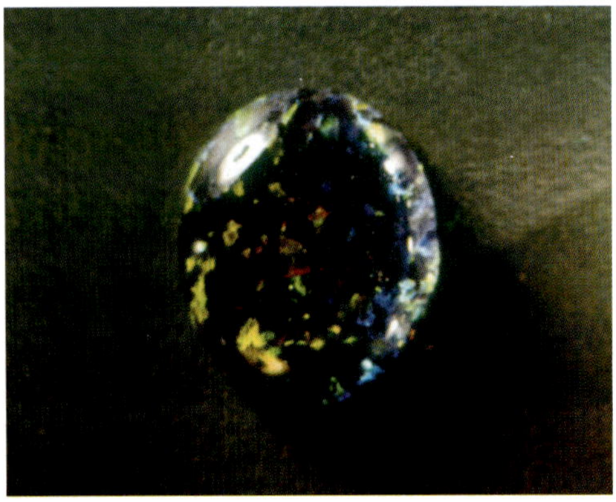

Figure 7.55 A 12 mm diameter synthetic black opal (diffraction) grown at Ets. Ceramiques Pierre Gilson.

SiO_2, containing a small amount of water, cemented together with more amorphous silica containing a different amount of water so that a small refractive index difference exists between the spheres and the cement.

Finally, there are 'liquid crystals,' organic compounds with a structure intermediate between those of a crystal and a liquid. These have twisted structures which can interact with light in a manner similar to diffraction to produce color, as in contact thermometers, thermography, as in Figure 7.57, and the 'mood' ring fad of a few years ago. Some beetle colors are derived from liquid crystal structures on the outer layers of their cuticles.

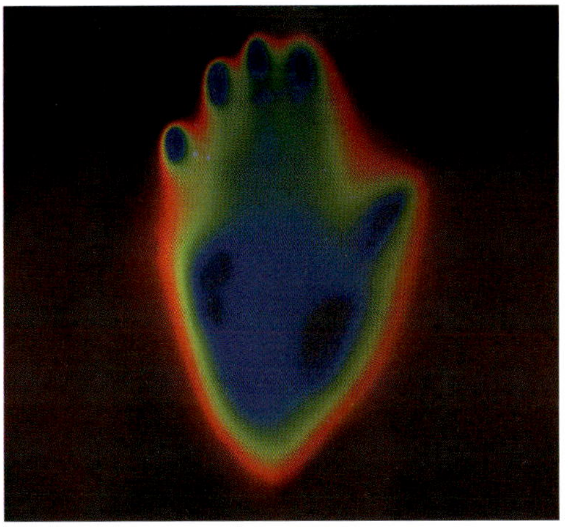

Figure 7.57 **Skin temperature revealed by thermography of a hand pressed against a black-backed cholesteric liquid crystal film giving iridescent metallic-like colors (multiple layer diffraction). Note that the metallic-like characteristic does not show in color printing.**

FURTHER READING

Apart from my own extended text on the subject (Nassau, 2001) (and my 'Colour' article, highly abbreviated, in the *Encyclopedia Britannica* since 1988), there appear to be no comprehensive modern discussions of the causes of color. Over 170 recommendations for further reading are given in Appendix 6 of my book (Nassau, 2001). The following selected items are accordingly representative rather than comprehensive.

A general source for many color-related topics is the 25-plus volume *Kirk–Othmer Encyclopedia of Chemical Technology* (Howe-Grant, 1991 onwards). Light and optics, usually including topics such as incandescence, dispersion, scattering, interference, and diffraction, are covered in optics textbooks (Wood, 1934; Ditchburn, 1976; Jenkins, 1976; Born and Wolf, 1980). Ligand-field (and crystal-field) theory is covered in advanced inorganic chemistry texts (Cotton and Wilkinson, 1988), as well as in specialized treatments (Figgis, 1966; Reinen, 1969; Burns, 1970). Color in organic molecules is covered to some extent in advanced organic chemistry texts (Streitweiser and Heathcock, 1981), and also in specialized treatments (Fabian and Hartman, 1980; Gordon and Gregory, 1983). There are only a few discussions of color derived from charge transfer (Burns, 1970; Smith and Strens, 1976; Cotton and Wilkinson, 1988). Band theory is covered in many solid state physics texts (Bube, 1974; Kittel, 1986), although color produced by this mechanism is not usually covered. There are several teatments of color centers (Farge and Fontana, 1979; Marfunin, 1979); most include some discussion of color caused by this mechanism. There are specific discussions of color in minerals and gemstones (Burns, 1970; Nassau, 1978, 1980, 2001; Marfunin, 1979; Fritsch and Rossman, 1987, 1988a, 1988b); in pigments and dyes (Nassau, 2001); in glass, glazes, and enamels (Bamford, 1977; Volf, 1984; Nassau, 1985, 2001); in plastics (Nassau, 1986, 2001); and in biological materials (Nassau, 2001), including six early but still definitive studies (with minor misattributions) of animal coloration (Mason, 1923a, 1923b, 1924, 1926, 1927a, 1927b).

REFERENCES

Bamford, C.R. (1977) *Color Generation and Control in Glass.* New York: Elsevier.

Born, M. and Wolf, E. (1999) *Principles of Optics*, 7th edn. New York: Pergamon Press.

Bube, R.H. (1974) *Electronic Properties of Crystalline Solids*. New York: Academic Press.

Burns, G.R. (1993) *Mineralogical Applications of Crystal Field Theory*, 2nd edn. Cambridge: Cambridge University Press.

Cotton, F.A. and Wilkinson, G. (1988) *Advanced Inorganic Chemistry*, 5th edn. New York: Wiley.

Ditchburn, R.W. (1976) *Light*, 3rd edn. New York: Academic Press; reprinted by Dover, New York, 1991.

Fabian, J. and Hartmann, H. (1980) *Light Absorption in Organic Colorants.* New York: Springer Verlag.

Farge, Y. and Fontana, M.P. (1979) *Electronic and Vibrational Properties of Point Defects in Ionic Crystals.* New York: North Holland.

Figgis, B.N. (1966) *Introduction to Ligand Fields*. New York: Wiley; reprinted by Krieger, Melbourne & Florida, 1986.

Fritsch, E. and Rossman, G.R. (1987) An update on color in gems, Part 1. *Gems and Gemology*, 23, 126–39.

Fritsch, E. and Rossman, G.R. (1988a) An update on color in gems, Part 2. *Gems and Gemology*, 24, 3–15.

Fritsch, E. and Rossman, G.R. (1988b) An update on color in gems, Part 3. *Gems and Gemology*, 24, 81–102.

Gordon, P.F. and Gregory, P. (1983) *Organic Chemistry in Color*. New York: Springer Verlag.

Howe-Grant, M. (ed.) (1991 on) *Kirk–Othmer Encyclopedia of Chemical Technology*, 4th edn. New York: Wiley.

Jenkins, F.A. (1976) *Fundamentals of Optics*, 4th edn. New York: McGraw-Hill.

Kittel, C. (1996) *Introduction to Solid State Physics*, 7th edn. New York: Wiley.

Marfunin, A.S. (1979) *Spectroscopy, Luminescence and Radiation Centers in Minerals.* New York: Springer Verlag.

Mason, C.W. (1923a) Structural colors in feathers, Part 1. *Journal of Physical Chemistry*, 27, 201–51.

Mason, C.W. (1923b) Structural colors in feathers, Part 2. *Journal of Physical Chemistry*, 27, 410–47.

Mason, C.W. (1924) Blue eyes. *Journal of Physical Chemistry*, 28, 498–501.

Mason, C.W. (1926) Structural colors in insects, Part 1. *Journal of Physical Chemistry*, 30, 383–95.

Mason, C.W. (1927) Structural colors in insects, Part 2. *Journal of Physical Chemistry*, 31, 321–54.

Mason, C.W. (1927) Structural colors in insects, Part 3. *Journal of Physical Chemistry*, 31, 1856–72.

Nassau, K. (1978) The origin of color in minerals. *American Mineralogist*, 63, 219–29.

Nassau, K. (1980) *Gems Made by Man.* Radnor, PA, Chilton, reprinted by Gemmological Institute of America, Santa Monica, CA, 1987.

Nassau, K. (1985) The varied causes of color in glass, in *Proceedings of the 1985 Defects in Glass Symposium*, Vol. 61. Materials Research Society, Pittsburgh, PA.

Nassau, K. (1986) Color in plastics: the varied causes, in *Proceedings 1986*, ANTEC, Society of Plastics Engineers, Stamford, CT.

Nassau, K. (2001) *The Physics and Chemistry of Color: The Fifteen Causes of Color*, 2nd edn. New York: Wiley.

Reinen, D. (1969) Ligand field spectroscopy and chemical bonding in Cr^{3+}-containing oxidic solids. *Structure and Bonding*, 6, 30–51.

Smith, G. and Strens, R.G.J. (1976) Intervalence transfer absorption in some silicate, oxide and phosphate minerals. In R.G.J. Strens (ed.), *Physics and Chemistry of Minerals and Rocks*. New York: Wiley, p. 583.

Streitweiser, A. *et al.* (1998) *Organic Chemistry*, 4th edn. New York: Macmillan.

Volf, M.B. (1984) *Chemical Approach to Glass.* New York: Elsevier.

Wood, R.W. (1934) *Physical Optics*, 3rd edn. New York: Macmillan; reprinted by Optical Society of America, Washington DC, 1988.

8 Digital Color Reproduction

Brian A. Wandell[1] and Louis D. Silverstein[2]

[1] Department of Psychology
Stanford University, Stanford, CA 94305-2130, USA

[2] VCD Sciences, Inc.
9695 E. Yucca Street, Scottsdale, AZ 85260-6201, USA

CHAPTER CONTENTS

The Science of Color
ISBN 0–444–512–519

8.1 INTRODUCTION

In this chapter we describe how principles of human vision are used to design image capture and display devices. The chapter is divided into four sections. First, we provide an overview of two properties of human vision that are essential in designing color imaging technologies. The next three sections describe the application of these and related principles along with the specific technologies. The second section reviews digital cameras and scanners. The third section reviews displays with a particular emphasis on cathode ray tube (CRT) and liquid crystal display (LCD) technologies. The fourth section describes aspects of color printing.

A number of topics in color technologies are not covered in this chapter. We do not include implementation details or discussions of any specific technology. This is a fascinating and rapidly developing area, but the advances are so rapid that our discussion would be out of date by the time an archival chapter is published or read. Also, we do not discuss image processing methods, such as compression standards or graphics rendering techniques, even though the color vision principles described here are fundamental to these methods. We have excluded this topic because this chapter is a compromise between breadth of coverage and existence.

Our focus is on the fundamental principles of color imaging technology that must be addressed in the design of capture and display technology. Quantitative methods useful for certain specific devices are described, and we expect that these methods will be useful for future generations of display and capture technologies as well. It is in this sense that we hope this chapter will serve as a practical reference for the general principles of color imaging technologies.

8.2 IMAGING AS A COMMUNICATIONS CHANNEL

In this review we emphasize the aspects of imaging devices that are important in characterizing their role within a communications channel. An overview of how imaging devices form a communications channel is shown in Figure 8.1. The input signal is the original scene. This scene is captured and communicated over a transmission channel. This transmission usually includes various computational operations that facilitate inter-device communication and efficient transmission and storage. The transmitted image is then converted to a form where it can be rendered by a display device. Finally, the displayed image is acquired by the human visual system. When the image communications channel works well, the visual experience of seeing the original image matches the visual experience of seeing the reproduction. Hence, channel metrics must be based on how well the system performs with respect to the human visual system.

From examining the imaging channel description, several requirements of the devices on the communications channel are evident. Capture devices must measure the original image over a range that matches the signals captured by the human visual system. Display devices must be

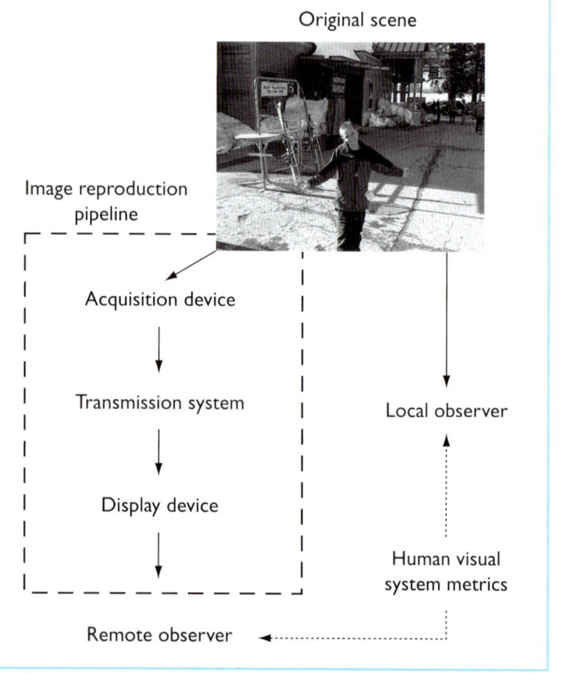

Figure 8.1 The image reproduction pipeline shares some properties with a general communications channel. The quality of the reproduction pipeline, the channel metrics, should be based on a comparison of the appearance of the original image with the appearance of the original scene. Hence, the visual significance of image features are an essential component in defining the quality of the channel.

able to deliver accurately controlled signals to the human visual system. Measures evaluating the quality of the communications channel must include comparisons of the *visual appearance*, a psychological quantity, associated with the original scene and the image delivered by the reproduction.

Two properties of human vision are central in the design of color imaging technologies. The first is trichromacy, a principle that has already been introduced in this book from the point of view of the behaviorist (see Chapter 3) and from the point of view of the physiologist (see Chapter 6). Here, we will introduce the principle from the point of view of the technologist. The second is the spatial resolution of the eye, and in particular spatial resolution limits for various types of colored stimuli. We briefly touch on each of these topics in the introduction. In the course of the chapter, we will return to explain how both aspects of human vision are important in the design of various technologies.

8.2.1 TRICHROMACY

The color-matching experiment coupled with the physiological and anatomical measurements of the three cone types (trichromacy) forms a beautiful story that relates brain and behavior. From the technologist's point of view, abstracting the story into mathematical terms, the color-matching experiment can be summarized by a very brief mathematical expression using simple linear algebra. Suppose the spectral power distribution of a light is $E(\lambda)$. Trichomacy tells us that the visual system makes a linear, three-dimensional measurement of this function. The three measurements can be expressed as the inner product of the cone photopigment absorption functions with the input spectral power distribution. For the L, M, and S cones the values are $<L(\lambda), E(\lambda)>$, $<M(\lambda), E(\lambda)>$ and $<S(\lambda), E(\lambda)>$. It is efficient to use matrix notation to express these three inner products. Create a matrix, $\mathbf{A}$, whose columns are the three cone absorption functions. The photopigments measure the three values $\mathbf{A}^t\,\mathbf{E}$. The photopigments do not change their absorption rates to any input signal in the null space of the matrix $\mathbf{A}^t$.

Seen from the technologist's viewpoint, the major goal of the image communications channel can be expressed by a *color-reproduction equation*. At a point in the original scene, the eye encodes three values, $\mathbf{A}^t\,\mathbf{E}$. When the ambient viewing conditions at the time of capture are the same as the ambient viewing conditions at the time of redisplay, the color-reproduction equation defines how to obtain a perfect color match: the transmission system must capture the original image and display a new image, with spectral composition, $E'(\lambda)$, such that $\mathbf{A}^t\,\mathbf{E} = \mathbf{A}^t\,\mathbf{E}'$. This simple equation is fundamental to the engineering of all color devices. Color engineers must analyze how design decisions influence the ability to satisfy the match in this equation.

Imaging systems never make a perfect match with respect to the color-reproduction equation. Consequently, color metrics (e.g., CIELAB) are an essential tool for analyzing how well the imaging pipeline succeeds. A few moments of thought suggest that certain types of errors are far worse than others. For example, if the original, $\mathbf{A}^t\,\mathbf{E}$, differs from the reproduction, $\mathbf{A}^t\,\mathbf{E}'$, only by a common scale factor across the entire image, the two scenes will look quite similar. In that case, the scenes will look rather like one another because it is as if we are looking at the original through dark glasses. If the original and reproduction differ by an additive offset, however, the color appearance in many color regions will be changed and the reproduction will not be satisfactory.

The color-reproduction equation is only accurate when the original and reproduction are viewed in the same general viewing conditions, including size and ambient lighting. If the reproduction covers a very large portion of the visual field, the reproduction context may not be important. On the other hand, if the reproduction covers only a small part of the visual field the context must be taken into account when considering the color-reproduction errors. Attempts to generalize the color-reproduction equation when the viewing conditions at time of image capture and redisplay differ are an important open problem in color engineering.

8.2.2 SPATIAL RESOLUTION AND COLOR

The spatial and temporal resolutions of human vision are also of great importance in the design of capture and reproduction devices. One reason for their importance is that there will be no improvement in image quality if the reproduction exceeds the spatial or temporal resolution of human vision. Hence, manufacturing cost is sensitive to these limits. There is a second subtler but equally important reason. The ability to control the acquisition and reproduction of spectral information is quite limited. Often, capture and display devices trade spatial and temporal information for color information. For example, color prints are often made by printing dots of colored inks adjacent to one another on the page (halftoning). When the dots are finely spaced, they blur together and are not individually resolved. Color is adjusted by varying the relative area covered by dots, effectively trading spatial resolution for color control. The spatial and temporal resolution limits of the human eye, and how these depend on color, are a key factor in designing this and other color imaging technologies.

The main properties of human spatial and temporal resolution are described in several reference sources (e.g., De Valois and De Valois, 1988; Wandell, 1995). An important feature of human vision is the poor spatial resolution for certain types of colors. The largest effect arises in the short-wavelength region of the spectrum. In this region, chromatic aberration of the human cornea and lens limits spatial resolution to 6 cycles per degree (cpd) (see Chapter 2; Wandell, 1995: ch. 2). But, there are other effects, too. Perceptual experiments show that certain patterns seen by the L and M cones can be difficult to detect as well. For example, if the sum of the L and M cone absorptions is constant across the image (L + M = constant), so that the pattern is defined only by a change in the difference (L − M) of the absorptions, spatial resolution is reduced to below 20 cpd (Mullen, 1985; Anderson *et al.*, 1991; Sekiguchi *et al.*, 1993a, 1993b). An intensity variation, however, in which the value of L + M varies, can be seen at spatial frequencies of 50 cpd or more.

Figure 8.2 compares human spatial resolution to several types of colored targets. The curves and data show the contrast sensitivity necessary to perceive harmonic patterns at different spatial frequencies. Measurements from several labs are plotted to describe the luminance and red–green spatial sensitivity. The luminance contrast sensitivity function shows a much higher spatial

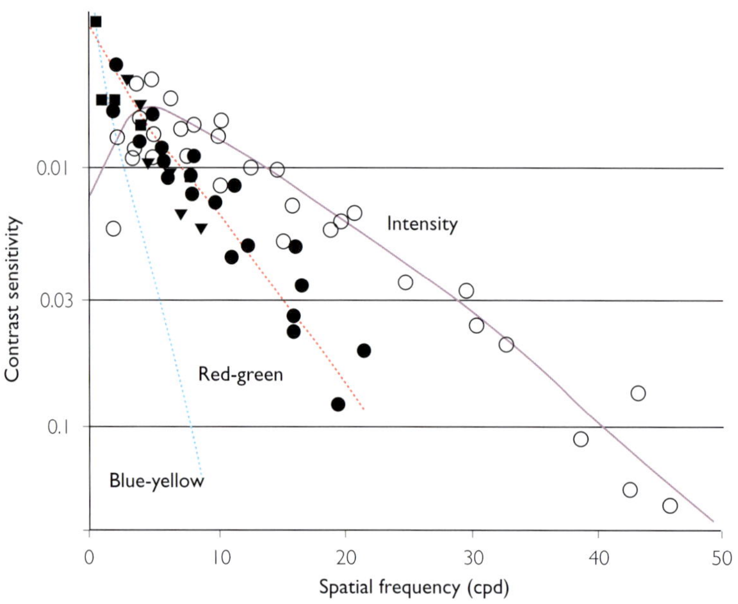

Figure 8.2 Human spatial contrast sensitivity depends on the color of the pattern. The lightly shaded curves show the general trends for stimuli containing mainly a luminance signal, a red–green signal, or a blue–yellow signal. The symbols are data reported in different papers from several groups (Anderson *et al.*, 1991; Sekiguchi *et al.*, 1993b; Poirson and Wandell, 1993). The figure is adapted from (Wandell, 1999), where further details are provided.

frequency limit and also a pronounced low-frequency decline. The spatial resolution to red–green stimuli falls off at higher spatial frequencies and has no low frequency fall off. The lowest resolution, limited to less than 8 cycles per degree, is for the blue–yellow stimuli. These values show that image capture, image coding, and image display devices require more spatial detail for luminance stimuli than red–green stimuli; very little spatial information about S cone (blue–yellow) image data is required.

8.3 IMAGE CAPTURE

8.3.1 OVERVIEW

In this section we review general principles of color image acquisition and how these principles are applied to the design of color cameras and scanners. We consider only image capture intended for subsequent display to a human observer, excluding devices designed for computer vision or other physical experiments. Our emphasis is on the capture of wavelength information, though we will consider how this interacts with spatial variables as well.

The general goal of wavelength capture for scanners and cameras is to acquire enough information about the input material to enable creation of a reproduction that will look similar and pleasing to the human eye. Because of the limited sensitivity of the human eye to variations in the wavelength composition, a complete spectral measurement of the image is unnecessary. The very existence of inexpensive color capture devices is possible only because of the savings that are possible because of human trichromacy: image capture devices achieve enormous efficiencies in representing the wavelength composition of the original source by measuring only those portions of the signal that human observers perceive. Capturing more wavelength information is wasteful of resources, needlessly driving up the cost of the device; capturing less will cause perceptually significant differences in the reproduction.

Figure 8.3 shows the physical factors that determine the wavelength composition of the image and thus the sensor absorptions. These factors are illustrated for capture by the human

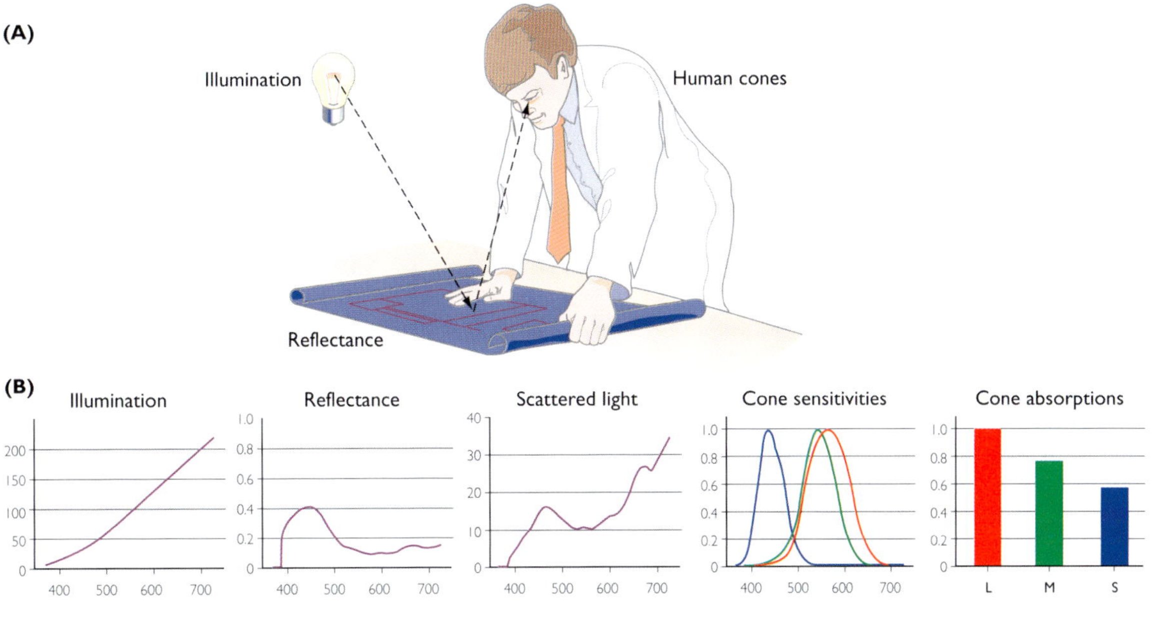

Figure 8.3 The physical factors governing sensor absorptions. The wavelength composition of the light sent to the eye (the color signal) depends on the ambient illumination and the surface reflectance. The number of photons absorbed in each of the eye's receptor types depends on the relative spectral absorption of the media of the eye and the photopigments within the receptors.

visual system, but the general formulation applies to other capture devices as well.

Suppose the illumination is diffuse and has radiance $E(\lambda)$ (measured in watts per square meter per steradian per nanometer). Given the particular viewing geometry, the illuminant radiance produces an irradiance at the surface that is specified in terms of watts per square meter per nanometer. The surface absorbs a portion of the irradiance and scatters a proportion back to the eye. The angular distribution of the scattered light depends on the imaging geometry and the properties of the surface. The angular distribution can be measured using goniophotometers (ASTM, 1991) or, more recently, conoscopic measurement systems (Fritsch and Mlynski, 1991; Leroux and Rossignol, 1995; Saleh, 1996). Fully predicting this geometry requires extensive theory and modeling of the surface properties. Because our emphasis is only the wavelength, and not the angular distribution of light, we restrict our calculations to Lambertian surfaces, that is surfaces that scatter uniformly in all directions. As a first approximation, the light emitted from CRTs and many printed materials follow Lambert's law. A somewhat better approximation, useful in some applications of illuminant estimation, is the dichromatic reflectance model (Lee, 1985; Shafer, 1985; Tominaga and Wandell, 1989).

Using a Lambertian model, the effect of the surface on the scattered wavelengths is described by the *surface reflectance function*, $S(\lambda)$, a dimensionless quantity. The scattered light is again defined by a radiance measurement, and it is given by the product $C(\lambda) = E(\lambda)S(\lambda)$ and (units of watts per steradian per meter squared per nanometer).

After passage through the optics of the eye, an image is formed at the retina. This can be expressed as irradiance at the retina (Rodieck, 1998). The sensor absorptions by the photoreceptors (or camera sensors) are calculated by an inner product between the image irradiance at the retina and the absorption function of the photoreceptor photopigment. For the ith receptor class this value is

$$a_i = \int_{370}^{730} A_i(\lambda)E(\lambda)S(\lambda)d\lambda \qquad (8.1)$$

where $A_i(\lambda)$ is the spectral absorption of the relevant sensor class.

For practical calculations, the wavelength functions are sampled and the integral is replaced by a summation. A matrix can then be used to find the predicted responses as follows. Place the three device spectral absorption functions, $A_i(\lambda)$, in the columns of an *absorption matrix*, **A**. To convert the continuous functions into discrete vectors, the CIE recommends using sampling intervals of 5 nm steps ranging from 380 to 780 nm. Most sensor absorption functions are smooth with respect to wavelength, so that the proper wavelength-sampling rate is limited by the expected variation in the irradiance signals, $C(\lambda)$. Expressing the image irradiance as a vector with the same sampling interval, **C**, the three response values are predicted by the matrix product $\mathbf{A}^t\,\mathbf{C}$.

8.3.1.1 Visible and hidden portions of the signal

Most cameras and scanners have three sensors. The three wavelength measurements, a_i, represent only a coarse sampling of the wavelength function $C(\lambda)$. Consequently, many different spectral power distributions can cause the same triplet of responses. A pair of lights, $(\mathbf{C}, \mathbf{C}')$, that cause the same responses in the capture device but that have different spectral power distributions are called *metamers*.

Once the sensor wavelength response functions of a device are known, it is straightforward to specify its metamers. Two lights C and C′ are metamers if $\mathbf{A}^t\,\mathbf{C} = \mathbf{A}^t\,\mathbf{C}'$, or equivalently if $\mathbf{A}^t\,(\mathbf{C}-\mathbf{C}') = \mathbf{0}$. That is, two lights are metamers if and only if their difference falls in the null space of $\mathbf{A}^t$.

Again using conventional linear algebra, the signal measured by any image capture device can be divided into two parts. One part of the signal influences the sensor response. We say this part is *visible* to the device. It can be expressed as a weighted sum of the columns of the sensor matrix, **A**. The part that is *hidden* from the device is orthogonal to the columns of **A**. Metamers differ only in their 'hidden' part.

Because image capture devices serve as a substitute for the visual system, it is desirable that they encode precisely the same part of the input signal as the visual system. An ideal image capture device must encode only those parts of the wavelength signal as the human visual system. Responding to portions of the signal to which humans are blind (e.g., infra-red), or failing to respond to portions the human visual system sees, usually will introduce errors into the image reproduction pipeline.

As a practical matter, the sensors in consumer devices do not align precisely, in the sense described above, with human vision. Much of the engineering of capture devices involves compensating for this basic difference in acquisition. These methods will be discussed after describing some of the basic features of practical capture devices.

8.3.2 SCANNERS FOR REFLECTIVE MEDIA

Figure 8.4 shows two designs of scanners used to capture signals from printed material. The scanners illuminate the page with an internal lamp. In the one-pass designs shown here, three sensors encode light scattered from the print surface. Most modern scanners use a one-pass design, though original designs were often based on three separate measurements acquired using one sensor and three different colored light sources.

Figure 8.4 shows an overview of the scanning elements in two patented designs. In the Canon design a small region in the image is focused onto an array of three parallel sensors (Tamura, 1983). In most modern implementations, the sensors are linear arrays of *charged-coupled devices* (CCDs) whose spectral sensitivities may be altered by the superposition of small colored filters. In this design, as the imaging element of the scanner moves across the document each line is focused, in turn, on one of the three different types of CCD arrays. By the time the entire document has been scanned all three arrays have scanned the entire page. By registering the signals acquired at different times, color images are obtained.

Hewlett–Packard has patented a design in which the capture device acquires signals through a set of dichroic mirrors (Vincent and Neuman, 1989). These mirrors reflect all wavelengths less than a cutoff wavelength and transmit all wavelengths above that cutoff. By arranging two sets of stacked mirrors, light in different wavebands is separated onto three identical linear CCD arrays. Using this method, all of the light analyzed at a single moment in time comes from the same source. Also, almost every photon in the visible range is acquired by one of the sensors. In this design the three sensor arrays are the same; the different spectral tuning of the sensors arises because of the properties of the dichroic mirrors along the light path.

The design of the Hewlett–Packard scanner forces the sensor wavelength responsivities to be essentially block functions, unlike the sensors in

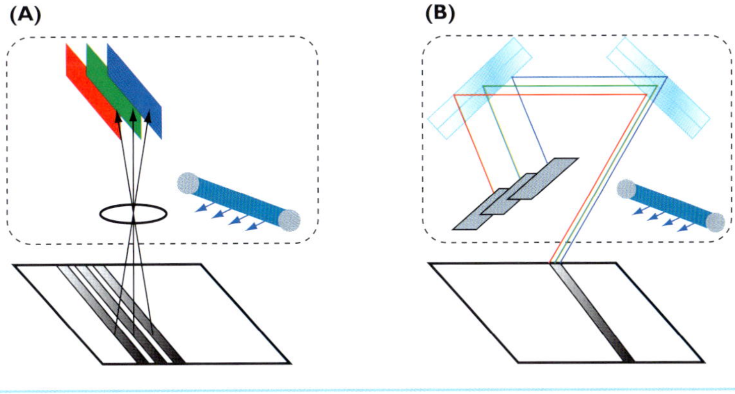

Figure 8.4 One-pass color scanner designs. In panel (A) the light from a line is measured three times as the three linear arrays pass. Because of this pipeline architecture, the total time to scan in three sensors is only slightly longer than the time to scan with a single (monochrome) sensor. In panel (B) light from a line is separated by means of dichroic mirrors into three wavelength regimes. Each of these separate wavelength regimes is imaged on a different sensor to produce the color image. See text for details.

the human eye. Consequently, it is impossible to use this design to measure the wavelength spectrum in the same way as the human eye. Even though it is impossible to guarantee that the color of the reproduction and original match, the simplicity and elegance of this engineering design has many practical advantages so that the design is still used in scanners and cameras. We will discuss how problems introduced by the mismatch between the acquisition device and the human eye can be minimized later in this section.

Finally, we conclude with a few of the properties of the capture environment that make the design of scanners relatively simple. First, scanners work in a closed environment: The illuminant is known, unlike the operating environment for cameras or the human eye. Knowledge of the illuminant simplifies color estimation and eliminates problems caused by the need to manage exposure duration and color balancing. Second, scanners mainly acquire data about a limited set of inputs: flat, printed material. It is possible to make a best guest, or even have the user specify, the type of printed material in the scanner. Knowledge about the source of the input can be a significant advantage for color processing. When the properties of the input material are known, better inferences about the input can be made. We will describe this principle at greater length after introducing color acquisition with digital cameras.

8.3.3 DIGITAL CAMERAS

There are two basic digital cameras designs. In one design, three or four color sensors are interleaved in mosaics within a single sensor array. Figure 8.5A shows a popular sensor in which four sensors are combined into three (R,G,B) signals. This is accomplished by forming weighted sums of the outputs in various combinations. Figure 8.5B illustrates the most commonly used mosaic for image acquisition, the *Bayer* pattern (Bayer, 1973). In this design (R,G,B) sensors are used and the middle-wavelength (G) sensor is present at twice the spatial sampling rate as the red and blue sensors. This design is effective because when the camera data are converted to a digital image, data from the green sensor are critical in defining the luminance representation. The human visual system is more sensitive to the luminance spatial component than the chromatic variations. The increased density of the green sensor improves the spatial sampling of the luminance signal and thus provides information that is better matched to the spatial resolution of the eye.

A design using prismatic optics is shown in Figure 8.5C. This design is analogous to the dichroic mirrors used in the Hewlett–Packard scanner. The prismatic optics form three images of the scene, separated by wavelength bands. These images are each captured by three independent sensor arrays. As in the dichroic mirror design, the three images represent non-overlapping portions of the spectrum so that, again, matching the human wavelength responsivity is not possible.

The sampling mosaic design is usually built with a single monochrome sensor with a superimposed color filter array (CFA). (For a novel development in which the sensor wavelength

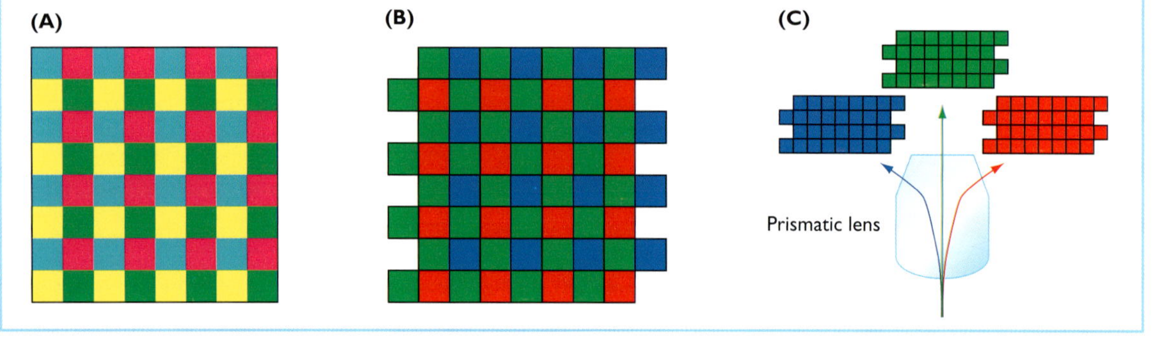

Figure 8.5 **Arrangements of the color sensors in digital cameras. (A) Four-color CMYG color filter array. (B) Three-color Bayer pattern color filter array. (C) Prismatic optics.**

responsivity is changed electronically see Silicon Vision, 2000.) In this design camera spatial resolution is traded for color information. To render images captured with this design, the data from the three types of color sensors must be interpolated to form an image with (R,G,B) values at every location. This interpolation process is called *demosaicing*, and a variety of demosaicing algorithms have been proposed (see, e.g., Adams *et al.*, 1998).

Demosaicing algorithms are a very important component of the digital camera system design. Some of the artifacts that can be introduced by using poor demosaicing algorithms are illustrated in Figure 8.6. The original image is shown in panel (A). This image was sampled to simulate an image acquired by a Bayer color filter array. The reconstructed image from a linear interpolation of the missing values is shown in panel (B). The reconstructed image formed by replicating pixel values is shown in (C). Neither method is acceptable and a variety of linear and nonlinear methods have been proposed and used in products (Brainard and Sherman, 1995; Adams *et al.*, 1998).

There are three advantages of the prismatic optics approach. First, for the same spatial resolution as the mosaic design, the sensor arrays can be smaller, and it is less expensive to build three smaller sensor arrays than one larger one. Second, nearly every photon is captured, producing a very efficient capture device. The mosaic design intentionally permits photons to fall on sensors that will not respond to them. Efficient photon capture is an important element of final image quality, giving the prismatic optics a design advantage. Finally, prismatic optics eliminates the need for demosaicing. The main disadvantage, of course, is the complexity of the prismatic optics, including the packaging and additional electronics needed to accommodate the additional sensor arrays.

8.3.4 CALIBRATION AND CHARACTERIZATION

In modern image capture applications, color characterization means finding a method to convert the measured (R,G,B) values into a description based on the CIE tristimulus values (or equivalently the human cone absorptions). For most image capture devices the conversion process will depend on the specific state of the device; calibration refers to the process of adjusting the device parameters so that the device is in a known state where the characterization is accurate. Because the (R,G,B) responses in a scanner or camera are unique to that device, the measured values are called *device-dependent*. Because the CIE values are not tied to the device, but rather to human vision, these are called *device-independent*.

The characterization process is usually divided into two parts. First, measurements are made of the relationship between light input intensity and scanner or camera output. The function relating these quantities is called the transduction function, also called the gamma function. In most systems, the output follows the same function of intensity no matter what the spectral composition of the input source. The sensors themselves respond linearly to the input signal, and any nonlinearities arise from processing after the initial capture. A simple model for this

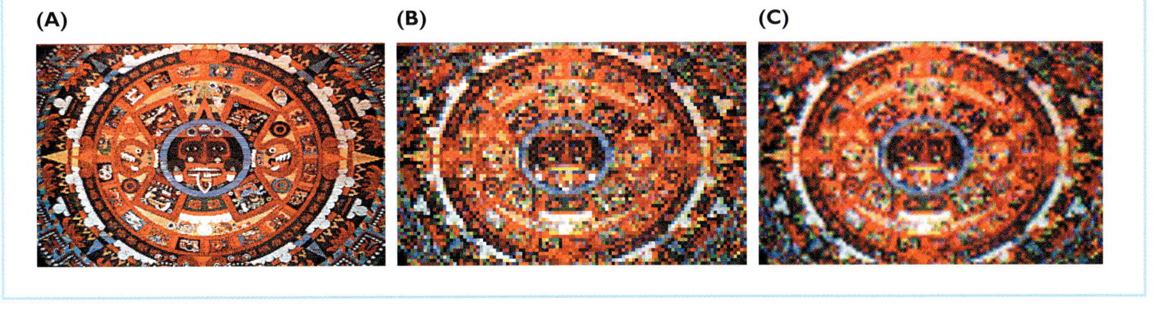

Figure 8.6 Spatial artifacts caused by demosaicing algorithms. The original image is shown in (A). Interpolation errors when using (B) linear interpolation and (C) pixel replication are shown.

type of system is given by the formula for a static nonlinearity:

$$d = F(\Sigma\, s(\lambda)r(\lambda)\delta\lambda)$$

where d is the digital value from the system, $s(\lambda)$ is the input signal spectral power distribution, $r(\lambda)$ is the sensor spectral responsivity, and F( ) is a monotonic function. Because F( ) is a fixed, monotonic, nonlinearity, it is possible to estimate the function and remove its effect. After correcting for F( ), the sensor wavelength responsivity can be estimated using standard linear methods. In the following sections, we describe some of the basic features of the nonlinear function used in most cameras. Then, we describe estimation methods for the sensor spectral responsivity.

8.3.4.1 Dynamic range and quantization

The dynamic range of a capture system is the ratio of the light level that produces a response just below system saturation and the light level needed to produce a response just above the dark noise. The device quantization describes how many intensity levels are classified in the digital output. For example, an 8-bit device classifies the input intensities into 256 levels. Each of these factors plays a significant role in determining the camera image quality.

The dynamic range and quantization properties are determined by different parts of the camera system. The dynamic range is an input-referred measurement; that is, its value is the ratio of two input light levels. Signal quantization is a description of the number of signal output levels and does not depend on the input signal at all. Despite this huge difference, one often hears the dynamic range of a device described in terms of the number of bits it codes. This is incorrect. A system that quantizes the output signal to 12 bits can have the same dynamic range as a system that quantizes the output to 8 bits. Two 8-bit systems can have very different dynamic ranges. To link the two measures, one must make a set of assumptions about how the camera designer chose the quantization levels, the properties of the sensor, and other system features. There is no guarantee that these assumptions will be met.

The *dynamic range* of commonly used CCD sensors is on the order of a factor of 500–1000 (60 dB), though devices with much higher dynamic range exist. Operationally, call one standard deviation of the sensor noise variability 1. Then, if the maximum response that we can read out prior to sensor saturation is 100, the dynamic range is 100. Photomultiplier tubes, an older but still important technology, have a dynamic range in excess of 1000. Dynamic range is commonly described in log units or decibels (20 log units). Hence, it is often said that CCD sensors have a dynamic range of 2–3 log units (40–60 dB) and photomultiplier tubes have a dynamic range of 3–4 log units (60–80 dB) (Janesick, 1997; dpreview.com, 2000). It is difficult to compare the dynamic range of these devices with that of the human eye; while the responses of these devices is roughly linear with input intensity, the visual system encodes light intensity using a nonlinear (compressive) transduction function (Cornsweet, 1970; Wandell, 1995).

How much is enough dynamic range? If we consider only the surface reflectances of objects, a range of two log units is quite large. This spans reflectances from that of white reflective paper (100%) to very black ink (1%). The dynamic range of a CCD sensor is adequate to encode the dynamic range of printed material. Slides can represent a somewhat larger range of densities, exceeding two log units, so that in these applications either specially cooled CCDs or photomultiplier tubes may be appropriate. Natural scenes may have even larger dynamic ranges due to (a) geometric relationship between the light source, surface, and viewer, and (b) shadows. Images containing a portion in direct sunlight and a second portion in dark shadow, or a shadow within a shade, can span 4 log units or more.

The analog-to-digital converters (ADCs) in the image capture system determine the signal quantization. In many early designs, uniform quantization steps were used, and the most frequently asked question was: How many bits of output are needed to capture the intensity differences seen by the human eye? The main principles of the answer are well understood: To match the intensity discrimination abilities of the human eye, the quantizer must classify intensities present at the finest discriminability. The finest human intensity resolution occurs at intensity levels somewhat lower than the mean image intensity. This demanding intensity region, then, determines the number of classification steps needed by a uniform quantizer, and a uniform quantizer must classify the image intensities into more than 1024 bins (more than 10 bits). Using this scheme, the quantization step at very high or low intensities is spaced more finely than the visual system can discriminate.

Although the inherent transduction of sensors used for digital imaging is linear, manufacturers often insert a nonlinear post-processing stage as shown in Figure 8.7A. The two-step process produces non-uniform quantization levels that approximate the discrimination capabilities of the human eye. In the method shown in panel (A), the image is first converted to 10 bits of quantization using a uniform conversion step. Then, a lookup table that produces a final result at 8 bits merges the quantization steps corresponding to high intensity levels. The design requires an extra lookup table beyond the ADC, but this results in an output that is only 8 bits and whose intensity classifications match the human eye more accurately. Reducing the number of bits to represent the image also has beneficial effects on signal storage and transmission. Finally, as we shall see later, this quantization scheme is useful when the camera data are combined with a CRT display.

8.3.4.2 Wavelength

Once the transduction function is known, the sensor responsivity, r( ), can be estimated from measurements with a variety of light sources, s( ). The corrected digital value is related to the signal and responsivity by the linear equation:

$$F^{-1}(d) = \Sigma\, s(\lambda) r(\lambda) d\lambda)$$

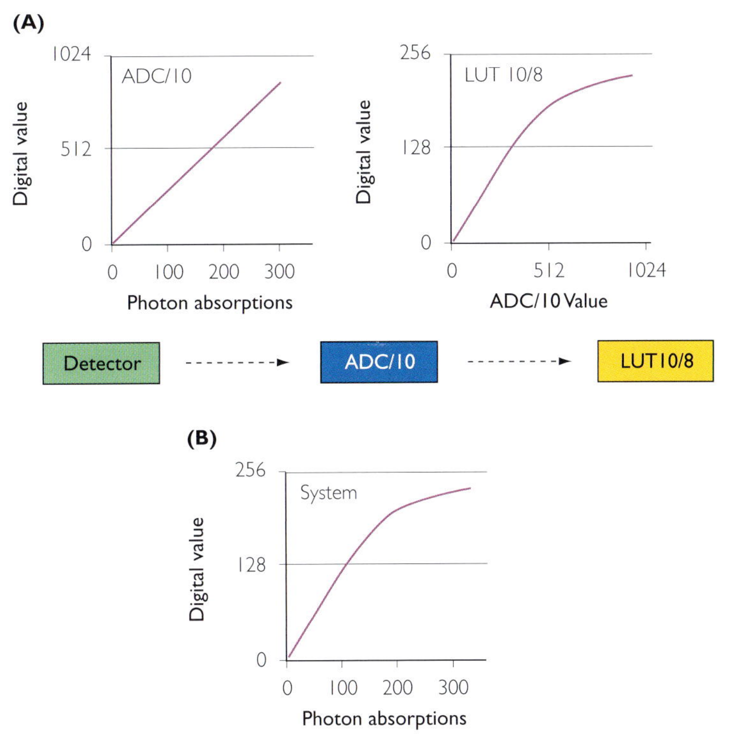

Figure 8.7 **Quantization architecture of a digital camera. (A) Quantization is often performed in two steps. A linear, 10-bit ADC step converts the analog sensor to digital form. Certain types of linear processing, including demosaicing and certain color transformations, are performed in this linear representation. The signal is then reduced to 8 bits by a nonlinear lookup table that compresses the high intensity quantization bins. (B) The overall camera transduction function is compressive, much as the visual sensitivity of the eye is a compressive function. Small differences in the dark regions are preserved, but these differences are not preserved in the light regions.**

One can only guarantee that the sensor response measures the same spectral image as the human cones if the sensor responsivities are linearly related to the human cones, or equivalently to the CIE Standard Observer functions $\bar{x}$, $\bar{y}$, and $\bar{z}$. That is, suppose there are three sensor responsivities, $r_i(\lambda)$. Then the image capture system will be guaranteed to see the same portion of the visible spectrum as the human eye if and only if there are weights, w_{ij}, such that

$$\bar{x} = w_{11}r_1 + w_{12}r_2 + w_{12}r_3$$

Two similar equations must hold for $\bar{y}$ and $\bar{z}$. When such a linear relationship exists, the sensors are *colorimetric*, and it is possible to guarantee that the sensor (R,G,B) responses can be converted to CIE tristimulus coordinates. The conversion step requires multiplying the (R,G,B) values by a 3×3 linear transformation comprised of the weights. It is possible to determine these weights from only a few measurements. Suppose that we know the (X,Y,Z) values of three color patches, and we know the linearized sensor values, F^{-1}(R,G,B). Then one can determine the linear transformation that maps the (X,Y,Z) values into the linear sensor values.

In general, limitations on the cost of manufacturing make it impractical for the spectral sensitivity of these sensors to match the spectral sensitivity of the cones or the tristimulus functions. It is straightforward to show that when the sensors are not within a linear transformation of the tristimulus functions, there will be pairs of surfaces such that: (a) the sensor responses to the two surfaces are identical, but (b) the tristimulus coordinates of the surfaces differ. For such a pair of surfaces, it is impossible to guarantee a correct estimate of the tristimulus coordinates from the measured responses.

Figure 8.8A shows the combined sensor and illuminant spectral responsivity of the MARC system, an elegant device used to digitize paintings (Martinez *et al.*, 1993; Cupitt *et al.*, 1996; Farrell *et al.*, 1999). These sensors are not colorimetric, that is they are not within a linear transformation of the human cones. Consequently, there are variations in the spectral power distribution that are visible to the human visual system, but not to the MARC system. Two such variations are shown in Figure 8.8B. Unless such stimuli can be eliminated from the set of input signals or inferred by other means, it is impossible to guarantee that the sensor values can be accurately transformed into tristimulus values.

8.3.4.3 Characterization of noncolorimetric sensors

When the wavelength responsivities of the color sensors do not match the human cones, characterization means making a best estimate of the tristimulus (X,Y,Z) values from the sensor responses, (R,G,B). There are two basic techniques that are used for making this best estimate.

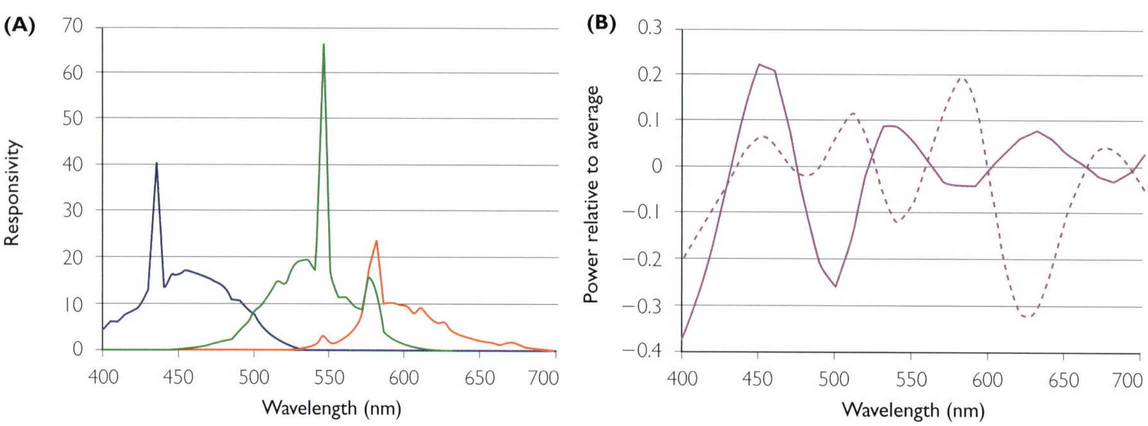

Figure 8.8 **The spectral responsivity of cameras and scanners rarely match that of the human cones. Consequently, differences in spectral variations visible to the human eye may not be visible to the device. (A) Combined illuminant and sensor spectral responsivities of the MARC scanner. (B) Examples of modulations of the spectral power distribution that differ to a human observer but result in the same response of the MARC scanner.**

First, characterization can involve making measurements of multiple stimuli to find a functional form that relates the measured (R,G,B) to the (X,Y,Z) values. The functional forms that are commonly used include simple global linear transformations (3×3 matrix), linear transformations that vary smoothly with the input data (interpolation), nonlinear polynomial functions, and methods based on simple neural networks.

Tetrahedral interpolation is an elegant computational method that can be reduced to very efficient hardware computation. This method applies a linear transformation to the measured data, but the linear transform coefficients vary as a function of the measured (R,G,B) values. The method is called tetrahedral because the input space is partitioned into a set of non-overlapping tetrahedra using a characterization data set. The linear transformation applied to any (R,G,B) value depends on the measured characterization values at the vertices of the tetrahedra (Hardeberg and Schmitt, 1997; Gill, 1999). The tetrahedral shape is preferred to cubes because tetrahedra are preserved across transformations from RGB to XYZ representations, so that transformations in either direction can be based on the same control points. Other geometric shapes, such as squares, can be transformed into curved shapes that are problematic when partitioning the response space. A patent has been obtained on the use of tetrahedral interpolation for color characterization (Sakamoto and Itooka, 1981).

The second technique that is helpful for characterization purposes is to specify the properties of the input signals. This can be a very powerful technique, particularly if the input signals fall in a sufficiently restricted set. For example, it is possible to use noncolorimetric camera sensors to estimate the tristimulus coordinates of a color display system that has only three independent primary lights (Horn, 1984; Wandell, 1986).

In many practical applications, for example when mainly processing a particular type of film print, the input material is restricted. Calibrating specifically for this print should lead to a relatively precise system compared to calibrating for arbitrary inputs. Hence, a target designed to span the color range of the print medium is helpful. Such a target, the ANSI (American National Standards Institute) IT8.7, has been standardized and is now provided by various vendors. These targets include examples of particular printed outputs and the manufacturer provides the tristimulus values of these prints. Hence, they form a good basis for calibrating a scanner or camera system that will be used regularly with one of a small set of targets. These targets may be purchased from a number of vendors.

8.3.5 COLOR RENDERING OF ACQUIRED IMAGES

Finally, we conclude this section with an observation about the role of camera characterization in the image systems pipeline. Often it is the case that an image is captured under one illumination condition and then rendered for an observer viewing the image under a different illumination. When this occurs, rendering the image with the same tristimulus coordinates as the original will not match the appearance of the original.

To understand the problem, consider that a black surface on a sunny beach may have a luminance of 200 cd/m^2. In a typical windowless office, a white surface will reflect on the order of 100 cd/m^2. Hence, to represent the color black on a display, one would not want to match the original scene tristimulus coordinates. The same principle holds for color variations as for luminance variations.

This issue is not important for scanners, which work in a fixed environment. However, digital cameras are used to acquire images under many different illuminants. One approach to solving this illuminant mismatch problem is to use algorithms that estimate the illuminant at the time of the image capture. If the illumination is known, then it is possible to make a rough guess of new tristimulus coordinates that will match the original in appearance. This process is called *color balancing*. Algorithms for color balancing are an important part of digital camera design, though a review of the issues is beyond the scope of this chapter. A second approach is to build a model of color appearance and to render the image so that the appearances of the original and rendered images match. The CIE has recently standardized one model in what will probably be a series of color appearance models (see Chapter 5; Fairchild, 1997; Luo and Hunt, 1998; TC1–34, 1998).

8.4 ELECTRONIC IMAGE DISPLAYS

8.4.1 OVERVIEW

Image rendering technologies can be divided into two major categories: electronic displays and printers. Electronic displays can be further subdivided into emissive and non-emissive types. Emissive displays are those in which the image-forming element also serves as the source of light, while non-emissive displays modulate some aspect of an extrinsic illumination source. There are currently a large number of display technologies for rendering an electronic image, but two types dominate the market: the cathode ray tube (CRT) is the dominant emissive technology while the liquid crystal display (LCD) is the pervasive non-emissive technology. Printing is a non-emissive rendering technology.

We have separated the discussion of image displays into emissive and non-emissive technologies because the methods used to control light intrinsic to the device and those used to control transmitted or reflected light from an external source differ significantly. In this section we describe the basic principles of CRTs and LCDs. While there are many ways to utilize liquid crystals to modulate light and create a display device, we focus our attention on the ubiquitous transmissive, twisted-nematic (TN) color LCD that contains a separate but integrated illumination source. The basic principles of color synthesis and color control for these LCDs and CRT devices are similar and will play a role in most, if not all, of the display technologies that are envisioned over the next decade. We show how these color synthesis principles are used to satisfy the color-reproduction equation, described in the introduction to this chapter. We also review the general methods and computational tools that are used to characterize such electronic display devices.

8.4.2 CRT DEVICES

The venerable CRT has dominated the display market for the past 45 years, despite repeated claims of its imminent demise. The principal technology for generating color in direct-view CRTs is the shadow-mask CRT, illustrated in Figure 8.9.

In this design, the three electron guns (one for each primary color phosphor) house a thermionic cathode that serves as a source of electrons. Video input voltages are applied to each electron gun assembly, which includes control grids for modulating the beam current flowing from the cathodes as well as electrodes to accelerate, shape and focus the electron beams on the phosphor-coated faceplate. The applied video

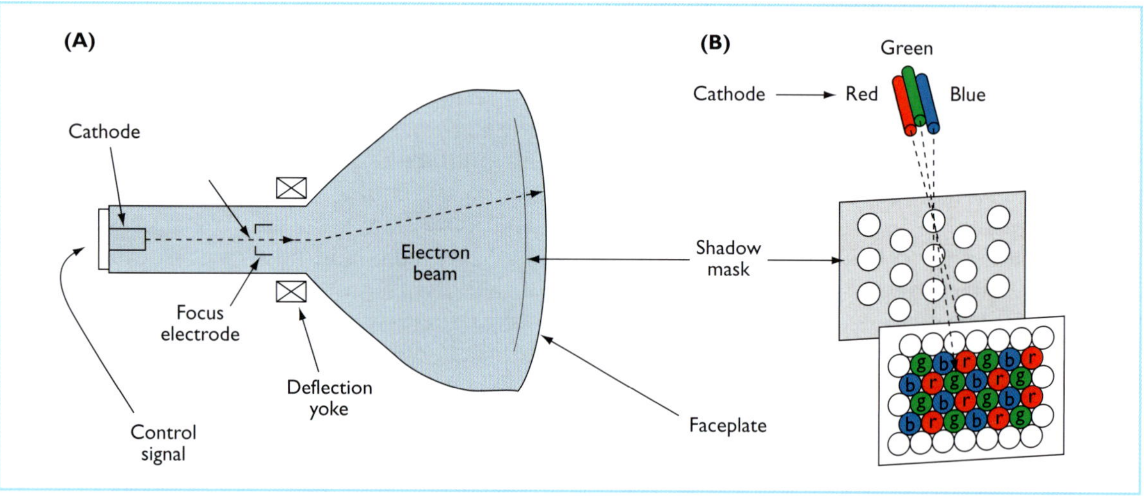

Figure 8.9 **The shadow-mask CRT. The basic architecture of a shadow mask color CRT display is shown in (A), and the geometric relations between the cathodes, shadow mask and phosphor-coated faceplate in determining color selection are shown in (B).**

signals cause the intensity of the electron beams to vary synchronously as the beams sweep out a raster path. The electrons that pass through the shadow-mask apertures excite the R, G, and B phosphors. The geometry of the apertures is coordinated with the phosphor pattern on the CRT faceplate. Electron absorptions cause the phosphors to emit light in a process called cathodoluminescence. As illustrated in Figure 8.9b, color selection and registration are determined by the position of the electron guns and their geometric relations to the shadow-mask and phosphor-coated faceplate.

Although there are several places in the CRT image pathway where sampling artifacts are introduced, sampling artifacts are minimized because the electron beam cross-section is approximately Gaussian and spans several groupings or triads of color phosphor dots. This shape imparts a low-pass spatial filter to the signal path so that the sampling rate does not introduce any appreciable spatial aliasing (Lyons and Farrell, 1989).

In designing CRTs, the positions of the electron guns, shadow-mask apertures and phosphors must all be taken into account and many configurations are currently available. In recent years there has been a trend toward the use of in-line configurations of electron guns, in which the electron beams are arrayed along a line rather than in a triangular configuration, due to their simpler alignment and deflection considerations (Silverstein and Merrifield, 1985; Sherr, 1993). In addition, slotted-mask and strip-mask (e.g., the familiar Sony Trinitron tube) color CRTs which use continuous vertical RGB phosphor stripes on the CRT faceplate have become popular. Current technology has enabled mask-pitch and associated phosphor component pitch (i.e., the center-to-center distance between RGB phosphor groupings or between like-color phosphor components) to be reduced to the range of 0.25 to 0.31 mm (Lehrer, 1985; Silverstein and Merrifield, 1985; Sherr, 1993).

The CRT design reduces spatial resolution and photon efficiency in exchange for color. It is important that the spatial patterning of the red, green, and blue phosphors be invisible under normal operation. At a nominal display viewing distance of 61.0 cm, this spacing translates into a range of subtended visual angles from approximately 1.41 to 1.75 arc minutes. Given the resolving capability of the chromatic channels of the human visual system (also see Chapters 2 and 6 of the present volume), this spacing is sufficient to ensure reliable spatial-additive color synthesis (Schade, 1958; VanderHorst and Bouman, 1969; Glenn *et al.*, 1985; Mullen, 1985).

Color CRTs are inefficient compared to monochrome displays because of the shadow mask. The presence of the mask reduces the percentage of electrons that result in an electron absorption and subsequent photon emission, and such masks are not needed in monochrome displays. The market has demonstrated that to most consumers the value of color information is worth the tradeoff.

8.4.3 LCD DEVICES

Direct-view color LCDs are commonplace in portable computer and miniature color television applications. They are beginning to penetrate the market for larger, high-resolution, high-performance color displays.

Figure 8.10 shows the major optical components of an active-matrix addressed transmissive TN LCD. The color LCD is composed of a backlight illumination source, diffuser, rear linear polarizer, glass sheets with transparent thin-film indium-tin-oxide (ITO) electrodes and thin-film transistors (TFTs), optically active layer of birefringent LC material, absorbing thin-film color selection filters, and a front polarizer. The operation of the LCD depends mainly on the polarization properties of light. Light from the illumination source is plane polarized by the rear (entrance) polarizer. The light passes through the liquid crystal (LC) layer where its polarization state can be altered. Depending on the polarization state after passing through the LC, the light is either absorbed or transmitted by the front (analyzing) polarizer.

Three components have the principal effects on the colorimetric and photometric characteristics of the emitted light: the spectral power distribution (SPD) of the illumination source; the spectral transmission of the thin-film color selection filters; and the spectral transmission of the LC cell (Silverstein, 2000). The largely clear optical elements, such as the glass containing the ITO electrodes, only modify the spectral

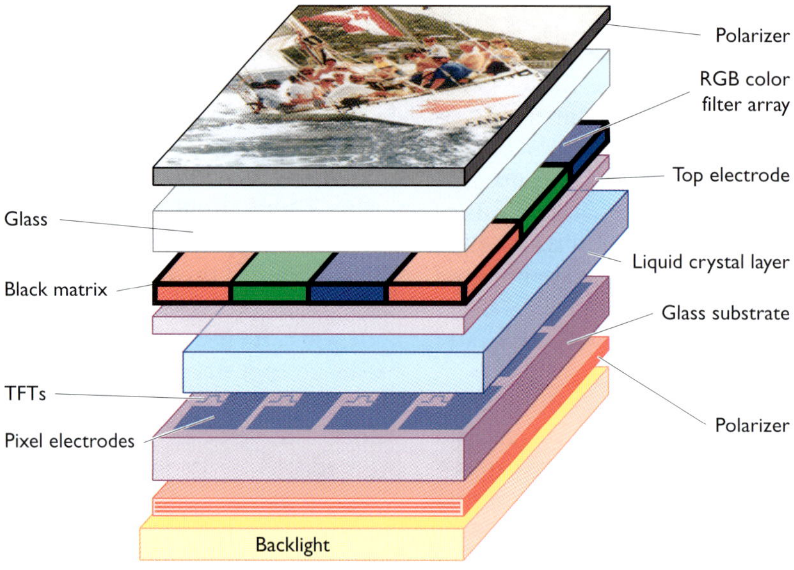

Figure 8.10 The architecture of a transmissive color LC display employing active-matrix addressing is shown. See text for details.

composition of the light by a small amount. Along the imaging path, prior to reaching the human observer, each optical component must be characterized by its full emission or transmission spectrum.

The backlight illumination for most direct-view color LCDs is either a hot-cathode (HCF) or a cold-cathode (CCF) fluorescent lamp. Fluorescent lamps have the advantages of high luminous efficiency and the ability to tailor the SPD of the lamp via the selection and mixture of individual phosphor components and their proportional contributions to the total phosphor blend. Tri-band phosphor mixtures are typically employed to improve color performance for these lamps. The final emission spectra are the weighted sum of the three phosphor emissions plus energy at the mercury emission lines.

Direct-view color LCDs typically use thin-film color absorption filters to determine the spectral composition of the three primary lights. Only a limited variety of dyes and pigments compatible with LC materials and the LCD manufacturing process exist. Once the filter materials are selected varying the filter thickness and dye concentration can make some adjustments to their spectral transmission, though the value of these parameters must fall within the limits of the thin-film deposition processes. If the spectral transmission of a set of reference filter materials is known, and the dye or pigment in concentration is known to follow Beer's Law within the range of concentrations used, then the spectral transmission of the filter material at other dye concentrations and film thickness may be estimated via the use of the Beer–Lambert Laws (Wyszecki and Stiles, 1982; Silverstein and Fiske, 1993).

The most complex spectral component of the system is the LC layer. The spectral properties of the LC cell depend on a variety of material parameters and the geometry of the LC cell. In addition, the spectral transmission depends on the display voltage (i.e. luminance or gray level) and the direction of light propagation (Silverstein and Fiske, 1993).

Liquid crystals (LCs) are complex, anisomeric organic molecules that, under certain temperature conditions, exhibit the fluid characteristics of a liquid and the molecular orientational order characteristics of a solid (Collings, 1990). A consequence of the ordering of anisomeric molecules is that LCs exhibit mechanical, electric, magnetic, and optical anisotropy (Penz, 1985; Scheffer and Nehring, 1992). Most LC materials are uniaxial and birefringent. Uniaxial materials possess one unique axis, the optic axis, which is parallel to the liquid crystal director (i.e., the long axis of the molecules). The anisotropic nature of LC materials gives them the optical property of birefringence, which refers to the phenomenon of light traveling with different velocities in crystalline materials depending on the propagation direction and the orientation of the light polarization relative to the crystalline axes (Collings, 1990). For a uniaxial LC, this implies different dielectric constants and refractive indices for the unique or 'extraordinary' direction and for other 'ordinary' directions in the LC material.

As mentioned above, the predominant LC cell configuration for high-performance color LCDs is the TN cell, whose basic principles of operation are illustrated in Figure 8.11. An entrance polarizer linearly polarizes the source light. In the field-off state (panel A), with no voltage applied, the LC layer optically rotates the axis of polarization of the incoming light. The typical twist or rotation angle used for most TN LCDs is 90°, although other twist angles may be used to achieve certain desired optical characteristics (Scheffer and Nehring, 1990, 1992). In the field-on state (panel B), the dielectric anisotropy of the LC material enables the applied electric field to deform the LC layer, destroying the twisted structure and eliminating the LC birefringence for normally incident incoming light. The LC layer does not rotate the axis of polarization of the incoming light. The difference in polarization state is the key variable for determining the display output.

After passage through the LC layer, the exit polarizer or 'analyzer' analyzes the polarization state of light exiting the LC layer. Light polarized parallel to the analyzer polarization vector is transmitted, light polarized perpendicular to the analyzer polarization direction is extinguished, and light polarized at intermediate angles follows Malus' Law; $I' = I \cos^2 \theta$, where (I) is the intensity of polarized incident light from a first linear polarizer, (I') is the intensity of light output and (θ) is the relative angle between the

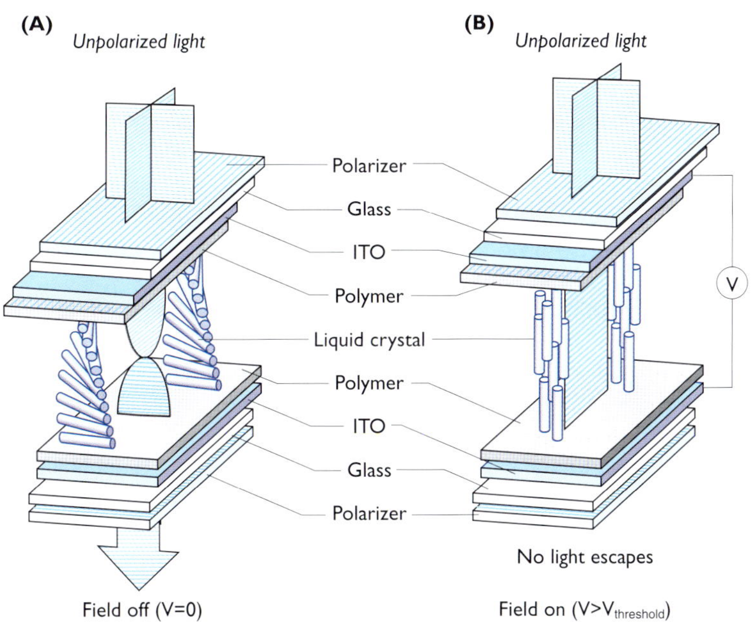

Figure 8.11 The composition of a TN LCD cell is shown. Applying voltage to the liquid crystal controls the transmission of light through the cell. These voltages alter the polarization of light passing through the cell. In (A), zero voltage is applied so that the twist structure is left undisturbed and rotates the polarization of the light 90° where it passes through the exit polarizer. In (B) a supra-threshold voltage is applied such that the LC twist structure is destroyed, leaving the initial polarization of light intact as it passes through the LC layer where it is finally absorbed by the orthogonal exit polarizer.

orientations of the two linear polarizers (Collett, 1993). Two configurations of TN cell entrance and exit polarizers are used. LCDs that use crossed rear and front polarizers operate in the normally white (NW) mode. LCDs with parallel polarizers operate in normally black (NB) mode. The TN cell of Figure 8.11 operates in the NW mode.

The precise polarization state of light exiting the LC cell depends on several liquid cell parameters, including the LC birefringence, LC layer thickness, twist angle, and importantly for us, the wavelength of the light. As a consequence of this dependence, the transmitted spectrum (and thus color appearance) of the display can vary with viewing angle. This variation is an important consideration in the ultimate color performance of LCDs and models of the influence of these parameters are an important element in LCD design (Silverstein, 1991; Silverstein and Fiske, 1993). Various methods for compensating for this wavelength-dependence have been developed.

8.4.3.1 Other LCD display technologies

There is increasing use of LCs in color projection systems. A major advantage of LCD color projectors over CRT-based systems is the ability to separate the image-forming elements and the illumination source. This permits the development of projectors with very high intensity output and thus extremely large projected images. Some of the key problems with LCD direct-view displays, such as viewing angle effects of the transmitted or reflected light, are eliminated in projection systems. The observer does not directly view the image, so LCD viewing angle effects are eliminated. Finally, the relatively small size of the LC image-forming elements permits a very compact optical design. Given the advantages of color projection systems based on LC technology, the market demand for these large-screen color displays continues to have substantial growth.

A second trend is the development of subtractive color displays. This approach offers the advantages of very high image resolution since each addressable pixel is capable of generating the full color gamut of the display, unlike typical color CRTs or LCDs which rely on additive spatial color synthesis of R, G, and B pixels and thus sacrifice two-thirds or more of the available pixels to serve the color synthesis function. The development of subtractive color LCDs is an important technology initiative for full-color head-mounted displays, in which the image source must be small and very high pixel densities are required to support good color image resolution across a wide field of view.

Current embodiments of subtractive color LCDs use three LC layers, each controlling the spectral transmission of a portion of the visible spectrum from a broadband illuminant. Thus, each LC layer acts as an electronically controlled color filter that is analogous to ink (see next section). Three different approaches to subtractive color LCDs have been developed. In the first, dichroic dye molecules are suspended within the LC material in what is typically called a guest–host LC cell (Silverstein and Bernot, 1991). Subtractive primaries (cyan, magenta, and yellow dyes) are used in the three respective LC cells. When the LC material is switched by the application of an applied electric field, the elongated dichroic dye molecules are reoriented along with the LC material, causing different degrees of spectral filtering in each cell as the LC director orientation is varied between alignment parallel and perpendicular to the cell surfaces. The second approach uses three TN LC cells with colored linear polarizers as the analyzers for each cell (Plummer, 1983). The cells are arranged such that each cell rotates the plane of polarization of light entering the cell into the entrance plane of the next cell in the stack. The linear polarizers employed as the analyzers in this novel configuration utilize cyan, magenta, and yellow dyes instead of the embedded iodine crystals found in standard, achromatic linear sheet polarizers. Each TN LC cell operates as a typical TN light valve, but instead of varying the transmission between an achromatic light and dark state the output of each cell varies from an achromatic state to the state produced by the spectral transmission of the respective dye. The stack of three such TN LC cells constitutes a full-color subtractive LCD. In a final approach, three LC cells configured as electrically controlled birefringence (ECB) cells are used to provide spectral shaping which approaches the subtractive color primaries (Conner, 1992).

Prototype subtractive LCDs yielding excellent color performance have been demonstrated for the guest–host configuration using appropriately selected dichroic dyes and for the stacked TN cell approach with high-quality color polarizers. The three-layer ECB cell configuration has been used in color projection panels for overhead projectors for a number of years, although good color saturation and precise color control have been difficult to achieve with ECB cells. Thus, while high-performance subtractive color LCDs are still in their early stages of development, their technical feasibility has been demonstrated. The potential advantages of subtractive color displays are compelling, and the technology will surely find a place in the future of electronic color imaging.

Color LCD technology is still relatively new and evolving at a rapid pace. Continuing advances in all key LCD technologies; LC materials, optical systems configurations, illumination sources, color filters, optical compensation techniques, driver chips, and LC controllers, promise to raise the level of performance for each successive generation of color LCDs. Research into the spatial and temporal imaging characteristics of color matrix displays, including the effects of color mosaic patterns and methods of luminance quantization, remains a highly active area of investigation (Silverstein *et al.*, 1990). As the evolution of color LCD technology progresses, those concerned with electronic color imaging can look forward to brighter, higher contrast displays that exceed the color performance and image quality of today's color workstation standards.

8.4.4 DISPLAY CHARACTERIZATION

The purpose of display characterization is to specify the relationship between the values that control the input to the display and the light emitted by the display (Brainard, 1989; Berns, Gorzynski, and Motta, 1993; Berns, Motta, and Gorzynski, 1993. Hence, while the device physics of CRTs and transmissive color LCDs are completely different, the principles and methods of display characterization are quite similar (Silverstein, 2000). In this section we describe the principles of characterization of a specific display at a specific point in time, and we provide example measurements.

A digital frame buffer controls most displays. The intensities emitted by the three primaries comprising each pixel are specified by three digital values (R,G,B). The potential scope of a complete characterization is enormous. The industry standard for color applications allocates 8 bits of intensity control for each display primary and a total of $2^{8\,(3)}$ or approximately 16.8 million combinations. Multiplied by roughly a million pixels on the screen, and taking into account interactions between pixels, makes it impossible to perform an exhaustive characterization. Instead, characterizations are always based on simple models of the device that make powerful assumptions about the relationships between the display primaries and the spatial interactions between pixels.

With respect to color control, the most important modeling assumption is that the primary intensities can be controlled independently. Specifically, a control signal to the red primary will produce the same emission no matter what state the green or blue primaries. This assumption, *primary independence*, can and should be empirically verified during characterization. We recommend working only with display systems that satisfy primary independence. A second important assumption is that the SPDs of the display primaries are invariant as their intensities are changed. If the SPDs of the primaries change with intensity level, characterization becomes more complex. If these two assumptions hold, the characterization task is simplified and only a few dozen measurements need to be made.

There are many other issues that one might be concerned about in characterization. The spatial and temporal distribution of the signals may interact with the primary levels; the display may not be perfectly stable across time or with temperature; there can be variations across the surface of the display or with viewing angle. In general, complete characterization is not possible and some assumptions about these effects must be made and hopefully evaluated.

In many scientific studies, experiments are often based on only a small number of stimuli. In such cases, it is best to measure each of the stimuli individually. If too large a set of stimuli is used to measure them all, the first question to check is primary independence. To evaluate independence, measure the light emitted by the

R primary alone, the G primary alone, and the sum of the R and G primaries (R + G). The sum of the R and G measurements alone should equal the measurement of R + G. Then, stimuli with spatial and temporal configurations similar to the ones that will be used in the experiments should be calibrated.

To specify the characterization process, we must measure the relationship between the digital control signals (frame buffers), the light emitted by each of the primaries (primary spectra and transduction), and the effect this light will have on the human observer (tristimulus and chromaticity values). An excellent review of the principles and issues of display characterization may be found in (Brainard, 1989). A discussion can also be found in (Wandell, 1995, Appendix B) and publications from the Rochester Institute of Technology (Berns, Gorzynski, and Motta, 1993; Berns, Motta, and Gorzynski, 1993), and CIE technical reports (CIE, 1996).

8.4.4.1 Frame buffers

The primary roles of the frame buffer are the storage, conditioning, and output of the video signals that drive the display device. The industry standard for color applications allocates 8 bits of intensity control for each display primary or approximately 16.8 million discretely addressable colors. The match between the sampled values and human color sensitivity is imperfect, however. Consequently, not all displayed colors can be discriminated from one another, and many colors that differ by a single bit in their digital representation are significantly above the threshold discriminability of the eye. This results in various types of color artifacts, such as contouring artifacts on shaded graphics. High-quality rendering and other demanding applications, such as psychophysical measurements, can require finer (10 or 12 bits) control over the primary intensity level.

Many of the features of the frame buffer are determined by cost considerations, and the primary costs relate to the size and speed of the frame buffer memory. Consider a display system with 1280 × 1024 addressable pixel resolution and each pixel controlled by a 24-bit value. This system requires 4 million bytes of (fast) memory to represent the frame. An economical alternative is the lookup table (LUT) architecture. In this design, the intensity levels of the primary colors are controlled by a list of entries in a lookup table. Hence, a single number represents the three voltage levels that control the primary intensities, say between 0 and 255. At display time, the system retrieves the primary values from the LUT. In this way, each pixel is represented by one 8-bit quantity. While the precision of intensity control is established by the 8-bit resolution of the digital-to-analog converters (DACs), the number of entries in the LUT limits the total number of colors available for simultaneous display.

One benefit of a LUT design is to reduce image memory. There are other benefits as well, for certain types of display conditions. For example, LUTs provide an efficient means for implementing image operations that depend only on display value, and not on display position. To alter the image luminance or contrast one can re-write the 256 LUT entries rather than the entire image buffer. In this way various image processing operations, spanning the control of drifting and flickering patterns, can be implemented by controlling only the LUT.

8.4.4.2 Primary spectra and transduction

Figure 8.12A shows the SPDs of the primary phosphor emissions in a modern, high-performance color CRT monitor. The phosphors in this particular display were from the P22 family. There are many different phosphors available to manufacturers. Notice that the red phosphor SPD has several discrete spikes. Such spikes are not commonly found in nature, and consequently the CRT emissions almost never match the spectral power distribution found in the original scene. The color match can only be arranged because of the analysis, based on the color-matching experiment, of the eye's inability to distinguish between different spectral power distributions (metamerism).

Figure 8.12B shows a typical transduction function for a CRT. The digital count, shown on the horizontal axis, is related to the primary luminance by a nonlinear function. The nonlinear relationship is a characteristic of the CRT tube itself, not the surrounding circuitry. Typically, the relationship is close to a power

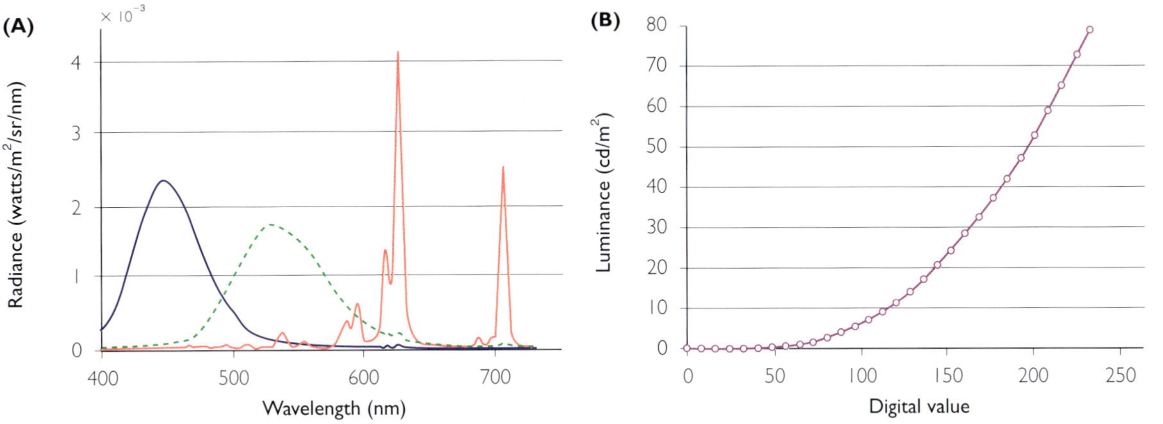

Figure 8.12 **(A) The spectral power distributions of the three primary phosphor emissions in a CRT display. (B) The transduction function relating digital value of the frame buffer to screen luminance for the same display is shown.**

function, Luminance = $\alpha(\text{Digital count})^{\gamma} + \beta$, or one of a set of other similar equations. Hence, because of the common use of gamma for the exponent, the transduction function is often called a 'gamma' curve. The value of the exponent differs between displays, but is generally between 1.7 and 2.2 for CRT displays, and its value is not under user control. User-controlled knobs manipulate the values of the gain (α) and offset (β) parameters. Extensive discussions of this curve and its implications for imaging can be found in the literature (Poynton, 1996).

Figure 8.13A shows the SPDs of three primaries in a particular LCD display. (Displays vary considerably.) The spikes in the distributions are due to materials placed in the fluorescent backlights. The peaks of the backlight emissions are designed to fall at the centers of the passbands of the thin-film color filters that are part of the LCD assembly. Notice that the shapes of the blue and green primary SPDs are narrower than the corresponding distributions for the CRT. This results in a larger range of displayable colors, as will be described below.

Figure 8.13B shows the transduction function of an LCD. The relation between the digital frame buffer value and the light intensity is nonlinear, as for the CRT. The relationship is not a natural consequence of the LCD display physics, but rather it is arranged by the manufacturer to be close to that of the CRT. For many years image data have been adjusted to appear attractive on

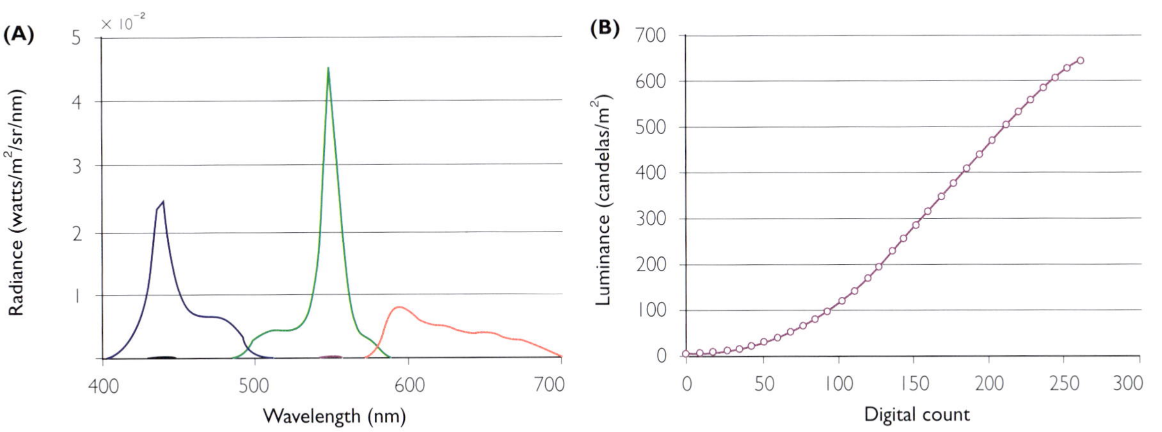

Figure 8.13 **(A) The spectral power distributions of the three primaries in an LC display. (B) The transduction function of the same display.**

CRT displays. Were the LCD transduction different from the CRT function, these images would not appear attractive, and customers would be dissatisfied.

The difference between the CRT and LCD properties raises the following question: How can one be sure that image data will appear as intended without knowing the display? An industry consortium, the International Color Consortium (ICC), has worked on proposals to solve this problem. The ICC recommends a solution in which display device characteristics are represented in a *device profile* file. Software manufacturers are urged to include routines that read and interpret the device profile. Hardware manufacturers and third-party vendors are urged to provide enough characterization data to permit accurate color rendering. The device profile is based on the CIE system (e.g., tristimulus coordinates or CIELAB coordinates) and several basic operators. Detail about these proposals, which continue to evolve, is available at <http://www.color.org>.

8.4.4.3 Tristimulus and chromaticity values

For most applications, it is not necessary to know the complete SPD of light emitted from a display. Rather, it is enough to know the effect of this light on the human cones. Usually, this is specified using CIE standard tristimulus coordinates. There are three major sets of color-matching functions (CMFs) used in display colorimetry (Wyszecki and Stiles, 1982). First, the CIE 1931 2° standard observer CMFs, which are appropriate for the calculation of tristimulus values when color fields spanning less than 4° are used. Second, the CIE 1964 10° degree supplementary standard observer CMFs, which are appropriate for color fields > 4° and reflect the shift toward increased short-wavelength sensitivity for large color fields. Finally, the Judd modification of the CIE 1931 2° CMFs correct for underestimates of the short-wavelength photopic sensitivity (i.e., < 460 nm) for the original 1931 CMFs. This last set of CMFs are important in basic color vision research and are the basis for a number of linear transformations to the cone absorption curves. They also serve as the basis for the CIE 1988 2° supplementary luminous efficiency function for photopic vision (CIE, 1990).

The tristimulus values of the three primary color phosphor emissions can be computed from the color rendering equation described in section 8.2.1. Suppose that the columns of the matrix $\mathbf{C}$ contain the color matching functions and the columns of the matrix $\mathbf{P}$ contain the spectral power distributions of the three primary lights at maximum intensity. The tristimulus coordinates of the three primaries are contained in the columns of the matrix product $\mathbf{C}^t\mathbf{P}$. To predict the tristimulus coordinates of a light emitted when the frame buffer values are $\mathbf{v}' = (r',g',b')$, first correct for the nonlinear transduction function, Fi( ). This produces three linear primary intensity values, $\mathbf{v} = (r,g,b) = (F_r(r), F_g(g), F_b(b))$. The tristimulus coordinates, $\mathbf{c}$, are $\mathbf{c} = \mathbf{C}^t\mathbf{P}\mathbf{v}$. To find the frame buffer values that will display a given set of tristimulus coordinates, $\mathbf{c}$, invert the calculation to find $\mathbf{v} = (\mathbf{C}^t\mathbf{P})^{-1}\,\mathbf{c}$ and then apply the inverse of the transduction value to obtain $\mathbf{v}'$. If the resulting values are negative or exceed the maximum intensity of one of the primaries, the desired color is called *out of gamut*.

The tristimulus calculations specify the part of the emitted light that is visible to the human observer. Two lights presented in the same context that have the same visible components will have the same color appearance. Even two lights with the same spectral power distribution may appear different when presented in different contexts (see Chapter 3).

It is common to express the tristimulus coordinates in a form that captures separately the luminance and color of the signal. To do this, the values (X,Y,Z), are converted to the form (Y,x,y) = (Y,X/(X + Y + Z), Y/(X + Y + Z)). The Y value is luminance and the values, (x,y), are *chromaticity coordinates*. These coordinates are invariant with the intensity of the signal. Doubling the intensity of a light doubles its Y (luminance) value, but leaves the (x,y) chromaticity coordinates unchanged.

The three pairs of chromaticity coordinates (one pair for each primary) define the range of colors that can be produced by the display. Figure 8.14 shows the chromaticity coordinates of each of the three primaries in a CRT display (panel A) and an LCD display (panel B). The triangle that connects these three points defines the device *color gamut*. The gamut represents the range of colors that can be displayed by the

(A)

(B)

(C)

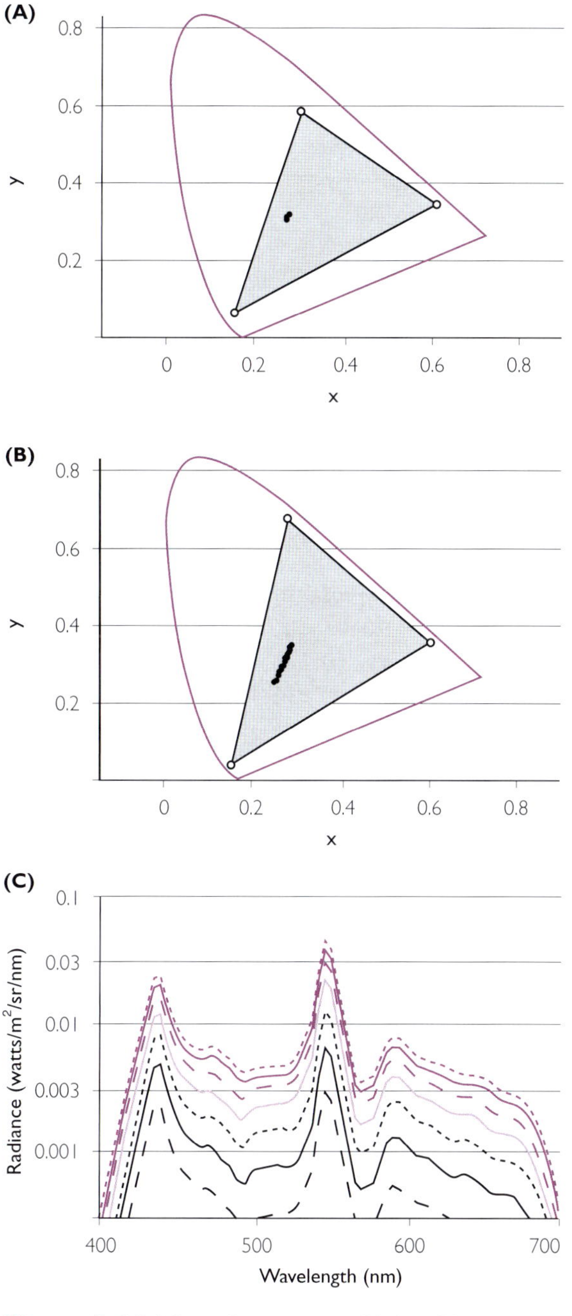

Figure 8.14 The color gamuts of (A) a CRT display and (B) an LC display plotted in the (x,y)-chromaticity diagram. The chromaticity coordinates of a series of grays are shown as the points in the middle of the graphs. (C) The spectral power distribution of the LCD gray series.

device. The smooth curve on the graph denotes the chromaticity coordinates of spectral lights. This curve is called the *spectrum locus* and all lights must have chromaticity coordinates within this area.

The color gamut of LCDs can be made larger than that of CRTs. This is because the choice of backlights and thin film color filters in LCDs offer display designers additional degrees of freedom, including primaries with narrower spectral distributions that fall closer to the spectrum locus than the broadband phosphors in CRTs. The difference in color gamuts between devices poses a problem for color reproduction. Suppose that an image is designed on an LCD, but we wish to display it on a CRT. It may be impossible to reproduce a light with the same tristimulus coordinates. This is called the *gamut-mapping* problem. How to compensate for mismatches in the gamut between display devices or between displays and printers is an active area of research.

Although direct-view LCDs are generally brighter and can have larger gamuts than CRTs, they do have one significant problem. A very desirable feature of a display is that scaling the digital counts of the frame buffer should preserve the chromaticity coordinates. Perhaps the most important values to preserve (for customer satisfaction) are the gray series, comprised of the digital values, say (10,10,10), (20,20,20) and so forth. Figure 8.14C shows the spectral power distribution of an LCD at a series of gray values. The chromaticity values of a gray series are shown in the center of the panels (A) and (B) for the CRT and LCD. The chromaticity shifts are much larger for the LCD than the CRT. This is caused by a change in the SPD passed by the liquid crystal layer and the polarizers. Panel (C) shows the SPD of the gray series at several mean levels. Were the SPDs invariant with level, the curves would be shifted copies of one another on this log radiance axis. The curves are not shifted copies, and notice that there are significant differences in the spacing in the long- and short-wavelength regions compared to the middle-wavelength regions. These differences occur because the LC polarization is not precisely the same for all wavelengths and also as a result of spectral variations in polarizer extinction. For the viewer, this results in a shift in display chromaticity of the primaries when they are presented at different intensity levels. It is possible to compensate for these changes using algorithms described by Spiegle and Brainard (1999).

8.5 PRINTING

8.5.1 OVERVIEW

Reflection prints are a convenient and flexible means of viewing and exchanging images. To view a reflection print, one needs no energy apart from the ambient light. The print itself is light and easy to transport. Printing can be applied to many different substrates, making it convenient to mark all kinds of objects. A look around any room will reveal printing on many objects, even on clothes. The printing industry is enormous, and managing the color appearance of printed copy is an important part of that industry.

Improvements in printing come from three basic sources: the ability to create papers and inks with improved ink absorption properties; the ability to control the placement of the inks on the page; and the ability to predict the perceptual consequences of the first two processes. Over the past two decades there have been advances in all three areas, though perhaps the most impressive advances have been in the ability to control the placement of ink on the page. In this chapter we will be concerned mainly with methods of creating colored prints under the control of digital computers, that is *digital printing*.

Our review of color printing is separated into two parts. First, we will introduce some of the concepts used by the color printing community. Because of their very separate historical developments, the color reproduction terminology used by the printing and display communities differs even when the concepts are closely related. We will introduce the concepts and terms used by the printing community but with an additional emphasis on showing how the emissive and reflective display methods are designed to obey the same color reproduction equations.

Second, we describe the ideas behind two printing methods, *continuous tone* and *halftone* printing. In continuous tone printing the printed page is covered with a very fine array of ink drops. The droplet density is controlled by the printing method. Hence, the control of continuous tone printing is conceptually similar to controlling the appearance of overlaid sheets of colored transparencies, a method called subtractive reproduction.

In halftone printing, the ink drops are larger and the printing process controls color by manipulating the dot position and size. The dots from different inks form several spatial mosaics, and color reproduction is more akin to an additive process: the reflected light is the sum of light scattered from the several mosaics.

8.5.2 INKS AND SUBTRACTIVE COLOR CALCULATIONS

Conventional color printing relies on three different types of colored ink: cyan, magenta, and yellow (CMY). A fourth ink, black, is also used in a special and important role that will be described later. In continuous tone printing, the amount and spectral composition of the light reflected from the page is controlled by superimposing these colored inks and controlling their density on the page.

The way in which the reflected light is controlled is illustrated using very simple, theoretical inks whose reflectance spectra are shown in Figure 8.15. These are called *block inks* because they divide the wavelength spectrum into three bands corresponding, roughly, to a red, green, and blue. Each of the inks is transparent to light

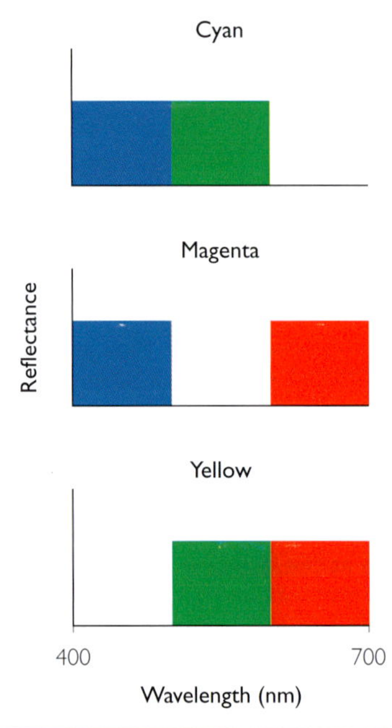

Figure 8.15 The reflectance functions of three (theoretical) block inks.

in two block regions, while absorbing light in a third block region. The inks take their names from the two regions in which they do not absorb. The cyan ink does not absorb in the blue and green bands, the magenta does not absorb in the red and blue, and the yellow does not absorb in the red and green.

The amount of light absorbed by ink is controlled by the amount of ink on the page. If a very thin layer of, say, cyan ink is placed down on white paper a small amount of the long wavelengths will be absorbed; the page will appear mainly white. If a great deal of cyan ink is placed on the page, a great deal of the long-wavelength region will be absorbed and the ink will take on its characteristic cyan appearance. Seen from this perspective, controlling the amount of the ink on the page is analogous to controlling the intensity of a display primary.

8.5.2.1 Density

To control any display technology, it is necessary to understand the relationship between the control variables and their action on the light arriving at the observer's eye. To understand the reflected light in the continuous tone process, we must predict the effect of altering the amount of ink on the page and the consequence of superimposing inks.

Suppose we place a very thin layer of ink, of thickness δ, on a piece of paper. The probability that a monochromatic ray of light, at wavelength λ, will be absorbed by the ink is proportional to the thickness of the layer, $a(\lambda)\delta$. Next, consider what will happen when the thickness of the ink is increased. Figure 8.16 shows some possible light paths as ambient light passes through the ink and is scattered towards an observer. Imagine that the average optical path length, including both passage towards the white page and passage back towards the eye, is D. Divide this path into N thin layers, each of thickness $\delta = D/N$. The absorption process follows the proportionality law within each thin layer. Consequently the chance that a ray will be reflected after traversing the entire optical path, D, is equal to the chance that it is not absorbed in any of the thin N layers, namely $(1 - \delta a(\lambda))^N$. As the thickness is subdivided into more layers, N, the probability of absorption is expressed as *Beer's law*:

$$\lim_{n\to\infty}\left(1 - a(\lambda)\frac{D}{N}\right)^N = e^{-Da(\lambda)} \qquad (8.2)$$

The proportion of reflected light depends on the optical path length, D, which is controlled by the amount of ink placed on the page. As D increases, the fraction of light reflected becomes zero (unless $a(\lambda) = 0$). The constant of proportionality, $a(\lambda)$, is the *absorption function* of the ink.

Conventionally, the ink is described using by an *optical density* function $od(\lambda) = -\log_{10}(a(\lambda))$. From equation 8.2 we find that optical density is proportional to the thickness,

$$od(\lambda) = 2.3Da(\lambda) \qquad (8.3)$$

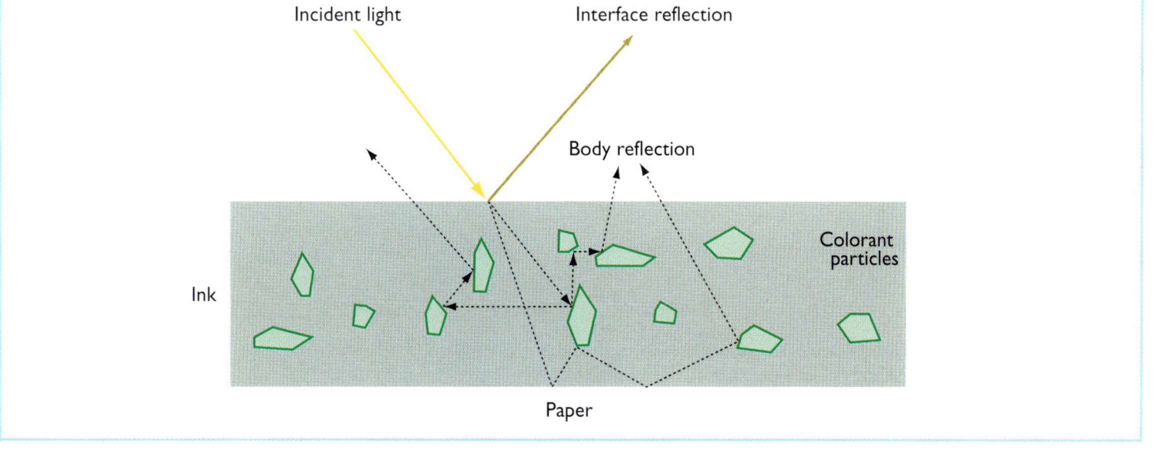

Figure 8.16 The scattered reflection from a layer of ink includes rays with different path lengths. Consequently, accurate prediction of the reflected light is a theoretically challenging problem.

Moreover, the optical density of two inks that are superimposed to form a single layer should add. Suppose the absorption functions of the inks are $a_i(\lambda)$. Then probability of absorption after traversing through the two layers is the product of the individual absorption functions, $\prod_{i=1,2}(1-a_i(\lambda))$. Since the absorption probabilities multiply, the optical densities add:

$$od(\lambda) = \log_{10}\left[\prod_{i=1,2}(1-a_i(\lambda))\right] = od_1(\lambda) + od_2(\lambda) \tag{8.4}$$

Equation 8.4 shows that when two inks are overlaid there is a linear relationship between density and the control variable (density of colorant in the ink) and the optical density. This is the key reason why it is convenient to use optical density, rather than reflectance, in describing inks. In meeting the requirements of the color reproduction equations, however, the observer sees the reflected light and the observer's cone absorptions must be predicted. The nonlinear relationship between the control variable (ink density) and the light absorption by the cones is significantly more complex than the parallel nonlinear relationship between frame buffer intensity and cone absorptions that must be addressed in display technology. In displays, the spectral shape of the phosphors does not change a great deal with level. In the case of ink reflections, however, the spectral reflectance function changes considerably with density level. Thus predicting and controlling the light signal in printing is a much more difficult computational challenge.

8.5.3 CONTINUOUS TONE PRINTING

The physical principles described above are only a general overview of the reflection process; they do not capture many of the details necessary to make a precise prediction of the properties of color prints. In practice, a number of factors arise that make the predictions based on these very simple calculations inaccurate. Figure 8.16 shows one aspect of the reflection process that we have omitted: the light that is scattered to the observer's eye from a single point on the page may have traversed one of many different optical paths. The optical path will depend on the viewing geometry and on microscopic details of the paper and surrounding inks. Hence, computing the true optical path is very difficult and the calculations we have reviewed only serve as a first order approximation to the true reflection.

Finally, there are a great many limitations on the inks that can be used. Many perfectly good inks are destroyed by exposure to the human environment and conversely perfectly good humans are destroyed by exposure to the ink's environment. Consequently, the supply of possible inks is limited and none is very close to the theoretical block inks. In addition, for all but the theoretical block inks, the shape of the reflectance function varies with density. Figure 8.17A shows the reflectance functions of four inks in a modern printer. The real inks overlap in their spectral reflection and absorption regions, unlike the perfect block inks. Panel (B) shows how the reflectance function of the magenta primary varies as a function of ink density. Notice that unlike the ideal block inks, the reflectance in both the short and middle wavelengths change as the magenta density varies.

The overlap in the absorption functions of the inks and the change in reflectance as a function of density make characterization calculations very difficult. We describe some of the basic methods later in this section. In addition, there are a great many ingenious efforts to understand and control such effects in order to make attractive prints. An excellent overview of these technologies, and many of the technologies described in this chapter, can be found in R.W. Hunt's book *The Reproduction of Colour* (Hunt, 1987).

Finally, we conclude with a discussion of the very important role of the black ink in printing. To form a black or gray color using the CMY inks requires mixing all three together. These inks are generally very expensive, and even worse, combining the three inks results in a very wet piece of paper. To reduce cost and to reduce bleeding within the paper, it is very effective to replace an equal mixture of the three colored inks with a single black ink in the appropriate density. The specific implementation of this will depend on the paper, colored inks, and black ink. The processes for substituting black ink for the colored inks are called *gray component removal* (GCR) or *undercolor removal* (UCR). Often, this process also improves the appearance of the print because

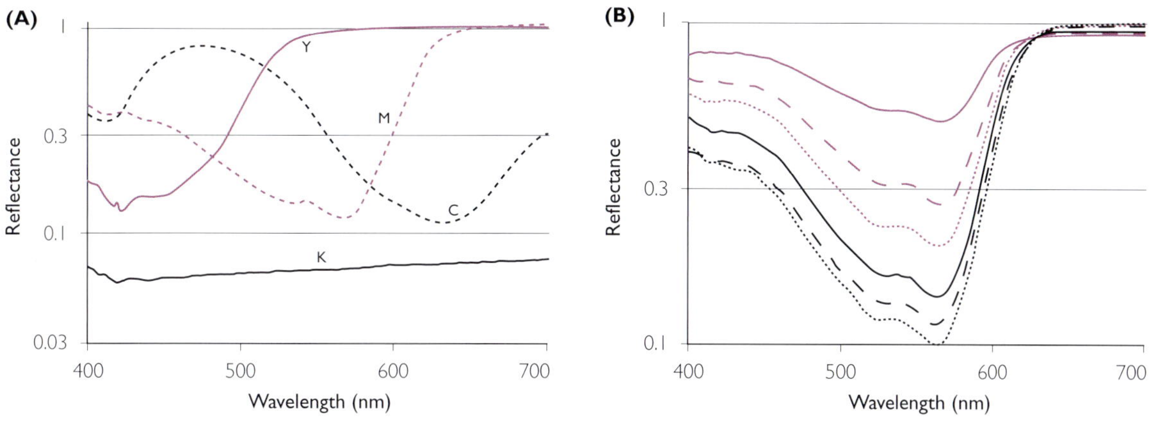

Figure 8.17 **(A) Reflectance functions of the four primaries of an ink jet printer measured at high density. (B) The reflectance function of the magenta ink at various densities.**

the black ink has higher contrast than the combination of cyan, magenta, and yellow.

8.5.4 HALFTONING

8.5.4.1 Traditional halftoning

Halftoning is a printing method that simulates continuous tone dots of varying size or position. In traditional halftoning, illustrated in Figure 8.18, intensity is adjusted by varying the size of the printed dot. The image shows light from an original being imaged onto a fine mesh screen, often called the halftone *screen*. The screen converts the original image into a collection of point sources whose intensities depend on the intensity of the original. These point sources form images on a high-contrast negative film. The fine screen mesh causes a set of pointspread images to be formed on the film.

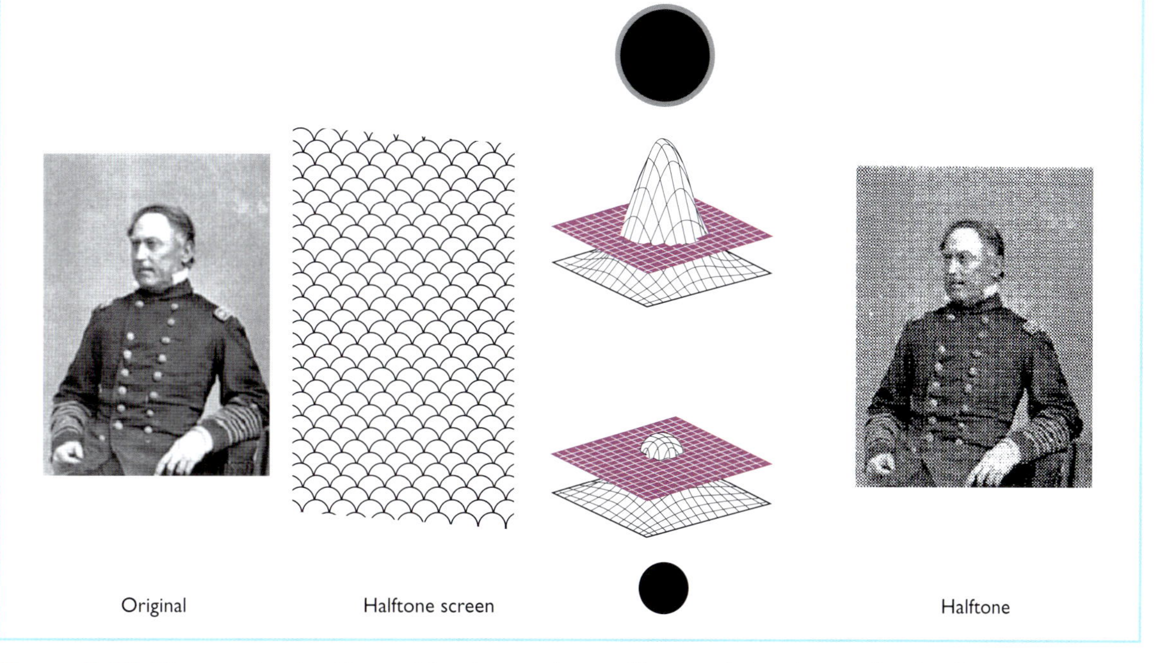

Figure 8.18 **The steps involved in traditional screening are illustrated. See the text for details.**

The pointspread images differ as shown in the intermediate levels of the figure. When the dot is low intensity, only a small amount of the dot area exceeds the threshold of the high-contrast film. When the dot is high intensity a large fraction of the dot area exceeds the threshold. Depending on the intensity of the original, a larger or smaller region of the high-contrast film is exposed. Hence, the halftone screen process converts intensity into dot area.

The negative high-contrast film is printed as a positive image. The dot sizes substitute for the original light levels, so that dark regions of the image have many large black dots and light regions have few. In a high-quality print, the dots themselves are below visible resolution. Even when they are visible, the regular pattern of dots does not interfere strongly with the content of most images.

To create a color halftone, the process is repeated for the CMY and black components. In traditional halftoning, regular screens are used and this can cause an additional problem. When overlaying images from different halftone screens, the separate images produce unwanted interference known as moiré patterns. To reduce such artifacts, the screens are rotated to different angles. Conventionally, the screen for black is oriented at 45° (straight up is 0°). The screen angles for the other inks are cyan (105), magenta (70), and yellow (90).

8.5.5 DIGITAL HALFTONING

Digital halftoning is a method for converting digital image files that represent the image intensity into an array of binary level values that represent dots in the printing process. The digital halftoning algorithms compute the positions where dots will be printed, and these are used to direct a digitally controlled printer. Both laser and ink jet technologies have evolved to a point where it is possible to control the dot placement with extraordinary accuracy and speed.

Three features of digital halftoning, that extend traditional halftoning, are of particular note. First, with digital techniques one does not need to place the dots in a perfectly regular array. Instead, it is possible to randomize the dot positions into disordered arrays. Using this method, it becomes harder for the eye to discern the screen pattern in monochrome printing and the problem of colored moiré is also reduced. Methods using randomized screen positions are sometimes called *stochastic screening, frequency modulated (FM) halftoning,* or *blue noise* methods (Ulichney, 1988; Mitsa *et al.*, 1991; Mitsa and Parker, 1992; Allebach and Lin, 1996). While it is technically possible to achieve these results with traditional screening methods, it is very easy to achieve these results with digital halftoning.

Second, in addition to computational methods for randomizing the dot placement, it is now commonplace to control the dot placement at a very fine level using piezo-electric positioning devices on the print head. A printer that emits 600 dots per inch (dpi) on a single line across the page may be able to place these dots at any of 1440 different positions.

Third, with digital control and computation it is possible to extend halftoning to a slightly more general process in which there is not just a single density level of, say, magenta ink printed on the page but one of two density levels. The multiple levels are achieved by including not just one source of magenta ink in the printer but also two sources, with different density. This process, often called *multi-level halftoning,* is in widespread use in digital printers such as the ink jet products.

There are two computational methods for implementing digital halftoning. One method, called dithering, is illustrated in Figure 8.19. This method approximates traditional screening and can be calculated at very high speeds. In this approach, the user selects a small matrix to serve as a *dither pattern,* also called a *mask,* for the calculation. Suppose the image and the mask are both represented at the resolution of the printer. Further suppose the mask is N × N. Digital halftoning begins by comparing the mask values with the intensity levels in an N × N region of the image. The image intensities are compared with the entries in the mask. Each of these is shown in the small surface plots in the figure. Suppose d_{ij} is a dither matrix entry and p_{ij} is an image intensity, then if $d_{ij} > p_{ij}$ set the printed point white, and otherwise set the point black. This process is repeated for each N × N block in the original picture until the entire image is converted from multiple intensity levels to a binary output suitable for printing as a halftone.

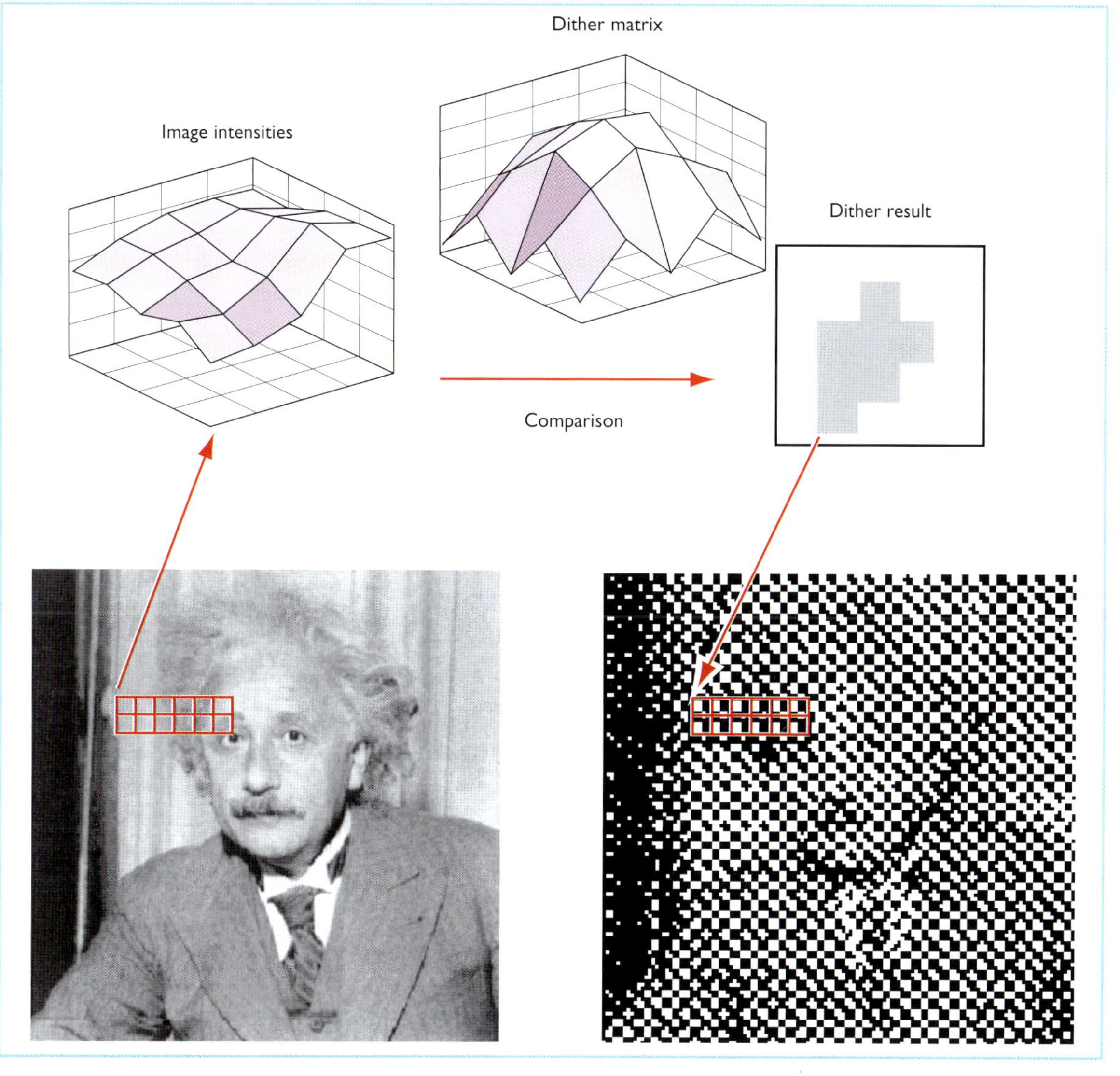

Figure 8.19 The steps involved in digital halftoning are illustrated. See the text for details.

The entries of the dither pattern partition the intensity levels in the original image. If the mask size is set to, say, N × N then the mask can partition the original image into $N^2 + 1$ intensity levels. Increasing the size of the dither pattern simulates more intensity levels, but reduces the effective spatial resolution of the printed picture. Several types of dither matrices are commonly used, and these are described below.

Digital halftoning algorithms are straightforward, but the terminology associated with digital halftoning and traditional screening has become intertwined and often very unclear. Printer dot density is usually specified in *dots per inch* (dpi). This describes the number of ink dots that can be placed on the page. Printer *addressability* refers to the number of positions where these dots can be placed. A printer may be able to place 300 dots per inch, but the center of these dots may fall at any of 1400 locations. Finally, the size of the dither pattern also influences the spatial resolution of the final print. A 3 × 3 mask reduces the spatial resolution of the print, and this is summarized by a quantity called the screen *lines*. A 300 dpi printer that uses a 3 × 3 mask is said to print at 100 screen lines per inch. A 300 dpi printer with a 6 × 6 mask is said to have 50 lines per inch.

8.5.5.1 Cluster dot dither

The *cluster dot* or *ordered dither* mask is designed to be similar to traditional screening. An example of a 5×5 dither pattern for a cluster dot is:

$$\begin{pmatrix} 1 & 9 & 16 & 8 & 7 \\ 10 & 17 & 21 & 20 & 15 \\ 2 & 22 & 25 & 24 & 6 \\ 11 & 18 & 23 & 19 & 14 \\ 3 & 12 & 4 & 13 & 5 \end{pmatrix} \left(\frac{255}{26}\right)$$

Consider the results of comparing this mask with uniform intensity patterns ranging from 0 to 255. The mask has twenty-five entries and can partition the input regions into 26 different levels. When the image intensity is very low ($<255/26$), all of the points are set black. As the image intensity increases the size of the dot shrinks, so that at a value just less than $25*(255/26)$ only a single dot is left in the middle.

A variant of this mask is shown in Figure 8.20A. While basically a cluster dot, the thresholds in the mask are arranged so that the growth in dot size occurs on a diagonal pattern. This has the effect of arranging the dots to fall on the 45° line, as in traditional screening. The result of applying this mask to an image is illustrated in Figure 8.20B.

8.5.5.2 Bayer dither and void and cluster dither

The Bayer (Bayer, 1973) dither pattern represented an early and important innovation that showed how digital halftoning might improve on traditional screening. The Bayer dither pattern was chosen so that the spatial structure of the printed dots would be less visible than the ordered dither dots. Figure 8.21A shows the result of applying an 8×8 Bayer dither mask to an image. The Bayer output compares favorably with the results of applying a traditional screening pattern, this time using an 8×8 digital dither pattern structured to give dots along the 45° diagonal (see Figure 8.20B).

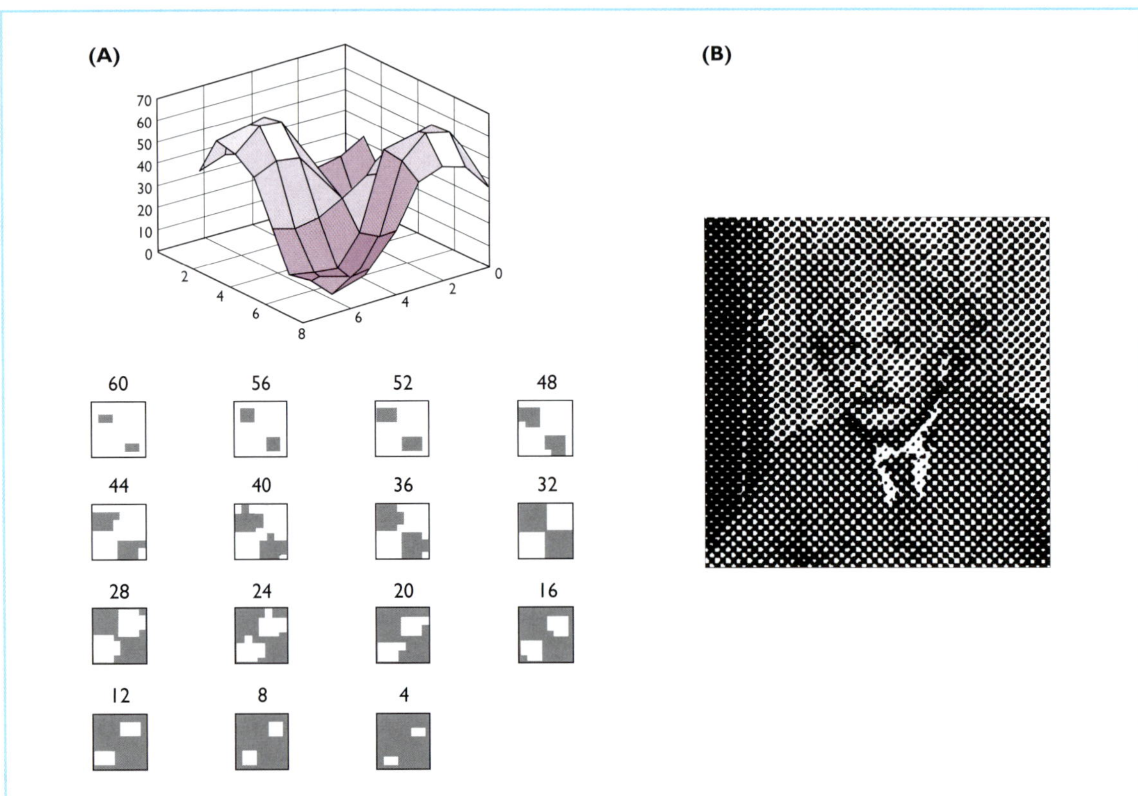

Figure 8.20 **Cluster dot halftoning is illustrated. The dot masks are shown in (A). The result of applying these masks to an image is shown in (B).**

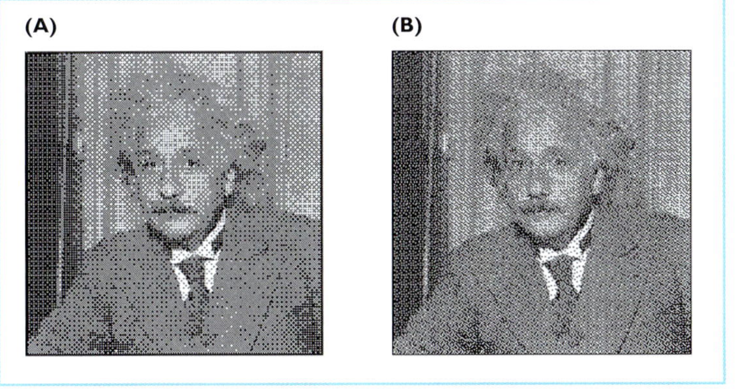

Figure 8.21 **Bayer dither (A) and void and cluster dither (B) applied to an image.**

For very low resolution printing, the Bayer dither mask results in images that are more appealing than ordered dither. Even so, the Bayer dither pattern contains a regular structure that is visible in the printed halftone. Ulichney (1993) proposed a method of creating dither patterns with locally random structure that are even less visible because they have most of their spatial structure in the high spatial frequencies. Because the spatial frequency power is in the high frequencies, these are called *blue-noise* masks. One computational method for implementing blue-noise masks is called the *void and cluster* method. In this method, a pattern is selected so that there are no very large voids or very large clusters.

Comparisons of the dither patterns from ordered dither, Bayer, void and cluster, and error diffusion are shown applied to simple intensity ramps (Figure 8.22). At low printer resolutions the Bayer and the void and cluster method are preferred to ordered dither. They are no more computationally expensive. Notice the similarity between the void and cluster pattern and the error diffusion pattern. The error diffusion process is explained in the next section. The pattern of dots created by this method is similar to the pattern created by void and cluster.

There is an analogy between the different halftoning methods and signal transmission methods in a communication channel. The cluster dot method modulates the light intensity by controlling the size of a dot, much like controlling the amplitude of a signal. The void and cluster method modulates the light intensity by varying the spatial structure of a complex pattern, much like controlling the frequency of a signal. Hence, sometimes cluster dot is described as an amplitude modulation (AM) screening technique while void and cluster is described as a frequency modulation (FM) screening technique.

8.5.5.3 Error diffusion

At low print resolutions, the best halftoning results are obtained using an adaptive algorithm in which the halftoning depends upon the data in the image itself. Floyd and Steinberg (1976) introduced the basic principals of adaptive halftoning methods in a brief and fundamental paper. Their algorithm is called *error diffusion*. The idea is to initiate the halftoning process by selecting a binary output level closest to the original intensity. This binary level will differ substantially from the original. The difference between the halftone output and the true image

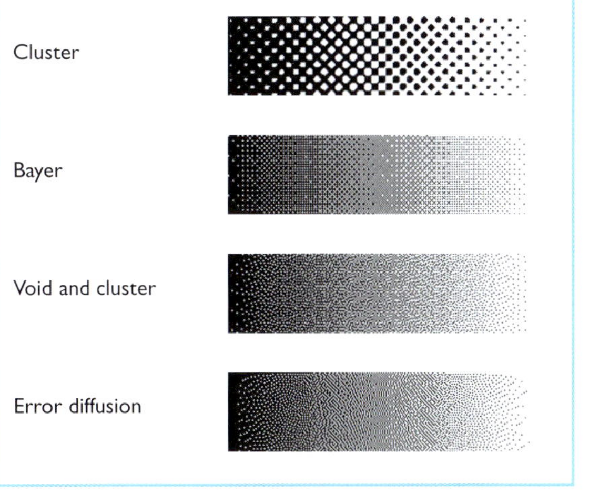

Figure 8.22 **Cluster dot, Bayer, void and cluster, and error diffusion applied to an intensity ramp.**

(i.e., the error) is added to neighboring pixels that have not yet been processed. Then, the binary output decision is made on the next pixel whose value now includes both the original image intensity and the errors that have been added from previously processed pixels. Figure 8.23 shows a flow chart of the algorithm (panel A) and a typical result (panel B).

The coefficients that distribute the error among neighboring pixels can be chosen depending on the source material and output device. Jarvis, Judice, and Ninke (1976) found the apportionment of error using the matrix

$$\begin{pmatrix} 0 & 0 & * & 7 & 5 \\ 3 & 5 & 7 & 5 & 3 \\ 1 & 3 & 5 & 3 & 1 \end{pmatrix} \left(\frac{1}{48}\right)$$

to be satisfactory, where * denotes the current image point being processed. Notice that the error is propagated forward to unprocessed pixels. Also, the algorithm works properly when applied to the linear intensity of the image. The algorithm should not be applied to images represented in a nonlinear space, such as the frame buffer values of a monitor. Instead, the image should be converted to a format that is linear with intensity prior to application of the algorithm.

For images printed at low spatial resolution, error-diffusion is considered the best method. Ulichney (1987) analyzed the spatial error of the method and showed that the error was mainly in the high spatial frequency regime. The drawback of error diffusion is that it is very time-consuming compared to the simple threshold operations used in dither patterns. For images at moderate to high spatial resolution (600 dpi), blue-noise masks are visually as attractive as error diffusion and much faster to compute. Depending on the nature of the paper, cluster dot can be preferred at high resolutions. The cluster dot algorithm separates the centroids of the ink so that there is less unwanted bleeding of the ink from cell to cell. In certain devices and at certain print resolutions, reducing the spread of the ink is more important than reducing the visibility of the mask.

8.5.5.4 Color digital halftoning

The principles of digital halftoning can be directly extended to making colored halftone prints. The most common extension to color for

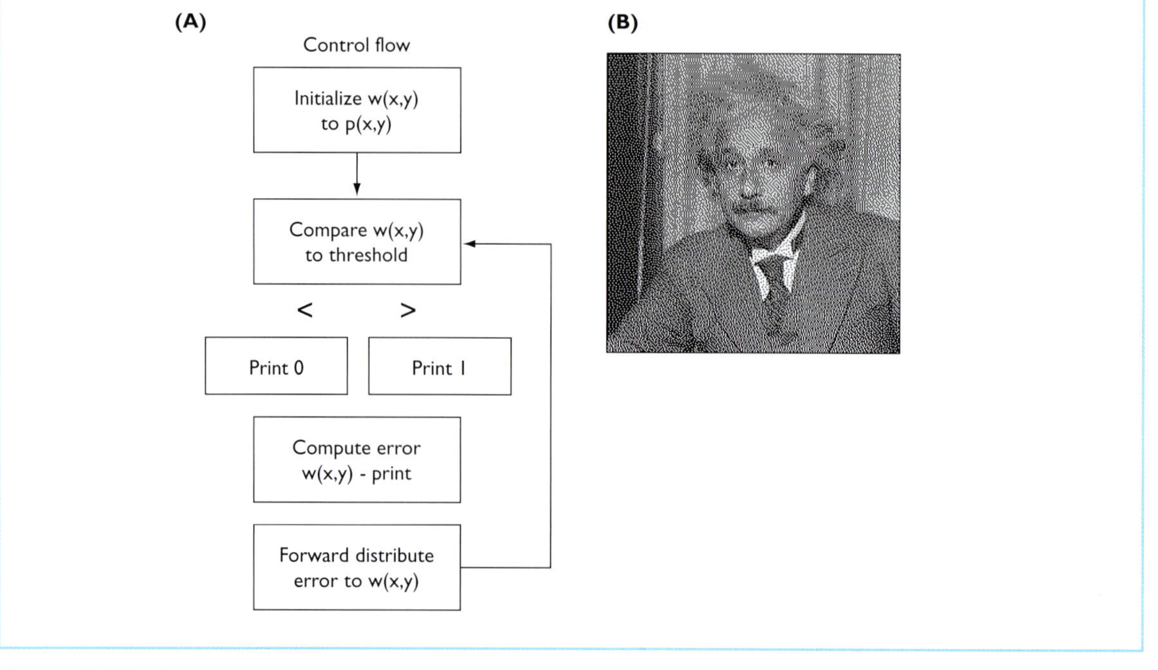

Figure 8.23 **The steps involved in error diffusion algorithm (A) and the resulting image (B). See text for details.**

dither patterns is to convert the original image into a CMY representation, and then to apply the digital halftoning algorithm separately to each of the color planes. This separable architecture is computationally efficient. The resulting output can be followed by a step of gray-component removal.

There are several technical issues that must be addressed when extending halftoning to color. First, the overlap between the dots comprising the colored planes can lead to undesirable spatial artifacts (moiré patterns). To minimize this spatial disturbance, the different color separations are printed with their dots arrays at different angles. By using these angles the effect of moiré between the dots in the separations is minimized. Typically, the dots comprising the black separation (K) are printed at 45°, and the CMY dots at 105°, 75°, and 90° respectively (vertical = 0). Second, depending on the type of printing process, the size of the dots may cause the mixture of halftones to overlap greatly or little. When the printing process produces sets of interleaved mosaics of dots, the characterization is similar to an additive system. When the printing process includes a great deal of overlap between the dots, the process is similar to a subtractive system characterized by the Neugebauer process described below. Hence, the color characterization needed to manage the different techniques will depend on the spatial structure of the printing process.

There are also issues that must be considered when extending to adaptive processing algorithms, such as error diffusion. In an adaptive process, the algorithm must decide which one of the usable dots should be printed next. Normally, the usable dots are one of the primaries alone (C,M,Y,K) or a mixture of the non-black primaries (CM,CY,MY,CMY). These algorithms can use the color error up to the current print position to decide which dot should be printed. The error can be a three-dimensional quantity, calculated jointly from all of the separation errors, which is far more complex than making a decision separately for each color separation.

8.5.6 PRINT CHARACTERIZATION

8.5.6.1 Transduction: the tone reproduction curve

The relationship between the device parameter that controls the ink density and the relative amount of reflected light is called the *tone reproduction curve* (TRC). This curve is the printer transduction function, analogous to the display transduction function. Figure 8.24A shows a tone reproduction curve measured for a monochrome laser printer. This printer achieves different gray levels by halftoning. Notice that the curve is similar to the curve measured on a CRT or LCD device. Figure 8.24Bb shows the tone reproduction curve for the magenta primary of an ink jet printer. This curve has the same general form as the black ink, but it never reaches as low a luminance level.

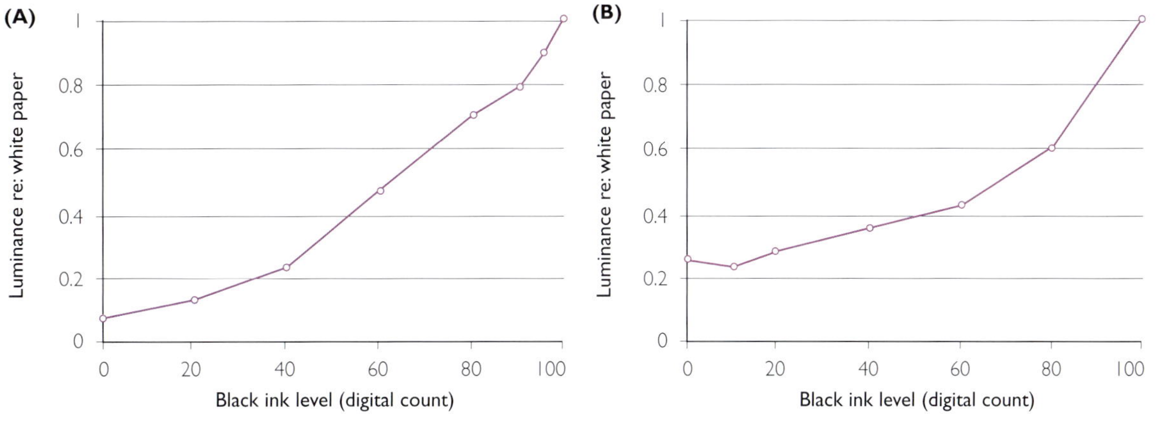

Figure 8.24 The printer tone reproduction curve. Curves are shown for (A) monochrome laser printer and (B) the magenta primary of an ink jet printer.

The TRC is a fundamental measurement of printer performance. For two reasons, however, the TRC cannot be combined easily with the ink primary reflectance functions to predict reflected light or solve the color-reproduction equation. First, the reflectance functions of the CMYK primaries do not combine additively. Overprinting inks and blending of the ink spots can cause light to follow optical paths whose spectral transmission is very complicated to predict. Second, even for pure ink, Beer's law (equation 8.4) shows that the ink reflectance function varies with density. Consequently, the tristimulus values of the reflected light will vary with density, making it impossible to use the simple principles that are applied to monitor characterization. Specifically, ink mixtures do not follow the rules of primary independence that are essential to the simple characterization of display devices.

An influential theory for predicting ink reflectance functions was provided by the brilliant color engineer Neugebauer (1937). The idea introduced in the *Neugebauer equations* is based on the following physical intuition. Imagine partitioning the printed page into extremely small areas over which each region contains only an infinitesimal (binary) amount of ink. At this spatial scale, we will find only eight possible combinations of ink (C,M,Y,CM, CY,MY,K); other combinations are eliminated because K combined with anything is equivalent to K. Any small region will contain many of these infinitesimal dots, and the reflectance function of the small region will be a weighted sum of these eight basic terms. The weights will depend on the area allocated to the infinitesimal dots, and any small region is predicted to have a reflectance function that is the weighted sum of eight possible basis terms. Predicting these basis terms from the ink primaries, and then predicting the ink reflectance functions is the main application of the theory. Practical difficulties in compensating for scatter into the paper and complicated light paths represent a continuing challenge to the theory, which continues to be an active area of investigation. For a modern update the reader may wish to consult the special symposium on this topic (Neugebauer, 1989).

Because of the difficulties in predicting the ink reflectance functions from first principles, printer characterization methods mainly rely on the use of extensive lookup tables. These tables are based on measurements of the tristimulus values measured from a variety of print samples on a variety of paper types. Tetrahedral lookup tables are often used for this purpose.

8.6 KEY WORDS

Color, displays, image capture, digital cameras, printing, scanning, LCD.

8.7 CONCLUSIONS

Color imaging technologies are central to many features of modern-day life. The breadth and vitality of the industry that creates these technologies is extraordinary. In reviewing a small part of these technologies, we have tried to explain how knowledge of the human visual system plays an important role in many design decisions. The widespread use of tristimulus coordinates for characterization represents one major contribution of vision science to imaging technology. Understanding when spatial and wavelength measurements can be safely traded for one another is a second contribution.

Equally, the contributions of color technology have propelled forward experiments in vision science. Improvements in color characterization and color displays have made new experimental methods and precise control possible. The interaction between these fields, as represented by the inclusion of this chapter in this volume, enriches both.

ACKNOWLEDGMENTS

We thank P. Catrysse, A. El Gamal, J. Farrell, and G. Starkweather. This work was supported in part by the Programmable Digital Camera project at Stanford University.

REFERENCES

Adams, J., Parulski, K., and Spaulding, K. (1998) Color processing in digital cameras. *IEEE Micro*, 18 (6), 20–30.

Allebach, J., and Lin, Q. (1996) FM screen design using DBS algorithm. Paper presented at the 1996 IEEE International Conference on Image Processing, ICIP'96. Part 1 (of 3), Lausanne, Switzerland.

Anderson, S., Mullen, K., and Hess, R. (1991) Human peripheral spatial resolution for achromatic and chromatic stimuli: limits imposed by optical and retinal factors. *Journal of Physiology*, 442, 47–64.

ASTM (1991) Standard recommended practice for goniophotometry of objects and materials. *ASTM Standards on Color and Appearance Measurement*, 3rd edn. Philadelphia: ASTM.

Bayer, B.E. (1973) An optimum method for two-level rendition of continuous-tone pictures. Paper presented at the IEEE Conference on Communications.

Berns, R.S., Gorzynski, M.E., and Motta, R.J. (1993) CRT colorimetry, Part I: Theory and practice. *Color Research and Application*, 18, 299–314.

Berns, R.S., Motta, R.J., and Gorzynski, M.E. (1993) CRT colorimetry, Part II: Metrology. *Color Research and Application*, 18, 315–25.

Brainard, D.H. (1989) Calibration of a computer controlled color monitor. *Color Research and Application*, 14, 23–34.

Brainard, D.H. and Sherman, D. (1995) Reconstructing images from trichromatic samples: from basic research to practical applications. *Proceedings of the Third IS&T/SID Color Imaging Conference: Color Science, Systems and Applications*, 4–10.

CIE (1990) *CIE 1988 2 deg Spectral Luminous Efficiency Function for Photopic Vision* (CIE 86). Commission Internationale de L'Eclairage (CIE).

CIE (1996) *The Relationship Between Digital and Colorimetric Data for Computer-Controlled CRT Display* (technical report 122–1996). Commission Internationale de L'Eclairage (CIE).

Collett, E. (1993) *Polarized Light: Fundamentals and Applications*. New York: Marcel Dekker, Inc.

Collings, P.J. (1990) *Liquid Crystals: Nature's Delicate Phase of Matter*. Princeton, NJ: Princeton University Press.

Conner, A.R. (1992) The evolution of the stacked color LCD. *Society for Information Display Applications Notes*, pp. 109–12.

Cornsweet, T.N. (1970) *Visual Perception*. New York: Academic Press.

Cupitt, J., Martinez, K., and Saunders, D. (1996) A methodology for art reproduction in colour: The MARC project. *Computers and the History of Art*, 6(2), 1–19.

DeValois, R.L. and DeValois, K.K. (1988) *Spatial vision*. New York: Oxford University Press.

dpreview.com. (2000) *Measuring Dynamic Range*. Available: http://www.dpreview.com/news/0011/00111608dynamicrange.aspThursday, 16 November.

Fairchild, M. (1997) *Color Appearance Models*. Reading, MA: Addison–Wesley Longman.

Farrell, J., Saunders, D., Cuppitt, J., and Wandell, B. (1999) Estimating spectral reflectance of art work. Paper presented at the Chiba Conference on Multispectral Imaging, Chiba, Japan.

Floyd, R.W. and Steinberg, L. (1976) An adaptive algorithm for spatial greyscale. *Proceedings of the Society for Information Display*, 17, 75–7.

Fritsch, M.W. and Mlynski, D.A. (1991) Faster contrast measurement of LCDs with improved conoscopic methods. *Proceedings of the Society for Information Display*, 32, 207–11.

Gill, G. (1999) *ICC profile I/O library (icclib), README file*. Available: http://web.access.net.au/argyll/icc_readme.html99/11/29.

Glenn, W.E., Glenn, K.G., and Bastian, C.J. (1985) Imaging system design based on psychophysical data. *Proceedings of the Society for Information Display*, 26, 71–8.

Hardeberg, J.Y. and Schmitt, F. (1997) Color printer characterization using a computational geometry approach. *Proceedings of the Fifth IS&T/SID Color Imaging Conference: Color Science, Systems and Applications*, 96–9.

Horn, B.K.P. (1984) Exact reproduction of colored images. *Computer Vision, Graphics and Image Processing*, 26, 135–67.

Hunt, R.W.G. (1987) *The Reproduction of Colour*, 4th edn. Tolworth: Fountain Press.

Janesick, J. (1997) CCD Transfer method – standard for absolute performance of CCDs and digital CCD camera systems. Paper presented at the Solid State Sensor Arrays: Development and Applications, San Jose.

Jarvis, J.F., Judice, C.N., and Ninke, W.H. (1976) A survey of techniques for the display of continuous tone pictures on bilevel displays. *Computer Graphics and Image Processing*, 5 (1), 13–40.

Lee, H.C. (1985) *Method for Determining the Color of a Scene Illuminant from a Color Image*. US: Kodak.

Lehrer, N.H. (1985) The challenge of the cathode-ray tube. In J.L.E. Tannas (ed.), *Flat-Panel Displays and CRTs*. New York: Van Nostrand Reinhold, pp. 138–76.

Leroux, T. and Rossignol, C. (1995) Fast analysis of contrast and color coordinates vs. viewing angle. *Society for Information Display Digest of Technical Papers*, 739–42.

Luo, M.R. and Hunt, R.W.G. (1998) The structure of the CIE 1997 color appearance model. *Color Research and Application*, 23, 138–46.

Lyons, N.P. and Farrell, J.E. (1989) Linear systems analysis of CRT displays, *Society for Information Display Digest of Technical Papers*, 220–3.

Martinez, K., Cupitt, J., and Perry, S. *High resolution colorimetric image browsing on the Web*. WWW.Elsevier. 30(1–7), 4 1998. http://www.ecs. soton.ac.uk.km/papers/www7/149.html.

Mitsa, T. and Parker, K.J. (1992) Digital halftoning technique using a blue-noise mask. *Journal of the Optical Society of America A*, 9 (11), 1920–9.

Mitsa, T., Ulichney, R., Parker, K.J., and Andre, J. (1991) The construction and evaluation of halftone patterns with manipulated power spectra. *Raster Imaging and Digital Typography II*. Cambridge: Cambridge University Press.

Mullen, K. (1985) The constrast sensitivity of human colour vision to red–green and blue–yellow chromatic gratings. *Journal of Physiology*, 359, 381–400.

Neugebauer, H.E.J. (1990) Neugebauer Memorial Seminar on Color Reproduction. *SPIE Proceedings Vol. 1184 14–15 Dec. 1989*. Tokyo, Japan. ISBN: 0-8194-0220-6.

Neugebauer, H.E.J. (1937) Die Theoretischen Grundlagen des Mehrfarbendruckes. In *Z. Wiss. Photogr.*, Volume 36, pages 73–89.

Penz, P.A. (1985) Nonemissive displays. In J.L.E. Tannas (ed.), *Flat-Panel Displays and CRTs*. New York: Van Nostrand Reinhold, pp. 415–57.

Plummer, W.T. (1983) Color filter. US Patent No. 4,416,514.

Poirson, A.B. and Wandell, B.A. (1993) The appearance of colored patterns: pattern-color separability. *Journal of the Optical Society of America A*, 10 (12): 2458–71.

Poynton, C. (1996) *A Technical Introduction to Digital Video*. New York: John Wiley and Sons.

Rodieck, R.W. (1998) *The First Steps in Seeing*. Sunderland, MA: Sinauer Press.

Sakamoto, T. and Itooka, A. (1981) Linear interpolator for color correction. US Patent No. 4,275,413.

Saleh, B.E.A. (1996) The Fourier scope: an optical instrument for measuring LCD viewing-angle characteristics. *Journal of the Society for Information Display*, 4 (1), 33–9.

Schade, O. (1958) On the quality of color-television images and the perception of colour detail. *Journal of the Society of Motion Pictures and Television Engineers*, 67, 801–19.

Scheffer, T. and Nehring, J. (1990) Twisted nematic and supertwisted nematic mode LCDs. In *Liquid Crystals: Applications and Uses, Volume I*. River Edge, NJ: World Scientific Publishing.

Scheffer, T. and Nehring, J. (1992) Twisted nematic (TN) and super-twisted nematic LCDs. *Society for Information Display Seminar Lecture Notes*, 1, M1/1?1/52.

Sekiguchi, N., Williams, D.R., and Brainard, D.H. (1993a) Aberration-free measurements of the visibility of isoluminant gratings. *Journal of the Optical Society of America A*, 10 (10), 2105–17.

Sekiguchi, N., Williams, D.R., and Brainard, D.H. (1993b) Efficiency in detection of isoluminant and isochromatic interference fringes. *Journal of the Optical Society of America A*, 10 (10), 2118–33.

Shafer, S.A. (1985) Using color to separate reflection components. *Color Research and Application*, 10, 210–18.

Sherr, S. (1993) *Electronic Displays*, 2nd edn. New York: John Wiley and Sons.

Silicon Vision (2000) *TFA Color Image Sensor (COSIMA)* Available: http://www.siliconvision.de/produkte/cosima-e. htm 2000.

Silverstein, L.D. (1991) Description of an on-axis colorimetric/photometric model for twisted-nematic color liquid crystal displays. Unpublished technical report for the NASA/ARPA Visual Display Engineering and Optimization System (ViDEOS) project. NASA/ARPA.

Silverstein, L.D. (2000) Color in electronic displays. Society for Information Display Seminar Lecture Notes, 1, M6/1–M6/88.

Silverstein, L.D. and Bernot, A.J. (1991) Apparatus and method for an electronically controlled color filter for use in information display applications. US Patent No. 5,032,007.

Silverstein, L.D. and Fiske, T.G. (1993) Colorimetric and photometric modeling of liquid crystal displays. *Proceedings of the First IS&T/SID Color Imaging Conference: Transforms & Transportability of Color*, 149–56.

Silverstein, L.D., Krantz, J.H., Gomer, F.E., Yei-Yu, Y., and Monty, R.W. (1990) Effects of spatial sampling and luminance quantization on the image quality of color matrix displays. *Journal of the Optical Society of America A*, 7 (10), 1955–68.

Silverstein, L.D. and Merrifield, R.M. (1985) The Development and Evaluation of Color Display Systems for Airborne Applications: Phase I – Fundamental Visual, Perceptual, and Display System Considerations. Technical Report DOT/FAA/PM-85-19. FAA.

Speigle, J.M. and Brainard, D.H. (1999) Predicting color from gray: the relationship between achromatic adjustment and asymmetric matching. *Journal of the Optical Society of America A*, 16 (10), 2370–6.

Tamura, Y. (1983) *Color Original Readout Apparatus*. Japan: Canon Kabushiki Kaisha.

TC1–34, C.C. (1998) Final CIE TC1–34 specification. Available: http://www.cis.rit.edu/people/faculty/fairchild/PDFs/CIECAM97s_TC_Draft.pdf.

Tominaga, S. and Wandell, B.A. (1989) The standard surface reflectance model and illuminant estimation. *Journal of the Optical Society of America A*, 6, 576–84.

Ulichney, R. (1987) *Digital Halftoning*. Boston, MA: MIT Press.

Ulichney, R. (1993) The void-and-cluster method for generating dither arrays. Paper presented to the SPIE, San Jose, CA.

Ulichney, R.A. (1988) Dithering with blue noise. *Proceedings of the IEEE*, 76 (1), 56–79.

VanderHorst, G.J.C. and Bouman, M.A. (1969) Spatiotemporal chromaticity discrimination. *Journal of the Optical Society of America*, 59, 1482–8.

Vincent, K. and Neuman, H. (1989) *Color Combiner and Separator and Implementations*. USA: Hewlett–Packard.

Wandell, B.A. (1986) Color rendering of camera data. *Color Research and Application (*Supplement), 11, S30–S33.

Wandell, B.A. (1995) *Foundations of Vision*. Sunderland, MA: Sinauer Press.

Wandell, B. (1999) Computational neuroimaging: color representations and processing. In M.S. Gazzaniga (ed.), *The New Cognitive Neurosciences*, 2nd edn. Cambridge, MA: MIT Press.

Wyszecki, G. and Stiles, W.S. (1982) *Color Science: Concepts and Methods, Quantitative and Formulae*. New York: Wiley.

Author Index

Subject Index